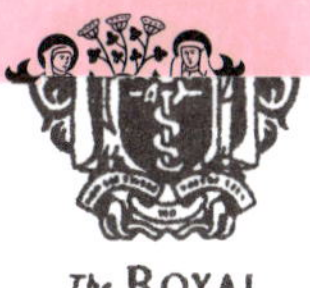

NEW AND EXPLORATORY THERAPEUTIC AGENTS FOR ASTHMA

LUNG BIOLOGY IN HEALTH AND DISEASE

1. Immunologic and Infectious Reactions in the Lung, *edited by C. H. Kirkpatrick and H. Y. Reynolds*
2. The Biochemical Basis of Pulmonary Function, *edited by R. G. Crystal*
3. Bioengineering Aspects of the Lung, *edited by J. B. West*
4. Metabolic Functions of the Lung, *edited by Y. S. Bakhle and J. R. Vane*
5. Respiratory Defense Mechanisms (in two parts), *edited by J. D. Brain, D. F. Proctor, and L. M. Reid*
6. Development of the Lung, *edited by W. A. Hodson*
7. Lung Water and Solute Exchange, *edited by N. C. Staub*
8. Extrapulmonary Manifestations of Respiratory Disease, *edited by E. D. Robin*
9. Chronic Obstructive Pulmonary Disease, *edited by T. L. Petty*
10. Pathogenesis and Therapy of Lung Cancer, *edited by C. C. Harris*
11. Genetic Determinants of Pulmonary Disease, *edited by S. D. Litwin*
12. The Lung in the Transition Between Health and Disease, *edited by P. T. Macklem and S. Permutt*
13. Evolution of Respiratory Processes: A Comparative Approach, *edited by S. C. Wood and C. Lenfant*
14. Pulmonary Vascular Diseases, *edited by K. M. Moser*
15. Physiology and Pharmacology of the Airways, *edited by J. A. Nadel*
16. Diagnostic Techniques in Pulmonary Disease (in two parts), *edited by M. A. Sackner*
17. Regulation of Breathing (in two parts), *edited by T. F. Hornbein*
18. Occupational Lung Diseases: Research Approaches and Methods, *edited by H. Weill and M. Turner-Warwick*
19. Immunopharmacology of the Lung, *edited by H. H. Newball*
20. Sarcoidosis and Other Granulomatous Diseases of the Lung, *edited by B. L. Fanburg*
21. Sleep and Breathing, *edited by N. A. Saunders and C. E. Sullivan*
22. *Pneumocystis carinii* Pneumonia: Pathogenesis, Diagnosis, and Treatment, *edited by L. S. Young*
23. Pulmonary Nuclear Medicine: Techniques in Diagnosis of Lung Disease, *edited by H. L. Atkins*
24. Acute Respiratory Failure, *edited by W. M. Zapol and K. J. Falke*
25. Gas Mixing and Distribution in the Lung, *edited by L. A. Engel and M. Paiva*

26. High-Frequency Ventilation in Intensive Care and During Surgery, *edited by G. Carlon and W. S. Howland*
27. Pulmonary Development: Transition from Intrauterine to Extrauterine Life, *edited by G. H. Nelson*
28. Chronic Obstructive Pulmonary Disease: Second Edition, *edited by T. L. Petty*
29. The Thorax (in two parts), *edited by C. Roussos and P. T. Macklem*
30. The Pleura in Health and Disease, *edited by J. Chrétien, J. Bignon, and A. Hirsch*
31. Drug Therapy for Asthma: Research and Clinical Practice, *edited by J. W. Jenne and S. Murphy*
32. Pulmonary Endothelium in Health and Disease, *edited by U. S. Ryan*
33. The Airways: Neural Control in Health and Disease, *edited by M. A. Kaliner and P. J. Barnes*
34. Pathophysiology and Treatment of Inhalation Injuries, *edited by J. Loke*
35. Respiratory Function of the Upper Airway, *edited by O. P. Mathew and G. Sant'Ambrogio*
36. Chronic Obstructive Pulmonary Disease: A Behavioral Perspective, *edited by A. J. McSweeny and I. Grant*
37. Biology of Lung Cancer: Diagnosis and Treatment, *edited by S. T. Rosen, J. L. Mulshine, F. Cuttitta, and P. G. Abrams*
38. Pulmonary Vascular Physiology and Pathophysiology, *edited by E. K. Weir and J. T. Reeves*
39. Comparative Pulmonary Physiology: Current Concepts, *edited by S. C. Wood*
40. Respiratory Physiology: An Analytical Approach, *edited by H. K. Chang and M. Paiva*
41. Lung Cell Biology, *edited by D. Massaro*
42. Heart–Lung Interactions in Health and Disease, *edited by S. M. Scharf and S. S. Cassidy*
43. Clinical Epidemiology of Chronic Obstructive Pulmonary Disease, *edited by M. J. Hensley and N. A. Saunders*
44. Surgical Pathology of Lung Neoplasms, *edited by A. M. Marchevsky*
45. The Lung in Rheumatic Diseases, *edited by G. W. Cannon and G. A. Zimmerman*
46. Diagnostic Imaging of the Lung, *edited by C. E. Putman*
47. Models of Lung Disease: Microscopy and Structural Methods, *edited by J. Gil*
48. Electron Microscopy of the Lung, *edited by D. E. Schraufnagel*
49. Asthma: Its Pathology and Treatment, *edited by M. A. Kaliner, P. J. Barnes, and C. G. A. Persson*
50. Acute Respiratory Failure: Second Edition, *edited by W. M. Zapol and F. Lemaire*
51. Lung Disease in the Tropics, *edited by O. P. Sharma*
52. Exercise: Pulmonary Physiology and Pathophysiology, *edited by B. J. Whipp and K. Wasserman*
53. Developmental Neurobiology of Breathing, *edited by G. G. Haddad and J. P. Farber*
54. Mediators of Pulmonary Inflammation, *edited by M. A. Bray and W. H. Anderson*

55. The Airway Epithelium, *edited by S. G. Farmer and D. Hay*
56. Physiological Adaptations in Vertebrates: Respiration, Circulation, and Metabolism, *edited by S. C. Wood, R. E. Weber, A. R. Hargens, and R. W. Millard*
57. The Bronchial Circulation, *edited by J. Butler*
58. Lung Cancer Differentiation: Implications for Diagnosis and Treatment, *edited by S. D. Bernal and P. J. Hesketh*
59. Pulmonary Complications of Systemic Disease, *edited by J. F. Murray*
60. Lung Vascular Injury: Molecular and Cellular Response, *edited by A. Johnson and T. J. Ferro*
61. Cytokines of the Lung, *edited by J. Kelley*
62. The Mast Cell in Health and Disease, *edited by M. A. Kaliner and D. D. Metcalfe*
63. Pulmonary Disease in the Elderly Patient, *edited by D. A. Mahler*
64. Cystic Fibrosis, *edited by P. B. Davis*
65. Signal Transduction in Lung Cells, *edited by J. S. Brody, D. M. Center, and V. A. Tkachuk*
66. Tuberculosis: A Comprehensive International Approach, *edited by L. B. Reichman and E. S. Hershfield*
67. Pharmacology of the Respiratory Tract: Experimental and Clinical Research, *edited by K. F. Chung and P. J. Barnes*
68. Prevention of Respiratory Diseases, *edited by A. Hirsch, M. Goldberg, J.-P. Martin, and R. Masse*
69. *Pneumocystis carinii* Pneumonia: Second Edition, *edited by P. D. Walzer*
70. Fluid and Solute Transport in the Airspaces of the Lungs, *edited by R. M. Effros and H. K. Chang*
71. Sleep and Breathing: Second Edition, *edited by N. A. Saunders and C. E. Sullivan*
72. Airway Secretion: Physiological Bases for the Control of Mucous Hypersecretion, *edited by T. Takishima and S. Shimura*
73. Sarcoidosis and Other Granulomatous Disorders, *edited by D. G. James*
74. Epidemiology of Lung Cancer, *edited by J. M. Samet*
75. Pulmonary Embolism, *edited by M. Morpurgo*
76. Sports and Exercise Medicine, *edited by S. C. Wood and R. C. Roach*
77. Endotoxin and the Lungs, *edited by K. L. Brigham*
78. The Mesothelial Cell and Mesothelioma, *edited by M.-C. Jaurand and J. Bignon*
79. Regulation of Breathing: Second Edition, *edited by J. A. Dempsey and A. I. Pack*
80. Pulmonary Fibrosis, *edited by S. Hin. Phan and R. S. Thrall*
81. Long-Term Oxygen Therapy: Scientific Basis and Clinical Application, *edited by W. J. O'Donohue, Jr.*
82. Ventral Brainstem Mechanisms and Control of Respiration and Blood Pressure, *edited by C. O. Trouth, R. M. Millis, H. F. Kiwull-Schöne, and M. E. Schläfke*
83. A History of Breathing Physiology, *edited by D. F. Proctor*
84. Surfactant Therapy for Lung Disease, *edited by B. Robertson and H. W. Taeusch*

85. The Thorax: Second Edition, Revised and Expanded (in three parts), *edited by C. Roussos*
86. Severe Asthma: Pathogenesis and Clinical Management, *edited by S. J. Szefler and D. Y. M. Leung*
87. *Mycobacterium avium*–Complex Infection: Progress in Research and Treatment, *edited by J. A. Korvick and C. A. Benson*
88. Alpha 1–Antitrypsin Deficiency: Biology • Pathogenesis • Clinical Manifestations • Therapy, *edited by R. G. Crystal*
89. Adhesion Molecules and the Lung, *edited by P. A. Ward and J. C. Fantone*
90. Respiratory Sensation, *edited by L. Adams and A. Guz*
91. Pulmonary Rehabilitation, *edited by A. P. Fishman*
92. Acute Respiratory Failure in Chronic Obstructive Pulmonary Disease, *edited by J.-P. Derenne, W. A. Whitelaw, and T. Similowski*
93. Environmental Impact on the Airways: From Injury to Repair, *edited by J. Chrétien and D. Dusser*
94. Inhalation Aerosols: Physical and Biological Basis for Therapy, *edited by A. J. Hickey*
95. Tissue Oxygen Deprivation: From Molecular to Integrated Function, *edited by G. G. Haddad and G. Lister*
96. The Genetics of Asthma, *edited by S. B. Liggett and D. A. Meyers*
97. Inhaled Glucocorticoids in Asthma: Mechanisms and Clinical Actions, *edited by R. P. Schleimer, W. W. Busse, and P. M. O'Byrne*
98. Nitric Oxide and the Lung, *edited by W. M. Zapol and K. D. Bloch*
99. Primary Pulmonary Hypertension, *edited by L. J. Rubin and S. Rich*
100. Lung Growth and Development, *edited by J. A. McDonald*
101. Parasitic Lung Diseases, *edited by A. A. F. Mahmoud*
102. Lung Macrophages and Dendritic Cells in Health and Disease, *edited by M. F. Lipscomb and S. W. Russell*
103. Pulmonary and Cardiac Imaging, *edited by C. Chiles and C. E. Putman*
104. Gene Therapy for Diseases of the Lung, *edited by K. L. Brigham*
105. Oxygen, Gene Expression, and Cellular Function, *edited by L. Biadasz Clerch and D. J. Massaro*
106. $Beta_2$-Agonists in Asthma Treatment, *edited by R. Pauwels and P. M. O'Byrne*
107. Inhalation Delivery of Therapeutic Peptides and Proteins, *edited by A. L. Adjei and P. K. Gupta*
108. Asthma in the Elderly, *edited by R. A. Barbee and J. W. Bloom*
109. Treatment of the Hospitalized Cystic Fibrosis Patient, *edited by D. M. Orenstein and R. C. Stern*
110. Asthma and Immunological Diseases in Pregnancy and Early Infancy, *edited by M. Schatz, R. S. Zeiger, and H. N. Claman*
111. Dyspnea, *edited by D. A. Mahler*
112. Proinflammatory and Antiinflammatory Peptides, *edited by S. I. Said*
113. Self-Management of Asthma, *edited by H. Kotses and A. Harver*
114. Eicosanoids, Aspirin, and Asthma, *edited by A. Szczeklik, R. J. Gryglewski, and J. R. Vane*
115. Fatal Asthma, *edited by A. L. Sheffer*
116. Pulmonary Edema, *edited by M. A. Matthay and D. H. Ingbar*

117. Inflammatory Mechanisms in Asthma, *edited by S. T. Holgate and W. W. Busse*
118. Physiological Basis of Ventilatory Support, *edited by J. J. Marini and A. S. Slutsky*
119. Human Immunodeficiency Virus and the Lung, *edited by M. J. Rosen and J. M. Beck*
120. Five-Lipoxygenase Products in Asthma, *edited by J. M. Drazen, S.-E. Dahlén, and T. H. Lee*
121. Complexity in Structure and Function of the Lung, *edited by M. P. Hlastala and H. T. Robertson*
122. Biology of Lung Cancer, *edited by M. A. Kane and P. A. Bunn, Jr.*
123. Rhinitis: Mechanisms and Management, *edited by R. M. Naclerio, S. R. Durham, and N. Mygind*
124. Lung Tumors: Fundamental Biology and Clinical Management, *edited by C. Brambilla and E. Brambilla*
125. Interleukin-5: From Molecule to Drug Target for Asthma, *edited by C. J. Sanderson*
126. Pediatric Asthma, *edited by S. Murphy and H. W. Kelly*
127. Viral Infections of the Respiratory Tract, *edited by R. Dolin and P. F. Wright*
128. Air Pollutants and the Respiratory Tract, *edited by D. L. Swift and W. M. Foster*
129. Gastroesophageal Reflux Disease and Airway Disease, *edited by M. R. Stein*
130. Exercise-Induced Asthma, *edited by E. R. McFadden, Jr.*
131. LAM and Other Diseases Characterized by Smooth Muscle Proliferation, *edited by J. Moss*
132. The Lung at Depth, *edited by C. E. G. Lundgren and J. N. Miller*
133. Regulation of Sleep and Circadian Rhythms, *edited by F. W. Turek and P. C. Zee*
134. Anticholinergic Agents in the Upper and Lower Airways, *edited by S. L. Spector*
135. Control of Breathing in Health and Disease, *edited by M. D. Altose and Y. Kawakami*
136. Immunotherapy in Asthma, *edited by J. Bousquet and H. Yssel*
137. Chronic Lung Disease in Early Infancy, *edited by R. D. Bland and J. J. Coalson*
138. Asthma's Impact on Society: The Social and Economic Burden, *edited by K. B. Weiss, A. S. Buist, and S. D. Sullivan*
139. New and Exploratory Therapeutic Agents for Asthma, *edited by M. Yeadon and Z. Diamant*

ADDITIONAL VOLUMES IN PREPARATION

Multimodality Treatment of Lung Cancer, *edited by A. T. Skarin*

Diagnostic Pulmonary Pathology, *edited by P. T. Cagle*

Cytokines in Pulmonary Disease: Infection and Inflammation, *edited by S. Nelson and T. R. Martin*

Asthma and Respiratory Infections, *edited by D. P. Skoner*

Particle–Lung Interactions, *edited by P. Gehr and J. Heyder*

Pulmonary and Peripheral Gas Exchange in Health and Disease, *edited by J. Roca, R. Rodriguez-Roisen, and P. Wagner*

Environmental Asthma, *edited by R. K. Bush*

Tuberculosis: A Comprehensive International Approach, Second Edition, *edited by L. B. Reichman and E. S. Hershfield*

Sleep and Breathing in Children: A Developmental Approach, *edited by G. M. Loughlin, J. L. Carroll, and C. L. Marcus*

Combination Therapy for Asthma and Chronic Obstructive Pulmonary Disease, *edited by R. J. Martin and M. Kraft*

NEW AND EXPLORATORY THERAPEUTIC AGENTS FOR ASTHMA

Edited by

Michael Yeadon
Pfizer Central Research
Sandwich, Kent, England

Zuzana Diamant
Erasmus University Medical Centre
Rotterdam, The Netherlands

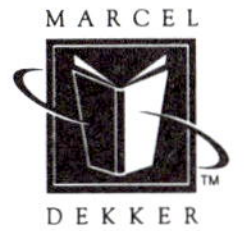

MARCEL DEKKER, INC. NEW YORK • BASEL

ISBN: 0-8247-7861-8

This book is printed on acid-free paper.

Headquarters
Marcel Dekker, Inc.
270 Madison Avenue, New York, NY 10016
tel: 212-696-9000; fax: 212-685-4540

Eastern Hemisphere Distribution
Marcel Dekker AG
Hutgasse 4, Postfach 812, CH-4001 Basel, Switzerland
tel: 41-61-261-8482; fax: 41-61-261-8896

World Wide Web
http://www.dekker.com

The publisher offers discounts on this book when ordered in bulk quantities. For more information, write to Special Sales/Professional Marketing at the headquarters address above.

Current printing (last digit):
10 9 8 7 6 5 4 3 2 1

PRINTED IN THE UNITED STATES OF AMERICA

For my wife Joanna and my daughters Becky and Holly.
M.Y.

For my husband Peter and my daughter Sharon.
Z.D.

INTRODUCTION

The Lord has created medicines out of the earth; and he that is wise will not abhor them.
Ecclesiastes 38:4

God has sent down a treatment for every ailment
Medicine of the Prophet by Ibn Qayyim al-Jawziyya

The search for new treatments is as old as medicine, irrespective of the civilization where it is practiced. Today, as one contemplates the multitude of medications that have been, and are being, developed, one can only marvel at what has been accomplished. It is well recognized that new drugs are essentially the result of basic and applied research. Early in this century, the advent of a chemical approach to medicine led to many extraordinary developments.

The past few decades have been characterized by a search to understand the mechanisms of disease—a quest spurred by the recognition that if pathogenic processes were known, new therapeutic opportunities would ensue. The validity of this concept is beautifully illustrated in the case of asthma. Here is a disease that has been known for more than two thousand years and that has a prevalence of considerable significance. Yet we had to wait for the latter part of this century to witness a better understanding of its mechanisms and, in turn, the development of new and effective pharmacotherapies. The work goes on giving us—and, more importantly, the patients—the prospect of even better treatment.

One could say that this new addition to the Lung Biology in Health and Disease series is the present and the future pharmacopeia of asthma. The editors, Michael Yeadon and Zuzana Diamant, bring years of experience in the pharmacology and clinical aspects of asthma; but, in addition, they have enrolled contributors who are at the forefronts of their fields of expertise. The result is a compendium of information and research outcomes that will help physicians to better serve their patients.

Moreover, it is also a window on the future for, indeed, research marches on and new opportunities develop. The advent of molecular genetics opens up new possibilities such as gene therapy and pharmacogenetics. Therefore, this book is a source of research ideas as well.

The Lung Biology in Health and Disease series includes many volumes on asthma, but this one is unique. As the executive editor, I am extemely grateful to all the contributors for adding this new volume to the series.

Claude Lenfant, M.D.
Bethesda, Maryland

PREFACE

In *New and Exploratory Therapeutic Agents for Asthma*, a volume in the Lung Biology in Health and Disease series, we have succeeded in obtaining contributions from a wide group of opinion-leading scientists recognized for their contributions to the field of asthma research. Although the authors have very diverse backgrounds and are from the four corners of the earth, they have in common a drive to understand asthma and the agents currently used to treat it and to take part in activities to discover, test, and develop further treatments. The range of skills that have been applied to reach the level of understanding we now have of this complex disease, and how much more there is to discover, is easily appreciated from a scan of the chapter subheads.

Asthma is a common, chronic disease of the airways (affecting 5% to 15% of the population) with a spectrum of severity of symptoms of (variable) airway obstruction that ranges from mild to life-threatening. Despite the availability of some effective therapies, in excess of 5000 deaths in the United States per year and 2000 deaths per year in the United Kingdom are directly attributed to asthma. In terms of patient numbers, chronic morbidity is much the greater problem—there remains a substantial unmet medical need, and the social and economic impact of asthma is high. Asthma has been described as the only major chronic, treatable disease of the developed world that is increasing in prevalence. In recognition of these factors, almost every major company within the pharmaceutical industry has active projects directed at finding novel, effective therapies for asthma. The total costs attributed to asthma research in the industry alone amount to many hundreds of millions of dollars in the last three decades. The challenges of finding novel, commercially viable therapies are increasing as good generic inhaled medicines from earlier research become available. Moderating this pessimism is the accelerating accumulation of information surrounding the genetics and molecular biology of asthma, which promises to herald a "golden age" of drug discovery.

Despite the intense research interest in asthma, a complete understanding of the fundamentals of the disease seems as distant as ever; however, over this period, the belief paradigm of the central features of asthma has been shifted by basic clinical and applied research from a disorder of airway smooth muscle to a disorder of the immune system. Recognition came in the 1980s that chronic eosinophilic inflammation of the airways was characteristic of asthma, and with it came a drive to understand the connection between episodic airway narrowing and other clinical symptoms as well as the immunopathology that produces the inflammatory response. Other fundamental questions remain: Why do some individuals develop allergy and why do a subset of these develop asthma? What drives symptoms of asthma in the apparently nonallergic sufferer? Are there really different types of asthma, and how should this affect current treatment and future research for new drugs?

Bronchodilator β_2 agonists and anticholinergics functionally antagonize the airflow restriction induced by agents that contract airway smooth muscle, and they continue to be a mainstay of rational, symptomatic treatment for asthma. In contrast, inhaled glucocorticoids were recognized to be effective before a basic rationale was available to explain their pharmacokinetic profile. It still remains far from clear which of the multiple actions of corticosteroids are responsible for clinical improvements in asthmatics and, indeed, how such corticosteroid-induced changes lead to benefit. The recent launch of antileukotriene agents represents the first new therapeutic class of drug in more than 20 years, and the full impact of these targeted drugs on the treatment of asthma and thought about it has yet to be felt. It is against this backdrop that basic asthma research continues in an effort to better understand the disease, to identify new targets, and to better understand the mechanisms of action of current drugs. In parallel, directed research continues in industry drug-discovery laboratories, with competition continuing to find, for example, the first broadly acceptable oral anti-inflammatory therapy for this disease, the first immunomodulator to lower antigen-specific IgE, the first anticytokine compound, or the first agent to combine bronchospasmolytic with anti-inflammatory properties in one well-tolerated therapeutic compound.

This distressing but fascinating disorder has been approached from many directions, and the products of this research are many molecules in clinical development as well as recently launched therapies. Although it is the nature of drug research that many attractive approaches are followed but few produce new drugs of clinically significant value, lessons are learned from each attempt. This is an evolving story. Although many of the narratives are by definition incomplete, this volume aims to cover these research products from bench to bedside, outlining their discovery and the rationale for their development, clinical development, and outcome.

This volume provides a thorough and up-to-date overview of the context for and position of newer and exploratory antiasthma drugs. The book begins with a trio of chapters giving a solid foundation of current thinking on the epidemiology, pathogenesis, pathophysiology, and pathohistology of the disease. Those reading into the area for the first time or those seeking an update will equally find that these chapters provide an excellent platform on recent and emerging developments in the pharmacotherapy of asthma. The next eight chapters address the status of the major therapeutic classes currently available for the treatment of asthma or in ongoing development: bronchodilators (''relievers''), anti-inflammatories (''controllers''), and antiallergics. The penultimate two chapters cover novel mechanisms for addressing the underlying pathology—for example, via immunomodulation and exploitation of numerous experimental approaches. The book finishes with a description of the current approaches to establishing the credentials of existing and future novel therapies in asthma. This is important, as regulators rightly expect evidence not only of objective improvements in laboratory endpoints but of clinical benefit as well.

In summary, the volume aims to provide quality coverage of the asthma area for the knowledgeable reader or the reader newly engaged in applying and/or developing asthma pharmacotherapies. Taken together, these chapters provide a rationale for the observed or anticipated therapeutic actions of current and emerging drugs in asthma and an introduction to future possible approaches. In particular, in the areas of emerging new information and potential novel therapies, the authors have succeeded in rendering complex material accessible to the interested but nonexpert reader who has a good working knowledge of asthma.

It has been an honor to be able to interact with the authors and we would like to take this opportunity to thank them for their fine contributions. We would also like to acknowledge the interest and support of Marcel Dekker, Inc., and Claude Lenfant, which have made this volume possible. We also beg their forgiveness for any errors and/or omissions that may have crept in and accept full responsibility for them.

Michael Yeadon
Zuzana Diamant

CONTRIBUTORS

Charles Advenier, M.D. Professor, Department of Pharmacology, Faculty of Medicine Paris West, University Paris V, Paris, France

Devendra K. Agrawal, Ph.D. Professor, Division of Allergy and Immunology, Department of Internal Medicine, Creighton University School of Medicine, Omaha, Nebraska

A. N. Banik, M.D., M.B.B.S., M.R.C.P.(UK) Department of University Medicine, Southampton General Hospital, Southampton, England

Peter J. Barnes, D.M., D.Sc., F.R.C.P. Professor and Head, Department of Thoracic Medicine, National Heart and Lung Institute, Imperial College, London, England

Richard Beasley, M.B.Ch.B.(Otago), D.M.(S'ton), F.R.A.C.P. Professor, Department of Medicine, Wellington School of Medicine, Otago University, Wellington, New Zealand

André Boonstra, Ph.D. Department of Immunology, Erasmus University, Rotterdam, The Netherlands

Carl D. Burgess, M.D., M.R.C.P.(UK), F.R.A.C.P. Associate Professor, Department of Medicine, Wellington School of Medicine, Otago University, Wellington, New Zealand

Richard W. Costello, M.D., M.R.C.P.I. Senior Lecturer, Department of Medicine, University of Liverpool, Liverpool, England

Julian Crane, M.B.B.S., M.R.C.P. Associate Professor, Department of Medicine, Wellington School of Medicine, Otago University, Wellington, New Zealand

Zuzana Diamant, M.D., Ph.D. Resident Pulmonologist, Department of Pulmonary Diseases, Erasmus University Medical Centre, Rotterdam, The Netherlands

Ratko Djukanović, M.D., D.M. Senior Lecturer in Medicine and Consultant Physician, Department of University Medicine, Southampton University, Southampton, England

John V. Fahy, M.D. Assistant Professor, Cardiovascular Research Institute and Department of Medicine, University of California, San Francisco, California

Allison D. Fryer, Ph.D. Associate Professor, Division of Physiology, Department of Environmental Health Sciences, School of Public Health, Johns Hopkins University, Baltimore, Maryland

Gerry Higgs, Ph.D. Head of Discovery Projects, Research Department, Celltech Therapeutics, Slough, Berkshire, England

Stephen T. Holgate, M.D., D.Sc., F.R.C.P. MRC Clinical Professor of Immunopharmacology, Department of University Medicine, School of Medicine, University of Southampton, Southampton, England

Bernadette Hughes, Ph.D. Manager, Cardiovascular Biology, Department of Discovery Biology, Pfizer Central Research, Sandwich, England

David B. Jacoby, M.D. Associate Professor, Division of Pulmonary and Critical Care Medicine, Department of Medicine, School of Medicine, and Division of Physiology, School of Public Health, Johns Hopkins University, Baltimore, Maryland

Guy F. Joos, M.D., Ph.D. Professor, Department of Respiratory Diseases, University Hospital Ghent, Ghent, Belgium

Johan C. Kips, M.D., Ph.D. Professor, Department of Respiratory Diseases, University Hospital Ghent, Ghent, Belgium

Romain A. Pauwels, M.D., Ph.D. Professor, Department of Respiratory Diseases, University Hospital Ghent, Ghent, Belgium

Anthony P. Sampson, M.A., Ph.D. Senior Lecturer in Immunopharmacology, Department of University Medicine, Southampton General Hospital, Southampton, England

Huub F. J. Savelkoul, Ph.D. Department of Immunology, Erasmus University, Rotterdam, The Netherlands

Joseph D. Spahn, M.D. Assistant Professor, Department of Pediatrics, University of Colorado Health Sciences Center, and Staff Physician, Department of Pediatrics, National Jewish Medical and Research Center, Denver, Colorado

Peter J. Sterk, M.D., Ph.D. Professor, Department of Pulmonology, Leiden University Medical Center, Leiden, The Netherlands

Stanley J. Szefler, M.D. Professor, Departments of Pediatrics and Pharmacology, University of Colorado Health Sciences Center, Helen Wohlberg and Herman Lambert Chair in Pharmacokinetics, and Director of Clinical Pharmacology, Department of Pediatrics, National Jewish Medical and Research Center, Denver, Colorado

Robert G. Townley, M.D. Professor, Department of Medicine, Creighton University School of Medicine, Omaha, Nebraska

CONTENTS

Introduction Claude Lenfant *v*
Preface *vii*
Contributors *xi*

1. Epidemiology of Asthma **1**
Stephen T. Holgate and A. N. Banik

I. Introduction 1
II. Defining the Asthmatic Phenotype 4
III. Gene–Environment Interaction in Pathogenesis of Asthma 5
IV. Transcription Factors: A Molecular Link Between the Environment and Genes 7
V. Twin Studies 8
VI. Family Studies 9
VII. IgE, Atopy, and Asthma 11
VIII. Early Life Origins of Asthma 11
IX. Breast-Feeding 13
X. Asthma Variants in Childhood 13
XI. Infections in Childhood 14
XII. The ‘‘Toxic’’ Environment 15
XIII. The Role of Allergens in Asthma 17
XIV. Diet and Lifestyle 19
XV. Conclusions 19
References 20

2. Pathophysiology of Asthma **27**
Peter J. Sterk

I. Introduction 27

II. Variable Airways Obstruction 29
III. Bronchoprovocation Tests 30
IV. What Protects Normal Subjects Against Bronchoconstriction? 31
V. Excessive Airway Narrowing in Asthma 33
VI. Hypersensitivity of the Airways 36
VII. Physiological Modulation of Airways Obstruction 39
VIII. Pharmacological Modulation 40
IX. Clinical Implications 41
X. Conclusions 43
References 44

3. Pathology of Asthma **57**
Ratko Djukanović

I. Introduction 57
II. The Inflammatory Cell Network 57
III. The Pathological Determinants of Asthma Severity 65
IV. The Process of Airways Restructuring in Asthma 68
V. Concluding Remarks 72
References 72

4. Muscarinic Receptor Subtypes and Anticholinergic Therapy **85**
Allison D. Fryer, Richard W. Costello, and David B. Jacoby

I. Introduction 85
II. General Overview of Muscarinic Receptor Subtypes 86
III. Parasympathetic Control of Airways 87
IV. Dysfunction of M_2 Muscarinic Receptors on the Cholinergic Nerves 94
V. Role of Parasympathetic Nerves in Asthma 96
VI. Anticholinergic Drugs 101
VII. Treatment of Airway Disease with Anticholinergics 104
VIII. Conclusion 105
References 105

5. Long-Acting β_2-Agonist Drugs **119**
Richard Beasley, Julian Crane, and Carl D. Burgess

I. Introduction 119
II. Pharmacology 119
III. Clinical Studies 125
IV. Airway Inflammation 133

V. Safety 135
VI. Recommended Use 145
References 146

6. Inhaled Glucocorticoids, Established and New **155**
Joseph D. Spahn and Stanley J. Szefler

I. Introduction 155
II. History 156
III. Mechanisms of Action 158
IV. Efficacy 159
V. Adverse Effects 161
VI. Fluticasone Propionate: The Newest Inhaled GC 168
References 172

7. Platelet-Activating Factor Antagonists in Bronchial Asthma **183**
Devendra K. Agrawal and Robert G. Townley

I. Introduction 183
II. Concluding Remarks 195
References 196

8. Tachykinin Receptor Antagonists **203**
Guy F. Joos and Charles Advenier

I. Introduction 203
II. Sensory Neuropeptides in Human Airways 205
III. Bronchoconstrictor Effect of Sensory Neuropeptides 209
IV. Classification of Tachykinin Receptor Antagonists 212
V. Effects of Tachykinin Receptor Antagonists on Airways 214
VI. Clinical Studies with Tachykinin Receptor Antagonists in Asthma 220
VII. Conclusions 221
References 222

9. Therapeutic Potential of Phosphodiesterase Type 4 Inhibitors in the Treatment of Asthma **237**
Bernadette Hughes and Gerry Higgs

I. Introduction 237
II. The Asthmatic Response 238
III. The Regulation by cAMP of Tissue Responses in Asthma 240
IV. Molecular Diversity of Phosphodiesterases 245

V. The Discovery of Novel PDE Inhibitors 248
VI. The Pharmacology of PDE4 Inhibitors 252
VII. Clinical Trials with PDE4 Inhibitors in Inflammatory Diseases 266
VIII. Conclusions 268
References 270

10. Leukotriene Modulators **285**
Anthony P. Sampson and Zuzana Diamant

I. Introduction 285
II. The Generation of Leukotrienes 287
III. Actions of Cysteinyl Leukotrienes Relevant to Asthma 292
IV. In Vivo Evidence for Cysteinyl-LT Production in Asthma 296
V. Antileukotriene Drugs 297
VI. Positioning of Leukotriene Modulators in Asthma Management 306
References 309

11. The Anti-IgE Treatment Strategy for Asthma **329**
John V. Fahy

I. Introduction 329
II. Development of Nonanaphylactogenic Anti-IgE Monoclonal Antibodies 330
III. The Role of IgE in Airway Inflammation: Lessons from Experiments Using Nonanaphylactogenic Anti-IgE 332
IV. Safety of the Anti-IgE Strategy 332
V. Effect of Anti-IgE Antibodies on Circulating Levels of IgE in Blood in Human Subjects 333
VI. Effect of Anti-IgE Antibody on Allergic Rhinitis 336
VII. Effect of Anti-IgE Antibodies on Early and Late Asthmatic Responses to Aerosolized Allergen 336
VIII. Dose Selection of Anti-IgE 339
IX. Summary 339
References 340

12. Activity of T-Cell Subsets in Allergic Asthma **343**
André Boonstra and Huub F. J. Savelkoul

I. Introduction 343
II. Th1-Th2 Subsets 344

III. Cytokines 346
IV. Genetics of Atopy and Asthma 348
V. Antigen Presentation 350
VI. Th2 Cells in the Airways of Patients with Asthma 352
VII. The Induction of Tolerance 353
VIII. Immunotherapy 354
References 355

13. New Targets for Future Asthma Therapy **361**
Peter J. Barnes

I. Introduction 361
II. New Bronchodilators 362
III. Mediator Antagonists 368
IV. New Anti-Inflammatory Drugs 373
V. Gene Therapy 380
VI. Conclusions 380
References 381

14. Current Practice and Future Trends in Clinical Trials in Asthma **391**
Johan C. Kips and Romain A. Pauwels

I. Introduction 391
II. Outcome Measures in Asthma 392
III. Conclusion 398
References 399

Author Index *405*
Subject Index *473*

NEW AND EXPLORATORY THERAPEUTIC AGENTS FOR ASTHMA

1

Epidemiology of Asthma

STEPHEN T. HOLGATE

University of Southampton
Southampton, England

A. N. BANIK

Southampton General Hospital
Southampton, England

I. Introduction

The epidemiology of a disease is a scientific approach to describing the distribution and determinants of the disease at a population level with the purpose of obtaining a better understanding of the forces driving the pathophysiology of the disease state (1). Asthma is a rapidly growing health problem in both the developed and developing world. This rapid increase, noted in most areas of the world, suggests that there are powerful environmental factors at work that are contributing to or driving the asthmatic disease process (1,2).

Almost identical studies in Aberdeen, the United Kingdom, repeated after a 25-year period showed that the prevalence of wheeze and diagnosed asthma had doubled from 1964 to 1989 (3). A similar trend was observed in children from Australia and New Zealand between 1982 and 1992 (4). Allergic diseases as a whole have also increased; a study in South Wales showed a doubling in the incidence of hay fever and eczema over the 15 years between 1973 and 1988 (5). Even in the same country, different regions can show significant differences in mortality and morbidity. A recent federal health survey in the United States found an estimated 15 million asthmatics. During the period from 1979 to 1994 the national increase for asthma mortality in the United States was 42% for the

5- to 34-year age group; over the same period in Illinois, however, the increase was a phenomenal 341%. This increase was confined almost exclusively to the nonwhite population (6).

The geographical heterogeneity of asthma can only be established if different countries follow identical methodologies in epidemiological surveys for identifying the asthmatic phenotype. Such an attempt has been made in both the European Community Respiratory Health Survey (ECRHS) study in Europe (7,8) and the International Study of Asthma and Allergy in Childhood (ISAAC) studies, where a common questionnaire/video is being used for the evaluation of childhood asthma (9). From these studies it is becoming apparent that differences between countries are real—with the United Kingdom, Ireland, New Zealand, and Australia having the highest prevalence of asthma, as opposed to Russia, China, and India, with the lowest asthma prevalence rates (Fig. 1). Of significance also is the finding that in countries with a low prevalence of allergic rhinoconjunctivitis or eczema, the prevalence of asthma symptoms was in the lowest quartile (10).

The ISAAC UK 1995 figures, based on self-administered questionnaires to schoolchildren, show a homogeneity of the asthma and allergy problem in the British isles (11). In the United Kingdom, about 19% of 13- to 14-year-olds were found to be on antiasthma medications and 33% of 13- to 14-year-olds claimed to have wheezed in the preceding 12 months. Within England and Wales, the 12-month prevalence of wheeze was relatively uniform in all regions (33%), with no significant urban-rural differences; however, it was somewhat higher in Scotland, at 37%. Thus the forces driving asthma can be regarded to be similar in all parts of the United Kingdom. This is in sharp contrast to the ISAAC-India figures, which show two- to threefold variation of 12-month asthma symptom prevalence as well as allergic rhinoconjunctivitis and atopic eczema symptoms between different Indian centers (10).

Higher prevalence rates have also been found among children of ''westernized'' countries than in the developing countries of Asia and Africa. In sub-Saharan Africa, the disease was almost nonexistent in the 1960s, but now its prevalence is approaching that in the Western world (12,13). An urban-rural divide can also be demonstrated in several studies, particularly from the ''developing'' world (14). Moreover, an increase in asthma prevalence has been observed in the offspring of first-generation migrants from rural to urban environments (15). Even among industrialized nations, the prevalence of asthma appears to be significantly higher in United Kingdom, Australia, and New Zealand than in Germany, the United States, or Canada despite similar living conditions (10).

The reasons behind this global epidemic of asthma are complex and probably multifactorial. An increasingly toxic environment combined with a more susceptible population has been postulated to be responsible for this trend (16).

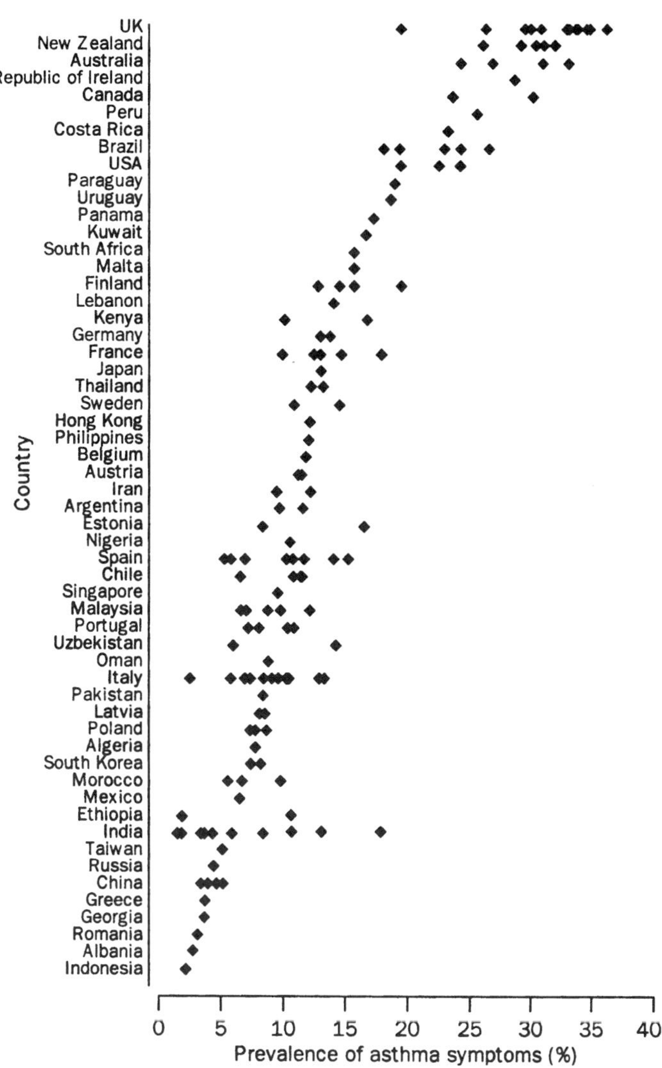

Figure 1 ISSAC 1998: 12-month prevalence of wheeze from written questionnaire.

Changing patterns of lifestyle, aeroallergens, diet, pollution, and a liberalization of diagnostic criteria—and even unrestricted use of antiasthma bronchodilator drug therapy—have all been suggested to contribute to this burgeoning problem. Epidemiological studies of asthma look into the spatial and temporal differences of the disease at a population level and thereby may provide insights into the etiology of this common but complex disorder.

II. Defining the Asthmatic Phenotype

Accurate epidemiological analysis of any disease condition requires a precise definition of the disease entity. To the clinician, asthma represents an obstructive airway disorder in which spontaneous or drug therapy–induced alterations in airflow limitation occur. Although the diagnosis of asthma seems relatively straightforward at the clinical level, numerous attempts at defining the asthma phenotype for epidemiological purposes have failed to reach a consensus (17). Neither is there a simple and specific laboratory test that reliably detects the asthmatic state. Questionnaires have been designed to detect characteristic asthma symptoms like breathlessness and wheeze, but unfortunately these are not specific for asthma. The 1995 defining statement of the National Institutes of Health (NIH) on asthma is more of a description than a strict definition and is unsuitable for epidemiological studies:

> . . . A chronic inflammatory disorder of the airways in which many cells play a role including mast cells and eosinophils. In susceptible individuals this causes recurrent episodes of wheezing, breathlessness, chest tightness and cough particularly at night and/or early in the morning. These symptoms are usually associated with widespread but variable airflow limitation reversible either spontaneously or with treatment and an associated increase in airway responsiveness to a variety of stimuli (18).

Many population studies have therefore looked into the period prevalence of "wheeze" rather than asthma. Reliance on subjective clinical data without objective studies can, however, lead to misdiagnosis. Another approach has been to look at "intermediate" asthma phenotypes—allergy/atopy and airway hyperresponsiveness (AHR) (19). Some studies have supplemented unverified subjective data from asthma/allergy questionnaires with some functional measurements—evidence of bronchial hyperresponsiveness (BHR) and "atopy" (7,20). BHR studies can demonstrate inducible airflow obstruction to wheeze-inducing substances like histamine, methacholine, or adenosine or to exercise-induced wheeze. These tests may be combined with 1–2 weeks of home peak-flow monitoring—showing labile airway function—such objective approaches have been shown to strengthen the diagnosis of asthma. In a study of 92 Dutch families—where 26% of the 320 children had "definite" asthma based on symptoms and

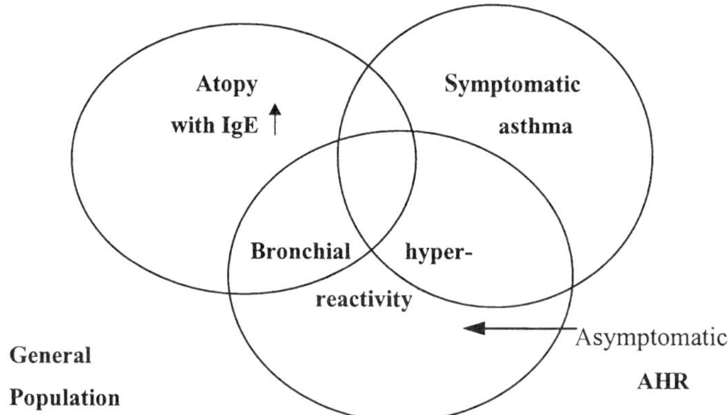

Figure 2 Overlapping intermediate phenotypes of asthma.

BHR—however, only 60% of these ''definite'' asthmatics had a prior physician diagnosis of asthma (21). BHR is also closely linked to an allergic diathesis, as shown by the association of serum IgE levels with BHR and asthma (22). Atopy is measured by serum IgE levels or by skin-prick responses to specific common environmental allergens. Asthma is more closely linked to serum IgE than to skin-test responses to allergens, while AHR is strongly related to total IgE even in nonasthmatic children. Symptomatic asthma, bronchial hyperreactivity, and atopy are distinct but overlapping phenotypes (Fig. 2); one can thus have asthma without atopy (i.e., nonatopic asthma) or airway hyperreactivity without asthma symptoms (asymptomatic airway hyperresponsiveness).

Other methods of substantiating the diagnosis of asthma include the use of surrogate diagnostic biomarkers. These include induced sputum cell and cytokine analysis and inflammatory cytokine measurements in urine (e.g., urinary leukotrienes) (23). Another indirect test of airway inflammation is measuring exhaled nitric oxide (NO) levels, which are abnormally increased in asthmatics but decline with inhaled steroid therapy and disease control (24). The relevance of these tests in the diagnosis and management of asthma remains to be substantiated. Bronchial biopsy evidence of allergic airway inflammation is useful in isolated cases; however, only noninvasive tests are applicable in population studies (25).

III. Gene–Environment Interaction in Pathogenesis of Asthma

While it is clear that the environment plays a dominant role in the development of asthma and allergic disorders, the genetic makeup of an individual appears to influence the initiation and perpetuation of these disease processes. Scientists are now paying increasing attention to studying the involvement of "genetic factors" in order to gain fresh insights into the etiology and pathogenesis of asthma and allergy (Fig. 3) (26).

There is compelling evidence demonstrating that asthma is a heritable disorder with a major genetic component (21). A child born to a family with one asthmatic parent has a risk of developing the disease several times greater than that of a child born into a nonasthmatic family. The risk is greater still if both parents have asthma (27,28). However, all children born to asthmatic parents do not develop the disease. It has been suggested that rather than directly causing asthma, the "asthma genes" create a susceptibility or vulnerability to asthma with which environmental factors interact, leading to the development of the asthma disease state (Fig. 4) (29). The identification of "culprit" genes involved in the asthma disease process should provide us with valuable clues into both the prevention and treatment aspects of asthma. As powerful tools of genetic analysis are brought to bear on the problem and the genes involved are identified, we expect to reap significant medical benefits over the next few years from this approach (30).

The mere presence of a gene does not guarantee its phenotypic expression, since the environment plays a critical role in controlling the degree of expression of one's genetic potential. A person's height, for example, is controlled by multiple genes; but unless the individual has good nutrition and enjoys good health, his or her final height may fall short of the inherent potential. Thus attaining one's genetic potential depends on gene–environment interaction.

The possibility also exists that genes that protect the lungs from environ-

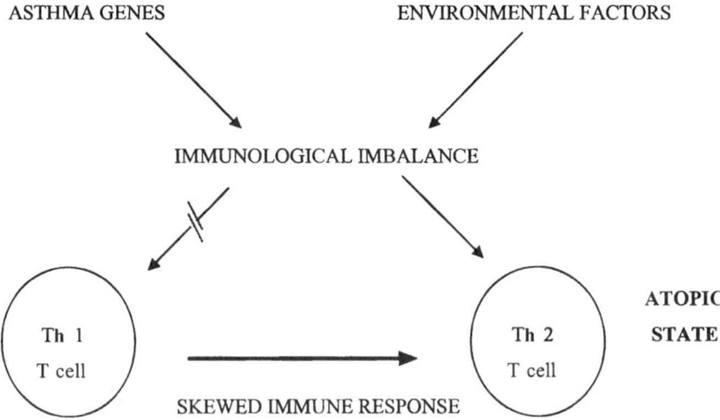

Figure 3 Immunological imbalance from gene–environment interaction creating a T-helper cell (type 2) skewing that favors the atopic/asthma state. Th1, T-helper type 1; Th2, T-helper type 2.

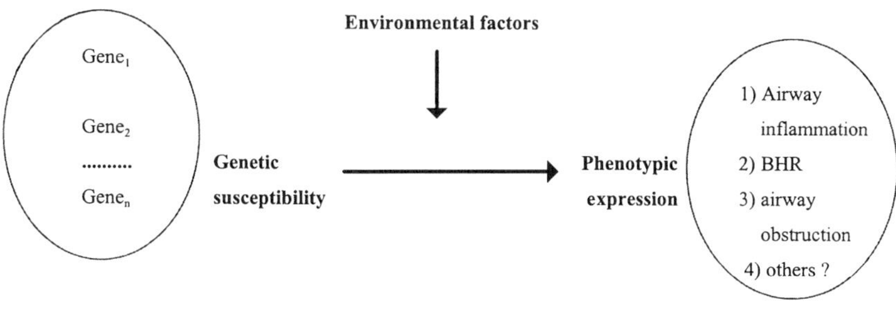

Figure 4 Environmental factors interacting with multiple asthma ''susceptibility'' genes (1–n) generating various elements of the asthma phenotype.

mental insults may be underactive, leading to cumulative lung dysfunction and damage. While the ZZ anomaly is well known in α_1 antitrypsin deficiency, defects in antioxidant system genes have been recently identified in chronic obstructive airway disease (COAD) subjects and might make the lungs more vulnerable to oxidant stress (31). Smith and Harrison from the University of Edinburgh have identified a relative deficiency (slow activity) in the protective microsomal epoxide hydrolase enzyme (mEPHX) in COAD and emphysema patients. Similar genes might play a role in asthmatics and need to be identified. Stress proteins are another potential protective pathway against cytotoxic stimuli and are expressed in both acute lung injury and in asthma (32). The stress response and stress proteins may confer protection against diverse forms of cellular and tissue injury. The stress response has been demonstrated to affect gene regulation mediated by nuclear factor–kappa B (NF-κB) by stabilizing I-kappa B alpha and inducing expression of I-kappa B alpha (see below). The composite result of these two effects is to decrease NF-kappa B nuclear translocation (33).

IV. Transcription Factors: A Molecular Link Between the Environment and Genes

How does the environment alter genetic expression? Multiple pathways are probably involved, and recently a great deal of interest has been devoted to a group of molecular messengers called *transcription factors*, a family of proteins that bind to the promoter region of target genes, thereby altering gene expression (34). Transcription factors act as nuclear messengers, converting cell-surface messages into alterations in gene activity by increasing or decreasing the rates

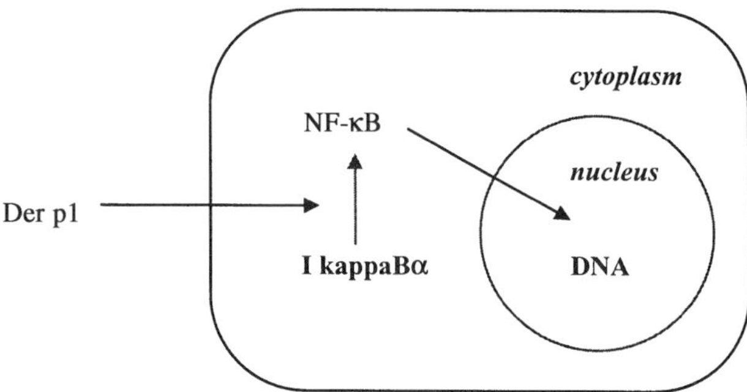

Figure 5 Nuclear transcription factors as a key molecular messenger between environmental agents and nuclear DNA. Der p1, house dust mite allergen; NF-κB, nuclear factor kappa B; IκBa, inhibitor to NF-κB.

of gene transcription. Transcription factors like AP-1, CREB, and NF-κB probably play a key role through gene modulation in the long-term regulation of cell function, growth, and differentiation.

When an allergen like Der p1 from dust mites is presented to a pulmonary epithelial cell, it activates—via surface receptors—the transcription factor NF-κB, which conveys the message to the nuclear DNA resulting in expression of several cytokine gene products (Fig. 5) (35). Researchers in Milan, Italy, have recently demonstrated that a house dust mite antigen called Der p1 can indeed promote activation of transcriptional factor NF-κB in bronchial epithelial cells of asthmatics by interfering with I-kappa B alpha activity (36). NF-κB can be activated by numerous cytokines including TNF-α and also by virus infections and by oxidants like hydrogen peroxide, leading to the activation of this pathway and thus to the genesis of proinflammatory cytokines. Steroids, on the other hand, inhibit both NF-κB and AP-1, direct interaction between the p65 subunit of NF-κB, and the activated glucocorticoid receptor has been demonstrated in the human lung. NF-κB is a transcriptional regulator of inducible nitric oxide synthase gene (iNOS) in human airway epithelium. This may explain the the inhibitory effects of steroids on iNOS gene expression. cAMP response element binding protein (CREB) appears to play a role in regulating beta$_2$-adrenoceptor expression. Transcription factors thus appear to play a major role at the cellular and subcellular levels in asthmatic lungs and can link environmental insults to the airways pathophysiological response.

V. Twin Studies

Research has already shown us that asthma is not a single-gene problem (37). Multiple genes are involved, each contributing to the total asthma "genetic load"

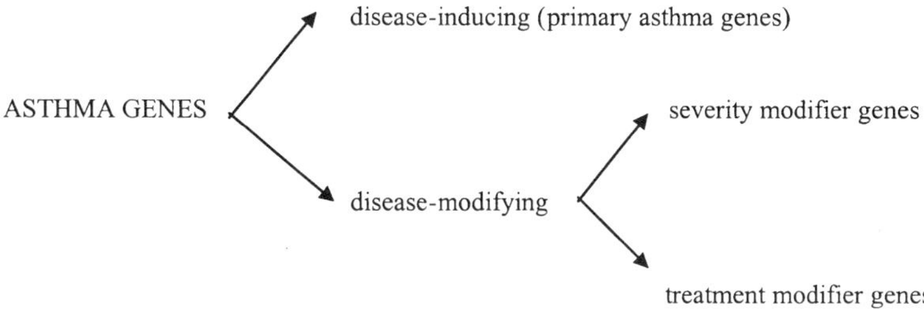

Figure 6 Classification of asthma genes.

(Fig. 6). One method used to discriminate between the environmental and genetic contributions in any complex disease like asthma has been the study of twins. Data from several monozygotic and dizygotic twin studies suggest that 50–60% of the asthma liability may be inherited. The assumption in such studies is that the twins have been reared in the same environment and therefore environmental factors are constant—or, conversely, in twin separation studies, that the influence of different environments on similar genotypes can be studied.

Lubs in 1971 analyzed data from the Swedish twin registry on 7000 pairs of adult twins (38). The concordance rate for asthma symptoms was 19% for monozygotic versus 4.8% for dizygotic twins. The relative risk of asthma/atopy in first-degree relatives was 1.3–3.1 times the risk of the general population. Moreover, the risk of developing a specific allergy was disease-specific in that relatives of an individual with asthma developed asthma rather than eczema or hay fever. Duffy, in a study on 3808 pairs of Australian twins, using self-reported data on asthma and hay fever, calculated a 60–70% heritability of these diseases, with a higher genetic correlation for women: 0.65 versus 0.52 for men (39). The largest population-based study was the 1991 Finnish twin cohort study on 27,776 individuals, which demonstrated an even more striking gender difference in the inheritance of asthma. While overall heritability was 35.6%, for women it was 67.8% and for men 0% (40).

Twin studies looking at twin pairs reared together and apart have also demonstrated a 50% contribution of genetic factors to total IgE levels; however, allergen-specific IgE appears to be largely controlled by one's environment rather than by one's genes (41). Basal serum IgE levels are thus not synonymous with symptomatic asthma or allergy.

VI. Family Studies

Thanks to the enormous effort devoted to making the human gene maps over the past few years and to technological advances, rapid strides can now be made to exploring the genetic basis of polygenic diseases like asthma (37). Several approaches are currently being employed in trying to identify the asthma and atopy genes (42). The whole-genome searches for linkage allow us to identify potential loci on chromosomes that are linked to the disease genes. The candidate-gene approach does not identify new genes but explores the importance of individual genes thought to play a role in the asthmatic disease process (43,44). This would allow us to concentrate our attention on the ''major'' asthma genes and would allow therapeutic strategies based on such studies to be more focused.

Family studies have been designed to determine whether the aggregation of a phenotypic trait is compatible with the existence of a putative major gene. The statistical techniques based on this approach is called *segregation analysis*. Evidence from such methods point to a handful of loci exerting most of the genetic control of asthma and atopy; this is referred to as the *polygenic model* with *oligogenic* influence.

The candidate-gene approach and whole-genome searches has thrown up several potential genes that appear to play a role in asthma and atopy (Table 1). Susceptibility genes involving the MHC II on chromosome 6p and the α chain of the T-cell receptor on chromosome 14q appear important at the allergen-

Table 1 Candidate Genes and Chromosomal Regions in Asthma and Atopy for Which Positive Linkage or Association Has Been Claimed

Chromosomal Location	Candidate(s)	Function
5q31	IL-3, IL-4, IL-5, IL-9 IL-13, GM-CSF	Cytokines upregulating IgE mast-cell, basophil, and eosinophil functions
5q32	β_2-Adrenoceptor (polymorphisms 16 and 27)	Bronchodilatation
6p	HLA complex	Antigen presentation
6p21.3	TNF-α(polymorphism E237G)	Pleiotropic inflammatory cytokine
11q13	Fc_eR1(polymorphism)	Transduction signaling on mast cells, basophils, and dendritic cells
12q	Interferon gamma	Inhibition of Th2 cells
	Constitutive form of nitric oxide synthase, mast-cell growth factor	Inflammatory mediators
13q	Esterase D protein	? function
14q	T-cell receptor α/γ complex	T-cell activation

Source: From Ref. 120.

specific level (45). Chromosome 11q13 is linked to the high-affinity IgE receptor and possibly to bronchial hyperreactivity (BHR) loci (46). Chromosome 5q31-33 appears especially promising, containing both the inflammatory cytokine cluster and the $beta_2$-adenoreceptor loci (47). The $beta_2$-adenoreceptor polymorphisms appear to be examples of asthma genes that are not primary causes of asthma but modify the course of the disease—possibly through effects on inflammation and BHR as well as response to beta-agonist therapy. (Fig. 3) (48). Variants of this receptor have been associated with nocturnal asthma as well as disease severity (49).

VII. IgE, Atopy, and Asthma

The majority of asthmatic individuals are atopic, with elevated total serum IgE levels. Atopy is the single most important risk factor for the development of asthma, increasing the risk by over 10-fold compared with those who are nonatopic (50). Atopy is a disorder of IgE responses to environmental allergens and is detected by elevations of total or antigen-specific serum IgE levels or by positive skin-prick testing. At IgE levels above 100 U/mL, the observed frequency of atopic diseases significantly increases; thus IgE levels > 100 U/mL are usually taken to signify presence of atopy (51).

In 1989, Burrows et al. showed a linear relation between log total serum IgE and prevalence of asthma in a large population study (52). While 11% of the children with no parental asthma had asthma, about one-third of children with one asthmatic parent and almost half of children with two asthmatic parents, respectively, had asthma. Highest rates of asthma were found in children of asthmatic parents who had high serum IgE levels. Xu and colleagues found, in a study of 92 Dutch families, that IgE inheritance appeared to favor a two-locus model, with the major locus linked to chromosome 5q. BHR also showed linkage to identical markers in 5q, suggesting the presence of an asthma ''causal'' gene in that region (53). Cookson, on the other hand, implicated chromosome 11q13 with the transmission of atopy, but only through the maternal line (54,55).

Evidence from family and twin studies suggests that while an individual may possess a predetermined genetic ability to produce excessive basal IgE, specific IgE responses are more influenced by exposure to specific environmental influences.

VIII. Early Life Origins of Asthma

A. Prenatal Influences

The predisposition of an individual to develop asthma and atopy begins early in life. The reasons are not merely genetic. Cord blood T lymphocytes from babies born to atopic mothers can respond to environmental allergens such as egg protein (ovalbumin) and milk protein (β-lactoglobulin) as well as those derived from house dust mites, cats, and birch pollen (56). This surprising finding might reflect a placental role in allowing the transmission of environmental allergens from mother to fetus, skewing the immune response antenatally toward the allergic T-lymphocyte Th2 pattern so characteristic of atopy and asthma. While the mechanisms are still unknown, they begin to appear around week 24–26 of pregnancy, when the fetus adopts a Th2 immune phenotype in order to prevent maternal rejection (57). In high-risk families, allergen avoidance should not only start early in life but should also include pregnancy, with a view to prevent such fetal programming. Fetal programming by the mother might explain several features that could contribute to the rising prevalence of allergy and asthma, including a link with cigarette smoking in pregnancy and the greater effect of maternal than paternal allergy on development of asthma in the offspring. Children who develop atopic diseases develop immunological changes early in life. In particular, a deficiency in secreting the allergy-damping cytokine interferon gamma has been observed in the peripheral blood mononuclear cells of these children (58). In the last trimester there is normally increased synthesis of interferon gamma, which allows a transition from the Th2 phenotype to the Th1 phenotype. Lack of this cytokine has been noted in atopic children 11 years of age or younger, including cord blood samples, leading to upregulation of cytokines associated with the allergic Th2 response. This suggests the existence of an impaired inhibitory mechanism for shutting down a Th2 response rather than one that primarily enhances it (59).

B. Tobacco Smoke and Maternal Cigarette Smoking

Maternal cigarette smoking is an important risk factor for childhood asthma (60,61). If the mother only smoked during pregnancy and quit before delivery, this effect could still be seen, and the newborn's cord blood would show elevated IgE levels (62,63). Both active and passive smoking may also lower the threshold for sensitization to environmental allergens. Babies born to smokers also have diminished lung function when compared with those born to nonsmoking mothers. In the Australian cohort study, infants with smoking mothers, as compared with controls, had increased airway responsiveness to histamine. This abnormal BHR induced by in utero exposure to cigarette smoke has been shown to persist in childhood for as long as 9 years (63,64). Tobacco smoke is strongly linked to both asthma and allergic sensitization. When parents smoke at home, there is an earlier onset of allergy in the children and up to five times more wheezy bronchitis than in nonsmoking households. Passive smoking is thus a significant risk factor in the development of childhood respiratory and allergic diseases (65).

IX. Breast-Feeding

Breast-feeding may have a protective role against atopic diseases and can certainly protect against wheezing illness in the first few months of life (66,67). Human milk is rich in long-chain fatty acids, which might have a role in preventing airway inflammation. In a 5-year follow-up study of 216 children in Canada, breast milk and whey-hydrolysate diets given in the first 4–6 months of life have both been shown to offer relative protection against the development of asthma and atopy in "high-risk" infants, unlike cow's milk or soya preparations (68). However, several long-term studies have failed to demonstrate significant protective effects of breast-feeding on asthma (69). Even when mothers adhered to hypoallergenic diets during 3 months of breast-feeding followed by 12 months of allergenic food avoidance for the infants, only short-term reductions in food allergy and eczema were noted (70,71). It is likely that to prevent allergen sensitization in potential asthmatics, avoidance of key aeroallergens might be more critical than dietary manipulation.

X. Asthma Variants in Childhood

All childhood wheeze is not representative of asthma. Children who predominantly wheeze during viral respiratory tract infections and who manifest neutrophilic responses during such episodes are quite distinct from the atopic asthmatics who have elevated eosinophil and mast-cell responses in bronchial lavages. It is the latter group who tend to develop the typical asthmatic pattern of episodic wheezing and bronchial hyperreactivity, whereas the former group tend to grow out of their "wheezing illness" (72). Children who have transient wheezing with symptoms before the age of 3 tend to have smaller airways and are more at risk from maternal cigarette smoking than maternal asthma or allergy (50). The Tucson study on childhood wheeze illustrated the benign nature of wheeze in the first 3 years of life—about 60% of this group had stopped wheezing by the age of 6. The "transient" wheezers—wheeze before 3 years but absent at 6 years—were characterized by persistently lower levels of lung function ($\dot{V}_{max}$ FRC) and normal levels of IgE; as opposed to children with persistent wheeze (about 14% of the group)—wheeze at both 3 and 6 years of age—who had atopy with raised IgE and normal initial airway function at 3 years, which diminished by 6 years of age (72). Overall, it appears that maternal asthma, maternal cigarette smoking, high IgE levels, and male sex are major risk factors for childhood wheeze. Conversely, absence of a family history of asthma/atopy, low levels of serum IgE, and male sex have a better prognosis. Girls with asthma are less likely to grow out of their disease and have a higher rate of hospital admissions with acute asthma than do boys (73).

XI. Infections in Childhood

Viral upper respiratory tract infections (RTIs) play an important role in asthma, both by exacerbating preexisting asthma and by influencing the disease's pathogenesis (Fig. 7). Viral RTIs have a potential to promote the development of airway inflammation and have also been found to contribute to enhanced airway responsiveness. The respiratory syncytial virus (RSV) agent and the parainfluenza virus have also been found to stimulate IgE antibody production (74) and eosinophilic inflammation (75).

Studies using the rhinovirus (RV16) to induce RTIs demonstrated both an enhancement of BHR as well as the induction of a late asthmatic response. Rhino-

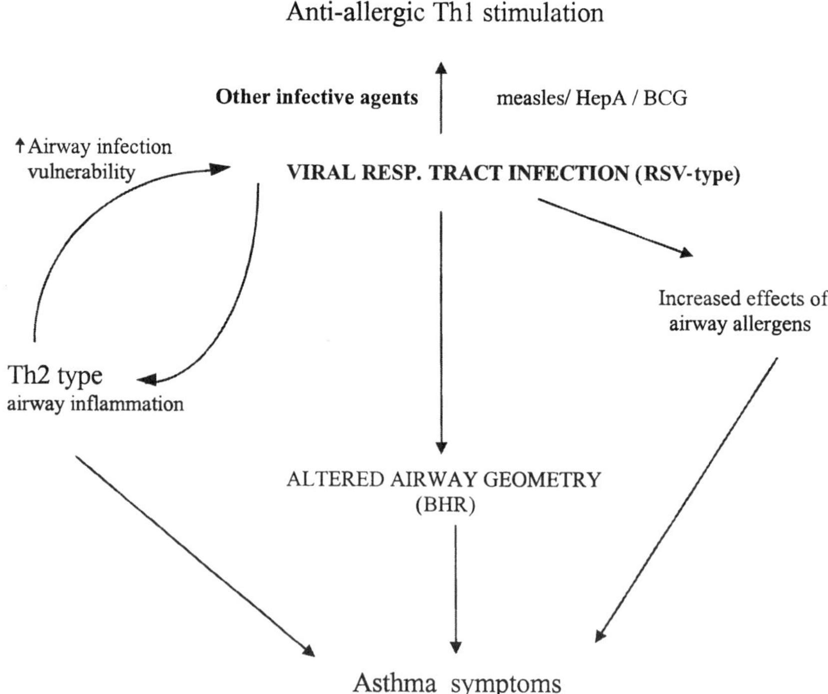

Figure 7 Dual role of infections in promoting or preventing a proallergic Th2 diathesis.

virus infection can also promote eosinophilic inflammation in the lower respiratory airways (76,77).

Some childhood infections seem to protect an individual from developing asthma and atopy. Measles infection in the first year of life has been shown to offer some protection against the development of asthma (78). The magnitude of delayed hypersensitivity to tuberculosis—as measured by skin BCG response—in 1-year-old Japanese children showed an inverse relationship to the development of later-life asthma (79). Recently hepatitis A seropositivity in 17- to 24-year-old male military recruits in Italy was shown to be inversely related to the incidence of atopy (80). Children with older siblings at home are also less likely to suffer from asthma. One study from the North of England showed a 1.7 times greater incidence of asthma in children with no older siblings as compared with those who had four older siblings, presumably because of greater exposure to infections especially in the first year of life (78). Conversely, viruses like RSV seem to augment the allergic Th2 response and might thus predispose an individual to developing asthma (50,81) The magnitude of RSV's effects on the lungs are highly variable but may be related to prior allergic sensitization of the subject, which increases airway vulnerability to virally, mediated damage (82).

It is possible that frequent childhood infections with pathogens of the non-RSV group could lead to a favorable immunological profile that might protect susceptible individuals from asthma and allergy—i.e., through an upregulated Th1 response. This might explain the inverse relationship between socioeconomic status and allergic conditions as well as the urban-to-rural decreasing gradient of asthma in developing countries. Whether significant Th1 activation by bacterial vaccines can modify the asthmatic process is currently being investigated at several centers (e.g., *Mycobacterium vaccae* studies) (83).

XII. The "Toxic" Environment

A. Air Pollution

Contrary to popular perception, the role of air pollution in the pathogenesis or amplification of asthma is still unresolved. A major problem is the difficulty of measuring the levels of an individual's exposure precisely. Not only are multiple pollutants probably involved but they can also interact with allergens in a synergistic manner (Fig. 8). This phenomenon has been observed with ozone and pollen allergens; prior ozone exposure can reduce the concentration of allergens required to provoke an asthmatic response (84,85). In vitro studies suggest that the critical protective barrier to airway allergens is an intact bronchial epithelium. When airways are exposed to "pollutants," epithelial permeability to antigens is enhanced (86). Ozone by itself can increase bronchial reactivity (87) and can

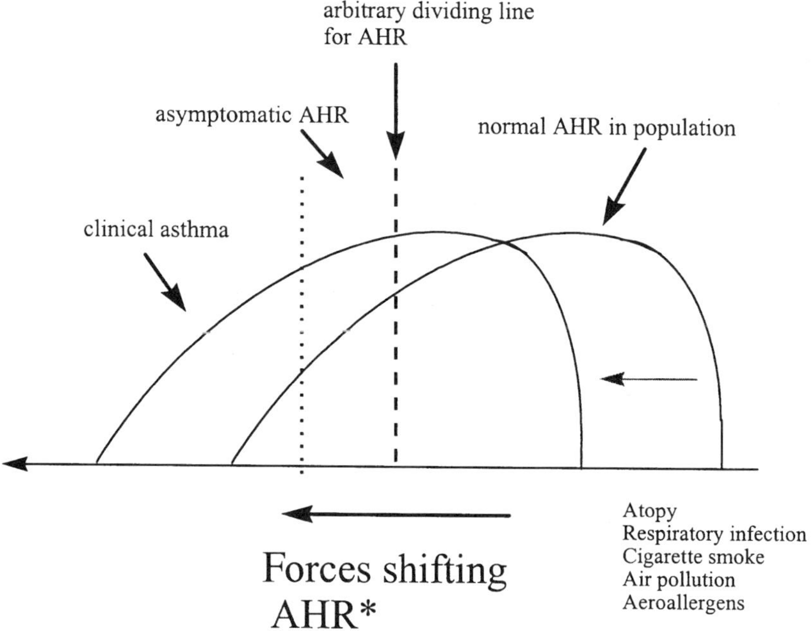

Figure 8 Population distribution of bronchial hyperresponsiveness (BHR); this can be skewed to the left by multiple environmental factors, resulting in increased prevalence of both asymptomatic and symptomatic BHR. *AHR = airway hyperresponsiveness.

significantly increase the production of inflammatory cytokines from bronchial epithelium of asthmatic subjects.

Airborne pollutants have been linked to dramatic asthma epidemics on several occasions; these include the Barcelona epidemic related to the unloading of soybeans and the castor bean–induced epidemics. Recently the role of thunderstorms in causing asthma "epidemics" has been described (89). Such storms have been linked to asthma exacerbations, probably by increasing atmospheric pollen levels (90). The infamous London smog of 1952, which caused up to 4000 excess cardiorespiratory deaths, illustrates the importance of weather in altering pollutant levels and dramatically increasing respiratory disease mortality and morbidity (91).

Urban smog is a complex cocktail of organic and inorganic particulate matter, aerosols, and gaseous pollutants. The paved road dust composition in Los Angeles/Pasadena, California, was found to include pollen, garden soil, plant fragments, and tire fragments (92). Of these, tire fragments are of interest because of their natural latex content, which acts both as an adjuvant and potent allergen capable of stimulating immediate hypersensitivity reactions (93). Particle size is critical in determining the pattern of particle deposition in the lungs, fine particles (PM10) <10 μm and ultrafine particles <0.1 μm being more ''toxic'' (94,95). Particles >2.5 μm in median diameter are deposited largely in the upper airways, while smaller particles <2.5 μm in median diameter can penetrate up to the alveolar spaces. ''Fine-particulate pollution'' has been linked to both a decrease in peak flow and an increase in respiratory symptoms (96,97).

Nonparticulate air pollutants like sulfur dioxide (SO_2) and fine particulate sulfates (SO_4) can directly provoke bronchospasm and asthma symptoms even at very low levels of exposure (98). Nitrogen dioxide from gas stoves appears to be the major nonparticulate indoor pollutant and has been linked to respiratory disease, but it has an inconsistent effect on pulmonary function (99,100). NO_2 levels of 400 ppb are not uncommon in households using gas stoves; there, levels are about 10 times higher than those in households not using gas (101). When the bronchial epithelia of asthmatics and non-asthmatics are exposed to NO_2 for 6 hr, the asthmatics' epithelial cells show a significant rise in cytokine generation; moreover, a clear threshold effect is seen with NO_2 levels below 200 ppb, which do not produce this effect (88,102).

Diesel fumes have also been suggested as a major respiratory irritant that can worsen airway inflammation. Diesel exhaust particles (DEPs) can induce allergic inflammation in both the upper and lower airways (with elevated levels of IgE and IL-4); moreover, DEPs can bind other allergens like the pollen antigen (Lol p1), forming small conglomerate particles of the critical size, 1–2 μm in diameter (103–105).

XIII. The Role of Allergens in Asthma

Environmental factors usually act as ''adjuvants'' or risk factors in the asthmatic disease process. While they can amplify preexisting disease, their causal role in asthma remains debatable. Major allergens that can aggravate airway inflammation include those of house dust mites, cats, cockroaches, alternaria, and pollen (101).

In many parts of the world, the house dust mite is the major source of indoor allergens. Rather than the mite itself being the major source of allergens, it is the fecal particles that contain the highest concentrations of allergenic digestive enzymes, including the cysteine protease Der p1. House dust mites thrive in hot and humid climates and produce multiple allergens that are predominantly concentrated in the bedding and blankets. In Papua New Guinea, highlanders' asthma was almost unknown until the introduction of blankets with their resident house dust mites (105). In colder, temperate climates, house dust mites have become a problem in recent years owing to the creation of a ''subtropical'' indoor climate by the improved heating systems and insulation. To survive and reproduce, the house dust mite requires an optimal temperature of 25°C and a relative humidity of 80%. Such households are also increasingly damp, and this could also favor fungal growth and spore production (106).

Der p1 is a relatively large particle in the 20-μm range; it can be effectively isolated by covering all bedding items in special fabrics with ultrafine pores (107). Howarth et al. (1992) demonstrated that such measures reduced the symptoms of asthma, allergic rhinitis, and eczema in university students with ongoing asthma and that it could also reduce bronchial reactivity (108,109). Another property of some allergens like Der p1 is the presence of enzymatic activity; this might facilitate antigen penetration across the bronchial epithelial barrier. In hot and dry climates like those of Tucson, Arizona, or Wagga Wagga, Australia, dust-mite levels are low; in spite of this, asthma and exercise-inducible wheeze prevalence are no lower here than in areas of high dust-mite allergen levels. Asthmatics in these regions demonstrate sensitization to alternaria, rye, and plantain; thus the culprit allergen depends on the geographical region (110).

Inner cities in America are another unique microenvironment, and asthmatics there have been sensitized to cockroach allergens (111). Cat allergens are potent irritants to asthmatic airways, and one explanation has been the smaller particle size of Fel d1, ~5 μm or less, which facilitates prolonged particle suspension times in room air and deeper penetration into the respiratory passages (112).

Several factors control the ability of an allergen to trigger an allergic immune response; these include the route of delivery, the quantity of antigen, particle size, presence of adjuvants, and special molecular attributes like enzymatic activity. Inhalation of allergens and direct immune stimulation of the bronchi are the dominant pathways in asthma, rather than ingested food allergens. The dose of antigen is also critical; low levels of Der p1 were not linked to asthma while levels >10 μg/g of dust were linked to an exponential increase in asthma (110). As discussed above, the presence of co-stimulants like ozone enhances the effects of aeroallergens.

The elimination of environmental allergens might reduce the development of asthma and allergies if initiated from early in a child's life. However the Isle of Wight study illustrates the inherent problems with such an approach: while asthma, eczema, and food allergies were reduced initially in the first 1–2 years of life in ''high-risk'' subjects, the benefits slowly wore off with time. By the age of 4 years, the rate of asthma was no longer statistically significant between the control group and intervention groups (71).

XIV. Diet and Lifestyle

Many workers feel that many of the ''environmental'' factors influencing asthma and allergy are linked to significant changes in diet and lifestyle. The higher incidence of asthma and allergy in adults and children of the former West Germany as opposed to those of the former East Germany has lent credence to this hypothesis (113). East German households have less insulation and wall-to-wall carpeting than West German households—hence less mites and molds. Moreover East German children are usually kept in day-care facilities from an early age—from the first year of life. This would increase the likelihood of exposure to recurrent childhood infections and could promote an antiallergic immune profile (114).

In another study looking at the prevalence of clinical allergy and sensitization in Germany, the East-West difference was most apparent in children and young adults born since the 1960s (115). This could be a reflection of the economic and cultural differences between the two halves of the country, which appeared following the Second World War.

Changing dietary habits may also be involved—a decline in the consumption of antioxidants such as vitamin C, manganese, and fish and an increase in consumption of high-salt foods, including ''fast'' foods—have been linked to increasing prevalence of asthma (116). In the United Kingdom, children who ate a ''westernized'' diet had significantly more asthma than those who ate an ''Asian'' diet, regardless of race (117). Children who eat fish at least once a week—with omega-3 fatty acids—are protected from having current asthma or airway hyperreactivity (118,119).

XV. Conclusions

Asthma and allergic disorders are increasing around the world and have become a major health burden especially in ''westernized'' countries and urbanized societies. Part of the predisposition in developing these disorders is undoubtedly genetic, and rapid progress is now being made in unraveling the details of the ''asthma gene'' pool. Most of the increase, however, appears to be linked to changes in the environment and lifestyle. Our environment has become considerably more ''toxic'' over the past few decades, and such pollution can certainly provoke or enhance inflammatory changes in our lungs. Such pollutants also can link up with allergens, leading to increased sensitization of susceptible individuals. Patterns of indoor allergens have also changed, thanks to improved heating and insulation. Childhood infections have declined significantly with a loss of their potential anti-allergic influence. Change in the ''early life'' environment appear to be especially critical, with maternal cigarette smoking and passive smoking appearing to increase asthma, while breast-feeding and non-RSV infections possibly protecting against it.

Although a precise definition of the asthma phenotype continues to evade us, the increasing use of standardized questionnaires—as in ISAAC and uniformity in procedures testing lung function, as in multicenter studies like ECRHS—will allow us to make accurate comparisons of asthma prevalence and distribution in different geographical regions. From such epidemiological data we hope to gain new insights into the complicated asthma paradigm.

References

1. Burney P. Why study the epidemiology of asthma? Thorax 1994; 49:171–174.
2. Anderson HR, Butland BK, Strachan DP. Trends in prevalence and severity of childhood asthma. BMJ 1994; 308:1600–1604.
3. Ninan TK, Russel G. Respiratory symptoms and atopy in Aberdeen schoolchildren: evidence from 2 surveys 25 years apart. BMJ 1992; 304:873–875.
4. Peat JK, Vanden bergh RH, Green WF, Mellis CM, Leederc SR, Woolcock AJ. Changing prevalence of asthma in Australian children. BMJ 1994; 308:1591–1596.
5. Burr M, Butland B, King S, Vaughan-Williams E. Changes in asthma prevalence: 2 surveys 15 years apart. Arch Dis Child 1989; 64:1452–1456.
6. CDC. Asthma mortality in Illinois: 1979–1994. MMWR 1997; 46:877–879.
7. Burney P, Chinn S, Luczynska C, Jarvis D, Lai E. Variations in the prevalence of respiratory symptoms, self-reported asthma attacks and use of asthma medications in the European Community Respiratory Health Survey (ECRHS). Eur Resp J 1996; 9:687–695.
8. Chinn S, Burney P, Jarvis D, Luczynska C. Variation in bronchial responsiveness in the European Community Respiratory Health Survey (ECRHS). Eur Respir J 1997; 10:2495–2501.
9. Pearce N, Weiland S, Keil U. Self reported prevalence of asthma symptoms in children in Australia, England, Germany and New Zealand: an International comparison using the ISAAC protocol. Eur Resp J 1993; 6:1455–1461.
10. Beasley R for ISAAC. Worldwide variation in prevalence of symptoms of asthma, allergic rhino-conjunctivitis and atopic eczema. Lancet 1998; 351:1225–1232.
11. Kaur B, Anderson HR, Austin J, Barr M, Strachan D, Warner JO. Asthma prevalence in UK: ISAAC (UK), Lancet conference on asthma, 1997.
12. Odhiambo J, Ng'ang'a L, Mungai M. Rural and urban respiratory health surveys in Kenya schoolchildren: Participation rates and prevalence of markers of asthma. Am J Resp Crit Care Med 1994; 149(pt 2):A385.
13. Ng'ang'a LW, Odhiambo JA, Omwega MJ, et al. Exercise-induced bronchospasm: a pilot survey in Nairobi school children. East Afr Med J 1997; 74:694–698.
14. Yermaneberham H, Bekele Z, Venn A, Lewis S, Parry E, Britton J. Prevalence of wheeze and asthma and relation to atopy in urban and rural Ethiopia. Lancet 1997; 350:85–90.

15. Newman-Taylor A. Environmental determinants of asthma. Lancet 1995; 345:296–299.
16. Seaton A, Godden D, Brown K. Increase in asthma: a more toxic environment or a more susceptible population? Thorax 1994; 49:171–174.
17. CIBA Foundation. CIBA symposia: Terminology, definition and classification of chronic pulmonary emphsema and related conditions. Thorax 1959; 14:286–299.
18. NIH/WHO National Institutes of Health. WHO/NIH 1995 Workshop Report—Global Strategy for Asthma Management and Prevention. Publication no. 95-3659. Bethseda, MD: NIH, 1995.
19. Weiss ST. Problems in the phenotypic assessment of asthma. Clin Exp Allergy 1995; 25 (suppl 2):12–14; discussion, 17–18.
20. Sears M, Jones D, Holdaway M. Prevalence of bronchial reactivity to inhaled methacholine in New Zealand school children. Thorax 1986; 41:283–289.
21. Bleecker ER, Postma DS, Meyers DA. Genetic susceptibility to asthma in changing environment. Ciba Found Symp 1997; 206:90–99.
22. Sears MR, Burrows B, Flannery EM, Herbison GP, Hewitt CJ, Holdaway MD. Relation between airway responsiveness and serum IgE in children with asthma and in apparently normal children. N Engl J Med 1991; 325:1067–1071.
23. Smith CM, Hawksworth RJ, Thien FC, Christie PE, Lee TH. Urinary leukotriene E4 in bronchial asthma. Eur Respir J 1992; 5:693–699.
24. Brynes C, Dinarevic S, Shinebourne E, Barnes P, Bush A. Exhaled nitric oxide measurements in normal and asthmatic children. Paed Pulmonol 1997; 24:312–318.
25. Djukanovic R, Roche WR, Wilson JW, et al. Mucosal inflammation in asthma. Am Rev Respir Dis 1990; 142:434–457.
26. Holgate S. Asthma genetics: waiting to exhale. Nature Genet 1997; 15:227–229.
27. ECRHS. Genes for asthma? An analysis of the European Community Respiratory Health Survey. Am J Respir Crit Care Med 1997; 156:1773–1780.
28. Bleecker ER, Postma DS, Meyers DA. Evidence for multiple genetic susceptibility loci for asthma. Am J Respir Crit Care Med 1997; 156:S113–S116.
29. Samet JM. Asthma and the environment: do environmental factors affect the incidence and prognosis of asthma? Toxicol Lett 1995; 82-83:33–38.
30. Panhuysen CI, Meyers DA, Postma DS, Bleecker ER. The genetics of asthma and atopy. Allergy 1995; 50:863–869.
31. Smith CA, Harrison DJ. Association between polymorphism in gene for microsomal epoxide hydrolase and susceptibility to emphysema (see comments). Lancet 1997; 350:630–633.
32. Wong HR, Wispe JR. The stress response and the lung. Am J Physiol 1997; 273: L1–L9.
33. Wong HR, Ryan M, Wispe JR. Stress response decreases NF-kappa B nuclear translocation and increases I-kappa B alpha expression in A549 cells. J Clin Invest 1997; 99:2423–2428.
34. Hunter T, Karin M. The regulation of transcription by phosphorylation. Cell 1992; 70:375–387.
35. Barnes PJ, Adcock IM. Transcription factors and asthma (in-process citation). Eur Respir J 1998; 12:221–234.

36. Stacey MA, Sun G, Vassalli G, Marini M, Bellini A, Mattoli S. The allergen Der p1 induces NF-kappaB activation through interference with I-kappa B alpha function in asthmatic bronchial epithelial cells. Biochem Biophys Res Commun 1997; 236:522–526.
37. CSGA. A genome-wide search for asthma susceptibility loci in ethnically diverse populations: the Collaborative Study on the Genetics of Asthma (CSGA). Nature Genet 1997; 15:389–392.
38. Lubs ML. Empiric risks for genetic counseling in families with allergy. J Pediatr 1972; 80:26–31.
39. Duffy D, Martin N, Battistutta D, Hopper J, Mathews JD. Genetics of asthma and hayfever in Australian twins. Am Rev Respir Dis 1990; 142:1351–1358.
40. Niemann M, Kaprio J, Koskenvou M. A population based study of bronchial asthma in adult twin pairs. Chest 1991; 100:70–75.
41. Hanson B, McGue M, Roitman-Johnson B, Segal NL, Bouchard TJ, Blumenthal M. Atopic disease and immunoglobulin E in twins reared apart and together. Am J Hum Genet 1991; 48:873–879.
42. Daniels S, Bhattacharya S, James A. A Genome wide search for quantitative loci underlying asthma. Nature 1996; 383:247–250.
43. Thomas NS, Wilkinson J, Holgate ST. The candidate region approach to the genetics of asthma and allergy. Am J Respir Crit Care Med 1997; 156:S144–S151.
44. Hall I. Candidate gene approaches: gene environmental interactions. Clin Exp Allergy 1998; 28(S1):74–76.
45. Moffatt MF, Cookson WO. Tumour necrosis factor haplotypes and asthma. Hum Mol Genet 1997; 6:551–554.
46. Young RP, Sharp PA, Lynch JR, et al. Confirmation of genetic linkage between atopic IgE responses and chromosome 11q13. J Med Genet 1992; 29:236–238.
47. Marsh DG, Neely JD, Breazeale DR, et al. Linkage analysis of IL4 and other chromosome 5q31. 1 markers and total serum immunoglobulin E concentrations. Science 1994; 264:1152–1156.
48. Hopes E, McDougall C, Christie G, et al. Association of glutamine 27 polymorphism of beta 2 adrenoceptor with reported childhood asthma: population-based study. BMJ 1998; 316:664.
49. Turki J, Pak J, Green S, Martin R, Liggett S. Genetic polymorphisms of the beta 2 adrenoceptor in nocturnal and non-nocturnal asthma: evidence that Gly 16 correlates with the nocturnal phenotype. J Clin Invest 1995; 95:1635–1641.
50. Martinez FD. Definition of pediatric asthma and associated risk factors. Pediatr Pulmonol Suppl 1997; 15:9–12.
51. Klink M, Cline MG, Halonen M, Burrows B. Problems in defining normal limits for serum IgE. J Allergy Clin Immunol 1990; 85:440–444.
52. Burrows B, Martinez F, Halonen M, Barbee R, Cline M. Association of asthma with serum IgE levels and skin test reactivity to allergens. N Engl J Med 1995; 320:271–277.
53. Postma DS, Bleecker ER, Amelung PJ, et al. Genetic susceptibility to asthma—bronchial hyperresponsiveness coinherited with a major gene for atopy. N Engl J Med 1995; 333:894–900.

54. Sandford AJ, Moffatt MF, Daniels SE, et al. A genetic map of chromosome 11q, including the atopy locus. Eur J Hum Genet 1995; 3:188–194.
55. Cookson WO, Young RP, Sandford AJ, et al. Maternal inheritance of atopic IgE responsiveness on chromosome 11q [published erratum appears in Lancet 1992; 340:1110 (see comments)]. Lancet 1992; 340:381–384.
56. Miles E, Warner J, Jones A, Colwell B, Bryant T, Warner J. Peripheral blood mononuclear cell proliferative responses in the first year of life in babies born of allergic parents. Clin Exp Allergy 1994; 24:223–230.
57. Warner JA, Jones AC, Miles EA, Colwell BM, Warner JO. Maternofetal interaction and allergy. Allergy 1996; 51:447–451.
58. Tang ML, Kemp AS, Thorburn J, Hill DJ. Reduced interferon-gamma secretion in neonates and subsequent atopy (see comments). Lancet 1994; 344:983–985.
59. Warner JA, Miles EA, Jones AC, Quint DJ, Colwell BM, Warner JO. Is deficiency of interferon gamma production by allergen triggered cord blood cells a predictor of atopic eczema? (see comments). Clin Exp Allergy 1994; 24:423–430.
60. Cook DG, Strachan DP. Health effects of passive smoking: 3. Parental smoking and prevalence of respiratory symptoms and asthma in school age children. Thorax 1997; 52:1081–1094.
61. Martinez FD. Maternal risk factors in asthma. Ciba Found Symp 1997; 206:233–239.
62. Taylor B, Wadsworth J. Maternal smoking during pregnancy and lower respiratory tract illness in early life. Arch Dis Child 1987; 62:785–791.
63. Martinez FD, Antognoni G, Macri F, et al. Parental smoking enhances bronchial responsiveness in nine-year-old children. Am Rev Respir Dis 1988; 138:518–523.
64. Bahna S. Concordance in atopic twins. J Allergy Clin Immunol 1983; 71:100.
65. Murray AB, Morrison BJ. Passive smoking by asthmatics: its greater effect on boys than on girls and on older than on younger children (see comments). Pediatrics 1989; 84:451–459.
66. Weiss ST. Diet as a risk factor for asthma. Ciba Found Symp 1997; 206:244–257.
67. McConnochie KM, Roghmann KJ. Breast feeding and maternal smoking as predictors of wheezing in children age 6 to 10 years. Pediatr Pulmonol 1986; 2:260–268.
68. Chandra RK. Five-year follow-up of high-risk infants with family history of allergy who were exclusively breast-fed or fed partial whey hydrolysate, soy, and conventional cow's milk formulas [see comments]. J Pediatr Gastroenterol Nutr 1997; 24:380–388.
69. Lewis S, Butland B, Strachan D, et al. Study of the aetiology of wheezing illness at age 16 in two national British birth cohorts. Thorax 1996; 51:670–676.
70. Lilja G, Dannaeus A, Foucard T, Graff-Lonnevig V, Johansson SG, Oman H. Effects of maternal diet during late pregnancy and lactation on the development of atopic diseases in infants up to 18 months of age—in vivo results. Clin Exp Allergy 1989; 19:473–479.
71. Hide DW, Matthews S, Tariq S, Arshad SH. Allergen avoidance in infancy and allergy at 4 years of age (see comments). Allergy 1996; 51:89–93.
72. Martinez FD, Wright AL, Taussig LM, Holberg CJ, Halonen M, Morgan WJ.

Asthma and wheezing in the first six years of life: The Group Health Medical Associates (see comments). N Engl J Med 1995; 332:133–138.
73. Weiss ST, Tosteson TD, Segal MR, Tager IB, Redline S, Speizer FE. Effects of asthma on pulmonary function in children: a longitudinal population-based study. Am Rev Respir Dis 1992; 145:58–64.
74. Welliver RC, Ogra PL. Respiratory syncytial virus. Comp Ther 1981; 7:34–40.
75. Schwarze J, Hamelmann E, Bradley KL, Takeda K, Gelfand EW. Respiratory syncytial virus infection results in airway hyperresponsiveness and enhanced airway sensitization to allergen. J Clin Invest 1997; 100:226–233.
76. Grunberg K, Smits HH, Timmers MC, et al. Experimental rhinovirus 16 infection. Effects on cell differentials and soluble markers in sputum in asthmatic subjects. Am J Respir Crit Care Med 1997; 156:609–616.
77. Johnston SL, Papi A, Bates PJ, Mastronarde JG, Monick MM, Hunninghake GW. Low grade rhinovirus infection induces a prolonged release of IL-8 in pulmonary epithelium. J Immunol 1998; 160:6172–6181.
78. Bodner C, Godden D, Seaton A. Family size, childhood infections and atopic diseases. The Aberdeen WHEASE Group. Thorax 1998; 53:28–32.
79. Shirakawa T, Enomoto T, Shimazu S, Hopkin JM. The inverse association between tuberculin responses and atopic disorder (see comments). Science 1997; 275:77–79.
80. Matricardi PM, Rosmini F, Ferrigno L, et al. Cross sectional retrospective study of prevalence of atopy among Italian military students with antibodies against hepatitis A virus (see comments). BMJ 1997; 314:999–1003.
81. Holgate ST. Asthma and allergy—Disorders of civilization? Q J Med 1998; 91: 171–184.
82. Robinson PJ, Hegele RG, Schellenberg RR. Allergic sensitization increases airway reactivity in guinea pigs with respiratory syncytial virus bronchiolitis. J Allergy Clin Immunol 1997; 100:492–498.
83. Erb KJ, Holloway JW, Sobeck A, Moll H, Le Gros G. Infection of mice with Mycobacterium bovis–bacillus Calmette-Guérin (BCG) suppresses allergen-induced airway eosinophilia. J Exp Med 1998; 187:561–569.
84. Jorres RD, Nowak D, Magnussen H. The effect of ozone exposure on allergen responsiveness in subjects with asthma or rhinitis. Am J Respir Crit Care Med 1996; 153:56–64.
85. Gielen MH, van der Zee SC, van Wijnen JH, van Steen CJ, Brunekreef B. Acute effects of summer air pollution on respiratory health of asthmatic children. Am J Respir Crit Care Med 1997; 155:2105–2108.
86. Rusznak C, Devalia JL, Davies RJ. Airway response of asthmatic subjects to inhaled allergen after exposure to pollutants. Thorax 1996; 51:1105–1108.
87. Lag M, Schwarze PE. Health effects of ozone in the environment. Tidsskr Nor Laegeforen 1997; 117:57–60.
89. Suphioglu C. Thunderstrom asthma due to grass pollen (in-process citation). Int Arch Allergy Immunol 1998; 116:253–260.
90. Newson R, Strachan D, Archibald E, Emberlin J, Hardaker P, Collier C. Effect of

thunderstorms and airborne grass pollen on the incidence of acute asthma in England, 1990–94 (see comments). Thorax 1997; 52:680–685.
91. Waller RE. Air pollution and community health. J R Coll Physicians Lond 1971; 5:362–368.
92. Glovsky MM, Miguel AG, Cass GR. Particulate air pollution: possible relevance in asthma. Allergy Asthma Proc 1997; 18:163–166.
93. Miguel AG, Cass GR, Weiss J, Glovsky MM. Latex allergens in tire dust and airborne particles. Environ Health Perspect 1996; 104:1180–1186.
94. Ostro B, Chestnut L. Assessing the health benefits of reducing particulate matter air pollution in the United States. Environ Res 1998; 76:94–106.
95. Timonen KL, Pekkanen J. Air pollution and respiratory health among children with asthmatic or cough symptoms. Am J Respir Crit Care Med 1997; 156:546–552.
96. Peters A, Wichmann H, Tuch T, Heinrich J, Heyder J. Respiratory effects are associated with the number of ultrafine particles. Am J Respir Crit Care Med 1997; 155:1376–1383.
97. Pope CAD, Dockery DW, Spengler JD, Raizenne ME. Respiratory health and PM10 pollution: A daily time series analysis. Am Rev Respir Dis 1991; 144:668–674.
98. Sheppard D. Sulfur dioxide and asthma—a double-edged sword? J Allergy Clin Immunol 1988; 82:961–964.
99. Moseler M, Hendel-Kramer A, Karmaus W, et al. Effect of moderate NO_2 air pollution on the lung function of children with asthmatic symptoms. Environ Res 1994; 67:109–124.
100. Kuhr J, Hendel-Kramer A, Karmaus W, et al. Air pollutant burden and bronchial asthma in school children. Soz Praventivmed 1991; 36:67–73.
101. Neas LM, Dockery DW, Ware JH, Spengler JD, Speizer FE, Ferris BG Jr. Association of indoor nitrogen dioxide with respiratory symptoms and pulmonary function in children. Am J Epidemiol 1991; 134:204–219.
102. Devalia JL, Rusznak C, Herdman MJ, Trigg CJ, Tarraf H, Davies RJ. Effect of nitrogen dioxide and sulphur dioxide on airway response of mild asthmatic patients to allergen inhalation. Lancet 1994; 344:1668–1671.
103. Knox RB, Suphioglu C, Taylor P, et al. Major grass pollen allergen Lol p 1 binds to diesel exhaust particles: implications for asthma and air pollution. Clin Exp Allergy 1997; 27:246–251.
104. Ormstad H, Johansen BV, Gaarder PI. Airborne house dust particles and diesel exhaust particles as allergen carriers (in-process citation). Clin Exp Allergy 1998; 28:702–708.
105. Sarpong SB, Karrison T. Skin test reactivity to indoor allergens as a marker of asthma severity in children with asthma. Ann Allergy Asthma Immunol 1998; 80: 303–308.
106. Leen MG, O'Connor T, Kelleher C, Mitchell EB, Loftus BG. Home environment and childhood asthma. Ir Med J 1994; 87:142–144.
107. Ehnert B, Lau-Schadendorf S, Weber A, Buettner P, Schou C, Wahn U. Reducing domestic exposure to dust mite allergen reduces bronchial hyperreactivity in sensitive children with asthma. J Allergy Clin Immunol 1992; 90:135–138.

108. Howarth P, Lunn A, Tomkin S. Study on 35 patients. J Br Allergy Clin Immunol 1992.
109. Denman AM, Cornthwaite D. Control of house dust mite antigen in bedding (letter, comment). Lancet 1990; 335:1038.
110. Peat JK, Tovey E, Toelle BG, et al. House dust mite allergens: a major risk factor for childhood asthma in Australia. Am J Respir Crit Care Med 1996; 153:141–146.
111. Kattan M, Mitchell H, Eggleston P, et al. Characteristics of inner-city children with asthma: the National Cooperative Inner-City Asthma Study. Pediatr Pulmonol 1997; 24:253–262.
112. Custovic A, Simpson A, Pahdi H, Green RM, Chapman MD, Woodcock A. Distribution, aerodynamic characteristics, and removal of the major cat allergen Fel d 1 in British homes. Thorax 1998; 53:33–38.
113. von Mutius E, Weiland SK, Fritzsch C, Duhme H, Keil U. Increasing prevalence of hay fever and atopy among children in Leipzig, East Germany. Lancet 1998; 351:862–866.
114. von Mutius E, Martinez FD, Fritzsch C, Nicolai T, Roell G, Thiemann HH. Prevalence of asthma and atopy in two areas of West and East Germany. Am J Respir Crit Care Med 1994; 149:358–364.
115. Weichmann H. Environment, lifestyle and allergy: the German answer. Allergology 1995; 4:315–316.
116. Soutar A, Seaton A, Brown K. Bronchial reactivity and dietary anti-oxidants. Thorax 1997; 52:166–170.
117. Carey OJ, Cookson JB, Britton J, Tattersfield AE. The effect of lifestyle on wheeze, atopy, and bronchial hyperreactivity in Asian and white children. Am J Respir Crit Care Med 1996; 154:537–540.
118. Hodge L, Salome CM, Peat JK, Haby MM, Xuan W, Woolcock AJ. Consumption of oily fish and childhood asthma risk (see comments). Med J Aust 1996; 164: 137–140.
119. Hodge L, Salome CM, Hughes JM, et al. Effect of dietary intake of omega-3 and omega-6 fatty acids on severity of asthma in children. Eur Respir J 1998; 11:361–365.
120. Holgate ST. Candidate genes and asthma. The cellular and mediator basis of asthma in relation to natural history. Lancet 1997: Oct; 350 Suppl 2:SII5–9.

2

Pathophysiology of Asthma

PETER J. STERK

Leiden University Medical Center
Leiden, The Netherlands

I. Introduction

Asthma is a clinical syndrome, descriptively defined according to abnormalities at the cellular, physiological, and clinical levels (1). These abnormalities include the presence of the cellular infiltrate within the airway wall, variable airways obstruction, and the occurrence of episodic symptoms of chest tightness and wheezing. In the absence of complete understanding of the pathogenesis of asthma, such a descriptive definition is inevitable and appropriate. This certainly does not mean that there is no progress in unraveling the causes of asthma and/or the best approaches for the management and prevention of the disease. In contrast, during the past decade, there has been an expanding growth in understanding of the fundamental abnormalities in the airways of patients with asthma (Table 1). In particular, this refers to the allergen-driven inflammation within the airway wall (2–4). The safe application of fiberoptic bronchoscopy in asthma has allowed pathologists, immunologists, and molecular biologists to investigate the interaction among the various resident cells and the inflammatory cells in the mucosa and lamina propria (5). At present, this approach seems to offer the best prospects for the gradual unraveling of the pathogenesis of asthma. In addition, it can be envisaged that monitoring of the cellular presence and activity during

Table 1 Characteristics of Asthma

Level of Abnormality	Characteristics		Stimulus
Clinical symptoms	Episodic	Dyspnea	Exercise
		Chest tightness	Cold, dry air
		Cough	Other irritants
		Wheezing	
		Nocturnal awakenings	
Lung function	Variable	Obstruction (reversible)	Allergens
		Hyperresponsiveness	Viruses
			Air pollutants
Airway inflammation	Infiltration	T lymphocytes	Cytokines
		Mast cells	Mediators
		Neutrophils	
		Eosinophils	
		Basophils	
	Neurogenic	NANC (e-NANC) nerves	Neuropeptides
Airway remodeling	Mucosa	Epithelial shedding	Mediators
		Subepithelial collagen deposition, goblet-cell hyperplasia	Cytokines
	Submucosa	Hyperemia, edema	Mediators
			Neuropeptides
	Smooth muscle	Hyperplasia, hypertrophy	Mediators
			Growth factors
	Adventitia	Hyperemia, edema, destruction of alveolar attachments	Enzymes

therapeutic interventions will provide a rationale for the development of a more causal treatment of the disease. Undoubtedly, major improvements in future asthma therapy and prevention will be based on respiratory cell and molecular biology (6,7).

A. From Inflammation to Airway Narrowing

Despite the rapidly increasing understanding of the genesis and modulation of airway inflammation in asthma, it is still largely unclear which are the main effector mechanisms causing the enhanced airways obstruction in the disease (8). This is rather unexpected, since this has been an area of physiological research for many decades. It is beyond doubt that airways obstruction remains the central characteristic responsible for the clinical expression of asthma (9). Even though the degree and variability of airways obstruction appear to be associated with many markers of airway inflammation in asthmatics, the physiological factors determining the severity of airway narrowing are far from being clarified.

The currently available models of asthma are almost invariably based on acute or subacute pathophysiology due to various inducers of airway inflammation (10). This applies for animal models as well as experimental human models of asthma. Such an approach is presently leading to the development of potentially powerful drugs in the prevention and reversal of acute inflammatory changes in the airways (6,7). However, asthma is a chronic disease, presenting in various clinical forms ranging from intermittent to severe, hence persistent (1); its pathophysiology might not be fully covered by these models.

Many tissue components appear to be able to contribute to the excessive and potentially life-threatening airway narrowing in asthma, including airway smooth muscle, airway nerves, bronchial vessels, connective tissue elements, mucosal or luminal exudates, and secretions (11). Each of these substrates can potentially be triggered by the various inflammatory pathways involved, but it has yet to be determined which of the effector mechanisms predominate in the various clinical presentations of asthma. This will be essential for the development of new and specific therapeutic agents for asthma, particularly those with more sustained activity than the ones currently available.

Hence, as long as asthma is characterized by difficult breathing, pathophysiology will be the cornerstone in the transition between the basic and clinical science aimed at improving the management and prevention of the disease.

II. Variable Airways Obstruction

The variability of the airways obstruction is a diagnostic criterion for asthma (1). This refers to spontaneous and transient episodes of measurable airflow limitation accompanied by symptoms of breathlessness. Such airflow limitation is often referred to as airways obstruction, despite the fact that—understandably—the basic measurement is usually based on airflow at the mouth as opposed to morphological techniques. The most common measurements for documenting variable airways obstruction include the following:

1. Daily home measurements of peak expiratory flow (PEF) (12). There are at least nine methods for analyzing morning and evening PEF readings (12), the current method of first choice being (highest-lowest value)/(highest value) (1), or the minimal morning PEF before bronchodilation in percentage of personal best or predicted value (12).

2. Laboratory measurement of reversibility of airways obstruction after inhaling a bronchodilator agent (13). This includes the recording of the forced

expiratory volume in one-second (FEV_1) (14) or PEF (15) after inhaling a short-acting bronchodilator (14,16), preferably a β_2-agonist as a functional antagonist. The response is usually expressed as the value obtained: (after-before value)/(predicted value) (13). A response in FEV_1 by >12% or >200 mL (in adults) or in PEF by >15% (1) or >60 L/min (15) is commonly regarded as indicative (but not fully specific) for asthma.

3. Laboratory provocation tests with inhaled bronchoconstrictor agents demonstrate the so-called airways hyperresponsiveness (17). Usually, these challenges are performed in a dose-response way by exposing the subject to increasing doses of the bronchoconstrictor stimulus while measuring an index of lung function. Hence, the essential outcome of the challenge is the bronchoconstrictor dose-response curve, which can be characterised by (a) the position (measuring *sensitivity*), (b) the slope (measuring *reactivity*), and (c) the plateau (measuring *maximal response*) (18). It must be emphasized that these three characteristics of the dose-response curve need to be carefully distinguished, because they can vary independently (18). It is mandatory to use strict terminology. The term *hyperresponsiveness* is recommended as a general description of the phenomenon. *Hypersensitivity* and *hyperreactivity* specifically refer to the leftward shift and the increase in slope of the dose-response curve, respectively. Unfortunately, the term *hyperreactivity* is often misused as being synonymous with *hypersensitivity*. Finally, *excessive airway narrowing* refers to an increase in maximal response, often leading to an unmeasurable plateau level. Since most investigators assume that the bronchi are the major component in these responses, the terms *airway hyperresponsiveness* and *bronchial hyperresponsiveness* are used interchangeably. Because of this confusing terminology, it is mandatory to specifically indicate the outcome measurements in describing the results of challenge tests.

In examining the pathophysiology of asthma in detail, it would be preferable, in principle, to concentrate on the spontaneous fluctuations of airways obstruction in patients. However, the unpredictable nature of such fluctuations and the rather simple lung function techniques available for home recordings are seriously limiting this approach. Alternatively, it has been widely acknowledged that mimicking the spontaneous airways obstruction by giving a strictly defined bronchoconstrictor challenge in the laboratory can be a strong investigational strategy in research on the pathophysiology of asthma.

III. Bronchoprovocation Tests

It is essential to specify the nature of the bronchoconstrictor applied (19). Some bronchoconstrictors act directly and predominantly on airway smooth muscle itself (e.g., methacholine, histamine), whereas other stimuli depend on the involvement of cellular or neurogenic mechanisms, indirectly leading to airway smooth muscle contraction and possibly to inflammatory changes in the airway wall (e.g., nonisotonic aerosols, cold/dry air, exercise, adenosine 5′-monophosphate (AMP), bradykinin, tachykinins, leukotrienes, sodium metabisulfite, etc.) (17,19).

Inflammatory mechanisms predominate after challenge with sensitizing agents, particularly during late asthmatic reactions (e.g., allergens, occupational sensitizers) (20,21). In addition, these challenges by themselves can also cause a temporary increase in airway responsiveness to other, nonsensitizing stimuli (so-called inducers), which also occurs after respiratory virus infection (22,23).

Therefore, it is not surprising that the results of the various challenge tests are only weakly correlated and not interchangeable, each test implicitly providing different and perhaps complementary information on the multiple pathophysiological pathways leading to airway narrowing.

Detailed guidelines for laboratory protocols on standardized bronchial challenge tests have been provided previously (17). Sensible usage of these tests is highly suited for pharmacological intervention studies on the mechanisms and treatment of variable airways obstruction in asthma.

IV. What Protects Normal Subjects Against Bronchoconstriction?

In 1986 Macklem challenged the generally accepted concept of airway hyperresponsiveness in asthma by pointing toward the unclarified airway *hypo*responsiveness in healthy subjects (24). Hence, why is not everyone having asthma (25)?

Woolcock et al. (26) were the first to recognize the potential importance of the limitation in the maximal degree of airway narrowing to bronchoconstrictor agents in normal subjects in vivo. When exposed to high doses of histamine or methacholine, normal subjects show a maximal response plateau on the dose-response curve at mild degrees of airway narrowing (26,27). The plateau in normal subjects represents limited bronchoconstriction in spite of supramaximal stimulation of the airways (28) and is usually reached at a 10–30% fall in FEV_1 from baseline (29,30). The presence and level of the plateau is reproducible within subjects between days, the coefficient of repeatability being about a 10–12% fall in FEV_1 (31–33). What protects them from severe airway narrowing in response to strong bronchoconstrictive stimuli? The determinants of the limited airway response in normal subjects are not fully understood (25,34).

A. Humoral or Neurogenic Inhibition

There is no evidence for humoral (e.g., cyclo-oxygenase products) or neurogenic inhibition of maximal airway narrowing in humans in vivo (35). However, inhibitory (neuro)peptides might be involved during specific bronchoconstrictor challenges, such as exercise (36). In addition, it is still unclear whether there is a role for endogenously released nitric oxide (NO) during bronchoconstriction in humans in vivo (37).

B. Limited Airway Smooth Muscle Contraction

Maximal airway smooth muscle shortening could be limited due to the intrinsic properties of the muscle itself or to mechanical interaction with its environment (38). With regard to the muscle, any deviation from the optimal resting length would attenuate its contractility (39). It is unknown whether, under physiological conditions in vivo, human airway smooth muscle is at optimal resting length, at which maximal active tension can be developed. From animal studies in vivo, it appears that optimal tracheal smooth muscle length is achieved at lung volumes close to functional residual capacity (FRC), even though a large variability has been observed in tracheal length/tension behavior between individual animals (40). Therefore, it cannot be excluded that limited bronchoconstriction in some subjects is due to nonoptimal resting smooth muscle length, particularly at low lung volumes (40). In addition, dynamic tidal volume oscillations may also reduce maximal bronchoconstriction. This can be explained by the hysteretic behavior of airway smooth muscle, which inhibits rapid, active development of transmural pressure during expiration (41). And finally, it has been postulated that smooth muscle orientation within the airway walls is a major determinant of maximal airway narrowing (42). This indicates that the change in airway resistance for a given degree of smooth muscle shortening is dependent on the angle of the smooth muscle helix together with the stiffness of the airway wall.

C. Mechanical Interdependence

The mechanical forces of interdependence between airways and their environment are likely to be a major determinant in the prevention of excessive airway narrowing in normal subjects (43). The elastic loads provided by cartilage and the surrounding lung parenchyma mechanically counterbalance muscle shortening, thereby potentially limiting maximal airway narrowing under physiological conditions (11,34,38,39). On the one hand, tracheal cartilage seems to promote maximal bronchoconstriction by providing a considerable preload, which stretches the muscle toward optimal length (44). However, on the other hand, cartilage supplies an afterload, thereby limiting maximal airway narrowing (45). A similar reasoning may hold for the elastic load of the parenchyma. When the muscle is stimulated, this load probably leads to a mixture of isometric and isotonic constriction (40,46), the net result being reduced maximal shortening with increasing load. The importance of the parenchymal elastic load has indirectly been established in studies in animals (47) and in normal humans in vivo (48). These experiments demonstrated that the level of maximal response plateau of lung resistance to inhaled methacholine increased with decreasing lung volume and thus with decreasing transpulmonary pressure (48). The association of the maximal response plateau with the afterload provided by the transpulmonary pressure has recently been confirmed by measuring the most negative transpulmonary pressure during tidal breathing throughout a methacholine challenge in normal subjects (49). Moreover, in isolated perfused rat lungs, the limited airway smooth muscle shortening with increasing lung volume could be confirmed morphometrically (50). Using both gas- and liquid-filled lungs, it appeared that lung tissue forces as well as surface forces act to oppose smooth muscle shortening in vivo (50).

Apparently, the major factor preventing excessive airway narrowing in normal subjects is the mechanical load limiting airway smooth muscle shortening. However, there must be other opposing forces involved. Even at relatively high transpulmonary pressures, methacholine is still able to induce airway closure in isolated dog lobes in vivo (51) or in rat lungs in vitro (50). These results are in accordance with carefully performed morphometric studies in excised dog lobes (52), indicating that the elastic load might not be the only contributor to limited airway smooth muscle shortening in vivo. This suggests that the forces of interdependence per se are insufficient to limit airway narrowing in intact lobes, whereas they might in whole lungs in situ. It is likely that parenchymal tissue distortion, as occurs secondary to airway narrowing (53), is one of the contributing factors under the latter conditions (54).

Hence, only recently, experimental data and quantitative model studies are gradually clarifying why normal subjects do not have the capability of having clinically significant degrees of airway narrowing. Such understanding seems to be essential and may have implications for therapeutic strategies toward restoring this physiological condition in patients with asthma who demonstrate excessive airway narrowing.

V. Excessive Airway Narrowing in Asthma

There is no doubt that the clinically most relevant aspect of airway hyperresponsiveness is the potential of excessive airway narrowing, which, implicitly, is a hazard to the patient (24,55). Theoretically, the mechanisms responsible for this phenomenon are airway smooth muscle shortening and any factor potentiating the effect of airway muscle shortening on luminal patency. It has been calculated that airway smooth muscle shortening by more than about 40% of its resting length would give loss of the in vivo plateau (38). What is the cause of that?

A. Airway Smooth Muscle Contractility and Velocity of Shortening

Increased contractility of airway smooth muscle has been observed in tracheal smooth muscle of hyperresponsive guinea pigs (56). This could be due either to enhanced intrinsic contractility (56) or to an increase in the mass of airway smooth muscle by hyperplasia or hypertrophy (57,58). Certainly, enhancement of intrinsic contractility has been observed in tracheal strips in asthma in vitro (59). This might be due to elevated actin-myosin adenosine triphosphate (ATP-ase) activity within the smooth muscle cells, leading to an increase in shortening velocity and in maximum shortening as observed after active sensitization in dogs (60) and after passive sensitization of human airways (61). The molecular basis of active force, stiffness and shortening velocity of airway smooth muscle has recently been addressed in further detail (62,63). While active force and stiffness are related to the number of actin-myosin interactions, the shortening velocity, mechanical friction, and hysteresivity of airway smooth muscle are governed by the rate of cross-bridge cycling (62,63). There is increasing evidence that asthma is characterized by reduced airway smooth muscle hysteresis (64). This means the impairment of the normally observed property of contracted airway smooth muscle to relax following mechanical stretch (41), which is presumably due to changes in the organization of contractile filaments or in plasticity of the smooth muscle cells (65). In normal subjects in vivo, this can be demonstrated by transient bronchodilation following a deep inspiration after challenges with bronchoconstrictor stimuli (64). Theoretically, there are two explanations for the loss of deep breath–induced bronchodilation in asthma. First, it might be related to the velocity of airway smooth muscle shortening. The relatively slow cross-bridge cycling and low velocity of shortening of smooth muscle would allow the stretch of a deep breath to cause a temporary bronchodilation in normal subjects (63). However, the rapid cross-bridge cycling rate and high velocity of shortening of airway smooth muscle in sensitized asthmatics (60,61) would lead to a quick restoration of airway smooth muscle tone following stretch, thereby preventing any transient relaxation or bronchodilation following a deep breath (63). Second, the impairment of airway hysteresis may also be explained by the development of a steady-state force maintaining ''latch-state'' of airway smooth muscle, secondary to the absence of periodic muscle stretch as caused by uncoupling of airway-parenchymal interdependence in asthma (11,62). The latter would be due to peribronchial swelling or destroyed alveolar attachments, and would strongly enhance excessive airway narrowing in response to bronchoconstrictor stimuli (11). Taken together, the factors leading to airway smooth muscle dysfunction are likely to contribute to airway hyperresponsiveness in asthma (63).

B. Airway Smooth Muscle Growth

Apart from airway smooth muscle contractility, increased airway smooth muscle thickness can be a major factor in determining excessive airway narrowing, as appears from recent mathematical model studies based on morphometrical dimensions of airways in asthma (66). Indeed, the mass of smooth muscle within the central and peripheral airways in asthma has been observed to be increased by hyperplasia and/or hypertrophy (67,68), even though this could not be confirmed in a recent morphometrical study (69). Airway smooth muscle proliferation can be caused by mechanical strain (70) as well as by multiple growth factors (57,58). The latter compounds will certainly be available in the microenvironment of the muscle during airways inflammation in asthma (2–4).

C. Reduction in Elastic Load

According to model predictions, any loss in elastic load and/or in shear modulus provided by the lung parenchyma will result in an increase in maximal response to bronchoconstrictive stimuli (54,66). This has indeed been observed in elastase-induced emphysema in rats (71) and in humans with α_1-antitrypsin deficiency (72). Even in asthma, there is a relationship between lung elasticity and the level of maximal airway narrowing (73). Since modification of elastic recoil pressure is by far the most successful way to change the maximal response to bronchoconstrictors in humans in vivo (48), it is not unlikely that many factors leading to excessive airway narrowing in asthma are mediated through a disturbance in the mechanical protection provided by the airway-parenchymal interdependence (11). Even the effects of airway wall swelling on the maximal bronchoconstrictive response are strongly related to the actual value of the elastic recoil pressure (11,54,74).

D. Airway Wall Swelling

Thickening of the airway wall, both internal (mucosal and submucosal) and external to the smooth muscle layer (adventitial or peribronchial), will strongly augment maximal airway narrowing in vivo (34,75). This can be due to swelling of the muscular and nonmuscular components within the airway wall (75) secondary to inflammatory processes (76), such as luminal plasma exudation, edema, and/or microvascular congestion. For a given degree of smooth muscle shortening, luminal patency is then more severely reduced by the increased wall area internal to the muscle layer (34), uncoupling of the interdependence between the airway wall and the surrounding elastic forces by an increased peribronchial radius in case of adventitial swelling (11,54), liquid filling of the interstices between luminal epithelial projections (77), decreased airway elastance (78), and/or a reduction in the number of epithelial folds (79). The latter remains uncertain, since mucosal folds may also be protective by their stiffness against severe airway narrowing (80,81). Again, from model studies (11,54) or experimental evidence (82), it appears that the effects of airway wall swelling on maximal airway narrowing are increasing with decreasing elastic recoil pressure or lung volume.

There is growing evidence for a role of airway wall thickness as a determinant of maximal airway narrowing in humans in vivo. These investigations have been made possible by combining modern physiological measurements with imaging techniques and careful morphometry (83,84). Experimental studies in humans in vivo have provided indirect evidence that inflammatory mechanisms indeed are the major determinants of excessive airway narrowing in asthmatics in vivo. The maximal response to inhaled histamine or methacholine in humans is increased 24 hr after challenge with the pro-inflammatory mediator leukotriene D_4 (85,86) and the tachykinin substance P (87). These observations are in keeping with increased microvascular permeability and airway wall swelling caused by mediators such as substance P, bradykinin, leukotriene C_4, and leukotriene D_4, as observed in studies in guinea pigs in vivo (88–90). Furthermore, the maximal response to methacholine in asthmatics is elevated after challenge with allergens in the laboratory (91) or after natural allergen exposure (92), after exposure to ozone (93), and up to 2 weeks following experimental infection with rhinovirus (94). The latter observation fits in with the role of viruses as the primary cause of exacerbations of asthma (23).

E. Relevance to Asthma

It must be emphasized that apart from edema, the chronic inflammatory swelling of the airway wall in asthma might also be due to collagen deposition (95–97), potentially secondary to chronic allergen exposure (98), and to an increase in the number and/or cross-sectional area of the bronchial vasculature (99–101). The most direct evidence of the relationship between excessive airway narrowing and airways inflammation comes from Möller et al., who showed the correlation of the maximal response to methacholine and the eosinophil counts in bronchial biopsies in asthma (102). Presumably, the peripheral airways are of major importance in determining these structure–function relationships in patients with asthma (103), as appears from physiological experiments (104) as well as from post mortem morphological data in asthma (105,106). When these factors are taken together, it is not surprising that chronic airway inflammation in asthma is associated with excessive airway narrowing to bronchoconstrictor stimuli (9,11).

VI. Hypersensitivity of the Airways

It is not easy to explain hypersensitivity of the asthmatic airways. Strictly speaking, we do not even know yet whether the airways in asthma really are hypersensitive to bronchoconstrictor stimuli in vivo. Traditionally, the lowered provocative concentration causing a 20% fall in FEV_1 (PC_{20}) is being interpreted as such (17). However, a leftward shift of a dose-response curve can be demonstrated only if the complete curve has been recorded (107). Then a leftward shift is expressed as the reduction in dose causing a half-maximal response (ED_{50}). Since in many circumstances, particularly in asthma, the maximal response in vivo cannot be measured (26,31), it remains unclear whether the PC_{20} adequately reflects the position of the dose-response curve. However, the more than 1000-fold range in PC_{20}, as observed between subjects, makes it plausible that it, at least in part, reflects real differences in airway sensitivity. Even though hypersensitivity of the airways per se should not be troublesome to the patient (24,55), it is easy to measure (17) and often associated with increases in maximal response (26,27,31,33). That is why most research studies on airway hyperresponsiveness in asthma are still using PC_{20} as the primary outcome (17). However, a recent study indeed indicates that PC_{20} does not provide the same information as ED_{50} (108). PC_{20} appears rather to be a complex variable, being affected by both the position and the shape of the dose-response curve to bronchoconstrictors in vivo (107,108).

The mechanisms determining hypersensitivity to bronchoconstrictors are principally those that amplify the stimulus given to the airways (55) and are addressed briefly below.

A. Epithelial Damage and Desquamation

Apart from being actively involved in airway inflammation (109), the bronchial epithelium can also be a target of the inflammatory stimuli leading to damage and desquamation (110). This could enhance any bronchoconstrictive stimulus to penetrate into the airway wall. Indeed, the severity of airway hyperresponsiveness (PC_{20}) is related to the extent of epithelial desquamation in patients with asthma (111–113). Such epithelial damage can be caused by chronic antigen exposure (114), virus infection (115), or environmental exposures, as to ozone (116). The associated increase in sensitivity to bronchoconstrictor stimuli might also be caused by impaired inhibitory activity of the epithelium—e.g., by the production of nitric oxide (NO) (117,118) or the neuropeptide degrading enzyme neutral endopeptidase (NEP) (see below).

B. Nonadrenergic, Noncholinergic Neural Activity

The involvement of the nonadrenergic noncholinergic nervous system (NANC) in increasing the sensitivity to inhaled bronchoconstrictors can be due to either impaired inhibition or augmented excitation (119). The impaired inhibition might be related to reduced NO synthesis (117,118) but might also be due to decreased production or availability of NEP, caused either by virus infection (120,121) or allergen exposure (121–125). Furthermore, when immunohistochemistry is used in bronchial biopsies, it appears that NEP expression is relatively low in asthmatic airways and that it is upregulated in patients on inhaled corticosteroids (126). Even though NEP dysfunction in asthma is an attractive hypothesis, this has thus far been difficult to confirm experimentally in vivo (127,128).

The excitatory NANC pathways are likely to be involved in airway hyperresponsiveness (129). Certainly, this has been established in experimental animals (130). However, the involvement of excitatory neuropeptides in airway hyperresponsiveness in asthma in vivo remains to be established and awaits experiments with powerful neurokinin receptor antagonists (131).

C. Cholinergic Activity

The role of the cholinergic nervous system in asthma and airway hyperresponsiveness has not been clarified yet (132). Even though the cholinergic system may not play a major role in the pathophysiology of stable asthma, it appears that anticholinergics are effective during exacerbations of the disease (132). The difficulty of establishing the involvement of the parasympathetic nerves in asthma is due to the only recent availability of specific antagonists of the various muscarinic receptor subtypes (133). There is no doubt that the cholinergic system can be activated in allergic airway inflammation (134). The most likely explanation is that this is due to a relative dysfunction of the inhibitory M_2 receptors, as has been established in vitro and in experimental animals in vivo (121,135,136) as well as indirectly in asthma in vivo (137). This might be due to allergen- (138) or virus-induced (136,139) M_2 receptor dysfunction, perhaps mediated by major basic protein (134) or interleukin-5 (140), thereby providing an explanation for the cholinergic activity during asthma exacerbations (132). It has also been postulated that allergen exposure can cause reduction in acetylcholine-esterase activity (141). Anyway, the response to the indirectly acting bronchoconstrictive stimulus hypertonic saline can be inhibited by atropine, ipratropium bromide, or lignocaïne in asthma (142). Hence, an increase in cholinergic tone seems to be an additional mechanism of airway hyperresponsiveness in asthma while being relatively more important in chronic obstructive pulmonary disease (COPD) (143).

D. Inflammatory Cell Influx and Activity

It is very likely that inflammatory cell influx (76) and activity (2–4) are important in the development of airway hyperresponsiveness in asthma. This evidence comes from various studies showing associations between the airway hyperresponsiveness to various stimuli and inflammatory cell numbers, particularly (activated EG^{2+}) eosinophils, in bronchoalveolar lavage fluid (144), bronchial biopsy specimens (145,146), and induced sputum (147) in asthma, even though this could not be established in all studies (148). In addition, the worsening in PC_{20}, e.g., after viral infection (149), or its improvement after treatment with inhaled corticosteroids (150) is related to the accompanying changes in eosinophil counts in sputum and bronchial biopsy specimens, respectively. Hence, there is a strong case for the involvement of inflammatory cell activity in inducing changes in the sensitivity to inhaled bronchoconstrictor stimuli in asthmatics in vivo.

VII. Physiological Modulation of Airways Obstruction

Most patients know how to modulate the severity of airways obstruction. The simplest modifiers in vivo appear to be based on well-known physiological principles. The patients take advantage of the mechanical airway-parenchymal interdependence (43,64). First, an increase in lung volume, and thereby in lung elastic recoil pressure, appears to be the most powerful way to prevent excessive airway narrowing (48). Second, a change in body posture from supine toward upright can also limit maximal airway narrowing (151), again, most probably due to a rise in lung volume. And third, a deep and rapid inspiration to total lung capacity gives transient bronchodilation during bronchoconstrictor challenges in normal and mildly asthmatic subjects (152–155). The effect of a deep breath affects the dose-response curve for up to 6 min (155), which seems to be due to changes in smooth muscle cell plasticity (65) and demonstrates the incomparability of indices of airway narrowing based on FEV_1 and airway resistance.

A. Impaired Deep Breath–Induced Bronchodilation

It is remarkable that the bronchodilation following a deep breath decreases when methacholine sensitivity increases (153), when airway inflammation is more severe (156), and when proinflammatory stimuli are being inhaled (85,87,157,158). This suggests that inflammation either increases parenchymal hysteresis (159,160) or blunts airway hysteresis by changing the smooth muscle itself (41,64) and/or that it acts by impairing the mechanical interdependence between the airways and the surrounding parenchyma (11,154,160). The latter uncoupling leads to unloading of airway smooth muscle and the absence of periodic stretch. This can enhance the secondary development of a contractile ‘‘latch state’’ of the muscle, that is difficult to overcome by stretching (62). Alternatively, based on animal experiments, it can also be postulated that the airway smooth muscle of sensitized asthmatics has an increased velocity of shortening (60,61) that can rapidly restore tone after stretch, thereby preventing the deep breath-induced relaxation and bronchodilation as observed in normals with relatively slow velocity of shortening (63).

Hence, both muscular and nonmuscular mechanisms are probably contributing to the loss of deep breath–induced bronchodilation in asthma (11,62,63). It can even be argued that loss of deep breath–induced bronchodilation might be a fundamental abnormality in asthma, because prohibiting deep breaths induces hyperresponsiveness in healthy humans (161,162). Even though such an abnormal response to a deep inspiration may not fully explain airway hyperresponsiveness (82), it seems to be clinically relevant, since it is related to the maximal degree of airway narrowing (163) and even to the degree of breathlessness in asthma (157). Hence, clarifying the impairment of deep breath–induced relief in our patients would be of great benefit for the future management of the disease.

VIII. Pharmacological Modulation

The effect of therapeutic intervention with drugs on airways obstruction in asthma has been an issue of extensive investigation (6,7,164) and is the general topic of the present book. In this chapter, I wish to concentrate briefly on the effects of drugs on bronchoconstrictor dose-response curves in vivo. In doing so, the various components of the response must be carefully distinguished. First, the treatment effects on responses to the ''direct'' stimuli (on airway smooth muscle) may differ from those on responses to ''indirect'' stimuli (mediated by airway inflammatory cells, resident cells, or nerves) (19). Second, drug-induced changes in sensitivity to certain stimuli are not necessarily accompanied by changes in maximal response to those stimuli (18).

A. Bronchodilators

Bronchodilators with functional antagonist properties, such as β_2-agonists, have an acute protective effect against bronchoconstrictor stimuli for their duration of action, thereby reducing the sensitivity to the stimulus (165). However, in patients with relatively severe asthma or COPD, excessive airway narrowing in response to bronchoconstrictors remains unchanged in spite of pretreatment with β_2-agonists (165). This is a serious disadvantage of these drugs in clinical practice. The other side of the coin is that the protective effects against bronchoconstrictor challenges are well suited for performing dose-finding experiments with β_2-agonists (166) and for studies aimed to examine the development of tolerance against β_2-agonists in humans in vivo (167).

B. Anti-inflammatory Drugs

Anti-inflammatory drugs have disease-modifying properties and thereby beneficial effects on bronchoconstrictor dose-response curves. It is well known that regular treatment with inhaled corticosteroids reduces the PC_{20} or PD_{20} to bronchoconstrictors in asthma, even though this rarely becomes normalized (168–170). However, in measuring a more adequate index of airway sensitivity, such as the EC_{50}, it appears that inhaled corticosteroids do not improve the sensitivity to bronchoconstrictors per se (107). More importantly, inhaled steroids are the only drugs leading to a decrease in maximal airway narrowing in the entire range of mild (171), moderate (108), and relatively severe asthma (172). On the other hand, sodium cromoglycate and nedocromil sodium, in spite of being effective in shifting the dose-response curve to direct and indirect stimuli to the right (169), do not reduce the maximal degree of airway narrowing in asthma (173). This fits in with the improvement by corticosteroids, and not by nedocromil, of the bronchodilation following a deep inspiration (169).

IX. Clinical Implications

The above developments in the understanding of the pathophysiology of asthma have implications for the (differential) diagnosis as well as the clinical management of the disease. It is now well recognized that the increase in ease and degree of airway narrowing in response to bronchoconstrictor stimuli in vivo constitutes the common physiological pathway of multiple cellular and biochemical abnormalities within the airways. The clinically most relevant component of the dose-response curve is the absence of a maximal response plateau, being indicative of the potential of unlimited, life-threatening airway narrowing. There is little doubt that this is one of the major pathways leading to fatal and near-fatal asthma after strong bronchoconstrictor stimuli are encountered (174).

Excessive airway narrowing is due to disturbances in airway mechanics. Potential explanations for this phenomenon in asthma include an increase in the mass or contractility of airway smooth muscle, mucosal and particularly adventitial swelling, reduction in elastic recoil pressure, and/or uncoupling of the forces of interdependence between airways and lung parenchyma. There is increasing evidence that the small airways play a major role in this (106). It should be noted that the accompanying closure of such small airways during bronchoconstriction might be detected at an early stage by a decrease in forced vital capacity without actually inducing potentially dangerous degrees of airway narrowing (175). The clinical applicability of such procedures needs further investigation.

A. Asthma Versus COPD

Bronchoprovocation tests in COPD have always been hard to interpret because it is felt that baseline airway caliber is a strong determinant of hyperresponsiveness in these patients. Indeed, the relationship between baseline FEV_1 and PC_{20} appears to be stronger in COPD than in asthma, both in clinical populations (176) and in epidemiological surveys (177–179). Certainly, this has a pathophysiological explanation: increased airway wall thickness (180) and/or reduced elastic recoil pressure (72). It can be recommended to statistically correct measurements of hyperresponsiveness for baseline lung function in COPD studies (181). It remains to be established whether the combined usage of ''direct'' and ''indirect'' bronchoprovocation tests can be used in the differential diagnosis between asthma and COPD (182,183). Again, in COPD patients, airway hyperresponsiveness seems to have prognostic meaning with regard to the annual decline in FEV_1 (184). This confirms results in the general population, also showing that hyperresponsiveness to histamine or methacholine is a prognostic determinant of the annual decline in lung function (185,186).

B. Therapeutic Strategies

The above observations suggest that it could be postulated that therapeutic strategies in asthma, and perhaps also in COPD, should be aimed to inhibit the pathophysiological processes within the airways. However, so far, this has not been recommended in the present international guidelines (1). In view of the above, it can be envisaged that (noninvasive) features of inflammation will be included in the monitoring of asthma in the near future. This may include, for example, inflammatory markers in induced sputum (147,187), or in exhaled air (188). Such an approach would add markers of *acute* inflammation to asthma management. We have recently argued that it would be most beneficial to normalize features of *chronic* airway inflammation. At present, it seems that integrative physiological markers, such as airway responsiveness to direct stimuli (histamine or methacholine), are most suitable for this purpose. This measure is less influenced by day-to-day variability of airway inflammation than sputum, exhaled air, and the so-called indirect hyperresponsiveness (e.g., AMP). In contrast to these last markers, airway hyperresponsiveness to direct stimuli responds relatively slowly but steadily to anti-inflammatory treatment (189,190). This is what one would expect from a marker associated with features of chronic airways inflammation, resulting in airway remodeling (83,95–97,191).

C. Treating Hyperresponsiveness?

We have recently addressed the issue of monitoring pathophysiology in asthma during a 2-year randomized parallel follow-up study in which we examined whether inclusion of airway hyperresponsiveness to the current guides of asthma treatment (symptoms and lung function) improves the clinical and histological outcome of the disease. It appeared that a treatment strategy including hyperresponsiveness as a guide for therapy adjustment led to a 50% reduction in cumulative incidence of exacerbations as compared with the group being treated according to the international consensus (150). Interestingly, this was accompanied by a decrease in subepithelial collagen thickness in the bronchial biopsies of the group with treatment aimed at improving hyperresponsiveness but not in the control group (150). The reduction in airway hyperresponsiveness in this study was correlated to the decrease in activated eosinophil counts in the bronchial lamina propria (150).

In summary, airway hyperresponsiveness to direct stimuli seems to be a useful surrogate marker of acute, and particularly chronic airway inflammation in asthma. It appears that this has implications for the clinical and histological outcome during long-term management of the disease.

X. Conclusions

During more than a century, it has been realized that variable airways obstruction represents the common pathophysiological pathway of multiple (cellular and biochemical) abnormalities within the airways, leading to an increase in ease and degree of airway narrowing in response to bronchoconstrictor stimuli in vivo. The clinically most relevant component of variable airways obstruction seems to be unlimited, potentially life-threatening airway narrowing, as shown by absence of a maximal response plateau on the in vivo dose-response curve.

The changes in airway mechanics are likely to be due to acute as well as chronic proinflammatory stimulation within the airways. Even though current asthma research is almost exclusively focused on the cells, cytokines, and mediators in allergic inflammation, there is increasing evidence that nonallergic stimuli (such as viral infections) play an important role in the development of airway hyperresponsiveness. Prolonged exposure to a variety of growth factors can potentially lead to structural changes and remodeling of the tissue elements within the airway wall. The limited improvement of airway hyperresponsiveness by long-term treatment with inhaled corticosteroids indicates that such chronic sequelae of inflammation might be important in the maintenance of this functional disorder (8). However, the good news is that long-term treatment strategies specifically aimed at improving airway hyperresponsiveness have now been shown to lead to a better clinical and pathological outcome in asthma (150).

A. New Pathophysiological Targets

Of course, the new developments in therapy with humanized monoclonal antibodies against the most relevant compounds in the pathophysiology of asthma are very promising. This refers not only to already existing antibodies against IgE (192) or IL-5 (193), but potentially also for similar strategies against cytokines or growth factors that might be involved in the chronic remodeling of the airways, such as transforming growth factor beta (TGF-β) (194,195).

Therefore, airways pathophysiology will be an essential part of future research on the pathogenesis and treatment of asthma as long as difficult breathing is considered to be the basic problem of this disease. It is now time to combine knowledge on the morphological, physiological, and molecular basis of asthma to develop a strategy for its future prevention and therapy. This might even be feasible by newly developed invasive techniques, such as high-resolution CT scans (83,196,197) or transbronchial biopsies (198), allowing studies on the relationship between the histopathology of the full cross-sectional area of the airway wall in relation to functional behavior of the airways in vivo. Then we will be following the lines already explored in more detail by our colleagues in cardiovascular research (199,200).

References

1. Global Initiative for Asthma. Global strategy for Asthma Management and Prevention. NHLBI/WHO Workshop Report, Publication no. 95-3659. Bethesda, MD: National Institutes of Health, National Heart, Lung and Blood Institute, 1995.
2. Holgate ST. Mediator and cytokine mechanisms in asthma. Thorax 1993; 48:103–109.
3. Barnes PJ. Cytokines as mediators of chronic asthma. Am J Respir Crit Care Med 1994; 150:s42–s49.
4. Borish L, Rosenwasser LJ. Update on cytokines. J Allergy Clin Immunol 1996; 97:719–734.
5. Jeffery PK. Bronchial biopsies and airway inflammation. Eur Respir J 1996; 9: 1583–1587.
6. Barnes PJ. New drugs for asthma. Clin Exp Allergy 1996; 26:738–745.
7. Holt PG, Sly PD. Allergic respiratory disease: strategic targets for primary prevention during childhood. Thorax 1997; 52:1–4.
8. Sterk PJ. Improving asthma treatment: the physiological message. Eur Respir J 1994; 7:220–222.
9. Paré PD, Bai TR. The consequences of chronic allergic inflammation. Thorax 1995; 50:328–332.
10. Wanner A, Abraham WM, James SD, Drazen JM, Richerson HB, Ram JS. Models of airway hyperresponsiveness. Am Rev Respir Dis 1990; 141:253–257.
11. Macklem PT. A theoretical analysis of the effect of airway smooth muscle load on airway narrowing. Am J Respir Crit Care Med 1996; 153:83–89.
12. Reddel HK, Salome CM, Peat JK, Woolcock AJ. Which index of peak expiratory flow is most useful in the management of stable asthma? Am J Respir Crit Care Med 1995; 151:1320–1325.
13. Brand PLP, Quanjer PH, Postma DS, Kerstjens HAM, Koeter GH, Dekhuijzen R, Sluiter HJ, and the Dutch CNSLD study group. Interpretation of bronchodilator response in patients with obstructive airways disease. Thorax 1992; 47:429–436.
14. Quanjer PhH, Tammeling GJ, Cotes JE, Perdersen OF, Peslin R, Yernault J-C. Lung volumes and forced ventilatory flows. Eur Respir J 1993; 6(suppl 16):5–40.
15. Dekker FW, Schrier AC, Sterk PJ, Dijkman JH. Validity of peak expiratory flow measurement in assessing reversibility of airflow obstruction. Thorax 1992; 47: 162–166.
16. American Thoracic Society. Guidelines for the evaluation of impairment/disability in patients with asthma. Am Rev Respir Dis 1993; 147:1056–1061.
17. Sterk PJ, Fabbri LM, Quanjer PhH, Cockcroft DW, O'Byrne PM, Anderson SD, Juniper EF, Malo J-L. Airway responsiveness: Standardized challenge testing with pharmacological, physical and sensitizing stimuli in adults. Eur Respir J 1993; 6(suppl 16):53–83.
18. Sterk PJ, Bel EH. The shape of the dose-response curve to inhaled bronchoconstrictor agents in asthma and in chronic obstructive pulmonary disease. Am Rev Respir Dis 1991; 143:1433–1437.

19. Pauwels R, Joos G, van der Straeten M. Bronchial hyperresponsiveness is not bronchial responsiveness is not bronchial asthma. Clin Allergy 1988; 18:317–321.
20. Weersink EJM, Postma DS, Aalbers R, de Monchy GJR. Early and late asthmatic reaction after allergen challenge. Respir Med 1994; 88:104–114.
21. Bentley AM, Kay AB, Durham SR. Human late asthmatic reactions. Clin Exp Allergy 1997; 27:71–86.
22. Sterk PJ. Virus-induced airway hyperresponsiveness in man. Eur Respir J 1993; 6:894–902.
23. Corne JM, Holgate ST. Mechanisms of virus induced exacerbations of asthma. Thorax 1997; 52:380–389.
24. Macklem PT. The clinical relevance of respiratory muscle research. Am Rev Respir Dis 1986; 134:812–815.
25. James A. Limited airway narrowing: why does not everyone have asthma? Eur Respir J 1994; 7:1210–1212.
26. Woolcock AJ, Salome CM, Yan K. The shape of the dose-response curve to histamine in asthmatic and normal subjects. Am Rev Respir Dis 1984; 130:71–75.
27. Sterk PJ, Daniel EE, Zamel N, Hargreave FE. Limited bronchoconstriction to methacholine using partial flow-volume curves in nonasthmatic subjects. Am Rev Respir Dis 1985; 132:272–277.
28. Sterk PJ, Timmers MC, Bel EH, Dijkman JH. The combined effects of histamine and methacholine on the maximal degree of airway narrowing in normal humans in vivo. Eur Respir J 1988; 1:34–40.
29. Sterk PJ, Timmers MC, Dijkman JH. Maximal airway narrowing in humans in vivo: Histamine compared with methacholine. Am Rev Respir Dis 1986; 134:714–718.
30. Moore BJ, Hilliam ChC, Verburgt LM, Wiggs BR. Vedal S, Pare PD. Shape and position of the complete dose-response curve for inhaled methacholine in normal subjects. Am J Respir Crit Care Med 1996; 154:642–648.
31. De Pee S, Timmers MC, Hermans J, Duiverman EJ, Sterk PJ. Comparison of maximal airway narrowing to methacholine between children and adults. Eur Respir J 1991; 4:421–428.
32. James A, Lougheed D, Pearce-Pinto G, Ryan G, Musk B. Maximal airway narrowing in a general population. Am Rev Respir Dis 1992; 146:895–899.
33. Lougheed MD, Pearce-Pinto G, de Klerk NH, Ryan G, Musk AW, James A. Variability of the plateau response to methacholine in subjects without respiratory symptoms. Thorax 1993; 48:512–517.
34. Moreno RH, Hogg JC, Paré PD. Mechanics of airway narrowing. Am Rev Respir Dis 1986; 133:1171–1180.
35. Sterk PJ, Daniel EE, Zamel N, Hargreave FE. Limited maximal airway narrowing in nonasthmatic subjects: Role of neural control and prostaglandin release. Am Rev Respir Dis 1985; 132:865–870.
36. De Gouw HWFM, Diamant Z, Kuijpers EA, Sont JK, Sterk PJ. Role of neutral endopeptidase in exercise-induced bronchoconstriction in asthmatic subjects. J Appl Physiol 1996; 81:673–678.
37. Taylor DA, Orr LM, McGrath JL, Jensen MW, Aikman SL, Barnes PJ, O'Connor

BJ. Nitric oxide is bronchoprotective to direct and indirect stimuli in asthmatic patients. Am J Respir Crit Care Med 1997; 155:A202.
38. Wiggs BR, Moreno R, Hogg JC, Hilliam C, Pare PD. A model of the mechanics of airway narrowing. J Appl Physiol 1990; 69:849–860.
39. Macklem PT. Mechanical factors determining maximum bronchoconstriction. Eur Respir J 1989; 2(suppl 6):516s–519s.
40. Okazawa M, Paré P, Road J. Tracheal smooth muscle mechanics in vivo. J Appl Physiol 1990; 68:209–219.
41. Gunst SJ, Stropp JQ, Service J. Mechanical modulation of pressure-volume characteristics of contracted canine airways in vitro. J Appl Physiol 1990; 68:2223–2229.
42. Bates JHT, Martin JG. A theoretical study of the effect of airway smooth muscle orientation on bronchoconstriction. J Appl Physiol 1990; 69:995–1001.
43. Hoppin FG. Parenchymal mechanics in asthma. Chest 1995; 107(3 suppl):140s–144s.
44. Moreno RH, Paré PD. Intravenous papain-induced cartilage softening decreases preload of tracheal smooth muscle. J Appl Physiol 1989; 66:1694–1698.
45. James AL, Paré PD, Moreno RH, Hogg JC. Quantitative measurement of smooth muscle shortening in isolated pig trachea. J Appl Physiol 1987; 63:1360–1365.
46. Ishida K, Pare PD, Blogg T, Schellenberg RR. Effects of elastic loading on porcine trachealis muscle mechanics. J Appl Physiol 1990; 69:1033–1039.
47. Sly PD, Brown KA, Bates JHT, Macklem PT, Milic-Emili J, Martin JG. Effect of lung volume on interruptor resistance in cats challenged with methacholine. J Appl Physiol 1988; 64:360–366.
48. Ding DJ, Martin JG, Macklem PT. Effects of lung volume on maximal methacholine-induced bronchoconstriction in normal humans. J Appl Physiol 1987; 62: 1324–1330.
49. Moore B, D'Yachkova Y, Ahmad HR, Paré PD. Mechanism of methacholine dose-response plateaus in normal subjects. Am Rev Respir Crit Care Med 1997; 155: A543.
50. James A, Pearce-Pinto G, Hillman D. Effects of lung volume and surface forces on maximal airway smooth muscle shortening. J Appl Physiol 1994; 77:1755–1762.
51. Warner DO, Gunst SJ. Limitation of maximal bronchoconstriction in living dogs. Am Rev Respir Dis 1992; 145:553–560.
52. Okazawa M, Bai TR, Wiggs BR, Pare PD. Airway smooth muscle shortening in excised canine lung lobes. J Appl Physiol 1993; 74:1613–1621.
53. Eidelman DH, Lei M, Ghezzo RH. Morphometry of methacholine-induced bronchoconstriction in the rat. J Appl Physiol 1993; 75:1702–1710.
54. Lambert RY, Paré PD. Lung parenchymal shear modulus, airway wall remodelling, and bronchial hyperresponsiveness. J Appl Physiol 1997; 83:140–147.
55. Sterk PJ, Bel EH. Bronchial hyperresponsiveness: the need for a distinction between hypersensitivity and excessive airway narrowing. Eur Respir J 1989; 2:267–274.
56. Ishida K, Paré PD, Thomson RJ, Schellenberg RR. Increased in vitro responses of tracheal smooth muscle from hyperresponsive guinea pigs. J Appl Physiol 1990; 68:1316–1320.

57. Hirst SJ, Twort CHC. The proliferative response of airway smooth muscle. Clin Exp Allergy 1992; 22:907–915.
58. Knox AJ. Airway re-modeling in asthma: role of airway smooth muscle. Clin Sci 1994; 86:647–652.
59. Bai TR. Abnormalities in airway smooth muscle in fatal asthma. Am Rev Respir Dis 1990; 141:552–557.
60. Jiang E, Rao K, Halayko AJ, Liu X, Stephens NL. Ragweed sensitization-induced increase of myosin light-chain kinase content in canine airway smooth muscle. Am J Respir Cell Mol Biol 1992; 7:567–573.
61. Mitchell RW, Rühlmann E, Magnussen H, Leff AR, Rabe KF. Passive sensitization of human bronchi augments smooth muscle shortening velocity and capacity. Am J Physiol 1994; 267:L218–L222.
62. Fredberg JJ, Jones KA, Nathan M, Raboudi S, Prakash YS, Shore SA, Butler JP, Sieck GC. Friction in airway smooth muscle: mechanism, latch and implications in asthma. J Appl Physiol 1996; 81:2703–2712.
63. Solway J, Fredberg JJ. Perhaps smooth muscle dysfunction contributes to asthmatic bronchial hyperresponsiveness after all. Am J Respir Cell Mol Biol 1997; 17:144–146.
64. Ingram RH, jr. Relationships among airway-parenchymal interactions, lung responsiveness, and inflammation in asthma. Chest 1995; 107(3 suppl):148s–153s.
65. Shen X, Wu MF, Tepper RS, Gunst SJ. Mechanisms for the mechanical response of airway smooth muscle to length oscillation. J Appl Physiol 1997; 83:731–738.
66. Lambert RK, Wiggs BR, Kuwano K, Hogg JC, Pare PD. Functional significance of increased airway smooth muscle in asthma and COPD. J Appl Physiol 1993; 74:2771–2781.
67. Ebina M, Takahashi T, Chiba T, Motomiya M. Cellular hypertrophy and hyperplasia of airway smooth muscles underlying bronchial asthma: A 3-D morphometric study. Am Rev Respir Dis 1993; 148:720–726.
68. Ebina M, Yaegashi H, Chiba R, Takahashi T, Motomiya M, Tanemura M. Hyperreactive site in the airway tree of asthmatic patients revealed by thickening of bronchial muscles: a morphometric study. Am Rev Respir Dis 1990; 141:1327–1332.
69. Thomson RJ, Bramley AM, Schellenberg R. Airway muscle stereology: implications for increased shortening in asthma. Am J Respir Crit Care Med 1997; 154: 749–757.
70. Smith PG, Janiga KE, Bruce MC. Strain increases airway smooth muscle cell proliferation. Am J Respir Cell Mol Biol 1994; 10:85–90.
71. Bellofiore S, Eidelman DH, Macklem PT, Martin RR. Effects of elastase-induced emphysema on airway responsiveness to methacholine in rats. J Appl Physiol 1989; 66:606–612.
72. Cheung D, Schot R, Zwinderman AH, Zagers H, Dijkman JH, Sterk PJ. Relationship between loss in parenchymal elastic recoil pressure and maximal airway narrowing in subjects with aplha-1-antitrypsin deficiency. Am J Respir Crit Care Med 1997; 155:135–140.
73. Woolcock AJ, Boonsawat W, Donnelly P, Salome C. Relationship between lung elasticity and the maximal response plateau. Am Rev Respir Dis 1992; 145:A461.

74. Wiggs SR, Bosken C, Pare PD, James A, Hogg JC. A model of airway narrowing in asthma and in chronic obstructive pulmonary disease. Am Rev Respir Dis 1992; 145:1251–1258.
75. James AL, Pare PD, Hogg JC. The mechanics of airway narrowing in asthma. Am Rev Respir Dis 1989; 139:242–246.
76. Djukanovic R, Roche WR, Wilson JW, Beasley CRW, Twentyman OP, Howarth PH, Holgate ST. Mucosal inflammation in asthma. Am Rev Respir Dis 1990; 142: 434–457.
77. Yager D, Butler JP, Bastacky J, Israel E, Smith G, Drazen JM. Amplification of airway constriction due to liquid filling of airway interstices. J Appl Physiol 1990; 69:2873–2884.
78. Bramley AM, Thomson RJ, Roberts CR, Schellenberg RR. Hypothesis: excessive bronchoconstriction in asthma is due to decreased airway elastance. Eur Respir J 1994; 7:337–341.
79. Lambert RK. Role of bronchial basement membrane in airway collapse. J Appl Physiol 1991; 71:666–673.
80. Lambert RK, Codd SL, Alley MR, Pack RJ. Physical determinants of bronchial mucosal folding. J Appl Physiol 1994; 77:1206–1216.
81. Okazawa M, Vedal S, Verburgt L, Lambert RK, Pare PD. Determinants of airway smooth muscle shortening in excised canine lobes. J Appl Physiol 1995; 78:608–614.
82. Brown RH, Mitzner W, Wagner EM. Interaction between airway edema and lung function on responsiveness of individual airways in vivo. J Appl Physiol 1997; 83: 366–370.
83. Boulet L-Ph, Belanger M, Carrier G. Airway responsiveness and bronchial-wall thickness in asthma with or without fixed airflow obstruction. Am J Respir Crit Care Med 1995; 152:865–871.
84. Michell HW, Sparrow MP. Video-imaging of lumen narrowing: muscle shortening and flow responsiveness in isolated bronchial segments of the pig. Eur Respir J 1994; 7:1317–1325.
85. Bel EH, van der Veen H, Kramps JA, Dijkman JH, Sterk PJ. Maximal airway narrowing to inhaled leukotriene D4 in normal subjects. Am Rev Respir Dis 1987; 136:979–984.
86. Bel EH, Van der Veen H, Dijkman JH, Sterk PJ. The effect of inhaled budesonide on the maximal degree of airway narrowing to leukotriene D_4 and methacholine in normal subjects in vivo. Am Rev Respir Dis 1989; 139:427–431.
87. Cheung D, van der Veen H, den Hartigh J, Dijkman JH, Sterk PJ. Effects of inhaled substance P on airway responsiveness to methacholine in asthmatic subjects in vivo. J Appl Physiol 1994; 77:1325–1332.
88. Lötvall JO, Lemen RJ, Pheng Lui K, Barnes PJ, Chung KF. Airflow obstruction after substance P aerosol: contribution of airway and pulmonary edema. J Appl Physiol 1990; 69:1473–1478.
89. Kurosawa M, Yodonawa S, Tsukakoshi H, Miyachi Y. Inhibition by a novel peptide leukotriene receptor antagonist ONO-1078 of airway wall thickening and airway hyperresponsiveness to histamine induced by leukotriene C_4 and leukotriene D_4 in guinea pigs. Clin Exp Allergy 1994; 24:960–968.

90. Kimura K, Inoue H, Ichinose M, Miura M, Kastumata U, Takahashi T, Takashima T. Bradykinin causes airway hyperresponsiveness and enhances maximal airway narrowing: Role of microvascular leakage and airway edema. Am Rev Respir Dis 1992; 146:1301–1305.
91. Boonsawat W, Salome CM, Woolcock AJ. Effect of allergen inhalation on the maximal response plateau of the dose-response curve to methacholine. Am Rev Respir Dis 1992; 146:565–569.
92. Prieto L, Berto JM, Lopez M, Peris A. Modifications of PC20 and maximal degree of airway narrowing to methacholine after pollen season in pollen sensitive asthmatic patients. Clin Exp Allergy 1993; 23:172–178.
93. Hiltermann TJN, Stolk J, Hiemstra PS, Fokkens PHB, Rombout PJA, Sont JK, Sterk PJ, Dijkman JH. Effect of ozone exposure on maximal airway narrowing in non-asthmatic and asthmatic subjects. Clin Sci 1995; 89:619–624.
94. Cheung D, Dick EC, Timmers MC, de Klerk EPA, Spaan WJM, Sterk PJ. Rhinovirus inhalation causes prolonged excessive airway narrowing in asthmatic subjects in vivo. Am J Respir Crit Care Med 1995; 152:1490–1496.
95. Sont JK, Willems LNA, Evertse CE, Neeskens P, van Krieken JHJM, Sterk PJ. Thickening of the airway subepithelial reticular layer is related to bronchial hyperresponsiveness to methacholine in subjects with atopic asthma. Am J Respir Crit Care Med 1995; 151(4, part 2):A833.
96. Chetta A, Foresi A, Del Donno M, Bertorelli G, Pesci A, Olivieri D. Airways remodelling is a distinctive feature of asthma and is related to severity of disease. Chest 1997; 111:852–857.
97. Boulet L-Ph, Laviolette M, Turcotte H, Cartier A, Dugas M, Malo J-L, Boutet M. Bronchial subepithelial fibrosis correlates with airway responsiveness to methacholine. Chest 1997; 112:45–52.
98. Gizycki MJ, Adelroth E, Rogers AV, O'Byrne PM, Jeffery PK. Myofibroblast involvement in the allergen-induced late response in mild atopic asthma. Am J Respir Cell Mol Biol 1997; 16:664–673.
99. Carroll NG, Cooke C, James AL. Bronchial blood vessel dimensions in asthma. Am J Respir Crit Care Med 1997; 155:689–695.
100. Li X, Wilson JW. Increased vascularity of the bronchial mucosa in mild asthma. Am J Respir Crit Care Med 1997; 156:229–233.
101. Sont JK, Willems LNA, Evertse CE, van Schadewijk WAAM, van Kieken JHJM, Sterk PJ. Bronchial blood vessel number and vascular cross-sectional area are determinants of variable airways obstruction. Eur Respir J 1996; 9(suppl 23):15s.
102. Möller GM, Overbeek SE, van Helden-Meeuwsen CG, Hoogsteden HC, Bogaard JM. Eosinophils in the bronchial mucosa in relation to indices from the methacholine dose-response curve in atopic asthmatics. J Appl Physiol 1999. In press.
103. Hogg JC. Pathology of asthma. J Allergy Clin Immunol 1993; 92:1–5.
104. Pellegrino R, Wilson O, Jenouri G, Rodarte JR. Lung mechanics during induced bronchoconstriction. J Appl Physiol 1996; 81:964–975.
105. Faul JL, Tormey VJ, Leonard C, Burke CM, Farmer J, Horne SJ, Poulter LW. Lung immunopathology in cases of sudden asthma death. Eur Respir J 1997; 10: 301–307.
106. Hamid Q, Song Y, Kotsimbos TC, Minshall E, Bai TR, Hegele RG, Hogg JC.

Inflammation of small airways in asthma. J Allergy Clin Immunol 1997; 100:44–51.

107. Jubber AS, Foster RW, Hassan NAGM, Carpenter JR, Small RC. Airway response to inhaled methacholine in normal human subjects. Pulm Pharmacol 1993; 6:177–184.
108. Overbeek SE, Rijnbeek PR, Vons C, Mulder PGH, Hoogsteden HC, Bogaard JM. Effects of fluticasone propionate on methacholine dose-response curves in non-smoking atopic asthmatics. Eur Respir J 1996; 9:2256–2262.
109. Raeburn D, Webber SE. Proinflammatory potential of the airway epithelium in bronchial asthma. Eur Respir J 1994; 7:2226–2233.
110. Montefort S, Herbert CA, Robinson C, Holgate ST. The bronchial epithelium as a target for inflammatory attack in asthma. Clin Exp Allergy 1992; 22:511–520.
111. Jeffery PK, Wardlaw AJ, Nelson FC, Collins JV, Kay AB. Bronchial biopsies in asthma: an ultrastructural, quantitative study and correlation with hyperreactivity. Am Rev Respir Dis 1989; 140:1745–1753.
112. Ohashi Y, Motojima S, Fukuda T, Makino S. Airway hyperresponsiveness, increased intracellular spaces of bronchial epithelium, and increased infiltration of cosinophils and lymphocytes in bronchial mucosa in asthma. Am Rev Respir Dis 1992; 145:1469–1476.
113. Boulet L-Ph, Turcotte H, Boutet M, Montmimy L, Laviolette M. Influence of natural antigenic exposure on expiratory flows, methacholine responsiveness, and airway inflammation in mild allergic asthma. J Allergy Clin Immunol 1993; 91:883–893.
114. Padrid Ph, Snook S, Finucane Th, Shiue P, Cozzi Ph, Solway J, Leff AR. Persistent airway hyperresponsiveness and histologic alterations after chronic antigen challenge in cats. Am J Respir Crit Care Med 1995; 151:184–193.
115. Wright PF, Ikizler M, Carroll KN, Endo Y. Interaction of viruses with respiratory epithelial cells. Semin Virol 1996; 7:227–235.
116. Koto H, Aizawa H, Takata S, Inoue H, Hara N. An important role of tachykinins in ozone-induced airway hyperresponsiveness. Am J Respir Crit Care Med 1995; 151:1763–1769.
117. Folkerts G, van der Linde HJ, Nijkamp FP. Virus-induced airway hyperresponsiveness in guinea pigs is related to a deficiency in nitric oxide. J Clin Invest 1995; 95:26–30.
118. De Gouw HWFM, Grünberg K, Schot R, Kroes ACM, Dick EC, Sterk PJ. Relationship between exhaled nitric oxide and airway hyperresponsiveness following experimental rhinovirus infection in asthmatic subjects. Eur Respir J 1998; 11:126–132.
119. Chung KF. Airway neuropeptides and neutral endopeptidase in asthma. Clin Exp Allergy 1996; 26:491–493.
120. Dusser DJ, Jacoby DB, Djokic TD, Rubinstein I, Borson DB, Nadel JA. Virus induces airway hyperresponsiveness to tachykinins: role of neutral endopeptidase. J Appl Physiol 1989; 67:1504–1511.
121. Elwood W, Lotvall JO, Barnes PJ, Chung KF. Airway hyperresponsiveness to acetylcholine and tachykinins after respiratory virus infection in the guinea pig. Ann Allergy 1993; 70:231–236.
122. Miura M, Ichinose M, Kimura K, Katsumata U, Takahashi T, Inoue H, Takishima

T. Dysfunction of nonadrenergic noncholinergic inhibitory system after antigen inhalation in actively sensitized cat airways. Am Rev Respir Dis 1992; 145;70–74.
123. Kawano O, Kohrogi H, Yamaguchi T, Araki S, Ando M. Neutral endopeptidase inhibitor potentiates allergic bronchoconstriction in guinea pigs in vivo. J Appl Physiol 1993; 75:185–190.
124. Bertrand C, Geppetti P, Graf PD, Foresi A, Nadel JA. Involvement of neurogenic inflammation in antigen-induced bronchoconstriction in guinea pigs. Am J Physiol 1993; 265:L507–L511.
125. Lilly CM, Kobzik L, Hall AE, Drazen JM. Effects of chronic airway inflammation on the activity and enzymatic inactivation of neuropeptides in guinea pig lungs. J Clin Invest 1994; 93:2667–2674.
126. Sont JK, van Krieken JHJM, van Klink HCJ, Roldaan AC, Apap CR, Willems LNA, Sterk PJ. Enhanced expression of neutral endopeptidase (NEP) in airway epithelium in biopsies from steroid- versus nonsteroid-treated patients with atopic asthma. Am J Respir Cell Mol Biol 1997; 16:549–556.
127. Diamant Z, van der Veen H, Kuijpers EAP, Bakker PF, Sterk PJ. The effect of inhaled thiorphan on allergen-induced airway responses in asthmatic subjects. Clin Exp Allergy 1996; 26:525–532.
128. Cheung D, Timmers MC, Bel EH, den Hartigh J, Dijkman JH, Sterk PJ. Neutral endopeptidase and airway hyperresponsiveness to neurokinin A in asthmatic subjects in vivo. Am Rev Respir Dis 1993; 148:1467–1474.
129. Baraniuk JN. The role of sensory neuropeptides in airway hyperresponsiveness. Pulmon Pharmacol 1996; 9:195–202.
130. Hsiue T-R, Garland A, Ray DW, Hershenson MB, Leff AR, Solway J. Endogenous sensory neuropeptide release enhances nonspecific airway responsiveness in guinea pigs. Am Rev Respir Dis 1992; 146:148–153.
131. Advenier C, Lagente V, Boichot E. The role of tachykinin receptor antagonists in the prevention of bronchial hyperresponsiveness, airway inflammation and cough. Eur Respir J 1997; 10:1892–1908.
132. Barnes PJ. Overview of neural mechanisms in asthma. Pulmon Pharmacol 1996; 9:151–159.
133. Barnes PJ. Muscarinic receptor subtypes in airways. Eur Respir J 1993; 6:328–331.
134. Tanaka DT, Ando RE, Larsen GL, Irvin ChG. Cholinergic mechanisms involved with histamine hyperreactivity in immune rabbit airways challenged with ragweed antigen. Am Rev Respir Dis 1991; 144:70–75.
135. Jacoby DB, Gleich GJ, Fryer AD. Human eosinophil major basic protein is an endogenous allosteric antagonist at the inhibitory muscarinic M_2 receptor. J Clin Invest 1993; 91:1314–1318.
136. Sorkness R, Clough JJ, Castleman WL, Lemanske RF. Virus-induced airway obstruction and parasympathetic hyperresponsiveness in adult rats. Am J Respir Crit Care Med 1994; 150:28–34.
137. Lammers JWJ, Minette P, McCusker M, Barnes PJ. The role of pirenzepine-sensitive (M1) muscarinic receptors in vagally mediated bronchoconstriction in humans. Am Rev Respir Dis 1989; 139:446–449.

138. Fryer AD, Wills-Karp M. Dysfunction of M2-muscarinic receptors in pulmonary parasympathetic nerves after antigen challenge. J Appl Physiol 1991; 71:2255–2261.
139. Kahn RM, Okaniami OA, Jacoby DB, Fryer AD. Viral infection induces dependence of neuronal M2 muscarinic receptors on cyclooxygenase in guinea pig lung. J Clin Invest 1996; 98:299–307.
140. Elbon CL, Jacoby DB, Fryer AD. Pretreatment with an antibody to interleukin-5 prevents loss of pulmonary M2 muscarinic receptor function in antigen-challenged guinea pigs. Am J Respir Cell Mol Biol 1995; 12:320–328.
141. Mitchell RW, Kelly E, Leff AR. Reduced activity of acetylcholinesterase in canine tracheal smooth muscle homogenates after active immune-sensitization. Am J Respir Cell Mol Biol 1991; 5:56–62.
142. Makker HK, Holgate ST. The contribution of neurogenic reflexes to hypertonic saline-induced bronchoconstriction in asthma. J Allergy Clin Immunol 1993; 92:82–88.
143. Gross NJ, Co E, Skorodin MS. Cholinergic bronchomotor tone in COPD: estimates of its amount in comparison with that in normal subjects. Chest 1989; 96:984–987.
144. Walker C, Kaegi MK, Braun P, Blaser K. Activated T cells and eosinophilia in bronchoalveolar lavages from subjects with asthma correlated with disease severity. J Allergy Clin Immunol 1991; 88:935–942.
145. Bentley AM, Menz G, Storz Chr, Robinson DS, Jeffery PK, Durham SR, Kay AB. Identification of T lymphocytes, macrophages, and activated eosinophils in the bronchial mucosa in intrinsic asthma. Am Rev Respir Dis 1992; 146:500–506.
146. Sont JK, van Krieken JHJM, Evertse ChE, Hooijer R, Willems LNA, Sterk PJ. Relationship between the inflammatory infiltrate in bronchial biopsy specimens and clinical severity of asthma in patients treated with inhaled steroids. Thorax 1996; 51:496–502.
147. Pizzichini E, Pizzichini MMM, Efthimiadis A, Evans S, Morris MM, Squillace D, Gleich GJ, Dolovich J, Hargreave FE. Indices of airway inflammation in induced sputum: reproducibility and validity of cell and fluid-phase measurements. Am J Respir Crit Care Med 1996; 154:308–317.
148. Djukanovic R, Wilson JW, Britten K, Wilson SJ, Walls AF, Roche WR, Howarth PH, Holgate ST. Quantitation of mast cells and eosinophils in the bronchial mucosa of symptomatic atopic asthmatics and healthy control subjects using immunohistochemistry. Am Rev Respir Dis 1990; 142:863–871.
149. Grünberg K, Smits HH, Timmers MC, de Klerk EPA, Dolhain RJEM, Dick EC, Hiemstra PS, Sterk PJ. Experimental rhinovirus 16 infection: effects on cell differentials and soluble markers in sputum in asthmatic subjects. Am J Respir Crit Care Med 1997; 156:606–616.
150. Sont JK, Willems LNA, Bel EH, van Krieken JHJM, Vandenbroucke JP, Sterk PJ, and the AMPUL Study Group. Clinical control and histopathological outcome of asthma when using airway hyperresponsiveness as an additional guide to long-term treatment. Am J Respir Crit Care Med 1999; 159:1043–1051.
151. Shardonofsky FR, Martin JG, Eidelman DH. Effect of body posture on concentra-

tion-response curves to inhaled methacholine. Am Rev Respir Dis 1992; 146:750–756.

152. Nadel JA, Tierney DF. Effect of a previous deep inspiration on airway resistance in man. J Appl Physiol 1961; 16:717–719.
153. Parham WM, Shepard RH, Norman PS, Fish JE. Analysis of time course and magnitude of lung inflation effects on airway tone: relation to airway reactivity. Am Rev Respir Dis 1983; 128:240–245.
154. Pellegrino R, Sterk PJ, Sont JK, Brusasco V. Assessing the effect of deep inhalation of airway caliber: a novel approach to lung function in asthma and COPD. Eur Respir J 1998; 12:1219–1227.
155. Malmberg P, Larsson K, Sundblad BM, Zhiping W. Importance of the time interval between FEV1 measurements in a methacholine provocation test. Eur Respir J 1993; 6:680–686.
156. Pliss LB, Ingenito EP, Ingram RH. Responsiveness, inflammation, and effects of deep breaths on obstruction in mild asthma. J Appl Physiol 1989; 66:2298–2304.
157. Sont JK, Booms P, Bel EH, Vandenbroucke JP, Sterk PJ. The severity of breathlessness during challenges with inhaled methacholine and hypertonic saline in atopic asthmatic subjects. Am J Respir Crit Care Med 1995; 151:360–368.
158. Bel EH, Timmers MC, Dijkman JH, Stahl EG, Sterk PJ. The effect of an inhaled leukotriene antagonist, L-648,051 on early and late asthmatic reactions and subsequent increase in airway responsiveness in man. J Allergy Clin Immunol 1990; 85: 1067–1075.
159. Pellegrino R, Violante B, Crimi E, Brusasco V. Effects of aerosol methacholine and histamine on airways and lung parenchyma in healthy humans. J Appl Physiol 1993; 74:2681–2686.
160. Dandurand RJ, Xu LH, Martin JG, Eidelman DH. Airway-parenchymal interdependence and bronchial responsiveness in two highly inbred rat strains. J Appl Physiol 1993; 74:538–544.
161. Skloot G, Permutt S, Togias A. Airway hyperresponsiveness in asthma: a problem of limited smooth muscle relaxation with inspiration. J Clin Invest 1995; 96:2393–2403.
162. Moore BJ, Verburgt LM, King CG, Pare PD. The effect of deep inspiration on methacholine dose-response curves in normal subjects. Am J Respir Crit Care Med 1997; 156:1278–1281.
163. Brusasco V, Pellegrino R, Violante B, Crimi E. Relationship between quasi-static pulmonary hysteresis and maximal airway narrowing in humans. J Appl Physiol 1992; 72:2075–2080.
164. Barnes PJ. New drugs for asthma. Clin Exp Allergy 1996; 26:738–745.
165. Bel EH, Zwinderman AH, Timmers MC, Dijkman JH, Sterk PJ. The protective effect of a β_2 agonist against excessive airway narrowing in response to bronchoconstrictor stimuli in asthma and chronic obstructive lung disease. Thorax 1991; 46:9–14.
166. Inman MD, Hamilton AL, Kerstjens HAM, Watson RM, O'Byrne PM. The utility of methacholine airway responsiveness measurements in evaluating anti-asthma drugs. J Allergy Clin Immunol 1998; 101:342–348.

167. Cheung D, Timmers MC, Zwinderman AH, Bel EH, Dijkman JH, Sterk PJ. The prolonged effects of a long-acting β_2-adrenoceptor agonist, salmeterol, on airway hyperresponsiveness in asthma. N Engl J Med 1992; 327:1198–1203.
168. Kraan J, Koëter GH, v/d Mark ThW, et al. Changes in bronchial hyperreactivity induced by 4 weeks of treatment with antiasthmatic drugs in patients with allergic asthma: a comparison between budesonide and terbutaline. J Allergy Clin Immunol 1988; 137:44–48.
169. Bel EH, Timmers MC, Hermans J, Dijkman JH, Sterk PJ. The long-term effects of nedocromil sodium and beclomethasone dipropionate on bronchial responsiveness to methacholine in nonatopic asthmatic subjects. Am Rev Respir Dis 1990; 141:21–28.
170. Waalkens HJ, van Essen-Zandvliet EE, Hughes MD, Gerritsen J, Duiverman EJ, Knol K, Kerrebijn KF, and the Dutch CNSLD Study Group. Cessation of long-term treatment with inhaled corticosteroid (budesonide) in children with asthma results in deterioration. Am Rev Respir Dis 1993; 148:1252–1257.
171. Bel EH, Timmers MC, Zwinderman AH, Dijkman JH, Sterk PJ. The effect of inhaled corticosteroids on the maximal degree of airway narrowing to methacholine in asthmatic subjects. Am Rev Respir Dis 1991; 143:109–111.
172. Booms P, Cheung D, Timmers MC, Sterk PJ. Protective effect of inhaled budesonide against unlimited airway narrowing to methacholine in atopic patients with asthma. J Allergy Clin Immunol 1997; 99:330–337.
173. Sont JK, Bel EH, Dijkman JH, Sterk PJ. The long-term effect of nedocromil sodium on the maximal degree of airway narrowing to methacholine in atopic asthmatic subjects. Clin Exp Allergy 1992; 22:554–560.
174. Molfino NA, Nannini LJ, Martelli AN, Slutsky AS. Respiratory arrest in near-fatal asthma. N Engl J Med 1991; 324:285–288.
175. Gibbons WJ, Sharma A, Lougheed D, Macklem PT. Detection of excessive bronchoconstriction in asthma. Am J Respir Crit Care Med 1996; 153:582–589.
176. Ramsdale EH, Hargreave FE. Differences in airway responsiveness in asthma and chronic airflow obstruction. Med Clin North Am 1990; 74:741–751.
177. O'Connor GT, Sparrow D, Segal MR, Weiss ST. Smoking, atopy, and methacholine airway responsiveness among middle-aged and eldery men: the normative aging study. Am Rev Respir Dis 1989; 140:1520–1526.
178. Josephs LK, Gregg I, Mullee MA, Campbell MJ, Holgate ST. A longitudinal study of baseline FEV_1 and bronchial responsiveness in patients with asthma. Eur Respir J 1992; 5:32–39.
179. Dirksen A, Madsen F, Engel T, Frolund L, Heinig JH, Mosbech H. Airway calibre as a confounder in interpreting bronchial responsiveness in asthma. Thorax 1992; 47:702–706.
180. Riess A, Wiggs B, Verbrugt L, Wright JL, Hogg JC, Pare PD. Morphologic determinants of airway responsiveness in chronic smokers. Am J Respir Crit Care Med 1996; 154:1444–1449.
181. Suppli Ch. Factors associated with increased bronchial responsiveness in adolescents and young adults: the importance of adjustment for prechallenge FEV_1. J Allergy Clin Immunol 1996; 97:761–777.

182. Oosterhoff Y, Jansen MAM, Postma DS, Koeter GH. Airway responsiveness to adenosine 5′-monophosphate in smokers and nonsmokers with atopic asthma. J Allergy Clin Immunol 1993; 92:773–776.
183. Oosterhoff Y, de Jong JW, Jansen MAM, Koeter GH, Postma DS. Airway responsiveness to adenosine 5′-monophosphate in chronic obstructive pulmonary disease is determined by smoking. Am Rev Respir Dis 1993; 147:553–558.
184. Tashkin DP, Altose MD, Connett JE, Kanner RE, Lee WW, Wise RA, for the Lung Health Study Research Group. Methacholine reactivity predicts changes in lung function over time in smokers with early chronic obstructive pulmonary disease. Am J Respir Crit Care Med 1996; 153:1802–1811.
185. Rijcken B, Schouten JP, Xu X, Rosner B, Weiss St. Airway hyperresponsiveness to histamine associates with accelerated decline in FEV_1. Am J Respir Crit Care Med 1995; 151:1377–1382.
186. O'Connor GT, Sparrow D, Weiss ST. A prospective longitudinal study of methacholine airway responsiveness as predictor of pulmonary function decline: the normative aging study. Am J Respir Crit Care Med 1995; 152:87–92.
187. In 't Veen JCCM, de Gouw HWFM, Smits HH, Sont JK, Hiemstra PS, Sterk PJ, Bel EH. Repeatability of cellular and soluble markers of inflammation in induced sputum from patients with asthma. Eur Respir J 1996; 9:2441–2447.
188. Kharitonov S, Alving K, Barnes PJ. Exhaled and nasal nitric oxide measurements: recommendations. Eur Respir J 1997; 10:1683–1693.
189. O'Connor BJ, Ridge SM, Barnes PJ, Fuller RW. Greater effect of inhaled budesonide on adenosine 5′-monophosphate-induced than on sodium-metabisulfite-induced bronchoconstriction in asthma. Am Rev Respir Dis 1992; 146:560–564.
190. Kerstjens HAM, Brand PLP, Hughes MD, Robinson NJ, Postma DS, Sluiter HJ, Bleecker ER, Dekhuyzen PNR, de Jong PM, Mengelers HJJ, Overbeek SE, Schoonbrood DFME, and the Dutch CNSLD Study Group. A comparison of bronchodilator therapy with or without inhaled corticosteroid therapy for obstructive airways disease. N Engl J Med 1992; 327:1413–1419.
191. Olivieri D, Chetta A, Del Donno M, Bertorelli G, Casalini A, Pesci A, Testi R, Foresi A. Effect of short-term treatment with low-dose inhaled fluticasone propionate on airway inflammation and remodelling in mild asthma: a placebo-controlled study. Am J Respir Crit Care Med 1997; 155:1864–1871.
192. Corne J, Djukanovic R, Thomas L, Warner J, Grandordy B, Gygax D, Heusser C, Patalano F, Richardson W, Kilchherr E, Staehelin T, Davis F, Gordon W, Sun L, Wang G, Chang T-W, Holgate ST. The effect of intravenous administration of a chimeric anti-IgE antibody on serum IgE levels in atopic subjects: efficacy, safety, and pharmacokinetics. J Clin Invest 1997; 99:879–887.
193. Leckie MJ, ten Brinke A, Jordan J, Khan J, Diamant Z, Walls CM, Cowley H, Hansel TT, Djukanovic R, Sterk PJ, Holgate ST, Barnes PJ. SB 240563, a humanized anti-IL-5 monoclonal antibody. Initial single dose safety and activity in patients with asthma. Am J Respir Crit Care Med 1999; 159(3part2):A624.
194. Vignola AM, Chanez R, Chiappara G, Merendino A, Pace E, Rizzo A, la Rocca AM, Bellia V, Bonsignore G, Bousquet J. Transforming growth factor-beta expression in mucosal biopsies in asthma and chronic bronchitis. Am J Respir Crit Care Med 1997; 156:591–599.

195. Minshall EM, Leung DYM, Martin RJ, Song YL, Cameron L, Ernst P, Hamid Q. Eosinophil-associated TGF-b1 mRNA expression and airway fibrosis in bronchial asthma. Am J Respir Cell Mol Biol 1997; 17:326–333.
196. Okazawa M, Muller N, McNamara AE, Child S, Verbrugt L, Pare PD. Human airway narrowing measured using high resolution computed tomography. Am J Respir Crit Care Med 1996; 154:1557–1562.
197. Paganin F, Seneterre E, Chanez P, Daures JP, Bruel JM, Michel FB, Bousquet J. Computed tomography of the lungs in asthma: influence of disease severity and etiology. Am J Respir Crit Care Med 1996; 153:110–114.
198. Kraft M, Djukanovic R, Wilson S, Holgate ST, Martin RJ. Alveolar tissue inflammation in asthma. Am J Respir Crit Care Med 1996; 154:1505–1510.
199. Dzau VJ, Gibbons GH, Cooke JP, Omoigui N. Vascular biology and medicine in the 1990s: scope, concepts, potentials, and perpectives. Circulation 1993; 87:705–719.
200. Page C, Black J, eds. Airways and Vascular Remodelling in Asthma and Cardiovascular Disease: implications for Therapeutic Intervention. London: Academic Press, 1994.

3

Pathology of Asthma

RATKO DJUKANOVIĆ

Southampton University
Southampton, England

I. Introduction

With the availability of research bronchoscopy as a tool to study the luminal and mucosal changes in the airways of asthmatic individuals, the pathology of asthma has been a subject of extensive research during the last 15 years. It is well established that airways inflammation is a feature of all forms of asthma, irrespective of whether they are related to atopy (1–6), occupation (7), or have no known cause (intrinsic or, more appropriately, nonatopic asthma) (8). Importantly, varying degrees of airways inflammation are seen across the range of asthma severity, although the characteristics of the cellular infiltrate may vary between mild and more severe forms. Following initial studies of individuals with mild asthma (1–5), there is now an increasing effort to improve the understanding of moderate and severe asthma, not least because of the relative ineffectiveness of the available anti-inflammatory drugs used in the treatment of this disease.

II. The Inflammatory Cell Network

A. Asthma: An Eosinophilic Bronchitis

Eosinophilia has long been associated with allergic diseases. Initially, these cells were believed to be beneficial in arresting allergic reactions through their ability to degrade histamine and stop its release in addition to inactivating leukotrienes and platelet activating factor (PAF) (9,10). However, there is now abundant information for these cells to be viewed as prominent effector cells responsible for many of the inflammatory responses in both asthma and allergic rhinitis (11). The combination of studies using induced sputum and bronchoalveolar lavage (BAL) (6,12–14) to study the products of cells residing in the airway lining fluid and bronchial biopsy (1,3) to characterize the cellular infiltrate in the epithelium and the deeper, submucosal layer have invariably shown increased numbers of eosinophils in asthma throughout the bronchus. This has led to the notion that asthma is a form of eosinophilic bronchitis (15).

The numbers of eosinophils in BAL are relatively low, rarely exceeding 5–10% of the total cell count due to dilution of the recovered cells from the bronchi by cells washed out from the alveoli, which contain few eosinophils and numerous macrophages (16,17). Eosinophil counts are much higher in sputum induced by inhalation of hypertonic saline (12–14), presumably because this technique predominantly samples the proximal airways (18). Eosinophils are also more abundant in the mucosa, where the extent of infiltration is expressed as cell numbers per surface area of the mucosa or length of the epithelium (1,3). Comparison of BAL and sputum eosinophil counts on the one hand and mucosal counts on the other shows at best a tendency toward correlation between these two compartments (18), possibly due to quantitative and/or qualitative differences between the mechanisms responsible for the accumulation and survival of these cells.

Importantly even the very mild, intermittent form of asthma, requiring only occasional use of bronchodilators, is characterized by high sputum eosinophil counts when compared with those of healthy control subjects (14). In biopsies, eosinophil counts are also raised in atopic nonasthmatics suffering from allergic rhinitis (2). This suggests that a low-grade degree of eosinophilic bronchial inflammation is a feature of atopy in general and that the degree of mucosal eosinophilia might determine the likelihood of functional impairment of the airways. However, the physiological relevance of subclinical eosinophilia is unclear, as these individuals are unlikely to develop any sequalae that would lead to restructuring of the airways and reduced lung function.

A number of studies employing BAL conducted in the mid-1980s have shown that stimulation with allergen using inhalation challenge leads to increased infiltration and degranulation of eosinophils in the lumen, especially in subjects who develop so-called dual-(early- and late-) phase asthmatic responses (19–21). These observations have now been confirmed in biopsy studies (22). The influx of eosinophils is associated with increased expression of intercellular adhesion molecule 1 (ICAM-1) and E-selectin (22) on mucosal post-capillary venules and an early accumulation of neutrophils and lymphocytes, all of which points to a complex upregulation of inflammatory processes involving a host of chemotactic factors and adhesion molecules.

In asthma, eosinophils are in an activated state, and secrete increased amounts of arginine-rich proteins, such as eosinophil cationic protein (ECP), eosinophil peroxidase (EPO), and major basic protein (MBP), which can be detected in BAL and induced sputum (14,17,21,23). All these proteins are stored in the granule matrix except for MBP, which is contained within the crystalline core identified as an electron-dense crystal structure by the electron microscope (11). In contrast to the healthy state, where sputum ECP levels rarely exceed 20 ng/mL, in asthma, concentrations as high as 650 ng/mL can be detected (14). Exposure to allergen in the laboratory leads to further elevations in ECP during the late-phase asthmatic response (21). These basic proteins are toxic to the epithelium (24,25); this, together with the pressure exerted by mucosal edema, is thought to lead to epithelial damage. Consistent with raised levels of ECP and MBP in the BAL fluid of asthmatic patients (17), electron microscopic investigation of the eosinophil's granule ultrastructure shows dissolution of both the granule matrix and the crystal core. This is seen as marked heterogeneity in the appearance of eosinophil granules (1,26). As further evidence of eosinophil degranulation, immunohistochemical analysis shows prominent deposits of both ECP and MBP in areas of epithelial damage of asthmatic lungs (27).

It is now appreciated that eosinophils also produce an array of cytokines and chemokines (reviewed in Ref. 28). Some of these (IL-3, IL-5, and GM-CSF) act in an autocrine manner to promote eosinophil maturation, activation, and survival (11). Others, such as IL-16 and RANTES, promote recruitment of eosinophils and T cells. Regulatory cytokines IL-2, IL-4, and IL-10 conceivably contribute to the control of T-cell activation, proliferation, and cytokine generation. Thus, in addition to causing immediate damage to the epithelium, bronchoconstriction, vasodilatation, and hypersecretion of mucus, eosinophils have their own ability to promote chronic inflammation.

B. Mast Cells: Central Effector Cells

Mast cells have long been associated with allergic diseases by way of their ability to respond specifically to allergens cross-linking IgE molecules bound to their cell surface via high-affinity FcεRI receptors. In nonasthmatic subjects, including patients with lung cancer, smokers, and nonasthmatic atopic individuals, mast cells recovered by BAL constitute a minority (0.04–0.6%) of the total nucleated cells (29–33). In asthmatics, these numbers can be increased up to three- to five-fold (30,33), which still constitutes only a minority of the inflammatory cells in the lumen. Although mast-cell numbers in the epithelium and submucosa are not necessarily raised in asthma (1,26), examination by electron microscopy shows extensive ultrastructural changes in their granules, which have been associated with mast-cell activation (1,26). Two patterns of degranulation have been described in vitro in experiments using isolated mast cells (34,35). The first, which is characterized by dissolution of granular contents and budding of granules on the cell membrane, is referred to as *piecemeal degranulation* (35). The second pattern, in which individual granules are seen to fuse and form channels through which the contents are released into the surrounding matrix, is described as the *anaphylactic type* (34). Both of these patterns are seen in asthmatic airways, in contrast to healthy airways, in which resting mast cells contain intact granules (1,26).

In support of ongoing mast cell mediator secretion, levels of mast cell–derived mediators are raised in the BAL and induced sputum in asthmatics (14,36–40). As with eosinophils, these changes are seen even in the mildest forms of the disease. Acute stimulation by allergen during an early asthmatic reaction (EAR) leads to mast-cell activation and release of histamine, which can be detected in BAL (37,41). The cellular provenance is confirmed by the associated rise in the 134-kDa neutral protease tryptase (37), a mediator found almost uniquely in mast cells. Other mast-cell mediators likely to play important roles as effectors of bronchoconstriction seen during the EAR are PGD_2 and the sulfidopeptide leukotrienes. In addition to being a direct spasmogen approximately 30 times more potent than histamine, PGD_2 is a potent vasodilator and increases vascular permeability (42). Mast cells are a major source of sulfidopeptide leukotrienes, which also increase vascular permeability and are between 100 and 1000 times more potent than histamine and methacholine as contractile agonists (43,44). The past few years have seen a particular interest in leukotrienes with the development of potent and selective inhibitors of the 5-lipoxygenase enzyme or antagonists of the LTD_4 receptor, which have been shown to be effective in abrogating the airways responses to exercise or allergen challenge (45) and to improve clinical symptoms (46). Their efficacy may be related to disease severity, in view of the limited evidence that the expression of the 5-lipoxygenase enzyme is normal in the airways mucosa of mild asthmatics but is raised in those with more severe disease (47,48).

Tryptase has recently generated significant interest both as an important mediator in asthma and as a therapeutic target. By comparison with control subjects, in whom tryptase is either undetectable or the levels are very low (less than 2 ng/mL), concentrations as high as 40 ng/mL can be detected in induced sputum of asthmatic individuals (14). However, the range of concentrations of tryptase in sputum from asthmatics is wide, suggesting that the extent of mast-cell involvement may vary, although there appears to be no relationship to disease severity. Tryptase has been shown to enhance airway smooth muscle responsiveness in dogs (49). It also degrades bronchodilator neuropeptides such as the vasoactive intestinal peptide (VIP) (50) and cleaves complement components to form anaphylatoxins (51) and kininogen, yielding bradykinin and lysylbradykinin (52). Tryptase also contributes to increased microvascular leakage in the mucosa (53), which, together with the capacity to chemoattract and activate eosinophils (54) and enhance the expression of ICAM-1 on epithelial cells (55), serves to promote mucosal eosinophilia. Of particular interest is the effect of tryptase on ICAM-1 expression, and it can be speculated that similar effects contribute to increased expression of this adhesion molecule on a number of other cell types (T cells, eosinophils, endothelial cells) (14,22,56). A close correlation can be demonstrated between the levels of tryptase and soluble ICAM-1 (sICAM-1) in induced sputum (14), which is in keeping with the described tryptase-induced upregulation of ICAM-1 and IL-8 in epithelial cells (55). These observations have pointed to tryptase as a major mediator of allergic reactions and have prompted the development of therapeutic agents that specifically target tryptase. One of these, APC366, a specific tryptase inhibitor, has been tested in a sheep model of allergic airways responses and has been shown to significantly attenuate the late-phase allergic response (LAR) (57). More recently, it has been shown that premedication of asthmatic volunteers with nebulized APC366 partially but significantly reduces the magnitude of the allergen-induced LAR in (58).

Bronchoalveolar lavage mast cells from atopic individuals with asthma as opposed to those from normal subjects contain and release more histamine both spontaneously and when stimulated with anti-IgE or allergen (30,31). Inverse correlations between the percentage of mast cells in the recovered BAL fluid and their histamine content and baseline spirometry suggest that histamine and other mast cell–derived mediators contribute to airflow obstruction (30). It has been known for many years that H_1-receptor antagonists have a minimal bronchodilator action (59) which is limited to very mild forms of asthma. This finding has been confirmed with the newer agents such as terfenadine (60). Other actions that may be relevant to the bronchoconstrictor action of this mediator are its capacity to dilate and increase the permeability of the bronchial vascular bed (61). By directly stimulating histamine H_2 receptors and acting indirectly through vagal reflexes and β-adrenergic stimulation, histamine is capable of stimulating the secretion of mucus (61); moreover, by action on H_1 receptors, it can modulate its viscosity (62), which may further contribute to airways obstruction. A positive correlation found between airways responsiveness, the relative numbers of mast cells recovered by BAL, and sputum levels of histamine implies a role for mast cells in perpetuating this pathophysiological abnormality (14,16,30). This observation has been extended in studies showing that increased spontaneous histamine release by BAL mast cells is seen only in those subjects with increased airways responsiveness (17) and that the concentration of histamine in the cell-free supernatant of BAL is related to the level of histamine responsiveness (41).

Mast cells are now also recognized for their capacity to produce cytokines—including IL-3, IL-4, IL-5, IL-6, granulocyte-macrophage colony stimulating factor (GM-CSF), and tumor necrosis factor alpha (TNF-α)—whose actions are of relevance to the initiation and maintenance of allergic responses (63). Importantly, IgE-mediated triggering of mast cells leads not only to secretion of stored cytokines but also results in their de novo generation (64). The extent to which mast cells contribute to the overall generation of cytokines in asthma is uncertain. Staining of adjacent 2-mm tissue sections embedded into glycol methacrylate (GMA) resin localizes the majority of IL-4 protein to mast cells and a lesser proportion to eosinophils but fails to detect IL-4 in T cells (64). This is in contrast to studies using hybridization to detect mRNA transcripts for IL-4 and other Th2-type cytokines, which show that the majority of cells positive for IL-4 mRNA are T cells (5). One interpretation is that there is a relatively high turnover of IL-4 produced by T cells, which, unlike mast cells, do not have a granular storage capacity and use this cytokine as an autocrine growth factor, promoting the development of Th2-type CD4+ T cells. An important consideration is the fact that only a minority of T cells in the airways are allergen-specific, in contrast to mast cells, which all bear IgE and can thus be directly stimulated by allergen.

It can be speculated that activation of IgE-bearing mast cells and release of IL-4 may promote the differentiation on Th0-type T cells into Th2-type T cells. However, it remains to be seen whether this happens in the mucosa or regional lymphoid tissue. The use of antibodies that distinguish between stored and secreted IL-4 for immunohistochemical staining has been helpful in demonstrating the ability of mast cells to generate cytokines as part of allergic inflammation (64). The finding of an increased proportion of mast cells displaying peripheral ring staining for IL-4 protein with antibody against the secreted form in stable asthma as well as further increases in this staining pattern in bronchial biopsies of pollen-sensitive asthmatics during the pollen season (65) point to allergen-induced activation of mast cells to secrete this central cytokine.

C. Immunoregulation of Airways Inflammation

Environmental allergens play a major role in both the initiation and maintenance of the allergic response. For an allergen (or indeed any antigen) to initiate an inflammatory response, it must be presented by an antigen-presenting cell (APC). Initially, this requires uptake of allergen, its processing (partial degradation) within the APC, physical association with the class II major histocompatibility complex (MHC) molecules, and exteriorization of the antigen/MHC class II complex on the surface of the APC. This is followed by an interaction between the complex and the antigen receptor on the T lymphocyte (TCR) and between a number of accessory cell-surface molecules (including LFA-1 and ICAM-1, CD40 and its ligand CD40L, CD28, and B7-1/B7-2) present on both cells, which recognize each other specifically and participate in the process of cellular costimulation (66–68). In addition, cytokines are produced, contributing to the overall response. The interaction between APCs and T cells during antigen presentation may determine not only the extent of T cell activation but also the differentiated phenotype of the T cell.

Naive T cells produce only IL-2 upon antigenic stimulation, after which they differentiate into either Th1- or Th2-type T cells as defined by the cytokines they produce (69,70). Thus, Th2 cells produce IL-2, IFN-γ and TNF-β and Th2 cells secrete IL-4, IL-5, IL-6, and IL-13 (71). Differentiation of naive T cells into Th2-type cells is believed to be central to the generation of allergen-specific IgE as well as the activation and maturation of mast cells and eosinophils. APCs are believed to play an important role in determining the differentiation of T-helper cells into one of the subsets. The presence of APC-derived IL-12 favors the development of Th1-type T cells (72), and preferential usage of the B7-2, as opposed to B7-1, costimulatory molecules promotes a Th2-type response, at least in animal models (73).

Antigen presentation in the lungs is believed to be conducted mainly by dendritic cells (74), which are considered by some researchers as the only true professional APCs (75). In both animal and human airways, dendritic cells, which express high levels of MHC class II, are most prominent within the airway epithelium, where they form an interdigitating network (76). The density of the intraepithelial dendritic cell population is maintained in a steady state by a balance between the recruitment of cells from the blood and their egress to local secondary lymphoid tissues, where antigen presentation is believed to occur. However, in response to a range of stimuli, including inhaled viruses and soluble antigens, the density of intraepithelial dendritic cells increases rapidly but transiently (77). Thus, even patients with stable asthma can be seen to have raised numbers of CD1α+ dendritic cells in the airways mucosa (78). It is of relevance to asthma therapy that the numbers of dendritic cells can be reduced by treatment with inhaled corticosteroids (79).

Pulmonary intraepithelial dendritic cells are ideally placed for the capture of inhaled antigens and are thought to act as sentinels of the immune system, sampling the antigens being delivered to the respiratory mucosal surface. The likely scenario that ensues is that these cells then migrate and present antigens to T cells within the local secondary lymphoid tissue. Once in the lymphoid tissues, dendritic cells are thought to be unique in their ability to induce primary responses of naive T cells to newly encountered antigens. However, the extent to which dendritic cells participate in the secondary response of memory T cells to an antigen and whether they are able to present antigen to memory T cells locally within the airways is unclear. In normal lungs, dendritic cells are often found in close association with macrophages, which appear to exert a suppressive effect on these cells (80), mediated, at least in part, through the release of NO. This downregulation of dendritic cell function by macrophages and possibly other cell types may be defective in some disease states, thus enhancing local antigen presentation. In the absence of local dendritic cell activity, antigen presentation during secondary immune responses could be carried out by B cells, but their frequency in the airways is low (81) and their role as APCs in the lungs unknown. Other cells present in the airway, including structural cells such as epithelial cells, carry MHC class II and may be capable of fulfilling some of the functions of antigen presentation. However, it is thought that antigen presentation by such cells may be incomplete, permitting only partial T-cell activation and possibly even inducing T-cell unresponsiveness.

Increased antigen presentation leads to activation of airway T cells in asthma. This is seen as enhanced expression of T-cell surface activation markers determined by flow cytometric analysis of cells retrieved by BAL (82) and immunohistochemical analysis of bronchial biopsies (3). As with mast cells and eosinophils, this is observed even in mild disease and is consistent with continuous antigenic stimulation, leading to overexpression of activation markers such as the IL-2 receptor (IL-2R), the class II major histocompatibility antigen, HLA-DR (3,82), and ICAM-1 (14). Further cell activation and transcription of genes for Th2-type cytokines occurs following allergen challenge (83). Allergen stimulation also results in an influx of T cells into the airways, both in the setting of natural exposure, such as the pollen season (65), and in association with laboratory-based allergen challenge (22). This involves combined effects of increased expression of adhesion molecules ICAM-1 and E-selectin (22) and increased production of T-cell chemotactic factors. A number of cytokines/chemokines are known to be chemoattractant for T cells (IL-1α and β; IL-2; IL-3; IL-4; IL-6; IL-8; RANTES; MIP-1α and β; MCP-1,2, and 3; IL-16; and, more recently, lymphotactin). Many of these are raised in unchallenged (IL-1, IL-2, IL-3, IL-4, IL-6) and allergen-challenged airways (IL-1, IL-6, Il-8, IL-16, RANTES, MIP-1α) of asthmatic individuals. Recent studies point to IL-16 (previously known as lymphocyte chemoattractant factor) as being an important if not the main chemoattractant for T cells in asthma, which, together with MIP-1α and RANTES, responds in an allergen-specific manner to attract T cells (84,85). Increased numbers of cells immunostaining and expressing transcripts for IL-16 have been shown recently in both the epithelium and submucosal inflammatory cells in asthmatic subjects when compared with both atopic nonasthmatic and nonatopic control subjects (86). IL-16 is produced in response to allergen (84,85), histamine, and serotonin (87). While allergen appears to require appropriate presentation by antigen-presenting cells via the costimulatory molecules B7 and CD28 (85), histamine and serotonin act by stimulating mast cells and CD8+ T cells, which have the capacity to store IL-16 (87).

Most of the research into the role of T cells in asthma has focused on the pro-inflammatory role of CD4+ T cells. More recently there has been increasing evidence that CD8+ T cells might also have a role in asthma pathogenesis. It is now widely appreciated that purified $CD8^+$ T cells possess the capacity to produce a wide range of cytokines and chemokines, which, in some instances (IFN-γ, GM-CSF, MIP-1α, IL-16, and RANTES) exceeds that of CD4+ T cells (88,89). Distinct cytokine-secreting subsets of $CD8^+$ T cells (Tc), similar to their CD4+ Th1- and Th2-type counterparts, have now been identified and designated Tc1 cells, which secrete predominantly IL-2 and IFN-γ, and Tc2, which secrete IL-4 and IL-5 (90–94). Circulating CD8+-positive T cells from asthmatic individual have increased intracellular concentrations of IL-4 as compared with cells from nonatopic healthy control subjects (95), although the mechanisms of activation of these cells and the release of IL-4 and its contribution to the overall allergic response remain unknown. CD8+ T cells might play an important role in the response to viral infection, which can influence the generation of cytokines by these cells (96). This may be of importance to both mild and, in particular, severe exacerbations of asthma in which increased numbers of CD8+ T cells accumulate in the airways mucosa (97).

III. The Pathological Determinants of Asthma Severity

Clinically, asthma is classified as being either intermittent or persistent, depending on the frequency and chronicity of symptoms. Intermittent asthma is characterized by infrequent asthma symptoms (less than once a week) and occasional use of β_2-agonists. Persistent asthma is further graded according to the frequency of symptoms and treatment requirements into mild (symptoms more often than once a week but less often than once a day), moderate (daily symptoms and use of inhaled bronchodilator and inhaled corticosteroids), and severe (with continuous symptoms and frequent exacerbations as well as regular use of oral corticosteroids). With increasing confidence in the safety of research bronchoscopy, an increasing number of researchers have conducted bronchoscopic studies in persons with severe asthma without any reports of serious side effects (6,98,99).

The first study that addressed the issue of determinants of asthma severity was conducted by Bousquet and colleagues (6). This study showed a close association between eosinophilia (both in blood and BAL) and ECP levels in BAL and the degree of asthma severity defined by the Aas score, which is based on symptoms and treatment requirements during the previous year (100). Importantly, none of the patients in this study had been on inhaled corticosteroids during the month preceding the study, thus controlling for the confounding effects of anti-inflammatory treatment. Subsequent studies have included patients on inhaled and oral corticosteroids. A proportion of patients remain symptomatic despite the use of anti-inflammatory treatment, and in these patients one continues to see raised eosinophil counts in sputum, (14,23,101). Treatment with inhaled corticosteroids alone also seems to be unable to abrogate the mucosal eosinophilia as seen in bronchial biopsies, which correlates with clinical disease severity (102). Significant reduction of mucosal eosinophilia to levels found in healthy individuals appears to be possible only with the use of oral corticosteroids, although in a minority of patients it persists regardless (98).

In an attempt to elucidate the mechanisms that determine asthma severity, a number of researchers have studied the events that occur during nocturnal asthma. While this form of asthma usually reflects poor disease control, genetic studies suggest that a Gly16 polymorphism of the β_2-adrenergic receptor, which may be responsible for downregulation of receptor numbers, is more frequent in nocturnal asthma. Bronchoscopic studies have shown an influx of eosinophils into the airways at night and their release of ECP, as demonstrated by BAL (103). Of particular interest has been the observation that prominent changes occur in the lung parenchyma, which has so far not been thought to be involved in asthma (104). Quantification of the cellular infiltrate shows an accumulation of eosinophils in the alveolar tissue in the early hours of the morning which is associated with increased expression of Th2-type cytokines (S.J. Wilson, unpublished observation).

As disease progresses, neutrophil counts are also seen to be increased as compared with those of healthy control subjects and patients with mild asthma, with severalfold increases in both BAL and transbronchial biopsies in the very severe forms of corticosteroid-dependent asthma (99). Neutrophils have so far not been thought to be important in asthma and have been viewed as being more characteristic of chronic bronchitis. Increased airways neutrophilia is seen in asthma exacerbations (105) and in asthma deaths (106). Because both of these have been linked with infections, neutrophilia has not been considered to be a feature of the chronic allergen-driven component of the pathogenesis of asthma. The mechanisms involved in recruiting and activating neutrophils remain to be elucidated, but initial studies point to raised LTB_4 (98), detected in BAL, and raised tissue levels of free IL-8 in the bronchial mucosa (107) in severe forms of asthma as being possibly implicated by attracting and activating neutrophils.

If neutrophils contribute to the disordered airways function, it is unclear which mechanisms are important. The levels of myeloperoxidase (MPO) are not raised in induced sputum in asthma, although both the neutrophil counts and MPO levels correlate with the levels of airways hyperresponsiveness (108), suggesting that they represent a marker of some other neutrophil function that contributes to this pathophysiological abnormality. It has been suggested that treatment with corticosteroids may be partly responsible for increased neutrophil numbers and function (109–111). However, short-term treatment with inhaled corticosteroids does not change neutrophil numbers in sputum (author's unpublished observation). It may be that longer-term corticosteroids may have an effect, although this remains to be demonstrated.

Corticosteroids have long been considered to be effective as anti-inflammatory agents, and detailed investigations have been conducted into the mechanisms involved (112–118). In addition to inhibiting IL-2 production and suppressing T-cell activation, corticosteroids reduce the numbers of cells expressing mRNA for Th2-type cytokines IL-4 and IL-5 in the BAL of asthmatic subjects; this reduction is associated with a fall in eosinophilic infiltration and improved symptom control (117). However, it is unclear why airways inflammation is not always fully responsive to corticosteroids. Although absolute corticosteroid resistance is rare, emerging data point to the existence of relative corticosteroid resistance in asthma patients, the extent of which may determine disease severity. Corticosteroid resistance is characterized by persistent T-cell activation and decreased ability of dexamethasone to suppress T-cell proliferative responses to the mitogen hemagglutinin (PHA) (119,120). Consistent with this abnormality, increased numbers of activated T cells expressing the IL-2R can be seen in bronchial biopsies of patients who continue to suffer from severe asthma despite treatment with high-dose inhaled corticosteroids and oral corticosteroids and despite residing in a hypoallergenic environment at high altitude (98). In these patients, the numbers of activated T cells correlate with the variability of peak expiratory flow (PEF), an indicator of airways hyperresponsiveness (98). In contrast to corticosteroid-sensitive patients, those who are corticosteroid-resistant have raised numbers of T cells expressing Th2-type cytokines (IL-4 and IL-5) in BAL, which are not reduced by treatment with prednisolone (121). Furthermore, corticosteroid-dependent asthma is characterized by increased serum levels of IL-5 (122) and increased immunostaining for this cytokine in bronchial biopsies (98).

At the extreme end of the spectrum of asthma severity are patients who die during an attack of asthma. At postmortem, their lungs are invariably hyperinflated and remain so upon opening of the chest wall, reflecting extensive bronchial obstruction. The presence of overwhelming bronchospasm in the absence of mucous plugging is probably rare, as suggested in a review of a large number of cases of fatal asthma (123,124). Abundant mucous plugs account for areas of atelectasis, which can lead to segmental and even lobar collapse following reabsorption of air distal to the site of bronchial obstruction. Mucous plugging leading to partial lung collapse can also be noted occasionally in living asthma patients, especially those suffering from allergic bronchopulmonary aspergillosis. The extent of mucous plugging in fatal asthma has been estimated to result in more than 50% occlusion of the peripheral airways (125). The pathophysiological implications of mucous plugging in severe asthma resulting in death are significant, and the presence of physical obstruction to airflow offers an explanation for the ineffectiveness of inhaled bronchodilator drugs.

In addition to containing desquamated epithelial cells, the mucous plugs seen in asthma deaths contain a prominent inflammatory cellular infiltrate, suggesting that the excessive production and secretion of mucus is associated with and probably preceded by inflammation that has not responded adequately to anti-inflammatory treatment. Alternatively, this finding may point to poor patient compliance. The epithelium is extensively damaged, leading to detachment of the columnar epithelial cells from the basal cells along a cleavage line that is susceptible to proinflammatory mediators and in particular the cationic proteins produced by eosinophils. Consistent with this, major basic protein (MBP) secreted by activated eosinophils is noted in areas of mucosal ulceration and within mucous plugs (27). In mild asthma, the effect of inflammation on epithelial desquamation appears to be predominantly one of detachment of the epithelial layer, sometimes in clumps, rather than direct cytotoxic damage to the cells (126,127). However, in asthma deaths, there is evidence of apoptosis within the shed epithelium, which is more prominent when compared with that in nonasthmatic subjects dying from other causes (128).

The implications of extensive epithelial damage in severe, fatal asthma have not been fully elucidated. In addition to loss of the physical barrier, which enables irritants to stimulate nerve endings and facilitate further stimulation of the deeper layers by inhaled allergen, epithelial damage is likely to impair mucociliary clearance significantly. Together with the loss of epithelium-derived bronchodilator substances (129), this is likely to contribute to fatal bronchospasm.

Among the infiltrating cells in asthma deaths, the eosinophil is the predominant cell type (130). Together with the mast cell, the eosinophil contributes to excessive secretion of mucus. Paradoxically, the numbers of mast cells are decreased (131). This can be explained by extensive degranulation, such that the granular contents responsible for the metachromatic staining of mast cells cannot be identified. Together, mast cells and eosinophils also contribute to microvascular leakage, resulting in airway edema and increased amounts of albumin in the mucus, which increases its viscosity via formation of viscous protein-glycoprotein complexes (132,133). By its ability to cause eosinophil activation and recruitment and tissue edema, tryptase, the mast-cell neutral protease, may be one of the many mediators contributing to the bronchoconstriction that eventually results in death.

IV. The Process of Airways Restructuring in Asthma

The outcome of any tissue injury is determined by the extent and duration of the insult that has resulted in morphological changes. Consistent with this notion, extensive morphological changes occur in asthmatic airways as a consequence of chronic inflammation. This gives rise to restructuring of the airway wall, which is also referred to as *airways remodeling*. The existence of these changes has long been known in cases of severe asthma (134) but is now seen to be typical of mild forms of the disease as well (135). Furthermore, it is now appreciated that the entire depth of the airway wall is affected and that the functional changes involve all the structural cells and the extracellular matrix.

The bronchial epithelium forms the first line of defense in the lungs by protecting the airways from environmental effects. It is composed of columnar ciliated, secretory, and basal cells. The epithelial cells are organized into a stratified layer (not pseudostratified, as previously thought), with the columnar cells resting upon the basal cells, which themselves are bound to the basement membrane (127). The cells are held together by junctional complexes between columnar cells, hemidesmosomal complexes between basal cells, and desmosomal contacts between columnar and basal cells. The existence of tight junctions renders the epithelium impermeable to macromolecules. Any loss of this protective barrier is likely to have significant implications for the deeper mucosal layers.

The interpretation of epithelial damage in biopsies obtained by bronchoscopy has been controversial because of possible damage to the epithelium during biopsy. Studies that have used rigid bronchoscopy and large biopsy forceps, which are less likely to cause artefactual damage than those used in fibreoptic bronchoscopy, have demonstrated widespread damage and shedding of the epithelium in asthmatic patients, although studies to date have been lacking in healthy control subjects (136). Artefactual damage notwithstanding, studies of bronchoscopic biopsies and BAL suggest an increase in the extent of epithelial sloughing as an integral part of the asthmatic process (17,26,137). These findings are consistent with epithelial clumps seen in sputum and described in the early literature as Creola bodies (138).

The mechanisms leading to epithelial damage have not been fully elucidated but probably involve a combination of mediators that are toxic to the epithelium, such as the arginine-rich eosinophil-derived cationic proteins and proteolytic enzymes (25,139), resulting in a fault line between the columnar and basal cells (126,127) and upward pressure from the edema of the submucosa. The damage inflicted on the epithelial layer is usually not due to cytotoxicity but appears to result from weakening of the junctional adhesion structures (126,127). This results in a more selective loss of columnar cells and relative preservation of the basal cell layer. As a consequence, an increased proportion of columnar cells is seen in clumps of two or more cells.

Among the spectrum of airways diseases, damage to the bronchial epithelium appears to be unique to asthma and is not seen in chronic bronchitis, where squamous-cell metaplasia may develop. While epithelial damage is associated with attempts at repair, as suggested by increased expression of the CD44 adhesion molecules in areas of regeneration (140,141), this apparently cannot lead to complete restitution. Whether this is due to repeated injury or an impaired repair mechanisms is unclear. The functionally altered epithelium expresses a wide range of adhesion molecules, including intercellular adhesion molecule-1 (ICAM-1) (142) and the $\alpha_3\beta_1$ (M. Vignola, personal communication) and $\alpha_v\beta_6$ integrins (143). The integrin $\alpha_3\beta_1$ is the counterreceptor for several extracellular matrix components involved in healing; furthermore, fibronectin and tenascin, which are restricted to epithelial cells and expressed only following injury, bind to $\alpha_v\beta_6$.

The implications of epithelial damage for asthma pathogenesis are not well understood. Theoretically, epithelial shedding should remove the protective barrier that prevents the allergens and microorganisms from damaging the deeper layers and at the same time reveal the nerve endings. In keeping with this notion, studies have shown that the degree of epithelial cell loss correlates with the measured level of airways hyperresponsiveness (17,26,137). In addition, the epithelium participates in the secretion of IgA to protect against microorganisms, but, if anything, the levels of IgA in sputum appear to be raised in asthma (J. Shute, personal communication). The loss of epithelial integrity results in increased permeability to macromolecules. The epithelium also inhibits the action of kinins via neutral endopeptidase effects and has antioxidant enzymes, which counter the effects of environmental oxidants such as ozone and nitrogen dioxide (144). Through their capacity to generate endothelins and lipoxygenase products of arachidonic acid, epithelial cells can contribute to smooth muscle tone, which is countered by the production of NO acting as a bronchodilator (145). However, an array of the mediators produced by the epithelium are proinflammatory (PGE_2, nitric oxide, 15HETE, endothelin, IL-1β, IL-6, IL-11, LIF, GM-CSF, IL-16, and IL-18, IL-8, MIP-1α, MCP-3, RANTES, and eotaxin) (146). Although theoretically sloughing of the layer of activated cells might act as a means of downregulating inflammation, it is unclear whether this is of physiological relevance.

As part of the response to chronic injury, the reticular layer of the basement membrane undergoes extensive changes. Interstitial collagen types III and V, products of myofibroblasts located beneath the true basement membrane upon which the epithelial cells rest, are deposited to form a dense and thickened layer (147). The extent of collagen deposition correlates with the increase in the numbers of myofibroblasts (148). Initially the thickening of the collagen was believed to be restricted to superficial layers of the submucosa (147). However, recent studies have shown that the deeper layers of the submucosa of asthmatic airways also contain significantly more collagen (149). The increased production and deposition of collagen involves a number of growth factors and cytokines, such as TGF, platelet-derived growth factor (PDGF), basic fibroblast growth factor (BFGF), TNF-α, IL-4, and endothelin in association with the mast-cell mediators tryptase and histamine (150–157). The relative importance of these factors to airways remodeling and their cellular source is unclear. A recent study has localized the major part of TGF-β to eosinophils (102). The increased numbers of eosinophils have been shown to correlate with reduced FEV_1, and the latter correlated with the extent of subepithelial fibrosis, pointing to a possible cause-and-effect relationship (102).

In parallel with collagen deposition, there are changes in the other components of the extracellular matrix indicating destruction of the elastic support. Furthermore, the appearance of α_2-laminin chains, which are normally seen during morphogenesis, points to an increased turnover of the tissue matrix (158). Immunohistochemical and electron microscopic analysis of elastin fibers in the bronchial mucosa shows evidence of lysis and fragmentation (159), even though the total content of elastic fibers appears not to differ between asthmatic and normal lungs (160). Degradation of elastase could result from activation of macrophages and eosinophils and their release of elastase and other metalloproteases (161–164). This change does not appear to be related to the use of corticosteroids, which are known to inhibit the generation of elastic fibers (165). The pathophysiological consequence of elastic fiber degradation are difficult to assess because the changes cannot be readily quantified and correlated with pulmonary function. The loss of elastic fibers is likely to make the airways less distensible (166). Whether similar changes occur in the bronchial adventitia and the parenchyma, where there is now evidence of inflammatory cell involvement (104), is uncertain, but the combination of airway and parenchymal changes could account for the loss of elastic recoil in asthma (167).

As a further component of airways restructuring due to chronic inflammation and possibly repeated bronchoconstriction, the airways smooth muscle layer undergoes hypertrophy and hyperplasia (134,168,169). In addition, prominent hyperplasia of mucous glands in the airway wall can be seen in cases of fatal asthma (170). Finally, recent studies show an increase in the numbers of blood vessels in the mucosa (171). How exactly this changes the airways physiology is unclear. Together with the edema of the mucosa, this results in an overall increase in wall thickness. The changes observed under the microscope find confirmation in studies employing computed tomography, which is able to demonstrate abnormalities of the airway wall in a significant proportion of asthmatics (172,173). In some studies the changes can be related to the duration and severity of asthma (174). It therefore seems logical that airways remodeling should be a target for asthma treatment, and indeed a number of studies have shown an increased rate of decline in lung function (175–177). However, it remains unclear which patients are at risk of developing structural changes that are of physiological relevance, and there are no cellular or physiological predictors for such a development. Nevertheless, long-term follow-up of patients with asthma treated with either β_2-agonists alone or with β_2-agonists and inhaled corticosteroids has shown a clear benefit of anti-inflammatory treatment in reducing the risk of loss of airways function (178,179).

V. Concluding Remarks

With the abundance of information on the pathology of asthma that we now possess there is no doubt that we have greatly improved our understanding of the pathogenesis of this disease. However, we are no closer to identifying the main factors that cause asthma and sustain the chronic inflammation. Indeed we do not know whether the mechanisms involved in initiating the disease and maintaining it are the same. Thus, elucidation of early events during the development of asthma is crucial if efforts are to result in preventive measures that might alter the susceptibility of atopic individuals to develop clinical asthma. Another main challenge is to identify which cell types, signal transduction mechanisms, and nuclear transcription factors are the main players in what is undoubtedly a complex cellular network. It is almost certain that targeting and neutralizing a single mediator or cell type is not going to arrest the asthmatic process. Finally, further attempts have to be made to improve our classification of asthma, which should be based not only on descriptive pathology but also on common intracellular defects so as to target the disease process more specifically.

Acknowledgments

The author gratefully acknowledges Mrs. K. Roberts for her excellent secretarial assistance with the preparation of this manuscript.

References

1. Djukanović R, Wilson JW, Britten KM, Wilson SJ, Walls AF, Howarth PH, Holgate ST. Quantitation of mast cells and eosinophils in the bronchial mucosa of atopic asthmatics and healthy control subjects using immunohistochemistry. Am Rev Respir Dis 1990; 142:863–871.
2. Djukanović R, Lai CKW, Wilson J, Britten KM, Wilson SJ, Roche WR, Howarth PH, Holgate ST. Bronchial mucosal manifestations of atopy: a comparison of markers of inflammation between atopic asthmatics, atopic nonasthmatics and healthy controls. Eur Respir J 1992; 5:538–544.
3. Azzawi M, Bradley B, Jeffery PJ, Frew AJ, Wardlaw AJ, Knowles G, Assoufi B, Collins JV, Durham S, Kay AB. Identification of activated T-lymphocytes and eosinophils in bronchial biopsies in stable atopic asthmatics. Am Rev Respir Dis 1990; 142:1407–1413.
4. Bradley BL, Azzawi M, Jacobson M, Assoufi B, Collins JV, Irani A-MA, Schwartz LB, Durham SR, Jeffery PK, Kay AB. Eosinophils, T-lymphocytes, mast cells, neutrophils and macrophages in bronchial biopsy specimens from atopic subjects without asthma and normal control subjects and relationship to bronchial hyperresponsiveness. J Allergy Clin Immunol 1991; 88:661–674.

5. Robinson DS, Hamid Q, Ying S, Tsicopoulos A, Barkans J, Bentley AM, Corrigan C, Durham SR, Kay AB. Predominant Th2-like bronchoalveolar T-lymphocyte population in atopic asthma. N Engl J Med 1992; 326:298–304.
6. Bousquet J, Chanez P, Lacoste JY, Barneon G, Ghavanian N, Enander I, Venge P, Ahlstedt S, Sinony-Lafontaine J, Godard P, Michel FB. Eosinophilic inflammation in asthma. N Engl J Med 1990; 323:1033–1039.
7. Saetta M, DiStefano A, Maestrelli P, DeMarzo N, Milani GF, Pivirotto F, Mapp CE, Fabbri LM. Airway mucosal inflammation in occupational asthma induced by toluene diisocyanate. Am Rev Respir Dis 1992; 145:160–168.
8. Bentley AM, Menz G, Storz C, Robinson DS, Bradley BL, Jeffery PK, Durham SR, Kay AB. Identification of T lymphocytes, macrophages, and activated eosinophils in the bronchial mucosa of intrinsic asthma: relationship to symptoms and bronchial hyperresponsiveness. Am Rev Respir Dis 1992; 146:500–506.
9. Goetzl EJ, Wasserman SI, Austen KF. Eosinophil polymorphonuclear function in immediate hypersensitity. Arch Pathol 1975; 99:1–4.
10. Wasserman SI, Goetzl EJ, Austen KF. Inactivation of slow reacting substance of anaphylaxis by human eosinophil arylsulfatase. J Immunol 1975; 114:645–649.
11. Djukanović R, Roche WR, Wilson JW, Beasley CRW, Twentyman OP, Howarth PH, Holgate ST. Mucosal inflammation in asthma: state of the Art. Am Rev Respir Dis 1990; 142:434–457.
12. Pin I, Gibson P, Kolendovic R, Girgis-Gabardo A, Denburg J, Hargreave F, Dolovich J. Use of induced sputum cell counts to investigate airway inflammation in asthma. Thorax 1992; 47:25–29.
13. Fahy J, Liu J, Wong H, Boushey H. Cellular and biochemical analysis of induced sputum from asthmatic and from healthy subjects. Am Rev Respir Dis 1993; 147: 1126–1131.
14. Louis R, Shute J, Biagi S, Stanciu L, Marrelli F, Tenor H, Hidi R, Djukanović R. Cell infiltration, ICAM-1 expression, and eosinophil chemotactic activity in asthmatic sputum. Am J Respir Crit Care Med 1997; 155:466–472.
15. Barnes PJ. A new approach to the treatment of asthma. N Engl J Med 1989; 321: 1517–1527.
16. Kirby JG, Hargreave FE, Gleich GJ, O'Byrne PM. Bronchoalveolar cell profiles of asthmatic and non-asthmatic subjects. Am Rev Respir Dis 1987; 136:379–383.
17. Wardlaw AJ, Dunnette S, Gleich GJ, Collins JV, Kay AB. Eosinophils and mast cells in bronchoalveolar lavage in mild asthma: relationship to bronchial hyperreactivity. Am Rev Respir Dis 1988; 137:62–69.
18. Grootendorst DC, Sont JK, Willems LNA, Kluin Nelemans JC, Van Krieken JHJM, Veselic Charvat M, Sterk PJ. Comparison of inflammatory cell counts in asthma: Induced sputum vs. bronchoalveolar lavage and bronchial biopsies. Clin Exp Allergy 1997; 27:769–779.
19. Metzger WJ, Zavala D, Richerson HB, Moseley P, Iwamota P, Monick M, Sjoerdsma K, Hunninghake GW. Local allergen challenge and bronchoalveolar lavage of allergic asthmatic lungs: description of the model and local airway inflammation. Am Rev Respir Dis 1987; 135:433–440.
20. Metzger WJ, Richerson HB, Worden K, Monick H, Hunninghake GW. Bronchoal-

veolar lavage of allergic asthmatic patients following allergen bronchoprovocation. Chest 1986; 89:477–483.

21. De Monchy JG, Kauffman HF, Venge P. Bronchoalveolar eosinophilia during allergen-induced late asthmatic reactions. Am Rev Respir Dis 1989; 131:373–376.
22. Montefort S, Gratziou C, Goulding D, Polosa R, Haskard DO, Howarth PH, Holgate ST, Carroll MP. Bronchial biopsy evidence for leukocyte infiltration and upregulation of leukocyte-endothelial cell adhesion molecules 6 hours after local allergen challenge of sensitised asthmatic airways. J Clin Invest 1994; 93:1411–1421.
23. in't Veen JCCM, de Gouw HWFM, Smits HH, Sont JK, Hiemstra PS, Sterk PJ, Bel EH. Repeatability of cellular and soluble markers of inflammation in induced sputum from patients with asthma. Eur Respir J 1996; 9:2441–2447.
24. Frigas E, Loegering DA, Gleich GJ. Cytotoxic effects of the guinea pig eosinophil major basic protein on tracheal epithelium. Lab Invest 1980; 42:25–42.
25. Frigas E, Loegering DA, Solley GO, Farrow GM, Gleich GJ. Elevated levels of eosinophil major basic protein in the sputum of patients with bronchial asthma. Mayo Clin Proc 1981; 56:345–353.
26. Beasley R, Roche WR, Roberts JA, Holgate ST. Cellular events in the bronchi in mild asthma and after bronchial provocation. Am Rev Respir Dis 1989; 139:806–817.
27. Filley WV, Holley LE, Kephart GM, Gleich GJ. Identification by immunofluorescence of eosinophil granule major basic protein in lung tissue of patients with bronchial asthma. Lancet 1982; 2:11–16.
28. Weller PF. Updates on cells and cytokines. Hum Eosinoph 1997; 100:283–287.
29. Agius RM, Godfrey RC, Holgate ST. Mast cell and histamine content of human bronchoalveolar lavage. Thorax 1985; 40:760–767.
30. Flint KC, Leung KBP, Hudspith BN, Brostoff J, Pearce FL, Johnson NM. Bronchoalveolar mast cells in extrinsic asthma: a mechanism for the initiation of antigen-specific broncho-constriction. Br Med J 1985; 291:923–926.
31. Pearce FL, Flint KC, Leung KBP, Hudspith BN, Seager K, Hammond MD, Brostoff J, Geraint-James D, Johnson NM. Some studies on human pulmonary mast cells obtained by bronchoalveolar lavage and by enzymatic dissociation of whole lung tissue. Int Arch Allergy Appl Immunol 1987; 82:507–512.
32. Flint KC, Leung KBP, Pearce FL, Hudspith BN, Brostoff J, Johnson NM. Human mast cells recovered by bronchoalveolar lavage: their morphology, histamine release and the effects of sodium cromoglycate. Clin Sci 1985; 68:427–432.
33. Tomioka M, Ida S, Shindoh Y, Ishihara T, Takishima T. Mast cells in bronchoalveolar lumen of patients with bronchial asthma. Am Rev Respir Dis 1984; 129: 1000–1005.
34. Dvorak AM, Schulman ES, Peters SP, MacGlashan DW, Newball HH, Schleimer RP, Lichtenstein LM. Immunoglobulin E–mediated degranulation of isolated human lung mast cells. Lab Invest 1985; 53:45–56.
35. Dvorak AM. The fine structure of human basophils and mast cells. In: Holgate ST, ed. Mast Cells, Mediators and Disease. Dodrecht, Boston, London: Kluwer, 1988: 29–97.
36. Wenzel SE, Westcott JY, Smith HR, Larsen GL. Spectrum of prostanoid release

after bronchoalveolar allergen challenge in atopic asthmatics and in control groups. Am Rev Respir Dis 1989; 139:450–457.
37. Wenzel SE, Fowler A, Schwartz LB. Activation of pulmonary mast cells by bronchoalveolar allergen challenge: in vivo release of histamine and tryptase in atopic subjects with and without asthma. Am Rev Respir Dis 1988; 137:1002–1008.
38. Broide DH, Gleich GJ, Cuomo AJ, Coburn DA, Federman EC, Schwartz LB, Wasserman SI. Evidence of ongoing mast cell and eosinophil degranulation in symptomatic asthma airway. J Allergy Clin Immunol 1991; 88:637–648.
39. Lam S, Chan H, LeRiche JC, Chan-Yeung M, Salari H. Release of leukotrienes in patients with bronchial asthma. J Allergy Clin Immunol 1988; 81:711–717.
40. Jarjour NN, Calhoun WJ, Schwartz LB, Busse WW. Elevated bronchoalveolar lavage fluid histamine levels in allergic asthmatics are associated with increase airway obstruction. Am Rev Respir Dis 1991; 144:83–87.
41. Casale TB, Wood D, Richerson HB, Zehr B, Zavala D, Hunninghake GW. Direct evidence of a role for mast cells in the pathogenesis of antigen-induced bronchoconstriction. J Clin Invest 1987; 80:1507–1511.
42. Beasley R, Hovel C, Mani R, Robinson C, Varley J, Holgate ST. Comparative vascular effects of histamine, prostaglandin (PG) D_2 and its metabolite 9α, 11β-PGF_2 in human skin. Clin Allergy 1988; 18:619–627.
43. Griffin M, Weiss WJ, Leitch GA, McFadden ER, Corey EJ, Austen FK, Drazen JM. Effects of leukotriene D on the airways in asthma. N Engl J Med 1983; 308: 436–439.
44. Adelroth E, Morris MM, Hargreave FE, O'Byrne PM. Airway responsiveness to leukotrienes C_4 and D_4 and to methacholine in patients with asthma and normal controls. N Engl J Med 1986; 315:480–484.
45. Finnerty JP, Wood-Baker R, Thomson H, Holgate ST. Role of leukotrienes in exercise-induced asthma: inhibitor effect of ICI 204219, a potent leukotriene D4-receptor antagonist. Am Rev Respir Dis 1992; 145:746–749.
46. Spector SL, Smith LJ, Glass M. Effects of 6 weeks of therapy with oral doses of ICI 204,219, a leukotriene D4 receptor antagonist, in subjects with bronchial asthma. Am J Respir Crit Care Med 1994; 150:618–663.
47. Bradding P, Redington AE, Djukanović R, Conrad DJ, Holgate ST. 15-Lipoxygenase immunoreactivity in normal and asthmatic airways. Am J Respir Crit Care Med 1995; 151:1201–1204.
48. Shannon VR, Chanez P, Bousquet J, Holtzman MJ. Histochemical evidence for induction of arachidonate 15-lipoxygenase in airway disease. Am Rev Respir Dis 1993; 147:1024–1028.
49. Sekizawa K, Caughey GH, Lazarus SC, Gold WM, Nadel JA. Mast cell tryptase causes airway smooth muscle hyperresponsiveness in dogs. J Clin Invest 1989; 83: 175–179.
50. Barnes PJ. Airway neuropeptides and asthma. Trends Pharm Sci 1987; 8:24–27.
51. Schwartz LB, Kawahara MS, Hugli TE, Vik DT, Fearon DT, Austen KF. Generation of C3a anaphylatoxin from human C3 by mast cell tryptase. J Immunol 1983; 130:1891–1895.
52. Proud D, Liekrerski ES, Bailey GS. Identification of human lung mast cell kinino-

genase as tryptase and relevance of tryptase kininogenase activity. Biochem Pharmacol 1988; 78:1473–1480.
53. Walls AF, He S, Teran L, Holgate ST. Mast cell proteases as mediators of vascular leakage and cell accumulation. J Allergy Clin Immunol 1993; 91:A256.
54. Jung, K, Shute J, Cairns J, Park H, Church MK, Walls A. Human mast cells tryptase: a mediator of eosinophil chemotaxis and degranulation (abstr). Am Rev Respir Crit Care Med 1995; 151:530.
55. Cairns J, Walls AF. Mast cell tryptase is a mitogen for epithelial cell stimulation of IL-8 production and ICAM-1 expression. J Immunol 1996: 156:275–283.
56. Hansel T, Braunstein J, Walker C, Blazer K, Bruijnzeel P. Sputum eosinophils from asthmatics express ICAM-1 and HLA-DR. Clin Exp Immunol 1991; 86:271–277.
57. Molinari JF, Moore WR, Clark J, Tanaka R, Butterfield JH, Abraham WM. Role of tryptase in immediate cutaneous responses in allergic sheep. J Appl Physiol 1995; 79:1966–1970.
58. Krishna MT, Chauhan AJ, Little L, Sampson K, Mant TGK, Hawksworth R, Djukanović R, Lee TH, Holgate ST. Effect of inhaled APC 366 on allergen-induced bronchoconstriction and airway hyperresponsiveness to histame in atopic asthmatics (abstr). Am J Respir Crit Care Med 1998; 157:456.
59. Popa V. Bronchodilator activity of an H_1 blocker, chlorpheniramine. J Allergy Clin Immunol 1977; 59:54–63.
60. Rafferty P, Holgate ST. Terfenadine (Seldane) is a potent and selective histamine H_1 receptor antagonist in asthmatic airways. Am Rev Respir Dis 1987; 135:181–184.
61. White MV, Slater JE. Kaliner MA. Histamine and asthma. Am Rev Respir Dis 1987; 135:1165–1176.
62. Marin MG, Davis B, Nadel JA. Effect of histamine on electrical and ion transport properties of tracheal epithelium. Am J Physiol 1977; 42:735–738.
63. Bradding P, Roberts JA, Britten KM, Montefort S, Djukanović R, Howarth PH, Holgate ST. Interleukins (IL)-4, -5, -6, and TNFα in normal and asthmatic airways: evidence for the human mast cell as an important source of these cytokines. Am J Respir Cell Mol Biol 1994; 10:471–480.
64. Okayama Y, Petit-Frére C, Kassel O, Semper A, Quint D, Tunon de Lara MJ, Bradding P, Holgate ST. Expression of messenger RNA for IL-4 and IL-5 in human lung and skin mast cells in response to FCε receptor cross-linkage and the presence of stem cell factor. J Immunol 1995; 155:1796–1808.
65. Djukanović R, Feather I, Gratziou C, Walls A, Peroni D, Bradding P, Judd M, Howarth PH, Holgate ST. The effect of natural allergen exposure during the grass-pollen season on airways inflammatory cells and asthma symptoms. Thorax 1996; 51:575–581.
66. Unanue ER. The concept of antigen processing and presentation. JAMA 1995; 274: 1071–1073.
67. Dougherty GJ, Murdoch S, Hogg N. The function of human intercellular adhesion molecule-1 (ICAM-1) in the generation of an immune response. Eur J Immunol 1988; 18:35–39.
68. June CH, Bluestone JA, Nadler LM, Thompson CB. The B7 and CD28 receptor families. Immunol Today 1994; 15:321–330.

69. Street NE, Mossmann TR. Functional diversity of T lymphocytes due to secretion of different cytokine patterns. FASEB J 1991; 5:171–177.
70. Mossmann TR, Cherwinski H, Bond MW, Giedlin MA, Coffman RL. Two types of murine helper T cell clone: 1. Definition according to profiles of lymphokine activities and secreted proteins. J Immunol 1986; 136:2348–2357.
71. Paul WE, Seder RA. Lymphocyte responses and cytokines. Cell 1994; 76:241–251.
72. Hsieh S-S, Macatonia SE, Tripp CS, Wolf SF, O'Garra A, Murphy KM. Development of Th1 CD4+ T cells through IL-12 produced by Listeria-induced macrophages. Science 1993; 260:547–549.
73. Keane-Myers AM, Gause WC, Finkelman FD, Xhou X-D, Wills-Karp M. Development of murine allergic asthma is dependent upon B7-2 costimulation. J Immunol 1998; 160:1036–1043.
74. Semper AE, Hartley JA. Dendritic cells in the lung: what is their relevance to asthma? Clin Exp Allergy 1996; 26:485–490.
75. Matzinger P. Tolerance, danger, and the extended family. Annu Rev Immunol 1994; 12:991–1045.
76. Holt PG, Schon-Hegrad MA, Phillips MJ, McMenamin PG. Ia-positive dendritic cells form a tightly meshed network within the human airway epithelium. Clin Exp Allergy 1989; 19:597–601.
77. Fokkens WJ, Vroom TM, Rijntjes E, Mulder PGH. Fluctuation of the number of CD-1(T6)-positive dendritic cells, presumably Langerhans cells, in the nasal mucosa of patients with an isolated grass-pollen allergy before, during and after the grass-pollen season. J Allergy Clin Immunol 1989; 84:39–43.
78. Tunon-de-Lara JM, Redington AE, Bradding P, Church MK, Hartley JA, Semper AE, Holgate ST. Dendritic cells in normal and asthmatic airways: expression of the α subunit of the high affinity immunoglobulin E receptor (FceRI-α). Clin Exp Allergy 1996; 26:648–655.
79. Möller GM, Overbeek SE, van Helden-Meeuwsen CG, van Haarst JMW, Prens EP, Mulder PG, Postma DS, Hoogsteden HC. Increased numbers of dendritic cells in the bronchial mucosa of atopic asthmatic patients: downregulation by inhaled corticosteroids. Clin Exp Allergy 1996; 26:517–524.
80. Holt PG, Degebrodt A, O'Leary C, Krska K, Plozza T. T cell activation by antigen-presenting cells from lung tissue digests: suppression by endogenous macrophages. Clin Exp Immunol 1985; 62:586–593.
81. Poston RN, Chanez P, Lacoste JY, Litchfield T, Lee TH, Bousquet J. Immunohistochemical characterization of the cellular infiltration in asthmatic bronchi. Am Rev Respir Dis 1992; 145:918–921.
82. Wilson JW, Djukanović R, Howarth PH, Holgate ST. Lymphocyte activation in bronchoalveolar lavage and peripheral blood in atopic asthma. Am Rev Respir Dis 1992; 145:958–960.
83. Robinson DS, Hamid Q, Bentley AM, Ying S, Kay AB, Durham SR. Activation of CD4+ T cells, increased Th2-type cytokine mRNA expression, and eosinophil recruitment in bronchoalveolar lavage after allergen inhalation challenge in patients with atopic asthma. J Allergy Clin Immunol 1993; 92:313–324.
84. Cruikshank WW, Long A, Tarpy RE, Kornfield H, Carroll MP, Teran L, Holgate

ST, Center DM. Early identification of interleukin-16 (lymphocyte chemoattractant factor) and macrophage inflammatory protein 1α (MIP1α) in bronchoalveolar lavage fluid of antigen-challenged asthmatics. Am J Respir Cell Mol Biol 1995; 13: 738–747.

85. Hidi R, Riches V, Djukanović R. Allergen-induced T cell chemotactic activity due to interleukin-16 and RANTES: role of B7-CD28/CTLA-4 costimulation and nuclear transcription factor NFκB (abstr). Eur Respir J 1998; 12:159s.
86. Laberge S, Ernst P, Ghaffar O, Cruikshank WW, Kornfield H, Center DM, Hamid Q. Increased expression of interleukin-16 in bronchial mucosa of subjects with atopic asthma. Am J Respir Cell Mol Biol 1993; 17:193–202.
87. Laberge S, Cruikshank WW, Kornfeld H, Center DM. Histamine-induced secretion of lymphocyte chemoattractant factor from $CD8^+$ T cells is independent of transcription and translation: Evidence for constitutive protein synthesis and storage. J Immunol 1995; 155:2902–2910.
88. Conlon K, Osborne J, Morimoto C, Ortaldo JR, Young HA. Comparison of lymphokine secretion and mRNA expression in the $CD45RA^+$ and $CD45RO^+$ subsets of human peripheral blood $CD4^+$ and $CD8^+$ lymphocytes. Eur J Immunol 1995; 25: 644–648.
89. Conlon K, Lloyd A, Chattopadhyay U, Lukacs N, Kunkel S, Schall T, Taub D, Morimoto C, Osborne J, Oppenheim J, Young H, Kelvin D, Ortaldo J. $CD8^+$ and $CD45RA^+$ human peripheral blood lymphocytes are potent sources of macrophage inflammatory protein 1α, interleukin-8 and RANTES. Eur J Immunol 1995; 25: 751–756.
90. Salgame P, Abrams JS, Clayberger C, Goldstein H, Convit J, Modlin RL, Bloom BR. Differing lymphokine profiles of functional subsets of human CD4 and CD8 T cell clones. Science 1991; 254:279–282.
91. Erard F, Wild M, Garcia-Sanz J, Le Gros G. Switch of CD8 T cells to noncytolytic CD8-CD4- cells that make Th2 cytokines and help B cells. Science 1993; 260: 1802–1805.
92. Croft M, Carter L, Swain SL, Dutton RW. Generation of polarized antigen-specific CD8 effector populations: reciprocal action of interleukin (IL)-4 and IL-12 in promoting type 2 versus type 1 cytokine profiles. J Exp Med 1994; 180:1715–1728.
93. Kemeny DM, Noble A, Holmes BJ, Diaz-Sanchez D. Immune regulation: a new role for the $CD8^+$ T cells. Immunol Today 1994; 15:107–110.
94. Maggi E, Giudizi MG, Biagiotti R, Annunziato F, Manetti R, Piccinni MP, Parronchi P, Sampognaro S, Giannarini L, Zuccati G, Romagnani S. Th2-like $CD8^+$ T cells showing B cell helper function and reduced cytolytic activity in human immunodeficiency virus type 1 infection. J Exp Med 1994; 180:489–495.
95. Stanciu LA, Shute J, Promwong C, Holgate ST, Djukanović R. Increased levels of IL-4 in $CD8^+$ T cells in atopic asthma. J Allergy Clin Immunol 1997; 100:373–378.
96. Coyle AJ, Erard F, Bertrand C, Walti S, Pircher H, le Gros G. Virus-specific $CD8^+$ cells can switch to interleukin 5 production and induce airway eosinophilia. J Exp Med 1995; 181:1229–1233.
97. Faul JL, Tormey VJ, Leonard C, Burke CM, Farmer J, Horne SJ, Poulter LW.

Lung immunopathology in cases of sudden asthma death. Eur Respir J 1997; 10: 301–307.

98. Vrugt B, Djukanović R, Bron A, Aalbers R. New insights into the pathogenesis of severe corticosteroid-dependent asthma. J Allergy Clin Immunol 1996; 98:S22–S26.
99. Wenzel SE, Szefler SJ, Leung DYM, Sloan SI, Rex MD, Martin RJ. Bronchoscopic evaluation of severe asthma: persistent inflammation associated with high dose glucocorticoids. Am J Respir Crit Care Med 1997; 156:737–743.
100. Aas K. Heterogeneity of bronchial asthma: sub-populations or different stages of the disease. Allergy 1981; 36:3–14.
101. Fujimoto K, Kubo K, Matsuzawa Y, Sekiguchi M. Eosinophil cationic protein levels in induced sputum correlate with the severity of bronchial asthma. Chest 1997; 112:1241–1247.
102. Minshall EM, Leung DYM, Martin RJ, Song YL, Cameron L, Ernst P, Hamid Q. Eosinophil-associated TGF-β_1 mRNA expression and airways fibrosis in bronchial asthma. Am J Respir Cell Mol Biol 1997; 17:326–333.
103. Mackay TW, Wallace WAH, Howie SEM, Brown PH, Greening AP, Church MK, Douglas JJ. Role of inflammation in nocturnal asthma. Thorax 1994; 49:257–262.
104. Kraft M, Djukanović R, Wilson S, Holgate ST, Martin RJ. Alveolar tissue inflammation in asthma. Am J Respir Crit Care Med 1996; 154:1505–1510.
105. Turner M, Hussack P, Sears M, Dolovich J, Hargreave FE. Exacerbations of asthma without sputum eosinophilia. Thorax 1995; 50:1057–1061.
106. Sur S, Crotty TB, Kephart GM, Hyma BA, Colby TV, Reed CE, Hunt LW, Gleich GJ. Sudden-onset fatal asthma—a distinct entity with few eosinophils and relatively more neutrophils in the airway submucosa? Am J Respir Crit Care Med 1993; 148:713–719.
107. Shute JK, Vrugt B, Lindley IJD, Holgate ST, Bron A, Aalbers R, Djukanović R. Free and complexed interleukin-8 in blood and bronchial mucosa in asthma. Am J Respir Crit Care Med 1997; 155:1877–1883.
108. Louis R, Holgate ST, Djukanović R. Induced sputum in asthma: comparison of asymptomatic vs symptomatic and steroid naive vs steroid treated patients (abstr). Eur Respir J 1996; 9:13.
109. Chanez P, Paradis L, Vignola AM, Vachier L, Vic P, Godard P, Bousquet J. Changes in bronchial inflammation of steroid (GCs) dependent asthmatics. Am J Respir Crit Care Med 1996; 153:212.
110. Cox G. Glucocorticoid treatment inhibits apoptosis in human neutrophils. J Immunol 1995; 154:4719–4725.
111. Schleimer RP, Freeland HS, Peters SP, Brown KE, Derse CP. An assessment of the effects of glucocorticoids on degranulation, chemotaxis, binding to vascular endothelium and formation of leukotriene B_4 by purified human neutrophils. J Pharmacol Exp Ther 1989; 250:598–605.
112. Kerstjens HAM, Brand PLP, Hughes MD, Robinson NJ, Postma DS, Sluiter HJ, Bleecker ER, Dekhuijzen PNR, Dejong PM, Mengelers HJJ, Overbeek SE, Schoonbrood DFME. A comparison of bronchodilator therapy with or without inhaled corticosteroid therapy for obstructive airways disease. N Engl J Med 1992; 327: 1413–1419.

113. Djukanović R, Homeyard S, Gratziou C, Madden J, Walls AF, Montefort S, Peroni D, Polosa R, Holgate ST, Howarth PH. The effect of treatment with oral corticosteroids on asthma symptoms and airways inflammation. Am J Respir Crit Care Med 1997; 155:826–832.
114. Wilson JW, Djukanović R, Howarth PH, Holgate ST. Inhaled beclomethasone dipropionate down-regulates airway lymphocyte activation in atopic asthma. Am J Respir Crit Care Med 1994; 149:86–90.
115. Djukanović R, Wilson JW, Britten KM, Wilson SJ, Walls AF, Roche WR, Howarth PH, Holgate ST. Effect of an inhaled corticosteroid on airway inflammation and symptoms in asthma. Am Rev Respir Dis 1992; 145:669–674.
116. Trigg CJ, Manolitsas ND, Wang J, Calderon MA, McAulay A, Jordan SE, Herdman MJ, Jhall N, Duddle JM, Hamilton SA, Devalia JL, Davies RJ. Placebo-controlled immunopathologic study of four months of inhaled corticosteroids in asthma. Am J Respir Crit Care Med 1994; 150:17–22.
117. Robinson DS, Hamid Q, Ying S, Bentley AM, Assoufi B, Durham SR, Kay AB. Prednisolone treatment in asthma is associated with modulation of bronchoalveolar lavage cell interleukin-4, interleukin-5 and interferon-γ cytokine gene expression. Am Rev Respir Dis 1993; 148:401–406.
118. Schleimer RP. Effects of corticosteroids on inflammatory cells relevant to their therapeutic applications in asthma. Am Rev Respir Dis 1990; 141:S59–S69.
119. Corrigan CJ, Brown PH, Barnes NC, Tsai J-J, Frew AJ, Kay AB. Glucocorticoid resistance in chronic asthma: Peripheral blood T lymphocyte activation and comparison of the T lymphocyte inhibitory effects of glucocorticoids and cyclosporin A. Am Rev Respir Dis 1991; 144:1026–1032.
120. Corrigan CJ, Brown PH, Barnes NC, Szefler SJ, Tsai J-J, Frew AJ, Kay AB. Glucocorticoid resistance in chronic asthma: glucocorticoid pharmacokinetics, glucocorticoid receptor characteristics and inhibition of peripheral blood T cell proliferation by glucocorticoids in vitro. Am Rev Respir Dis 1991; 144:1016–1025.
121. Leung DYM, Martin RJ, Szefler SJ, Sher ER, Ying S, Kay AB, Hamid Q. Dysregulation of interleukin-4, interleukin-5, and interferon-γ gene expression in steroid-resistant asthma. J Exp Med 1995; 181:33–40.
122. Alexander AG, Barkans J, Moqbel R, Barnes NC, Kay AB, Corrigan CJ. Serum interleukin 5 concentrations in atopic and not-atopic patients with glucocorticoid-dependent asthma. Thorax 1994; 49:1231–1233.
123. Messer JW, Peters GA, Bennett WA. Causes of death and pathologic findings in 304 cases of bronchial asthma. Dis Chest 1960; 38:616–624.
124. Reid LM. The presence or absence of bronchial mucus in fatal asthma. J Allergy Clin Immunol 1987; 80:415–416.
125. Saetta M, di Stefano A, Rosina C, Thiene G, Fabbri LM. Quantitative structural analysis of peripheral airways and arteries in sudden fatal asthma. Am Rev Respir Dis 1991; 143:138–143.
126. Montefort S, Djukanović R, Holgate ST, Roche WR. Ciliated cell damage in the bronchial epithelium of asthmatics and non-asthmatics. Clin Exp Allergy 1993; 23: 185–189.
127. Montefort S, Roberts JA, Beasley R, Holgate ST, Roche WR. The site of disruption

of the bronchial epithelium in asthmatic and non-asthmatic subjects. Thorax 1992; 47:499–503.

128. Holloway L, Beasley R, Roche WR. The pathology of fatal asthma. In: Busse WW, Holgate ST, eds. Asthma and Rhinitis. Boston: Blackwell, 1995:109–117.
129. Vanhoutte PM. Epithelium-derived relaxing factor(s) and bronchial reactivity. J Allergy Clin Immunol 1989; 83:855–861.
130. Synek M, Beasley R, Frew AJ, Goulding D, Holloway L, Lampe FC, Roche WR, Holgate ST. Cellular infiltration of the airways in asthma of varying severity. Am J Respir Crit Care Med 1996; 154:224–230.
131. Heard BE, Nunn AJ, Kay AB. Mast cells in human lungs. J Pathol 1989; 157:59–63.
132. Forstner JF, Jabbal I, Findlay GG. Interaction of mucins with calcium, H^+ ion and albumin. Mod Probl Paedatr 1977; 19:54–65.
133. List SJ, Findlay BP, Forstner GG, Forstner JF. Enhancement of the viscosity of mucin by serum albumin. Biochem J 1978; 175:565–571.
134. Dunnill MS, Massarella GR, Anderson GA. A comparison of the quantitative anatomy of the bronchi in normal subjects, in status asthmaticus, in chronic bronchitis, and in emphysema. Thorax 1989; 24:175–179.
135. Bousquet J, Vignola AM, Chanez P, Campbell AM, Bonsignore GB, Michel FB. Airways remodelling in asthma: no doubt, no more? Int Arch Allergy Immunol 1995; 107:211–214.
136. Laitinen LA, Heino M, Laitinen A, Kava T, Haahtela T. Damage of the airway epithelium and bronchial reactivity in patients with asthma. Am Rev Respir Dis 1985; 131:599–606.
137. Jeffery PK, Wardlaw AJ, Nelson FC, Collins JC, Kay AB. Bronchial biopsies in asthma: an ultrastructural, quantitative study and correlation with hyperreactivity. Am Rev Respir Dis 1989; 140:1745–1753.
138. Naylor B. The shedding of the mucosa of the bronchial tree in asthma. Thorax 1962; 17:69–72.
139. Redington AE, Polosa R, Walls AF, Howarth PH, Holgate ST. Role of mast-cells and basophils in asthma. Chem Immunol 1995; 61:22–59.
140. Lackie PM, Baker JE, Günthert U, Holgate ST. Expression of CD44 isoforms is increased in the airway epithelium of asthmatic subjects. Am J Respir Cell Mol Biol 1997; 16:14–22.
141. Peroni DG, Djukanović R, Bradding P, Feather IH, Montefort S, Howarth PH, Jones DB, Holgate ST. Expression of CD44 and integrins in bronchial mucosa of normal and mildly asthmatic subjects. Eur Respir J 1996; 9:2236–2242.
142. Manolitsas ND, Trigg CJ, McAulay AE, Wang JH, Jordan SE, Dardenne AJ, Davies RJ. The expression of intracellular-adhesion molecule-1 and the beta-1 integrins in asthma. Eur Respir J 1994; 7:1439–1444.
143. Huang X-Z, Wu JF, Cass D, Erle DJ, Corry D, Young SG, Farese RV, Sheppard D. Inactivation of the integrin β_6 subunit gene reveals a role of epithelial integrins in regulating inflammation in the lung and skin. J Cell Biol 1996; 133:921–928.
144. Frossard N, Rhoden KJ, Barnes PJ. Influence of epithelium on guinea pig airway

responses to tachykinins: role of endopeptidase and cyclooxygenase. J Pharmacol Exp Ther 1989; 144:292–298.
145. Lindsay G, Diamond L, Thompson DC, Cibulsky SM, Altiere RJ. Nitric oxide. Role as a relaxant agonist and transmitter of nonadrenergic noncholinergic inhibitory nerves in guinea pig trachea (abstr). Chest 1995; 107:125.
146. Holgate ST. Asthma: a dynamic disease of inflammation and repair. In: The Rising Trends of Asthma (Ciba Foundation Symposium 206). Chichester, UK: Wiley, 1997:5–34.
147. Roche WR, Beasley R, Williams JH, Holgate ST. Subepithelial fibrosis in the bronchi of asthmatics. Lancet 1989; 1:520–524.
148. Brewster CE, Howarth PH, Djukanović R, Wilson JW, Holgate ST, Roche WR. Myofibroblasts and subepithelial fibrosis in bronchial asthma. Am J Respir Cell Mol Biol 1990; 3:507–511.
149. Wilson JW, Li X. The measurement of subepithelial and submucosal collagen in the asthmatic airways. Clin Exp Allergy 1997; 27:363–371.
150. Redington AE, Madden J, Frew AJ, Djukanović R, Roche WR, Holgate ST, Howarth PH. Transforming growth factor-β1 in asthma: measurement in bronchoalveolar lavage fluid. Am J Respir Crit Care Med 1997; 156:642–647.
151. Redington AE, Springall DR, Ghatei MA, Holgate ST, Polak JM, Howarth PH. Endothelin in bronchoalveolar lavage fluid and its relation to airflow obstruction in asthma. Am J Respir Crit Care Med 1995; 151:1034–1039.
152. Redington AE, Howarth PH. Airway wall remodelling in asthma. Thorax 1997; 52:310–312.
153. Postlethwaite AE, Holness MA, Katai H, Raghow R. Human fibroblasts synthesize elevated levels of extracellular matrix proteins in response to interleukin 4. J Clin Invest 1992; 90:1479–1485.
154. Raines EW, Bowen-Page DF, Ross R. Platelet-derived growth factor. In: Sporn MB, Roberts, AB, eds. Handbook of Experimental Pharmacology: Peptide Growth Factors and Their Receptors. Heidelberg: Springer-Verlag, 1990:173–262.
155. Ruoss SJ, Hartmann R, Caughey GH. Mast cell tryptase is a mitogen for cultured fibroblasts. J Clin Invest 1991; 88:493–499.
156. Springall DR, Howarth P, Counihan H, Djukanović R, Holgate ST, Polak JM. Endothelin immunoreactivity of airway epithelium in asthmatic patients. Lancet 1991; 337:697–701.
157. Vilcek J, Palombella VJ, Henrikson-DeStefano D, Swenson C, Feinman R, Hirai M, Tsujimoto M. Fibroblast growth enhancing activity of tumour necrosis factor and its relationship to other polypeptide growth factors. J Exp Med 1986; 163:632–643.
158. Altraja A, Laitinen A, Virtanen I, Kämpe M, Simonsson BG, Karlsson S-E, Håkansson P, Venge P, Sillastu H, Laitinen LA. Expression of laminins in the airways in various types of asthmatic patients: a morphometric study. Am J Respir Cell Mol Biol 1996; 15:482–488.
159. Bousquet J, Lacoste J-Y, Chanez P, Vic P, Godard P, Michel F-B. Bronchial elastic fibers in normal subjects and asthmatic patients. Am J Respir Dis 1996; 153:1646–1654.
160. Godfrey R, Lorimer S, Majumdar S, Adelroth E, Johansson S, Jeffery P. Airway

and lung parenchymal content of elastic fiber is not reduced in asthma (abstr). Am Rev Respir Dis 1992; 145:463.
161. Rodriguez R, White R, Senior R, Levine E. Elastase release from human alveolar macrophages: comparison between smokers and nonsmokers. Science 1977; 198: 313–314.
162. Senior RM, Connolly NL, Cury JD, Welgus HG, Campbell EJ. Elastin degradation by human alveolar macrophages: A prominent role of metalloproteinase activity. Am Rev Respir Dis 1989; 139:1251–1256.
163. Lungarella G, Menegazzi R, Gardi C, Spessotto P, de-Santi MM, Bertoncin P, Patriarca P, Calzoni P, Zabucchi G. Identification of elastase in human eosinophils: immunolocalization, isolation, and partial characterization. Arch Biochem Biophys 1002; 292:128–135.
164. Shapiro S, Kobayashi DK, Ley TJ. Cloning and characterization of a unique elastolytic metalloproteinase produced by human macrophages. J Biol Chem 1993; 268: 23824–23829.
165. Kahari VM. Dexamethasone suppresses elastin gene expression in human skin fibroblasts in culture. Biochem Biophys Res Commun 1994; 201:1189–1196.
166. Wilson JW, Li X, Pain MC. The lack of distensibility of asthmatic airways. Am Rev Respir Dis 1993; 148:806–809.
167. McCarthy DS, Sigurdson M. Lung elastic recoil and reduced airflow in clinically stable asthma. Thorax 1980; 35:298–302.
168. Huber HL, Koessler KK. The pathology of bronchial asthma. Arch Intern Med 1922; 30:689–760.
169. Heard BE, Hossain S. Hyperplasia of bronchial smooth muscle in asthma. J Pathol 1972; 110:319–321.
170. Takizawa T, Thurlbeck WM. Muscle and mucous gland size in the major bronchi of patients with chronic bronchitis, asthma, and asthmatic bronchitis. Am Rev Respir Dis 1971; 104:331–336.
171. Li X, Wilson JW. Increased vascularity of the bronchial mucosa in mild asthma. Am J Respir Crit Care Med 1997; 156:229–233.
172. Lynch DA, Newell JD, Tschomper BA, Cink TM, Newman LS, Bethal R. Uncomplicated asthma in adults: comparison of CT appearances of the lungs in asthmatic and healthy subjects. Radiology 1993; 188:829–833.
173. Paganin F, Séneterre E, Chanez P, Daurés JP, Bruel JM, Michel FB, Bousquet J. Computed tomography of the lungs in asthma: influence of disease severity and etiology. Am J Respir Crit Care Med 1996; 153:110–114.
174. Boulet L-P, Bélanger M, Carrier G. Airway hyperresponsiveness and bronchial wall thickness in asthma with or without fixed airflow obstruction. Am J Respir Crit Care Med 1995; 152:865–871.
175. Schachter EN, Dlyle CA, Beck GJ. A prospective study of asthma in a rural community. Chest 1984; 85:623–630.
176. Peat JK, Woolcock AJ, Cullen K. Rate of decline of lung function in subjects with asthma. Eur J Respir Dis 1987; 70:171–179.
177. Ulrik CS, Lange P. Decline of lung function in adults with bronchial asthma. Am J Respir Crit Care Med 1994; 150:629–634.
178. Laitinen LA, Laitinen A, Haahtela T. A comparative study of the effects of an

inhaled corticosteroid, budesonide, and a β_2-agonist, terbutaline, on airway inflammation in newly diagnosed asthma: a randomized double-blind, parallel-group controlled trial. J Allergy Clin Immunol 1992; 90:32–42.
179. Haahtela T. Airway remodelling takes place in asthma—what are the clinical implications? Clin Exp Allergy 1997; 27:351–353.

4

Muscarinic Receptor Subtypes and Anticholinergic Therapy

ALLISON D. FRYER and DAVID B. JACOBY

Johns Hopkins University
Baltimore, Maryland

RICHARD W. COSTELLO

University of Liverpool
Liverpool, England

I. Introduction

The parasympathetic nerves provide the dominant autonomic control of airway smooth muscle. These nerves release acetylcholine onto muscarinic receptors on the airway smooth muscle and glands, stimulating bronchoconstriction and hypersecretion, respectively. The earliest treatments for asthma were anticholinergic drugs, demonstrating that airway hyperreactivity was originally thought to result from some abnormality of the cholinergic, parasympathetic control of the airways. However, in the 1970s, the cholinergic hypothesis of asthma was largely discarded, since a series of clinical trials had not been able to demonstrate that anticholinergic drugs were very effective bronchodilators. Finally, with the introduction of corticosteroids, which were effective in asthma, the focus of research into mechanisms of airway hyperreactivity switched from studying the parasympathetic nerves to studying the role of inflammation in asthma.

However, the cholinergic hypothesis of asthma may have been discarded prematurely. This chapter reviews the parasympathetic control of the airways and the distribution of muscarinic receptor subtypes within the lungs. The evidence for increased parasympathetic drive to the lungs of asthmatics is evaluated and the clinical trials with anticholinergics are assessed. The role of beneficial muscarinic receptors is described, as is the effect of inflammatory cells upon the function of these muscarinic receptors. Finally, the treatment of airway disease with anticholinergic drugs, including the newer, selective anticholinergics, and the potential of anti-inflammatory drugs to alter muscarinic receptor expression and function is discussed.

II. General Overview of Muscarinic Receptor Subtypes

In 1914, Sir Henry Dale divided receptors for acetylcholine into 2 families on the basis of whether they could be stimulated by nicotine or by muscarine. Although acetylcholine stimulated receptors in both skeletal and smooth muscle, receptors in the skeletal muscle responded only to nicotine while the receptors in smooth muscle responded only to muscarine. Atropine blocked only the effects of muscarine. Dale subsequently coined the names *muscarinic* and *nicotinic* receptors to describe these cholinoreceptors (1).

Although muscarinic receptors were not formally divided into subtypes until 1980, evidence for the presence of subtypes had been in the literature for 30 years. A neuromuscular blocking drug, gallamine (Flaxedil®), was reported to induce substantial tachycardia in patients. It was subsequently demonstrated that gallamine-induced tachycardia arose from selective blockade of muscarinic receptors in the heart (gallamine eventually fell out of clinical use because of this side effect). Gallamine did not block muscarinic receptors in smooth muscle (2). Additional, selective antagonists for the cardiac muscarinic receptors versus other muscarinic receptors were later reported (3). Official recognition of the existence of muscarinic receptor subtypes, however, did not come until 1980, with the development of the selective muscarinic receptor antagonist pirenzepine. Muscarinic receptors with a high affinity for pirenzepine (in the cerebral cortex) were termed *M_1 receptors*, while all other muscarinic receptors, including those in the heart, glands and smooth muscle were termed *M_2 receptors* (4). This classification did not, however, take into account the earlier data demonstrating that cardiac muscarinic receptors were different from muscarinic receptors in smooth muscle and glands. Eventually, as additional, selective antagonists were introduced, the M_2 receptors were further divided into additional subtypes (M_2–M_4).

Muscarinic receptors have now been classified into five subtypes, and atropine blocks all five with equal affinity. Five muscarinic receptor genes, termed m_1–m_5, have now been cloned and the proteins isolated. However, only four muscarinic receptors (M_1–M_4) can be distinguished pharmacologically using selective antagonists (5). At this time, selective agonists are not available to characterize muscarinic receptor subtypes. M_1 receptors are located in the central nervous system, autonomic ganglia, and in some peripheral organs and are selectively blocked by pirenzepine. M_2 receptors are located in the heart, smooth muscle, central nervous system, and autonomic nerves and are selectively blocked by gallamine and methoctramine. M_3 receptors are present in glands and smooth muscle and are selectively blocked by darifenacin. There are some functional data suggesting that M_3 receptors may eventually be further divided into additional subclasses (5). Classification of M_4 receptors is still difficult due to a lack of more selective antagonists. With the exceptions of himbacine and para-fluoro-hexahydrosiladifenidol, which have a higher affinity for the M_4 than for the M_2 receptors, M_4 receptors share many of the same affinities for selective antagonists as M_2 receptors.

This chapter focuses on M_1, M_2, and M_3, since these three muscarinic receptors predominate in the lungs. Although muscarinic receptors in the lungs are generally supplied by the parasympathetic nerves, some muscarinic receptors are present in the absence of any detectable nerve supply, and it may be that these receptors are either stimulated by nonneuronal acetylcholine (see below) or are constitutively active even in the absence of acetylcholine. At this point, however, the physiological function of these noninnervated receptors is unknown.

III. Parasympathetic Control of Airways

In the absence of any sympathetic nerve supply to the airway smooth muscle, the autonomic control of the airways is provided by the parasympathetic nerves. Electrical stimulation of these nerves results in bronchoconstriction. At rest, airway tone is also controlled by these nerves, since either sectioning or pharmacological blockade of the parasympathetic nerves results in bronchodilation in animals and in humans (6). Reflex bronchoconstriction, initiated either centrally or locally, is also mediated via the parasympathetic nerves (7).

A. Distribution of Parasympathetic Nerves in the Lungs

The cell bodies of the parasympathetic nerves that supply the lungs are located in the medulla. The axons travel in the vagus nerves (the tenth cranial nerves) to the lungs and other peripheral organs. The parasympathetic nerves supplying the trachea loop up from the vagi in the recurrent laryngeal and the pararecurrent laryngeal nerves. Other branches of the vagi enter the lungs and synapse with the postganglionic nerves in the bronchial smooth muscle. The cell bodies of the postganglionic nerves lie in clusters of cells in two parallel chains along the smooth muscle in the trachea (8). Some of these ganglia are very small, made up of only two cell bodies. The postganglionic fibers from these cell bodies release acetylcholine and directly supply the airway smooth muscle and glands.

The cholinergic innervation of the lungs is increased at points of branching of the bronchi, with the hilus being the site of the densest collection of ganglia. From the hilus down, the ganglia decrease in density, as do the numbers of postganglionic fibers and of muscarinic receptors. Although in most species there are muscarinic receptors in the peripheral lungs (9–12), cholinergic nerves have not been demonstrated below the terminal bronchi, and functional studies cannot demonstrate an effect of stimulation of the vagus nerves on the respiratory bronchioles and alveoli.

B. Distribution of Muscarinic Receptors in the Lungs

The lungs express predominantly M_1, M_2, and M_3 receptors. The distribution of muscarinic receptors within the lungs has been quantified using radioligand binding to slide-mounted tissue sections. Within the trachea and bronchi, muscarinic receptors have been localized to the smooth muscle, submucosal glands, epithelium, and parasympathetic nerves. Functional and pharmacological studies have identified which subtypes of receptors are present in these tissues and are responsible for the various functions of the lungs (Fig. 1).

Muscarinic Receptors on Airway Epithelial Cells

Although there are muscarinic receptors on the epithelium, the parasympathetic nerves do not supply the airway epithelial cells. However, acetylcholine is present in airway epithelial cells, as is the enzyme choline α-acetyl-transferase (13); thus

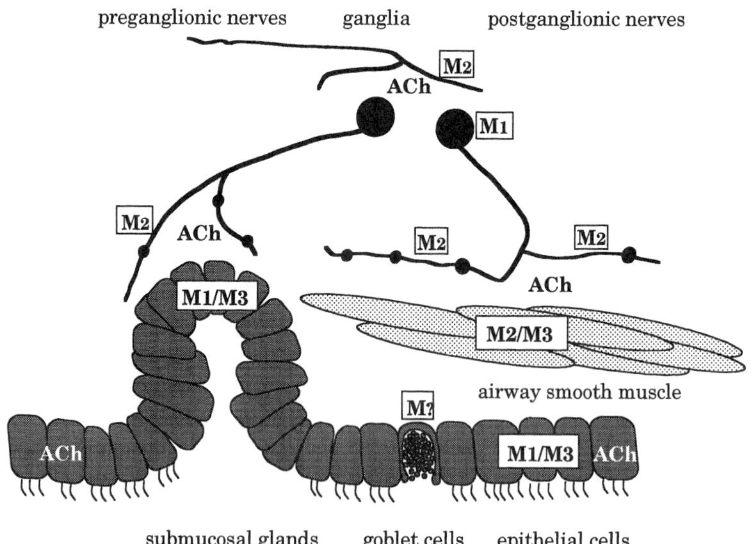

Figure 1 Location of muscarinic receptor subtypes in the lungs.

acetylcholine may serve as an autocoid in the epithelium. Nothing is known about the mechanisms of acetylcholine storage in or release from the epithelial cells. The possibility exists that it is local nonneuronal acetylcholine rather than neuronal acetylcholine that may influence the epithelium.

In the trachea and lungs, the presence of muscarinic receptors on the epithelium is regional and species-specific. The airway epithelium secretes chloride and absorbs sodium. Both of these processes may induce passive movement of water and are therefore determinants of the volume and character of airway secretions. Acetylcholine stimulates chloride secretion (and also, presumably, water secretion) in the trachea of dogs (14,15) but not of rabbits (16), and this effect is blocked by atropine. Whether the airway epithelium responds to endogenous cholinergic stimulation is not known. Muscarinic receptors have not yet been demonstrated in human tracheal epithelium.

Airway secretions are moved up the airway by the movement of cilia on the epithelial cells. Muscarinic agonists increase ciliary beat frequency (17) via stimulation of M_1 and M_3 receptors in epithelial cell explants from human nose (18,19) and by stimulation of M_3 receptors in epithelial cell explants from pig trachea (20). Mucociliary clearance is decreased by atropine but not by ipratropium (21); the clinical significance of this is not known.

In human bronchial epithelium, mRNA for M_3 receptors has been detected (22), but autoradiography has not confirmed the presence of muscarinic receptors on human airway epithelium, suggesting either that they are not expressed, or that there is a high rate of turnover of the protein (11,23). In guinea pig, the tracheal epithelium is also devoid of muscarinic receptors, while the bronchial epithelium expresses M_3 receptors (11). In ferrets, both tracheal and bronchial epithelium has muscarinic receptors (10). Thus, the presence of muscarinic receptors in epithelial cells varies with airway generation and with species.

Muscarinic Receptors on Glands in the Lungs

There is a dense population of muscarinic receptors in the airway glands (10,11,23), and these glands are cholinergically innervated (24,25). Stimulation of parasympathetic nerves or administration of cholinergic agents causes mucus secretion via stimulation of muscarinic receptors (26–28). Mechanical stimulation of the airway also results in gland secretion, which is a reflex mediated via the parasympathetic nerves (29,30). Atropine inhibits reflex-induced secretion (29).

There is fairly good agreement across a variety of species, including humans, that both M_1 and M_3 receptors are present in the mucosal glands (11,28,31,32). However, functional studies carried out in feline, ferret, and human isolated tissues have demonstrated that it is the M_3 receptors that mediate mucus secretion (28,32,33).

In the lungs, it has been demonstrated that release of acetylcholine from the parasympathetic nerves supplying the glands is inhibited by neuronal M_2 receptors (32). Since neuronal M_2 receptors on the nerves supplying the airway smooth muscle are dysfunctional in animal models of hyperreactivity and in asthma (see below), they may also be dysfunctional on the nerves supplying the glands, increasing acetylcholine release and thus increasing mucus secretion. This may be relevant, since chronic cholinergic stimulation can cause glandular hypertrophy (34,35), as is seen in asthma and chronic bronchitis.

Mucus secretion from goblet cells is also mediated by the cholinergic nerves. Electrical stimulation of the vagus nerves induces mucus secretion from the goblet cells in anesthetized guinea pigs, and this effect is blocked by atropine (28). Muscarinic agonists also increase mucus secretion in cultured hamster goblet cells (36). The subtype of muscarinic receptor that mediates goblet cell secretion is not yet characterized.

The clinical significance of inhibition of gland secretion by muscarinic antagonists is uncertain. Treatment of patients with either chronic bronchitis or diffuse panbronchiolitis with the anticholinergic medication oxitropium decreased the volume of sputum volume by about one-third but increased the concentration of protein in the sputum by one-third (37). Thus, anticholinergic agents appear to inhibit water secretion. Whether the source of this water is the glands or the surface epithelium is not known. In addition, oxitropium is a nonselective antagonist and may have blocked several muscarinic receptor subtypes.

Muscarinic Receptors on Airway Smooth Muscle

Electrical stimulation of the vagus nerves releases acetylcholine onto muscarinic receptors on airway smooth muscle, causing immediate contraction of the muscle and bronchoconstriction. Both contraction and bronchoconstriction are dependent upon the strength of the stimulus and both are rapidly reversible with cessation of stimulation (38,39).

Acetylcholine induces bronchoconstriction by stimulating muscarinic receptors on smooth muscle within the trachea and bronchi. Muscarinic receptor density decreases with airway size. Within the airway smooth muscle, the greatest density is within the lower trachea, with significantly fewer muscarinic receptors in the bronchial smooth muscle (10,11). In most species there are muscarinic receptors in the parenchyma, but they are not supplied by cholinergic nerves and their function is not known (11,22). The alveoli of some species—for example, ferret and guinea pig—have no apparent muscarinic receptors (9–11,40).

There are two muscarinic receptor binding sites in the airway smooth muscle in all species studied. Since neither has a high affinity for pirenzepine, they are not of the M_1 subtype (41,42). Binding studies and Northern blot analysis have demonstrated that the airway smooth muscle expresses M_2 and M_3 receptors

(43–45). Although this was initially demonstrated in the cow by Roffel and colleagues (43,45), it has subsequently been confirmed in all species studied.

In most species, M_2 receptors predominate over the M_3 receptors in the upper airways by 70–90% (42,43,46–51), although the proportions are closer to equal in the guinea pig (52,53). However, the relative proportions of M_2 to M_3 receptors is not homogenous throughout the lungs. M_2 receptors outnumber M_3 receptors by 7.6:1 in the dog trachea, while in the bronchi this proportion has decreased to 1.5:1. In the parenchyma, there are M_3 receptors but no M_2 receptors at all, although there is also no smooth muscle (40).

There are few studies examining which muscarinic receptor subtypes are present in human airway smooth muscle, and there are no studies on the proportion of M_2/M_3 receptors in human tracheal smooth muscle. As in other animal species, it is known that the muscarinic receptors are not M_1 (54) and are presumed to be either M_2 or M_3 based on the presence of mRNA for these two subtypes in the lungs (22). As in all other species (see below), contraction of human airway smooth muscle is mediated by the M_3 receptors (55).

M_3 Muscarinic Receptors on Airway Smooth Muscle

Although it appears that both M_2 and M_3 receptors are present on the airway smooth muscle, functional studies in animals (45,53,56–61) and in humans (55) have demonstrated that smooth muscle contraction is mediated via the M_3 receptors. Thus, the receptor mediating contraction in airway smooth muscle is the same as that mediating contraction in ileal, uterine, and bladder smooth muscle (62).

It is believed that the M_3 receptors are coupled via pertussis toxin–insensitive GTP binding regulatory proteins (G proteins) to phospholipase C and the turnover of membrane phosphoinositides (63,64). Phospholipase C catalyzes the breakdown of the membrane phospholipid phosphatidylinositol 4,5-bisphosphate to inositol triphosphate and diacylglycerol, ultimately leading to phosphorylation of proteins via activation of protein kinases, increased release of intracellular Ca^{2+}, and bronchoconstriction (65–67). This muscarinic receptor–mediated pathway is initiated by stimulation of M_3 receptors on airway smooth muscle (63,64) and has been demonstrated in all species studied, including humans (67,68).

M_2 Muscarinic Receptors on Airway Smooth Muscle

Although the majority of muscarinic receptors on airway smooth muscle are M_2, the function of these receptors is not clear. Stimulation of M_2 receptors in airway smooth muscle leads to inhibition of adenylyl cyclase activity via inhibitory, pertussis-sensitive G proteins (Gi) (64,69,70). Thus, M_2 receptors on smooth muscle do not contribute directly to smooth muscle contraction but may inhibit relaxation by inhibiting β-adrenoceptor–mediated increases in adenylate cyclase (40,71).

Muscarinic Receptors in the Alveoli and Peripheral Lung

While the presence of muscarinic receptors has been reported in the alveoli, they are far less dense there than in other regions of the lungs (56). Both M_2 and M_3 receptor protein has been detected in rat peripheral lung (72,73) whereas in human parenchyma M_1 and M_3 receptors have been reported (22,56,74–76). However, it is unclear whether muscarinic receptors in the peripheral lung are associated with the airway muscle or with the vasculature. Although M_3 receptors in the peripheral lung mediate contraction (77) and increase cAMP (78), M_2 receptors mediate vasoconstriction while M_1 receptors mediate vasodilatation (79).

C. Autocontrol of Acetylcholine Release in the Airways

In 1984, Fryer and Maclagan first demonstrated that functional muscarinic receptors were present in the parasympathetic nerves supplying the lung (80). Muscarinic receptors have since been described in the autonomic nerves supplying the lungs of all species studied, including humans. Autoradiographic binding to tissue sections of bovine, guinea pig, and human lung as well as cultures of postganglionic, parasympathetic nerves from the trachea demonstrate dense labeling of muscarinic receptors in airway ganglia and nerve axons (11,23,81,82). Of these tissues, muscarinic receptors are most dense in the parasympathetic ganglia. In human lung, the parasympathetic ganglia contain three times the density of muscarinic receptors as the smooth muscle (10,11,23).

Muscarinic Receptors in Airway Ganglia and on Preganglionic Nerves

The greatest density of muscarinic receptors in the lungs is found in the parasympathetic ganglia. Neurotransmission through the ganglia is mediated by nicotinic receptors, which initiate a fast excitatory postsynaptic potential (fast epsp). However, ganglia modulate the frequency at which postganglionic nerves fire (83); thus the nicotinic fast epsp can be modulated by M_1 receptors, which initiate a slow excitatory postsynaptic potential (74,84–86), and by M_2 receptors, which can initiate a slow inhibitory postsynaptic potential (87,88).

In the lungs, excitatory M_1 receptors have been characterized in the parasympathetic ganglia in animals (84,86) and in humans (89). Blockade of the excitatory M_1 receptors with the selective antagonist pirenzepine inhibits parasympathetically mediated reflex bronchoconstriction at doses that do not inhibit methacholine induced-bronchoconstriction (89). Thus, these muscarinic receptors alter the ability of the postganglionic parasympathetic nerves to generate an action potential.

In addition to the ganglionic receptors, there are preganglionic receptors. M_2 receptors are located presynaptically and inhibit release of acetylcholine from the preganglionic nerves (90). These preganglionic M_2 receptors function in a manner similar to that of the prejunctional receptors on the postganglionic nerves (see below).

Muscarinic Receptors on Postganglionic Parasympathetic Nerves

M_2 receptors on postganglionic parasympathetic nerves inhibit release of acetylcholine from these nerves (Fig. 2) (80). Stimulation of these receptors with a muscarinic receptor agonist, such as pilocarpine, decreases release of acetylcholine from the vagus nerves and inhibits bronchoconstriction induced by electrical stimulation of the vagus nerves. Conversely, blockade of these neuronal M_2 receptors with gallamine potentiates vagally induced bronchoconstriction.

These inhibitory neuronal muscarinic receptors were initially classified as M_2 receptors on the basis of the selectivity of gallamine. It has been suggested that the inhibitory neuronal receptors are not identical to the M_2 receptors in the heart but are like either M_2 or M_4 (91). However, since only M_2 receptor RNA has been demonstrated in cultured parasympathetic nerves from the trachea (92), these neuronal receptors will be referred to as M_2 receptors. Neuronal M_2 receptors have now been described in the parasympathetic nerves supplying the lungs of all species studied thus far, including guinea pigs (80,86,93–95), cats (96,97), rats (98), mice (99), dogs (58,100), horses (101), rabbits (102), and humans (103).

The neuronal M_2 receptors function under physiological conditions and are critical to maintaining normal release of acetylcholine from the vagus nerves. In vivo, pharmacological blockade of these receptors increases vagally induced bronchoconstriction by 5–10 fold (500–1000%), while stimulation of the neu-

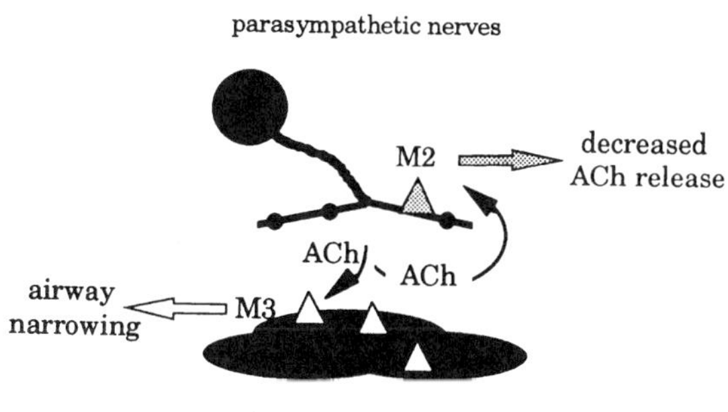

Figure 2 Neuronal M_2 receptors (shaded triangles) inhibit release of acetylcholine from the parasympathetic nerves. Contraction of airway smooth muscle is mediated by M_3 receptors (open triangles). While the function of the M_3 receptors is unchanged in animal models of hyperreactivity, the neuronal M_2 receptors are dysfunctional, leading to increased release of acetylcholine from the vagus nerves (see text).

ronal M_2 receptors with selective agonists inhibits vagally induced bronchoconstriction by 80% (80,91). In human bronchi contracted by electrical field stimulation, pilocarpine inhibits the contraction by 96%, demonstrating that the M_2 receptors also exert a marked degree of inhibition in human lung (103). These pharmacological studies have now been complemented by studies measuring acetylcholine released from the nerves in the presence of muscarinic agonists and antagonists (92,104).

The importance of these receptors can be seen when they are not functioning normally. Bronchoconstriction induced by electrical stimulation of the vagus nerves is increased 5-fold when the neuronal M_2 receptors are blocked with selective antagonists (92,104). Conversely, in certain conditions when the neuronal M_2 receptors are hyperfunctional, the bronchoconstriction induced by electrical stimulation of the vagus nerves is almost abolished (105).

IV. Dysfunction of M_2 Muscarinic Receptors on the Cholinergic Nerves

Sensitization to and challenge with an antigen increases release of acetylcholine from the vagus nerves and vagally induced bronchoconstriction in guinea pigs, dogs, mice, and rats (99,106–110). Likewise, vagally induced bronchoconstriction is also potentiated in dogs, rats, and guinea pigs exposed to ozone or acutely infected with influenza virus (111–121). As in human asthma, there was no evidence in any of these animal models that the M_3 receptors on airway smooth muscle were altered. Thus an important component of airway hyperresponsiveness is increased release of acetylcholine from the nerves. (For a complete review, see Ref. 122.)

In animals acutely infected with parainfluenza virus, exposed to ozone, or sensitized and challenged with antigen, the function of the neuronal M_2 receptors is impaired (109,119,120,123). Thus, in three different models of airway hyperreactivity, the function of the neuronal M_2 receptors is markedly decreased.

Airway hyperresponsiveness in all three of these models is associated with increased release of acetylcholine from the vagus nerves. Since the function of the M_3 receptors on airway smooth muscles, which are responsible for contraction, is not altered, increased acetylcholine release leads to enhanced bronchoconstriction. In addition, reflex bronchoconstriction, which can be triggered by both intravenous histamine or intravenous methacholine, is also potentiated in these models of airway hyperreactivity. Since these neuronal M_2 receptors are so important in controlling vagally induced bronchoconstriction, loss of function of the neuronal muscarinic receptors may be a mechanism for the increased release of acetylcholine from the vagus nerves that is seen in these animal models of airway hyperreactivity.

In the antigen-challenged guinea pigs, decreased function of the neuronal M_2 receptors is mediated by eosinophils. Following antigen challenge of guinea pigs, eosinophils are recruited to the airway nerves (124). If eosinophils are depleted with an antibody to interleukin-5 (125) or if migration is inhibited with an antibody to the adhesion molecule very late activation antigen (VLA)-4 prior to antigen challenge, the function of the M_2 receptors can be protected and antigen challenge–induced airway hyperreactivity prevented (126).

Eosinophils release eosinophil major basic protein, which is an antagonist for M_2 but not for M_3 receptors (127). Airway hyperreactivity in antigen-challenged guinea pigs can be acutely reversed if major basic protein is removed from the neuronal M_2 receptors in vivo by the administration of negatively charged compounds such as heparin, desulfated heparin, and poly-l-glutamate (128,129). Since M_2 receptor function can also be protected and hyperreactivity prevented with an antibody to eosinophil major basic protein (despite the presence of eosinophils in the lungs) (130), it is blockade of the neuronal M_2 receptors with major basic protein that causes airway hyperreactivity in antigen-challenged guinea pigs (Fig. 3). Our observation that eosinophils are recruited to the nerves, and that major basic protein is associated with the nerves in the airways of patients who died of severe asthma (124), underscores the potential importance of this mechanism.

In addition to major basic protein–mediated loss of neuronal M_2 receptor function, there are additional mechanisms for decreased function of neuronal M_2 receptors. Loss of receptor function in ozone-exposed animals is due to the presence of inflammatory cells (131), but it is not yet known whether eosinophils or some other inflammatory cell is responsible for decreased M_2 receptor function. In animals infected with parainfluenza virus, the virus itself may alter receptor

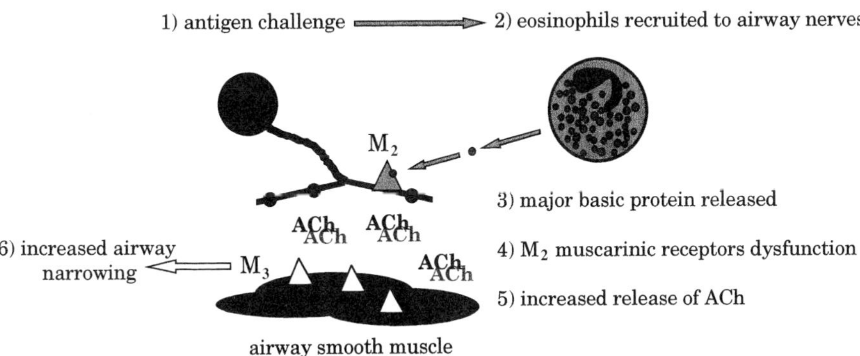

Figure 3 Mechanism of airway hyperreactivity in antigen-challenged guinea pigs.

function via the production of viral neuraminidase, which cleaves sialic acid from the receptor, thus reducing the affinity of acetylcholine for the M_2 receptors (132). In addition, viral infection of nerves in vitro decreases expression and function of the M_2 receptors. Finally, viruses also alter neuronal M_2 receptor function by recruitment or activation of some inflammatory cell that is not an eosinophil (133); thus other inflammatory cells have the means to inhibit neuronal M_2 receptor function.

In summary, M_2 receptor function is inhibited in animal models of asthma and in patients with asthma. Decreased M_2 receptor function is associated with increased vagally mediated bronchoconstriction, including reflex bronchoconstriction mediated via the vagus nerves. In antigen-sensitized and challenged guinea pigs, loss of M_2 receptor function is mediated by eosinophil major basic protein. However, there are additional mechanisms for loss of M_2 receptor function, and which mechanism is important in ozone-exposed and virus-infected animals is still not known. In patients with asthma, the function of the inhibitory neuronal M_2 receptors is also impaired (134,135). While mechanisms for loss of M_2 receptor function in human disease are not known, a role for eosinophils is suggested, since there is a significant increase in the number of eosinophils associated with the nerves in sections of human lung from patients who have died of asthma (124).

V. Role of Parasympathetic Nerves in Asthma

It was long assumed that asthma resulted from overactivity of the parasympathetic nerves; thus several studies have been carried out in which the vagi were surgically sectioned in asthmatics (136–138). Although all of these studies were uncontrolled, all reported some benefit to the majority of patients, with additional ''brilliant cures'' (136) or ''very good improvement'' (137) in some. The opposing argument for the importance of the vagi arises from lung transplants. It has been argued that since patients receiving lung transplants, which would necessitate sectioning the vagus nerves, from an asthmatic donor may develop asthma, the vagus is not required for the development of asthma (139). However, transplanted lungs can be reinnervated with preganglionic vagal fibers, as has been demonstrated in dogs (140). In addition, the postganglionic parasympathetic fibers are transplanted along with the lungs, and it is from these fibers that release of acetylcholine is thought to be increased (134,135).

One of the earliest herbal treatments for asthma was pharmacological blockade of the parasympathetic nerves with anticholinergic drugs such as stramonium from the *Datura* plant. Newer anticholinergic drugs, such as atropine and ipratropium, are also effective bronchodilators (122,141–147). The increased airway tone characteristic of asthma can be completely blocked by ipratropium bromide, demonstrating that it is vagally mediated (148).

A. Problems with Interpretation of Anticholinergic Efficacy

Cholinergic control of the airways is clearly abnormal in asthmatics (149,150). However, confusion surrounding the role of the vagus nerves in asthma has arisen for several reasons. First, the contribution of the vagus nerves to airway hyperresponsiveness varies with the type of provocation; second, the methods used to determine the role of the vagus have not always been adequate. Since it is not feasible either to stimulate the vagus nerves directly or to inhibit the vagus nerves by vagotomy, it is not possible to directly assess the role of the cholinergic nerves. Thus, vagal blockade can only be induced pharmacologically using muscarinic receptor antagonists. However, interpretation of these studies is complicated by the inability to test the degree of blockade achieved.

Since muscarinic receptor subtypes in the heart and lungs are different, it is not valid to infer blockade of muscarinic receptors in the lungs from inhibition of tachycardia in the heart. Likewise, innervation of the lungs and glands is also different; thus blockade of salivation may not reflect blockade of bronchoconstriction. Thus is it not necessarily valid to assume that blockade of cholinergic activity in one organ applies to another.

Many studies have tried to demonstrate adequate anticholinergic blockade by showing that they have blocked bronchoconstriction induced by inhaled acetylcholine (151–153). However, it was shown in dogs that this is not comparable. When inhaled, the dose of atropine required to block vagally induced bronchoconstriction is significantly greater than the dose of atropine required to block acetylcholine-induced bronchoconstriction (154). (However, it is notable that the same dose of atropine given intravenously blocks both acetylcholine and vagally induced bronchoconstriction.) Similarly, a much larger dose of inhaled atropine is required to block cold air–induced bronchoconstriction than to block methacholine-induced bronchoconstriction (155). Thus, pharmacological inhibition of the cholinergic nerves using inhaled anticholinergics, may not adequately block the receptors, and without dose-response curves or use of intravenous anticholinergics, which produce a more complete and uniform dilation than does inhaled atropine (156–157), it is difficult to draw any conclusions concerning the degree of pharmacological blockade of the vagus nerves in humans.

Further complicating the interpretation of studies with anticholinergic drugs is the fact that although the anticholinergics used are classified as nonselective and should block both the M_3 receptors, which mediate smooth muscle contraction, and the M_2 receptors, which inhibit the release of acetylcholine from the nerve endings, both atropine and ipratropium (at low doses) preferentially block M_2 receptors. Thus, at low doses, both atropine and ipratropium block the neuronal M_2 receptors, increasing acetylcholine release and potentially overcoming any postjunctional antagonism of M_3 receptors on airway smooth muscle. Perhaps more importantly, ipratropium can actually potentiate vagally induced bronchoconstriction by 100% at doses lower than those required to block the postjunctional M_3 receptor (Fig. 4) (158). This may explain why the dose of atropine required to block vagally induced bronchoconstriction is greater than the dose required to block acetylcholine-induced bronchoconstriction (94). Thus the effects of any nonselective antimuscarinic drugs will depend upon a balance between blockade of the inhibitory neuronal M_2 receptors and blockade of the postjunctional M_3 receptors.

In light of these studies, it has been important to develop selective M_3 receptor antagonists as the next generation of anticholinergic bronchodilators.

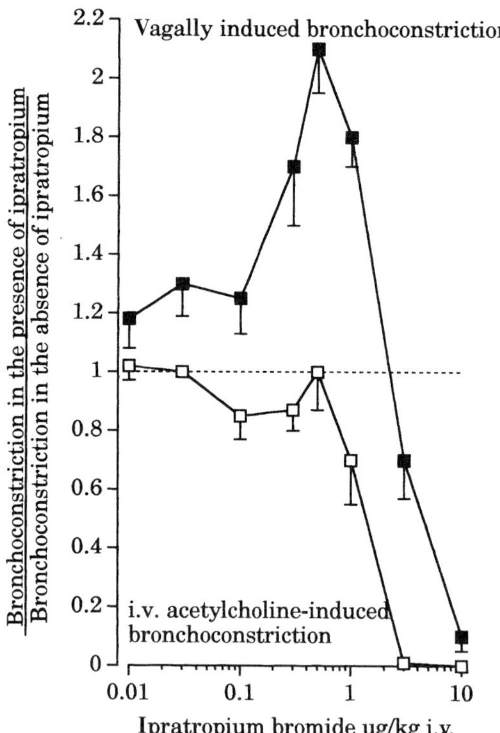

Figure 4 Ipratropium bromide binds to both M_2 receptors on the airway nerves, increasing vagally induced bronchoconstriction, and to M_3 receptors on the airway smooth muscle, decreasing the contractile response to acetylcholine in vagotomized guinea pigs. Note that doses of ipratropium that have little effect on M_3 receptors potentiate vagally induced bronchoconstriction. (From data in Ref. 158.)

Although the M_2 receptors are dysfunctional in patients with asthma (134,135), it has been demonstrated in animal models that M_2 receptors can be dysfunctional without being entirely nonfunctional (109). Thus nonselective anticholinergics have the capacity to further inhibit any remaining M_2 function, leading to further increased release of acetylcholine. It is important, then, to use the selective M_3 receptor antagonists—such as tiotropium bromide, darifenacin, and revatropate—to better define the role of the cholinergic nerves in asthma (see below).

Therefore, studies on the role of the cholinergic nerves in asthma, particularly studies using inhaled anticholinergics, should be interpreted with caution in the light of these confounding problems. A definite role for the cholinergic nerves has been demonstrated in animal models of asthma, in which vagal cooling or sectioning overcomes the methodological problems of human studies.

B. Role of Parasympathetic Nerves in Airway Hyperresponsiveness

A characteristic of most patients with asthma is airway hyperresponsiveness to many nonspecific stimuli, including sulfur dioxide, dust, citric acid, exercise, and cold air. In humans, nonspecific airway hyperresponsiveness is at least partially vagally mediated, since it can be blocked by intravenous atropine, or by high, adequate doses of inhaled anticholinergic agents (159–165). In experimental animals, these responses can be abolished by cutting the vagus nerves (166–168).

It has long been thought that airway hyperresponsiveness to an inhaled muscarinic agonist, such as methacholine, is due to a direct effect on the airway smooth muscle bypassing the vagi. However, it now appears that airway hyperreactivity to methacholine is also vagally mediated. Infusion of methacholine into the bronchial artery of anesthetized sheep, which supplies the bronchi and distal airways but not the trachea, induces smooth muscle contraction in an isolated segment of the trachea. This response is abolished by bilateral vagotomy. Furthermore, aerosolized methacholine delivered into the lower airways also induces contraction of the trachea. Vagotomy not only blocks this tracheal response but also substantially attenuates the lower airway response (169). A similar effect has been demonstrated in rats, where intravenous methacholine–induced bronchoconstriction is significantly potentiated in antigen-challenged rats but is returned to normal in these animals by vagotomy (170). Likewise, airway hyperreactivity to methacholine in virus-infected rats could only be demonstrated in the presence of intact vagus nerves (121). Thus, the usual assumptions concerning the lack of a vagal component to the response to methacholine need to be reassessed.

C. Role of the Parasympathetic Nerves in Allergic Asthma

Studies Using Anticholinergic Agents in Animals

The increase in airway resistance that follows inhaled antigen challenge is blocked by vagotomy, by intravenous atropine, or by cooling the vagus nerves in dogs (171). In guinea pigs, intravenous atropine partially reverses and bilateral vagotomy completely blocks antigen-induced bronchoconstriction (172). Similar results have been found in many other studies of both guinea pigs (173) and primates (174,175). Not all studies have shown that atropine protects against antigen-induced bronchoconstriction (176,177). However, many of these studies used relatively low doses of atropine, and none attempted to demonstrate adequate vagal blockade.

Studies Using Anticholinergic Agents in Humans

In humans, many studies have concluded that the cholinergic nerves are not important in allergic asthma (151,178–181). However, most of these studies used only single low doses of inhaled anticholinergic drugs without testing higher doses or attempting to demonstrate adequate vagal blockade, which is especially important when administering an anticholinergic agent by inhalation (as discussed above). On the other hand, intravenous atropine (1.5–2.5 mg) or high doses of inhaled atropine inhibit antigen-induced increases in airway resistance in allergic asthmatics (177,179,182–184). Similar findings have been reported using ipratropium bromide and its analogue oxitropium bromide (182–184). Thus, it is likely that increased release of acetylcholine from the vagus nerves contributes to antigen-induced airway hyperreactivity in humans.

D. Role of the Parasympathetic Nerves in Virus-Induced Asthma

Viral infections of the airways commonly exacerbate asthma (185–190), especially in children (190). Airway hyperresponsiveness to histamine in subjects with naturally occurring viral infections is vagally mediated and blocked by atropine (191–192). It was initially postulated that the afferent limb of the reflex arc was potentiated by viral infections through damage to the epithelium and exposure of irritant receptors. However, Buckner et al. subsequently demonstrated that the response to electrical stimulation of the vagus nerve was increased by parainfluenza virus infection in guinea pigs, demonstrating that it is the efferent, parasympathetic limb of the reflex arc that is potentiated by viral infection (114).

Increased release of acetylcholine from the parasympathetic nerves may be the result of neuronal M_2 receptor dysfunction, as we have demonstrated in parainfluenza virus–infected guinea pigs (119). Inflammatory cells may contribute to M_2 receptor dysfunction but are not the only mechanism (133). Viral neuraminidase (which is found in both influenza and parainfluenza viruses) can significantly decrease agonist affinity for M_2 receptors by cleaving sialic acid residues from the receptor (119). Furthermore, we have recently shown that both viral infection and exposure to interferon gamma (which is produced by lymphocytes in response to viral infections) markedly decrease M_2 receptor gene expression in parasympathetic neurons (193).

Thus, viral airway infections potentiate vagally mediated reflex bronchoconstriction in both humans and experimental animals. Increased release of acetylcholine from the vagus may be due to loss of the negative feedback normally provided by inhibitory M_2 receptors on the nerve endings. Finally, viruses are capable of inhibiting neuronal M_2 receptor function by several different mechanisms and it is not yet clear which of these mechanisms is important in vivo.

E. Role of the Parasympathetic Nerves in Nocturnal Asthma

In patients with nocturnal asthma, intravenous atropine almost completely inhibits the fall in peak flow at night, while inhaled anticholinergic agents attenuate the fall in peak flow at night in a dose-dependent manner (194,195). Thus, nocturnal asthma is mediated by a cholinergic reflex. At the same time, patients with nocturnal asthma have increased circulating eosinophils and neutrophils at 4.00 a.m. compared to themselves at 4.00 p.m. and compared to patients without nocturnal asthma at 4.00 a.m. (196). It is tempting to speculate that increased eosinophils and subsequent loss of M_2 receptor function may contribute to nocturnal asthma.

F. Role of the Parasympathetic Nerves in Psychogenic Asthma

Bronchoconstriction can be triggered by stress in some patients with asthma (197). Likewise, bronchoconstriction can be initiated by asking a subject to inhale an inert substance that the subject believes to be a bronchoconstrictor (198). Both psychogenic and emotionally induced bronchoconstriction are blocked by anticholinergics (199).

G. Other Forms of Asthma

Although multiple mechanisms are likely to be involved in exercise-induced asthma, a role for vagally mediated reflexes is suggested, since anticholinergics are effective bronchodilators in this type of asthma (162,164,192). Likewise, asthmatics who develop bronchospasm after taking β_2-blockers also respond to treatment with anticholinergics (200–202).

VI. Anticholinergic Drugs

A. Nonselective Muscarinic Receptor Antagonists

Atropine and Scopolamine

Atropine is a naturally occurring anticholinergic, extracted from *Atropa belladonna* (''deadly nightshade''), and named for Atropos, the third of the three fates, who had the responsibility of cutting the thread of life. Atropine is also found in *Datura stramonium*. Scopolamine, another anticholinergic agent that has been used to treat a number of conditions including motion sickness, is found in the plant henbane.

Atropine and other naturally occurring anticholinergics were originally administered in the form of cigarettes in the early part of the nineteenth century. Atropine has been used orally, parenterally, and by nebulization in the treatment of airway disease. The therapeutic use of atropine is limited by its toxicity and side effects. Dry mouth and urinary retention are common side effects, while atropine poisoning leads to coma and extremely high fever, delirium, and finally death.

Ipratropium Bromide

Because of the systemic and central nervous system toxicity of atropine, ipratropium—a poorly absorbed quaternary ammonium derivative—was synthesized. Ipratropium is the most widely used anticholinergic medication and is effective in the treatment of asthma and COPD and in the symptomatic relief of rhinitis (see below).

The effectiveness of ipratropium in treating airway diseases is limited by the fact that it is nonselective between M_2 and M_3 receptors (Fig. 4). Thus, while it decreases the bronchoconstrictive effects of acetylcholine, ipratropium increases the release of acetylcholine from the vagus by blocking the inhibitory M_2 receptor on the nerves (158).

B. Selective M_3 Receptor Antagonists

Tiotropium Bromide

Tiotropium bromide (Ba 679 BR; Fig. 5) is a recently developed anticholinergic agent that has two advantages in the treatment of airway disease: it has an extremely long duration of activity (203,204), and it is functionally selective for the M_3 receptor. In fact, the binding affinity of tiotropium for M_2 and M_3 receptors is approximately equal; however, the dissociation of this compound from the M_2 receptor is relatively rapid ($t_{1/2}$ = 3.6 hr), while the dissociation from the M_3 receptor is very prolonged ($t_{1/2}$ = 34.7 hr). Thus, after several hours, the effect at the M_2 receptor dissipates, while the bronchoconstriction resulting from the binding of acetylcholine to the M_3 receptor on the airway smooth muscle is antagonized for many hours.

Darifenacin and Revatropate

Two newer anticholinergic medications, revatropate and darifenacin, are structurally quite different from atropine (205). Both are M_3 receptor–selective, revatro-

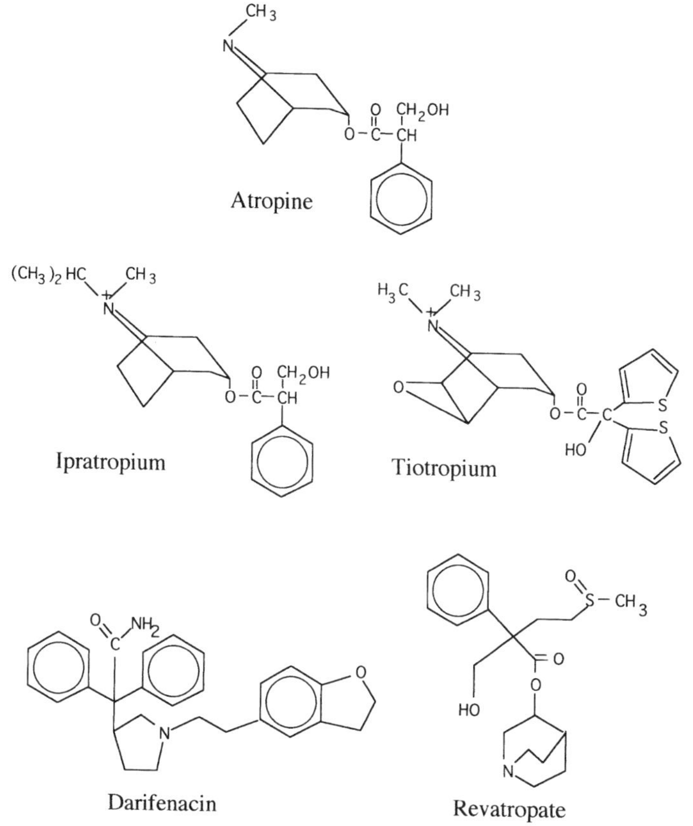

Atropine

Ipratropium

Tiotropium

Darifenacin

Revatropate

Figure 5 Structures of five anticholinergic medications. Note that both ipratropium and tiotropium have the quaternary ammonium structure, markedly decreasing absorption from the gastrointestinal tract and from other mucous membranes.

pate having a 50-fold higher affinity for M_3 receptors than for M_2 receptors, while darifenacin has an 16-fold higher affinity for M_3 than for M_2 receptors.

C. Novel Approaches for Reducing Parasympathetic Drive

Since release of acetylcholine is controlled by the neuronal M_2 receptors, it may be possible to manipulate the activity of these receptors with medication. In animal models of airway hyperreactivity, a specific inflammatory cell protein blocks these beneficial receptors (see above). If dysfunction of these neuronal M_2 receptors is also mediated via inflammatory cell products in asthma, this would be an additional mechanism by which corticosteroids, which inhibit inflammation, may inhibit vagally induced hyperreactivity. Heparin analogues, which are nonanticoagulant, have been shown to completely reverse airway hyperreactivity in animal models of asthma by restoring the function of the neuronal M_2 receptors (129). Thus, in the future, it may also be possible to inhibit parasympathetic nerve activity by removing inflammatory cell products with novel compounds such as the heparin analogues.

VII. Treatment of Airway Disease with Anticholinergics

A. Anticholinergics in Asthma

Early studies in stable asthmatics showed that anticholinergics, including atropine (149,206–210) and ipratropium bromide (211), were comparable to β_2-agonists as bronchodilators. However, these studies were criticized because they did not attempt to compare the effects of maximal doses of the two classes of medications. It was subsequently demonstrated that if albuterol was given repeatedly until no further bronchodilation could be achieved, ipratropium caused a small further dilatation. In contrast, albuterol caused substantial dilation after maximal doses of ipratropium, especially in younger patients (211). This was interpreted as showing that β_2-agonists reverse bronchoconstriction resulting from mechanisms other than cholinergic, while anticholinergics are limited to this latter class of mechanisms. Alternatively, it may also be the case that anticholinergics were less effective because the currently available anticholinergics are suboptimal for the reasons discussed above.

In the acute setting, several studies have suggested that greater bronchodilation and decreased need for hospitalization can be achieved using a combination of anticholinergics and β_2-agonists when compared with β_2-agonists alone (141,212–214), particularly in the pediatric age group. Other studies have not found a difference between repeated treatment with β_2-agonists versus the combination with anticholinergics (145,215,216).

B. Anticholinergics in Chronic Obstructive Pulmonary Disease

Because of the relative ineffectiveness of β_2-agonists in patients with Chronic Obstructive Pulmonary Disease (COPD), the effects of anticholinergic treatment has been studied in these patients. Patients who are unresponsive to β_2-agonists may have a significant bronchodilation response to atropine (149,217). Furthermore, after treatment with the β_2-agonist, addition of atropine may bring further relief of bronchoconstriction (149). A recent study demonstrated the effectiveness of tiotropium in patients with COPD (218). Chronic treatment with anticholinergics may also decrease the volume of airway secretions (37).

In the acute setting, the role of anticholinergics in the treatment of COPD is unclear. Adding ipratropium to β_2-agonist treatment may shorten the duration of emergency room treatment (219), although not all studies have confirmed this (147). Inadequate doses of anticholinergics may have contributed to this finding.

C. Anticholinergics in Rhinitis

Naclerio and colleagues (220–223) demonstrated in nonasthmatics that when histamine, antigen, or cold, dry air is applied in only one nostril, there is a vagally mediated increase in secretions in the contralateral nostril that is blocked by atropine. A substantial cholinergic component to the ipsilateral response is also present.

In several large, controlled clinical trials, nasal ipratropium was effective in relieving symptoms in patients with allergic rhinitis (224), nonallergic rhinitis (225), and the common cold (226). In these studies ipratropium was administered daily for 4–8 weeks and was effective at inhibiting rhinorrhea compared to placebo. Nasal ipratropium bromide treatment was well tolerated.

VIII. Conclusion

The cholinergic nervous system clearly plays an important role in asthma, COPD, and rhinitis. Dysfunction of inhibitory M_2 receptors on the vagal nerve endings may contribute to increased acetylcholine release in these diseases as well as after viral infection, exposure to ozone, or inhalation of antigen. Future studies need to clarify the role of these receptors in human airway disease. Improved anticholinergic medications, including selective M_3 antagonists, may offer more effective interruption of these reflexes. Furthermore, understanding the effects of inflammatory cells and their products on the cholinergic control of the airways may suggest new ways to address this component of the pathophysiology of airway disease.

References

1. Dale HH. The action of certain esthers and ethers of choline and their relation to muscarine. J Pharmacol Exp Ther 1914; 6:147–190.
2. Riker WF, Wescoe WC. The pharmacology of flaxedil with observations on certain analogues. Ann NY Acad Sci 1951; 54:373–392.
3. Barlow RB, Franks FM, Pearson JDM. A comparison of the affinities of antagonists for acetylcholine receptors in the ileum, bronchial muscle and iris of the guinea-pig. Br J Pharmacol 1972; 46:300–314.
4. Hammer R, Berrie CP, Birdsall NJM, Burgen ASV, Hulme EC. Pirenzepine distin-

guishes between different subclasses of muscarinic receptors. Nature 1980; 283: 90–92.
5. Eglen RM, Hegde SS, Watson N. Muscarinic receptor subtypes and smooth muscle function. Pharmacol Rev 1996; 48:531–565.
6. Severinghaus JW, Stupfel M. Respiratory dead space increase following atropine in man, and atropine, vagal or ganglionic blockade and hypothermia in dogs. J Appl Physiol 1955; 8:81–87.
7. Widdicombe J. The parasympathetic nervous system in airways disease. Scand J Respir Dis 1979; 103:38S–43S.
8. Baker DG, McDonald DM, Basbaum CB, Mitchell RA. The architecture of nerves and ganglia of the ferret trachea as revealed by acetylcholinesterase histochemistry. J Comp Neurosci 1986; 246:513–526.
9. Cheng JB, Townley RG. Comparison of muscarinic and beta adrenergic receptors between bovine peripheral lung and tracheal smooth muscles: a striking difference. Life Sci 1982; 30:2079–2086.
10. Barnes PJ, Nadel JA, Roberts JM, Basbaum CB. Muscarinic receptors in lung and trachea: autoradiographic localization using [3H]Quinuclidinyl benzylate. Eur J Pharmacol 1983; 86:103–106.
11. Mak JCW, Barnes PJ. Autoradiographic visualization of muscarinic receptor subtypes in human and guinea-pig lung. Am Rev Respir Dis 1990; 141:1559–1568.
12. Emala C, Aryana A, Levine M, Yasuda R, Satkus S, Wolfe B, Hirshman C. Basenji-greyhound dog: increased m_2 muscarinic receptor expression in trachealis muscle. Am J Physiol 1995; 268:L935–L940.
13. Klapproth H, Reinheimer T, Metzen J, Munch M, Bittinger F, Kirkpatrick C, Hohle K, Schnemann M, Racke K, Wessler I. Non-neuronal acetylcholine, a signaling molecule synthesized by surface cells of rat and man. Naunyn Schmiedebergs Arch Pharmacol 1997; 355:515–523.
14. Marin M, Davis B, Nadel J. Effect of acetylcholine on Cl- and NA^+fluxes across dog tracheal epithelium in vitro. Am J Physiol 1976; 231:1546–1549.
15. Boucher RC, Gatzy JT. Regional effects of autonomic agents on ion transport across excised canine airways. J Appl Physiol 1982; 52:893–901.
16. Jarnigan F, Davis JD, Bromberg PA, Gatzy JT, Boucher RC. Bio electric properties and ion transport of excised rabbit trachea. J Appl Physiol 1983; 55:1884–1892.
17. Wong L, Miller I, Yeates D. Regulation of ciliary beat frequency by autonomic mechanisms in vitro. J Appl Physiol 1988; 65:1895–1901.
18. Yang B, McCaffrey T. The roles of muscarinic receptor subtypes in modulation of nasal ciliary action. Rhinology 1996; 34:136–139.
19. Yang B, Schlosser R, McCaffrey T. Signal transduction pathways in modulation of ciliary beat frequency by methacholine. Ann Otol Rhinol Laryngol 1997; 106: 230–236.
20. Salathe M, Lipson E, Ivonnet P, Brookman R. Muscarinic receptor signaling in ciliated tracheal epithelial cells: dual effects on Ca^{2+} and ciliary beating. Am J Physiol 1997; 272:L301–L310.
21. Wanner A. Effect of ipratropium bromide on airway mucociliary function. Am J Med 1986; 81:23–27.

22. Mak JCW, Baraniuk JN, Barnes PJ. Localization of muscarinic receptor subtype mRNAs in human lung. Am J Respir Cell Mol Biol 1992; 7:344–348.
23. van Koppen CJ, Blanksteijn M, Klaassen BM, Rodrigues de Miranda JF, Beld AJ, van Ginneken CAM. Autoradiographic visualization of muscarinic receptors in human bronchi. J Pharmacol Exp Ther 1988; 244:760–764.
24. Bensch K, Gordon G, Miller L. Studies on the bronchial counterpart of the Kultschitzky (argentaffin) cell and innervation of bronchial glands. J Ultrastruct Res 1965; 12:668–686.
25. Meyrick B, Reid L. Ultra structure of cells in the human bronchial submucosal glands. J Anatomy 1970; 107:281–299.
26. Borson DB, Chinn RA, Davis B, Nadel JA. Adrenergic and cholinergic nerves mediate fluid secretion from tracheal glands of ferrets. J Appl Physiol 1980; 49: 1027–1031.
27. Culp D, Marin M. Characterization of muscarinic cholinergic receptors in cat tracheal gland cells. J Appl Physiol 1986; 61:1375–1382.
28. Okayama M, Mullol J, Baraniuk J, Hausfeld J, Feldman B, Merida M, Shelhammer J, Kaliner M. Muscarinic receptor subtypes in human nasal mucosa: characterization, autoradiographic localization, and function in vitro. Am J Respir Cell Mol Biol 1993; 8:176–187.
29. Phipps R, Richardson P. The effects of irritation at various levels of the airway upon tracheal mucus secretion in the cat. J Physiol 1976; 261:563–581.
30. German V, Ueki I, Nadel J. Micropipette measurement of airway submucosal gland secretion: laryngeal reflex. Am Rev Respir Dis 1980; 49:1027–1031.
31. Yang CM, Farley JM, Dwyer TM. Muscarinic stimulation of submucosal glands in swine trachea. J Appl Physiol 1988; 64:200–209.
32. Ramnarine S, Haddad E, Khawaja A, Mak J, Rogers D. On muscarinic control of neurogenic mucus secretion in ferret trachea. J Physiol (Lond) 1996; 494:577–586.
33. Ishihara H, Shimura S, Satoh M, Masuda T, Nonaka H, Kase H, Sasaki T, Sasaki H, Takishima T, Tamura K. Muscarinic receptor subtypes in feline tracheal submucosal gland secretion. Am J Physiol 1992; 262:L223–L228.
34. Baker A, Chakrin L, Wardell J. Chronic cholinergic stimulation of canine respiratory tissue: its effect on the activities of glycosyltransferases and release of macromolecules. Am Rev Respir Dis 1975; 111:423–431.
35. Sturgess J, Reid L. The effect of isoprenaline and pilocarpine on a) bronchial mucus secreting tissue and b) pancreas, salivary glands, heart, thymus, liver and spleen. Br J Exp Pathol 1973; 54:388–403.
36. Steel D, Hanrahan J. Muscarinic-induced mucin secretion and intracellular signaling by hamster tracheal goblet cells. Am J Physiol 1997; 272:L230–L237.
37. Tamaoki J, Chiyotani A, Tagaya E, Sakai N, Konno K. Effect of long term treatment with oxitropium bromide on airway secretion in chronic bronchitis and diffuse panbronchiolitis. Thorax 1994; 49:545–548.
38. Nadel J, Barnes P. Autonomic regulation of the airways. Ann Rev Med 1984; 35: 451–467.
39. Undem BJ, Myers AC, Barthlow H, Weinreich D. Vagal innervation of guinea-pig bronchial smooth muscle. J Appl Physiol 1990; 69:1336–1346.
40. Emala CW, Aryana A, Levine MA, Yasuda RP, Satkus SA, Wolfe BB, Hirshman

CA. Expression of muscarinic receptor subtypes and M_2 muscarinic inhibition of adenylyl cyclase in lung. Am J Physiol 1995; 268:L101–L107.

41. Yang CM, Farley JM, Dwyer TM. Biochemical characteristics of muscarinic cholinoreceptors in swine tracheal smooth muscle. J Auton Pharmacol 1986; 6:15–24.
42. Madison JM, Jones CA, Tom-Moy M, Brown JK. Affinities of pirenzepine for muscarinic cholinergic receptors in membranes isolated from bovine tracheal mucosa and smooth muscle. Am Rev Respir Dis 1987; 135:719–724.
43. Roffel AF, in't Hout WG, de Zeeuw RA, Zaagsma J. The M_2 selective antagonist AF-DX 116 shows high affinity for muscarine receptors in bovine tracheal membranes. Naunyn Schmiedebergs Arch Pharmacol 1987; 335:593–595.
44. Maeda A, Kubo T, Mishina M, Numa S. Tissue distribution of mRNAs encoding muscarinic acetylcholine receptor subtypes. FEBS Lett 1988; 239:339–342.
45. Roffel AF, Elzinga CR, Van Amsterdam RG, de Zeeuw RA, Zaagsma J. Muscarinic M_2 receptors in bovine tracheal smooth muscle: discrepancies between binding and function. Eur J Pharmacol 1988; 153:73–82.
46. Roffel AF, Elzinga CR, Meurs H, Zaagsma J. Allosteric interactions of three muscarine antagonists at bovine tracheal smooth muscle and cardiac M_2 receptors. Eur J Pharmacol 1989, 172:61–70.
47. Fryer AD, El-Fakahany EE. Identification of three muscarinic receptor subtypes in rat lung using binding studies with selective antagonists. Life Sci 1990; 47:611–618.
48. Lucchesi A, Scheid CR, Romano FD, Kargacin ME, Mullikin-Kilpatrick D, Yamaguchi H, Honeyman TW. Ligand binding and G protein coupling of muscarinic receptors in airway smooth muscle. Am J Physiol 1990; 258:C730–C738.
49. Mahesh VK, Nunan LM, Halonen M, Yamamura HI, Palmer JD, Bloom JW. A minority of muscarinic receptors mediate rabbit tracheal smooth muscle contraction. Am J Respir Cell Mol Biol 1992; 6:279–286.
50. Haddad E, Mak J, Hislop A, Haworth S, Barnes P. Characterization of muscarinic receptor subtypes in pig airways: radioligand binding and Northern blotting studies. Am J Physiol 1994; 266:L642–L648.
51. Schaefer O, Ethier M, Madison J. Muscarinic regulation of cyclic AMP in bovine trachealis cells. Am J Respir Cell Mol Biol 1995; 13:217–226.
52. Yang CM. Characterization of muscarinic receptors in dog tracheal smooth muscle cells. J Auton Pharmacol 1991; 11:51–61.
53. Haddad E-B, Landry Y, Gies J-P. Muscarinic receptor subtypes in guinea-pig airways. Am J Physiol 1991; 261:L327–L333.
54. van Koppen CJ, Rodrigues de Miranda JF, Beld AJ, Hermanussen MW, Willem J, Lammers J, vanGinneken CAM. Characterization of the muscarinic receptor in human tracheal smooth muscle. Naunyn Schmiedebergs Arch Pharmacol 1985; 331:247–252.
55. Roffel AF, Elzinga CRS, Zaagsma J. Muscarinic M_3 receptors mediate contraction of human central and peripheral airway smooth muscle. Pulm Pharmacol 1990; 3: 47–51.
56. Gies JP, Bertrand C, Vanderheyden P, Waeldele F, Dumont P, Pauli G, Landry Y. Characterization of muscarinic receptors in human, guinea-pig and rat lung. J Pharmacol Exp Ther 1989; 250:309–315.

57. Janssen LJ, Daniel EE. Pre- and postjunctional muscarinic receptors in canine bronchi. Am J Physiol 1990; 259:L304–L314.
58. Brichant JF, Warner DO, Gunst SJ, Rehder K. Muscarinic receptor subtypes in canine trachea. Am J Physiol 1990; 258:L349–L354.
59. Itabashi S, Aikawa T, Sekisawa K, Ohrui T, Sasaki H, Takishima T. Pre- and postjunctional muscarinic receptor subtypes in dog airways. Eur J Pharmacol 1991; 204:235–241.
60. Howell RE, Laemont K, Gaudette R, Raynor M, Warner A, Noronha-Blob L. Characterization of the airway smooth muscle muscarinic receptor in vivo. Eur J Pharmacol 1991; 197:109–112.
61. vanNieuwstadt R, Henricks P, Hajer R, van der Meer van Roomen W, Breukink H, Nijkamp F. Characterization of muscarinic receptors in equine tracheal smooth muscle in vitro. Vet Quarterly 1997; 19:54–57.
62. Mitchelson F. Muscarinic receptor differentiation. Pharmacol Ther 1988; 37:357–423.
63. Roffel AF, Meurs H, Elzinga CRS, Zaagsma J. Characterization of the muscarinic receptor subtype involved in phosphoinositide metabolism in bovine tracheal smooth muscle. Br J Pharmacol 1990; 99:293–296.
64. Yang CM, Chou SP, Sung TC. Muscarinic receptor subtypes coupled to generation of different second messengers in isolated tracheal smooth muscle cells. Br J Pharmacol 1991; 104:613–618.
65. Grandordy BM, Cuss FM, Sampson AS, Palmer JB, Barnes PJ. Phosphatidylinositol response to cholinergic agonists in airway smooth muscle: relationship to contractile and muscarinic receptor occupancy. J Pharmacol Exp Ther 1986; 238:273–279.
66. Meurs H, Roffel AF, Postema JB, Timmermans A, Elzinga CR, Kauffman HF, Zaagsma J. Evidence for a direct relationship between phosphoinositide metabolism and airway smooth muscle contraction induced by muscarinic agonists. Eur J Pharmacol 1988; 156:271–274.
67. Meurs H, Timmermans A, Van Amsterdam GM, Brouwer F, Kauffman HF, Zaagsma J. Muscarinic receptors in human airway smooth muscle are coupled to phosphoinositide metabolism. Eur J Pharmacol 1989; 156:271–274.
68. Widdop S, Daykin K, Hall I. Expression of muscarinic M_2 receptors in cultured human airway smooth muscle cells. Am J Respir Cell Mol Biol 1993; 9:541–546.
69. Jones CA, Madison JM, Tom-Moy M, Brown JK. Muscarinic cholinergic inhibition of adenylate cyclase in airway smooth muscle. Am J Physiol 1987; 253:C97–C104.
70. Sankary RM, Jones CA, Madison JM, Brown JK. Muscarinic cholinergic inhibition of cyclic AMP accumulation in airway smooth muscle. Am Rev Respir Dis 1988; 57:801–807.
71. Fernandes LB, Fryer AD, Hirshman CA. M_2 muscarinic receptors inhibit isoproterenol-induced relaxation of canine airway smooth muscle. J Pharmacol Exp Ther 1992; 262:119–126.
72. Yasuda R, Ciesla W, Flores L, Wall S, Li M, Satkus S, Weisstein J, Spagnola B, Wolfe B. Development of antisera selective for m_4 and m_5 muscarinic cholinergic receptors: distribution of m_4 and m_5 in rat brain. Mol Pharmacol 1993; 43:149–157.

73. Wall S, Yasuda R, Li M, Wolfe B. Development of an antiserum against m_3 muscarinic receptors: distribution of m_3 receptors in rat tissues and clonal cell lines. Mol Pharmacol 1995; 40:783–789.
74. Bloom JW, Halonen M, Yamamura HI. Characterization of muscarinic cholinergic receptor subtypes in human peripheral lung. J Pharmacol Exp Ther 1988; 244:625–632.
75. Casale TB, Ecklund P. Characterization of muscarinic receptor subtypes on human peripheral lung. J Appl Physiol 1988; 65:594–600.
76. Mak JCW, Barnes PJ. Muscarinic receptor subtypes in human and guinea-pig lung. Eur J Pharmacol 1989; 164:223–230.
77. Post M, TeBiesebeek J, Doods H, Wemer J, Van Rooij H, Porsius A. Functional characterization of the muscarinic receptor in rat lungs. Eur J Pharmacol 1991; 202: 67–92.
78. Esqueda E, Gerstin E, Griffen M, Ehlert F. Stimulation of cyclic AMP accumulation and phosphoinositide hydrolysis by M_3 muscarinic receptors in the rat peripheral lung. Biochem Pharmacol 1996; 52:643–658.
79. Wilson P, Khimenko P, Barnard J, Moore T, Taylor A. Muscarinic agonists and antagonists cause vasodilation in isolated rat lung. J Appl Physiol 1995; 78:1401 1411.
80. Fryer AD, Maclagan J. Muscarinic inhibitory receptors in pulmonary parasympathetic nerves in the guinea-pig. Br J Pharmacol 1984; 83:973–978.
81. van Koppen CJ, Blanksteijn M, Klaassen BM, Rodrigues de Miranda JF, Beld AJ, van Ginneken CAM. Autoradiographic visualization of muscarinic receptors in pulmonary nerves and ganglia. Neurosci Lett 1987; 83:237–240.
82. James S, Bailey D, Burnstock G. Autoradiographic visualization of muscarinic receptors on rat paratracheal neurons in dissociated cell culture. Brain Res 1990; 513: 74–80.
83. Mitchell RA, Herbert DA, Baker DG, Basbaum CB. In vivo activity of tracheal parasympathetic ganglion cells innervating tracheal smooth muscle. Brain Res 1987; 437:157–160.
84. Bloom JW, Yamamura HI, Baumgarttener C, Halonen M. A muscarinic receptor with high affinity for pirenzepine mediates vagally induced bronchoconstriction. Eur J Pharmacol 1987; 133:21–27.
85. Beck KC, Vetterman J, Flavahan NA, Rehder K. Muscarinic M_1 receptors mediate the increase in pulmonary resistance during vagus nerve stimulation in dogs. Am Rev Respir Dis 1987; 136:1135–1139.
86. Yang KJ, Biggs DF. Muscarinic receptors and parasympathetic neurotransmission in guinea-pig trachea. Eur J Pharmacol 1991; 193:301–308.
87. Gallagher JP, Griffith WH, Shinnick-Gallagher P. Cholinergic transmission in cat parasympathetic ganglia. J Physiol 1982; 332:473–486.
88. Ashe JH, Yaroshe CA. Differential and selective antagonism of the slow inhibitory post-synaptic potential by gallamine and pirenzepine. Neuropharmacology 1984: 23:1321–1329.
89. Lammers JWJ, Minette P, McCusker M, Barnes P. The role of pirenzepine sensitive muscarinic receptors in vagally mediated bronchoconstriction in humans. Am Rev Respir Dis 1989; 139:446–449.

90. Myers A, Undem B. Muscarinic receptor regulation of synaptic transmission in airway parasympathetic ganglia. Am J Physiol 1996; 270:L630–L636.
91. Kilbinger H, Schneider R, Siefken H, Wolf D, D'Agostino G. Characterization of prejunctional muscarinic autoreceptors in guinea-pig trachea. Br J Pharmacol 1991; 103:1757–1763.
92. Fryer AD, Elbon CL, Kim AL, Xiao HQ, Levey AI, Jacoby DB. Cultures of airway parasympathetic nerves express functional M2 muscarinic receptors. Am J Respir Cell Mol Biol 1996; 15:716–725.
93. Faulkner D, Fryer AD, Maclagan J. Post-ganglionic muscarinic receptors in pulmonary parasympathetic nerves in the guinea-pig. Br J Pharmacol 1986; 88:181–188.
94. Fryer AD, Maclagan J. Pancuronium and gallamine are antagonists for pre- and postjunctional muscarinic receptors in the guinea-pig lung. Naunyn Schmiedebergs Arch Pharmacol 1987; 335:367–371.
95. Doelman CJA, Sprong RC, Nagtegaal JE, Rodrigues de Miranda JF, Bast A. Prejunctional muscarinic receptors on cholinergic nerves in the guinea-pig airway are of the M_2 subtype. Eur J Pharmacol 1991; 193:117–119.
96. Blaber LC, Fryer AD, Maclagan J. Neuronal muscarinic receptors attenuate vagally induced contraction of feline bronchial smooth muscle. Br J Pharmacol 1985; 86: 723–728.
97. Killingsworth CR, Mingfu Y, Robinson NE. Evidence for the absence of a functional role for muscarinic M_2 inhibitory receptors in cat trachea in vivo: contrast with in vitro results. Br J Pharmacol 1992; 105:263–270.
98. Aas P, Maclagan J. Evidence for prejunctional M_2 muscarinic receptors in pulmonary cholinergic nerves of the rat. Br J Pharmacol 1990; 101:73–76.
99. Larsen GL, Fame TM, Renz H, Loader JE, Graves J, Hill M, Gelfand EW. Increased acetylcholine release in tracheas from allergen-exposed IgE-immune mice. Am J Physiol 1994; 266:L263–L270.
100. Ito Y, Yoshitomi T. Autoregulation of acetylcholine release from vagus nerves terminals through activation of muscarinic receptors in the dog trachea. Br J Pharmacol 1988; 93:636–646.
101. Wang Z, Yu M, Robinson N, Derksen F. Acetylcholine release form airway cholinergic nerves in horses with heaves, an airway obstructive disease. Am J Respir Crit Care Med 1995; 151:830–835.
102. Matsumoto S, Nagayama T, Kanno T, Yamasaki M, Shimizu T. Evidence for the presence of function of the inhibitory M_2 muscarinic receptors in rabbit airways and lungs. J Auton Nerv System 1995; 53:126–136.
103. Minette P, Barnes PJ. Prejunctional inhibitory muscarinic receptors on cholinergic nerves in human and guinea-pig airways. J Appl Physiol 1988; 64:2532–2537
104. Baker DG, Brown JK. Potent muscarinic cholinergic regulation of acetylcholine release from nerve endings in airway smooth muscle (abstr). Am Rev Respir Dis 1991; 143:A358.
105. Belmonte KE, Jacoby DB, Fryer AD. Increased function of inhibitory neuronal M_2 muscarinic receptors in diabetic rat lungs. Br J Pharmacol 1997; 121:1287–1294.
106. McCaig DJ. Comparison of autonomic responses in the trachea isolated from normal and albumin-sensitive guinea-pigs. Br J Pharmacol 1987; 92:809–816.

107. Mitchell RW, Kroeger EA, Kepron W, Stephens NL. Local parasympathetic mechanisms for ragweed-sensitized canine trachealis hyperresponsiveness. J Pharmacol Exp Ther 1987; 243:907–914.
108. Tanaka D, Ando R, Larsen G, Irvin C. Cholinergic mechanisms involved with histamine hyperreactivity in immune rabbit airways challenged with ragweed antigen. Am Rev Respir Dis 1991; 144:70–75.
109. Fryer AD, Wills-Karp M. Dysfunction of M_2 muscarinic receptors in pulmonary parasympathetic nerves after antigen challenge in guinea-pigs. J Appl Physiol 1991; 71:2255–2261.
110. Mitchell R, Ndukuw I, Ikeda K, Arbetter K, Leff A. Effect of immune sensitization on stimulated ACh release from trachealis muscle in vitro. Am J Physiol 1993; 265:L13–L18.
111. Lee LY, Bleeker ER, Nadel JA. Effect of ozone on bronchomotor response to inhaled histamine aerosol in dogs. J Appl Physiol 1977; 43:626–631.
112. Buckner CK, Clayton DE, Ain-Shoka AA, Busse WW, Dick EC, Shult P. Parainfluenza 3 infection blocks the ability of a beta adrenergic receptor to inhibit antigen-induced contraction of guinea pig isolated airway smooth muscle. J Clin Invest 1981; 67:376–384.
113. Holtzman MJ. Inflammation of the airway epithelium and the development of airway hyperresponsiveness. Prog Respir Res 1985; 19:165–172.
114. Buckner CK, Songsiridej V, Dick EC, Busse WW. In vivo and in vitro studies of the use of the guinea pig as a model for virus-provoked airway hyperreactivity. Am Rev Respir Dis 1985; 132:305–310.
115. Walters EH, O'Byrne PM, Graf PD, Fabbri LM, Nadel JA. The responsiveness of airway smooth muscle in vitro from dogs with airway hyperresponsiveness in vivo. Clin Sci 1986; 71:605–611.
116. Jacoby DB, Ueki IF, Loegering DA, Gleich GJ, Widdicombe JH, Nadel JA. Effect of human eosinophil major basic protein on ion transport in canine tracheal epithelium. Am Rev Respir Dis 1988; 137:13–16.
117. Jacoby DB, Tamaoki J, Borson DB, Nadel JA. Influenza infection causes airway hyperresponsiveness by decreasing enkephalinase. J Appl Physiol 1988; 64:2653–2658.
118. Killingsworth CR, Robinson NE, Adams T, Maes RK, Berney C, Rozanski E. Cholinergic reactivity of tracheal smooth muscle following infection with feline herpesvirus-I. J Appl Physiol 1990; 69:1953–1960.
119. Fryer AD, Jacoby DB. Parainfluenza virus infection damages inhibitory M_2 muscarinic receptors on pulmonary parasympathetic nerves in the guinea-pig. Br J Pharmacol 1991; 102:267–271.
120. Schultheis A, Bassett D, Fryer A. Ozone-induced airway hyperresponsiveness and loss of neuronal M_2 muscarinic receptor function. J Appl Physiol 1994; 76:1088–1097.
121. Sorkness R, Clough J, Castleman W, Lemanske Jr R. Virus-induced airway obstruction and parasympathetic hyperresponsiveness in adult rats. Am J Respir Crit Care Med 1994; 150:28–34.
122. Costello R, Fryer A. Cholinergic mechanisms in asthma. In: Barnes P, Grunstein M, eds. Asthma. Philadelphia: Lippincott-Raven, 1997:965–984.

123. Fryer AD, Jacoby DB. Effect of inflammatory cell mediators on M_2 muscarinic receptors in the lungs. Life Sci 1993; 52:529–536.
124. Costello R, Schofield B, Kephart G, Gleich G, Jacoby D, Fryer A. Localization of eosinophils to airway nerves and the effect on neuronal M_2 muscarinic receptor function. Am J Physiol 1997; 273:L93–L103.
125. Elbon CL, Jacoby DB, Fryer AD. Pretreatment with an antibody to interleukin-5 prevents loss of pulmonary M_2 muscarinic receptor function in antigen challenged guinea-pigs. Am J Respir Cell Mol Biol 1995; 12:320–328.
126. Fryer AD, Costello RW, Yost BY, Lobb RR, Tedder TF, Steeber AS, Bochner BS. Antibody to VLA-4, but not to L-selection, protects neuronal M_2 muscarinic receptors in antigen challenged guinea pig airways. J Clin Invest 1997; 99:2036–2044.
127. Jacoby DB, Gleich GJ, Fryer AD. Human eosinophil major basic protein is an endogenous allosteric antagonist at the inhibitory muscarinic M_2 receptor. J Clin Invest 1993; 91:1314–1318.
128. Fryer AD, Jacoby DB. Function of pulmonary M_2 muscarinic receptors in antigen challenged guinea-pigs is restored by heparin and poly-1-glutamate. J Clin Invest 1992; 90:2292–2298.
129. Fryer A, Huang Y, Rao G, Jacoby D, Mancilla, E, Whorton R, Piantadosi C, Kennedy T, Hoidel J. Selective O-desulfation produces non anticoagulant heparin that retains pharmacological activity in the lung. J Pharmacol Exp Ther 1997; 282:208–219.
130. Evans CM, Jacoby DB, Gleich GJ, Fryer AD, Costello RW. Antibody to eosinophil major basic protein protects M2 receptor function in antigen challenged guinea pigs in vivo. J Clin Invest 1997; 100:2254–2262.
131. Gambone LM, Elbon CL, Fryer AD. Ozone-induced loss of neuronal M_2 muscarinic receptor function is prevented by cyclophosphamide. J Appl Physiol 1994; 77: 1492–1499.
132. Fryer AD, El-Fakahany EE, Jacoby DB. Parainfluenza virus type 1 reduces the affinity of agonists for muscarinic receptors in guinea-pig heart and lung. Eur J Pharmacol 1990; 181:51–58.
133. Fryer AD, Yarkony KA, Jacoby DB. The effect of leukocyte depletion on M2 muscarinic receptor function in parainfluenza virus-infected guinea-pigs. Br J Pharmacol 1994; 112:588–594.
134. Ayala LE, Ahmed T. Is there loss of a protective muscarinic receptor in asthma? Chest 1989; 96:1285–1291.
135. Minette PJ, Lammers JWJ, Dixon CMS, McCusker MT, Barnes PJ. A muscarinic agonist inhibits reflex bronchoconstriction in normal but not asthmatic subjects. J Appl Physiol 1989; 67:2461–2465.
136. Phillips E, Scott W. The surgical treatment of bronchial asthma. Arch Surg 1929; 19:1425–1456.
137. Dimitrov-Szokodi D, Husveti A, Balogh G. Lung denervation in the therapy of intractable bronchial asthma. J Thorac Surg 1957; 33:166–184.
138. Overholt R. Pulmonary denervation and resection in asthmatic patients. Ann Allergy 1959; 17:534–545.
139. Corris P, Dark J. Aetology of asthma: lessons from lung transplantation (see comments). Lancet 1993; 341:1369–1371.

140. Edmunds L, Nadel J, Graf P. Reinnervation of the re implanted canine lung. J Appl Physiol 1971; 31:722–727.
141. O'Driscoll BR, Taylor RJ, Horsley MG, Chambers DK, Bernstein A. Nebulized salbutamol with and without ipratropium bromide in acute airflow obstruction. Lancet 1989; 1:1418–1420.
142. Louw SJ, Goldin JG, Isaacs S. Relative efficacy of nebulized ipratropium bromide and fenoterol in acute severe asthma. S Afr Med J 1990; 77:24–26.
143. Bruderman I, Cohen-Aronovski R, Smorzik J. A comparative study of various combinations of ipratropium bromide and metaproterenol in allergic asthmatic patients. Chest 1983; 83:208–210.
144. van Schayck CP, Folgering H, Harbers H, Maas KL, van Weel C. Effects of allergy and age on responses to salbutamol and ipratropium bromide in moderate asthma and chronic bronchitis. Thorax 1991; 46:355–359.
145. Summers QA, Tarala RA. Nebulized ipratropium in the treatment of acute asthma. Chest 1990; 97:430–434.
146. Leahy BC, Gomm SA, Allen SC. Comparison of nebulized salbutamol with nebulized ipratropium bromide in acute asthma. Br J Dis Chest 1983; 77:159–163.
147. Petrie GR, Palmer KNV. Comparison of aerosol ipratropium bromide and salbutamol in chronic bronchitis and asthma. Br Med J 1975; 1:430–432.
148. Molfino N, Slutsky A, Julia-Serda G. Assessment of airway tone in asthma: comparison between double lung transplant patients and healthy subjects. Am Rev Respir Dis 1993; 148:1238–1243.
149. Gross NJ, Skorodin MS. Anticholinergic antimuscarinic bronchodilators. Am Rev Respir Dis 1984; 129:856–870.
150. Barnes PJ. Neural control of human airways in health and disease. Am Rev Respir Dis 1986; 134:1289–1314.
151. Fish JE, Rosenthall RR, Summer WR, Menkes H, Norman PS, Permutt S. The effect of atropine on acute antigen-mediated airway constriction in subjects with allergic asthma. Am Rev Respir Dis 1977; 115:371–379.
152. Cockcroft DW, Ruffin RE, Hargreave FE. Effect of SCH 1000 in allergen-induced asthma. Clin Allergy 1978; 8:361–372.
153. Boulet L, Latimer K, Roberts R, Juniper E, Cockcroft D, Thompson N, Daniel E, Hargreave F. The effect of atropine on allergen induced increases in bronchial responsiveness to histamine. Am Rev Respir Dis 1984; 130:368–372.
154. Holtzman M, McNamara P, Sheppard D, Fabbri L, Hahn H, Graf P, Nadel J. Intravenous versus inhaled atropine for inhibiting bronchoconstrictor responses in dogs. J Appl Physiol 1983; 54:134–139.
155. Sheppard D, Epstein J, Holtzman M, JA N, Boushey H. Effect of route of atropine delivery on bronchospasm from cold air and methacholine. J Appl Physiol 1983; 54:130–133.
156. DeToyer A, Yernault J, Rodenstein D. Effects of vagal blockade on lung mechanics in normal man. J Appl Physiol 1979; 46:217–226.
157. Weiss ST, McFadden E, Ingram R. Parenteral vs. inhaled atropine: density dependence of maximal expiratory flow. J Appl Physiol 1982; 53:392–396.
158. Fryer AD, Maclagan J. Ipratropium bromide potentiates bronchoconstriction in-

duced by vagal nerve stimulation in the guinea-pig. Eur J Pharmacol 1987; 139: 187–191.

159. Smith L, McFadden E. Bronchial hyperreactivity revisited. Ann Allergy Asthma Immunol 1995; 74:454–469.
160. Nadel JA, Salem H, Tamplin B, Tokiwa Y. Mechanism of bronchoconstriction during inhalation of sulfur dioxide. J Appl Physiol 1965; 20:164–167.
161. Simonsson B, Jacobs F, Nadel J. Role of autonomic nervous system and the cough reflex in the increased responsiveness of airways in patients with obstructive lung disease. J Clin Invest 1968; 46:1812–1818.
162. Simonsson B, Skoogh BE, Ekstrom-Jodal B. Exercise induced airways constriction. Thorax 1972; 27:169–180.
163. Gayrard P, Orehek J, Charpin J. The prevention of the bronchoconstrictor effects of deep inspiration or of cigarette smoking in asthmatic patients by SCH 1000. Postgrad Med J 1975; 51:102.
164. Tinkelman DG, Cavanaugh MJ, Cooper DM. Inhibition of exercise-induced bronchospasm by atropine. Am Rev Respir Dis 1976; 114:87–94.
165. Sheppard D, Epstein J, Holtzman MJ, Nadel JA, Boushey HA. Dose-dependent inhibition of cold air-induced bronchoconstriction by atropine. J Appl Physiol 1982; 53:169–174.
166. Widdicombe JG, Kent DC, Nadel JA. Mechanism of bronchoconstriction during inhalation of dust. J Appl Physiol 1962; 17:613–616.
167. Boushey HA, Richardson PS, Widdicombe JG. Reflex effects of laryngeal irritation on the pattern of breathing and total lung resistance. J Physiol (Lond) 1972; 224: 501–513.
168. Gertner A, Bromberger-Barnea B, Kelly L, Traystman R, Menkes H. Local vagal responses in the lung periphery. J Appl Physiol 1984; 57:1079–1088.
169. Jacoby D, Wagner E. Airway smooth muscle reflex responses to methacholine (abstr). Am J Respir Crit Care Med 1996; 153:A628.
170. Belmonte K, Fryer A, Costello R. Role of insulin in antigen induced airway eosinophilia and neuronal M_2 muscarinic receptor dysfunction in rats. J Appl Physiol 1998; 85:1708–1718.
171. Gold WM, Kessler GF, Yu DYC. Role of vagus nerves in experimental asthma in allergic dogs. J Appl Physiol 1972; 33:719–725.
172. Koller E. Respiratory reflexes during anaphylactic bronchial asthma in guinea pigs. Experientia 1969; 25:368–369.
173. Mills JE, Widdicombe JG. Role of the vagus nerves in anaphylaxis and histamine-induced bronchoconstriction in guinea-pigs. Br J Pharmacol 1970; 39:724–731.
174. Zimmermann I, Islam M, Lanser K, Ulmer W. Antigen-induced airway obstruction and the influence of vagus blockade. Respiration 1976; 33:95–103.
175. Miller M, Patterson R, Harris K. A comparison of immunologic asthma to two types of cholinergic responses in the rhesus monkey. J Lab Clin Med 1976; 88: 995–1007.
176. Hirshman C, Downes H. Basenji-greyhound dog model of asthma: Influence of atropine on antigen-induced bronchoconstriction. J Appl Physiol 1981; 50:761–765.

177. Eiser N, Guz A. Effect of atropine on experimentally induced airway obstruction in man. Bull Eur Physiol Pathol Respir 1982; 18:449–460.
178. Ruffin R, Cockcroft D, Hargreave F. A comparison of the protective effect of fenoterol and SCH 1000 on allergen-induced asthma. J Allergy Clin Immunol 1978; 61: 42–47.
179. Rosenthal R, Norman P, Summer W, Permutt S. Role of the parasympathetic system in antigen induced bronchospasm. J Appl Physiol 1977; 42:600–606.
180. Cockcroft DW, Ruffin RE, Dolovich J, Hargreave FE. Allergen-induced increases in non-allergic bronchial reactivity. Clin Allergy 1977; 7:505–513.
181. Schiller I, Lowell F. the effects of drugs in modifying the response of asthmatic subjects to inhalation of pollen extracts as determined by vital capacity measurements. Ann Allergy 1947; 5:564–566.
182. Kresten W. Protective effect of metered aerosol SCH 1000 (ipratropium bromide) against bronchoconstriction by allergen inhalation. Respiration 1974; 31:412–417.
183. Orehek J, Gayard P, Grimaud C, Charpin J. Allergen-induced bronchoconstriction in asthma: antagonistic effect of a synthetic anticholinergic drug. Bull Physiol Pathol Resp Nancy 1975; 11:193–201.
184. Schultz-Weringhaus G. Anticholinergic versus beta adrenergic therapy in allergic airways obstruction. Respiration 1981; 41:239–247.
185. Little JW, Hall WJ, Douglas RG, Mudholkar GS, Speers DM, Patel K. Airway hyperreactivity and peripheral airway dysfunction in influenza A infection. Am Rev Respir Dis 1978; 118:295–303.
186. Frick OL, German DF, Mills J. Development of allergy in children: I. association with virus infections. J Allergy Clin Immunol 1979; 63:228–241.
187. Henderson FW, Clyde WA, Collier AM, Denny FW, Senior RJ, Sheaffer CI, Conley WG, Christian RM. The etiologic and epidemiologic spectrum of bronchiolitis in pediatric practice. J Pediatr 1979; 95:183–190.
188. Welliver RC. Upper respiratory infections in asthma. J Allergy Clin Immunol 1983; 72:341–346.
189. Frick WE, Busse WW. Respiratory infections: Their role in airway responsiveness and pathogenesis of asthma. Clin Chest Med 1988; 9:539–549.
190. Johnston S, Pattemore P, Sanderson G. Community study of role of viral infections in exacerbations of asthma in 9–11 year old children. Br Med J 1995; 310:1225–1229.
191. Empey DW, Laitinen LA, Jacobs L, Gold WM, Nadel JA. Mechanisms of bronchial hyperreactivity in normal subjects following upper respiratory tract infection. Am Rev Respir Dis 1976; 113:523–527.
192. Aquilina AT, Hall WJ, Douglas RG, Utell MJ. Airway reactivity in subjects with viral upper respiratory tract infections: the effects of exercise and cold air. Am Rev Respir Dis 1980; 122:3–10.
193. Jacoby DB, Xiao HQ, Lee NH, Fryer AD. Virus- and interferon-induced loss of inhibitory M_2 muscarinic receptor function and gene expression in cultured airway parasympathetic neurons. J Clin Invest 1998; 102:242–248.
194. Catterall J, Rhind G, Shapiro C, Douglas N. Is nocturnal asthma caused by changes in airway cholinergic activity? Thorax 1988; 43:720–724.

195. Morrison J, Pearson S, Dean H. Parasympathetic nervous system in nocturnal asthma. Br Med J 1988; 296:1427–1429.
196. Martin R, Cicutto L, Smith H, Ballard R, Szefler S. Airways inflammation in nocturnal asthma. Am Rev Respir Dis 1991; 143:351–357.
197. Smith L, Shelhammer J, Kaliner J. Cholinergic nervous system and immediate hypersensitivity: an analysis of pupillary responses. J Allergy Clin Immunol 1980; 66:374–378.
198. McFadden ER, Luparello T, Lyons H, Bleeker E. The mechanism of action of suggestion in the introduction of acute asthmatic attacks. Psychosom Med 1969; 31:134–143.
199. Neild JE, Cameron IR. Bronchoconstriction in response to suggestion: its prevention by an inhaled anticholinergic agent. Br Med J 1971; 290:674.
200. Grieco M, Pierson R. Mechanism of bronchoconstriction due to beta adrenergic blockade: studies with practolol, propranolol and atropine. J Allergy Clin Immunol 1971; 48:143–152.
201. Giulekas D, Georgopoulos D, Papakosta D, Antoniadou H, Sotiropoulou E, Vamvalis C. Influence of pindolol on asthmatics and effect of bronchodilators. Respiration 1986; 50:158–166.
202. Barnes P. Muscarinic receptors in airways: recent developments. J Appl Physiol 1990; 68:1777–1785.
203. Takahashi T, Belvisi M, Patel H, Ward J, Tadjkarimi S, Yacoub M, Barnes P. Effect of Ba679BR, a novel long-acting anticholinergic agent, on cholinergic neurotransmission in guinea pig and human airways. Am J Respir Crit Care Med 1994; 150:1640–1645.
204. O'Connor B, Towse L, Barnes P. Prolonged effect of tiotropium bromide on methacholine-induced bronchoconstriction in asthma. Am J Respir Crit Care Med 1996; 154:876–880.
205. Alabaster V. Discovery and development of selective M_3 antagonists for clinical use. Life Sci 1997; 60:1053–1060.
206. Cavanaugh M, Cooper D. Inhaled atropine sulphate: dose response characteristics. Am Rev Respir Dis 1976; 114:517–524.
207. Chick T, Jenne J. Comparative bronchodilator responses to atropine and terbutaline in asthma and chronic bronchitis Chest 1977; 72:719–723.
208. Crompton G. A comparison of responses to bronchodilator drugs in chronic bronchitis and acute asthma. Thorax 1968; 23:46–55.
209. Cropp G. The role of the parasympathetic nervous system in the maintenance of chronic airway obstruction in asthmatic children. Am Rev Respir Dis 1975; 112: 599–605.
210. Larsen G, Barron R, Cotton E, Brooks J. A comparative study of inhaled atropine sulphate and isoproterenol hydrochloride in cystic fibrosis. Am Rev Respir Dis 1979; 119:399–407.
211. Ullah MI, Newman GB, Saunders KB. Influence of age on response to ipratropium and salbutamol in asthma. Thorax 1981; 36:523–529.
212. Reisman J, Galdes-Sebalt M, Kazim F, Canny G, Levison H. Frequent administration by inhalation of salbutamol and ipratropium bromide in the initial management of severe acute asthma in children. J Allergy Clin Immunol 1988; 81:16–20.

213. Schuh S, Johnson D, Callahan S, Canny G, Levinson H. Efficacy of frequent nebulized ipratropium bromide added to frequent high dose albuterol therapy in severe childhood asthma. J Pediatr 1995; 126:639–645.
214. Patrick D, Dales R, Stark R, Laliberte G, Dickinson G. Severe exacerbations of COPD and asthma: Incremental benefit of adding ipratropium to the usual therapy. Chest 1990; 98:295–297.
215. Young G, Freitas P. A randomized comparison of atropine and metaproterenol inhalation therapies for refractory status asthmatics [published erratum appears in Ann Emerg Med 1991; 20:1031]. Ann Emerg Med 1991; 20:513–519.
216. Karpel J, Schacter E, Fanta C. A comparison of ipratropium and albuterol vs. albuterol alone for treatment of acute asthma. Chest 1996; 110:611–616.
217. Marini J, Lakshminarayan S. The effect of atropine inhalation in ''irreversible'' chronic bronchitis. Chest 1980; 77:591–596.
218. Maeson F, Smeets J, Sledsens T, Wald F, Cornelissen P. Tiotropium bromide, a new long acting antimuscarinic bronchodilator: a pharmacodynamic study in patients with chronic obstructive pulmonary disease (COPD). Eur J Respir Dis 1995; 8:1506–1513.
219. Shrestha M, O'Brian T, Haddox R, Gourlay H, Reed G. Decreased duration of emergency department treatment of chronic obstructive pulmonary disease exacerbations with the addition of ipratropium bromide to beta-agonist therapy. Ann Emerg Med 1991; 20:1206–1209.
220. Cruz A, Togias A, Lichtenstein L, Kagey-Sobotka A, Proud D, Naclerio R. Local application of atropine attenuates the upper airway reaction to cold, dry air. Am Rev Respir Dis. 1992; 146:340–346.
221. Baroody F, Wagenmann M, Naclerio R. Comparison of the secretory response of the nasal mucosa to methacholine and histamine. J Appl Physiol 1993; 74:2661–2671.
222. Philip G, Jankowski R, Baroody F, Naclerio R, Togias A. Reflex activation of nasal secretion by unilateral inhalation of cold dry air. Am Rev Respir Dis 1993; 148:1616–1622.
223. Baroody F, Ford S, Lichtenstein L, Kagey-Sobotka A, Naclerio R. Physiologic responses and histamine release after nasal antigen challenge: effect of atropine. Am J Respir Crit Care Med 1994; 149:1457–1465.
224. Meltzer EO, Orgel HA, Bronsky EA, Findlay SR, Georgitis JN, Grossman J, Ratner P, Wood CC. Ipratropium bromide aqueous nasal spray for patients with perennial allergic rhinitis: a study of its effect on their symptoms, quality of life, and nasal cytology. J Allergy Clin Immunol 1992; 90:242–249.
225. Bronsky EA, Druce H, Findlay SR, Hampel FC, Kaiser H, Ratner P, Valentine MD, Wood CC. A clinical trial of ipratropium bromide nasal spray in patients with perennial non allergic rhinitis. J Allergy Clin Immunol 1995; 95:1117–1122.
226. Hayden F, Diamond L, Wood P, Korts D, Wecker M. Effectiveness and safety of intranasal ipratropium bromide in common colds: a randomized, double-blind, placebo-controlled trial. Ann Intern Med 1996; 125:89–97.

5

Long-Acting β_2-Agonist Drugs

RICHARD BEASLEY, JULIAN CRANE, and CARL D. BURGESS

Wellington School of Medicine
Otago University
Wellington, New Zealand

I. Introduction

It is nearly 10 years since the introduction of the inhaled long-acting β_2-agonists formoterol and salmeterol. They have become an integral part of the pharmaceutical management for patients with moderate to severe persistent asthma whose disease is not controlled with regular use of inhaled corticosteroids. In contrast to the short-acting β_2-agonists, long-acting agents are used regularly, with the therapeutic endpoint being better overall control of the patient's symptoms and improved lung function. Studies that have examined their efficacy and safety have provided insight not only into the optimal ways in which these agents can be used in the management of asthma but also into issues relating to the use of β_2-agonist drugs in general. In this chapter, we examine the role of long-acting β_2-agonists in the treatment of asthma, highlighting issues where clinical uncertainty still exists.

II. Pharmacology

Although there are similarities between the two drugs, salmeterol has a longer side chain than formoterol, and both have longer side chains than the short-acting

β_2-agonists (such as salbutamol). Salmeterol is more lipid-soluble than formoterol, but both drugs have a higher degree of lipophilicity than the short-acting β_2-agonists (1). This latter property may be the reason for their long duration of action (see below).

A. Receptor Properties

A number of studies have been performed investigating the potency, efficacy, selectivity, and affinity of salmeterol and formoterol using in vitro techniques with both animal and human tissues. Both drugs have been compared with one another and with other β_2-agonists (2–5). In essence, the species used did not seem to affect the results. In a comparative study of different β_2-agonists, Naline et al. showed in isolated human bronchus that formoterol was the most potent, followed by fenoterol, salmeterol, isoprenaline, salbutamol, adrenaline, and terbutaline, respectively (Table 1) (2). The study showed that all the agents acted as partial agonists at the β_2-receptor when compared to isoprenaline, but formoterol had much greater efficacy than salmeterol, salbutamol, and terbutaline, all of which had about equal efficacy, proving that these latter agents are partial agonists when compared with formoterol (2). In these (2) and in similar experiments using guinea pig trachea (3,4), formoterol was approximately 200 times more potent than salmeterol (3,4). Roux et al. examined the effects of formoterol,

Table 1 Potency, Efficacy, and Intrinsic Activity of β_2-Agonists in Isolated Human Bronchus[a]

	Resting Tone			ACh 10^{-3}M		
	-log EC_{50}	E_{max}	IA	-log EC_{50}	E_{max}	IA
Isoprenaline	7.31	98	1.00	6.56	85	1.00
Adrenaline	6.85	95	0.97	6.29	87	1.02
Salbutamol	7.12	83[b]	0.85	—	55[b]	0.64
Terbutaline	6.48	94	0.96	—	56[d]	0.66
Fenoterol	8.02	97	0.99	6.96	64[d]	0.75
Formoterol	9.63	94[c]	0.96	8.74	71	0.84
Salmeterol	7.60	70[b]	0.71	—	53[b]	0.62

[a]The potency (-log EC_{50}), efficacy (E_{max}) and intrinsic activity (IA) of various β_2-agonists compared with isoprenaline in isolated human bronchus at resting tone or precontracted with acetylcholine (ACh).

[b]$p < 0.001$, significantly different from isoprenaline.

[c]$p < 0.05$

[d]$p < 0.01$

Source: From Ref. 2.

salmeterol, salbutamol, fenoterol, and isoprenaline in guinea pig tissues precontracted with histamine (5). Both long-acting agents were 10 times as potent as isoprenaline and fenoterol and 100 times more potent than salbutamol in minimally contracted tissues (Fig. 1). However, when the tissue was maximally contracted, although salmeterol was equally potent with formoterol, it acted as a partial agonist when compared to formoterol or salbutamol, which showed equal efficacy in this model.

Selectivity studies have shown that formoterol and salmeterol are more selective for the β_2 receptor than other β_2-receptor agonists, such as salbutamol and terbutaline (5–7). Furthermore, both long-acting agents have a higher affinity for the β_2-receptor than the other β_2-agonists (5).

In summary, both formoterol and salmeterol are more potent and more selective for the β_2-receptor than the commonly used short-acting β_2-agonists, such as salbutamol and terbutaline, and salmeterol acts as a partial agonist when compared with formoterol in animal models. Whether all of these properties are important in the clinical situation is open to question, particularly the role of partial agonism, because this property becomes evident only at tissue concentrations well above those attained in clinical use.

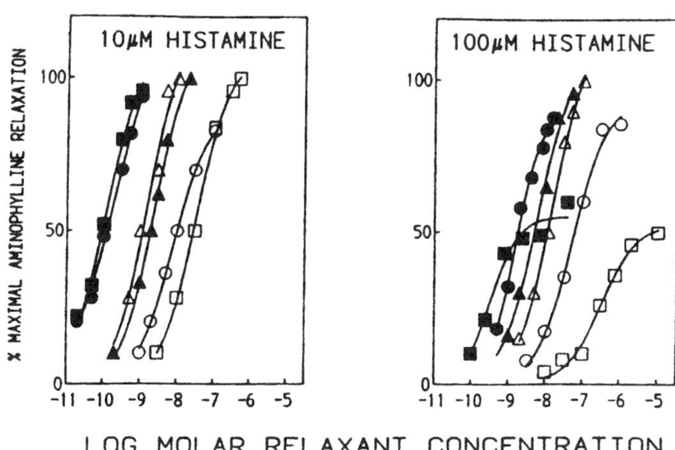

Figure 1 Concentration-response curves to β_2-agonists in guinea pig tracheal spirals precontracted with 10 and 100 μm histamine. Relaxation relative to a maximal effect of aminophylline is plotted against the negative log molar concentration of the relaxant. Values are mean ± SEM from three to six spirals. Formoterol (solid circles), salmeterol (solid squares), fenoterol (open triangles), salbutamol (open circles), isoprenaline (solid triangles), soterenol (open squares). (From Ref. 5.)

B. Duration of Action

In vitro studies have shown that both formoterol and salmeterol relax tracheal smooth muscle for a longer period of time than other β_2-agonists that are commonly used as bronchodilators, independent of the species used; salmeterol has a longer duration of action than formoterol (Table 2) (2,8,9). In vitro studies have also demonstrated differences between salmeterol and the other β_2-agonists in that the duration of smooth muscle relaxation, onset of relaxation, and maximum relaxation attained in the trachea with isoprenaline, fenoterol, salbutamol, and formoterol is dose-dependent, whereas such dose-dependence could not be demonstrated with salmeterol (8,9). The reason for this lack of dose-response with salmeterol is unknown but it is probably due to the fact that ''low doses'' cause a maximum effect. The only effect that is dose-related in in vitro studies with salmeterol is that increasing the dose administered results in a more rapid onset of action (8).

C. Mechanism of Action

Two major theories have been proposed to explain the long duration of action of these β_2-agonists. The first is the exosite theory, which broadly states that there is an exosite (or exoreceptor site) where the inactive chain (or tail) of these agonists bind (10). This holds the drug in place and allows the active head to

Table 2 Duration of Action of β_2-Agonists on Isolated Human Bronchus

	$tE/_2$ Recovery,[a] min	
Isoprenaline 3×10^{-7}M	4.22	±0.63
Adrenaline 10^{-7}M	2.15	±0.54[b]
Salbutamol 3×10^{-7}M	7.59	±2.30
Terbutaline 10^{-6}M	9.44	±1.90[b]
Fenoterol 3×10^{-8}M	7.21	±0.88[b]
Formoterol 3×10^{-9}M	33.9	±4.9[c]
Salmeterol 3×10^{-7}M	102.2	±24.7[d]

[a] $tE/_2$ is calculated as the time from washing the preparation to attainment of 50% of basal tone.
[b] $p < 0.05$, significantly different from isoprenaline
[c] $p < 0.001$
[d] $p < 0.01$
Source: From Ref. 2.

engage with the β_2-receptor. Theoretically, this would account for a longer duration of action and may also account for the reassertion of the relaxant effects when the drug is displaced from the β_2-receptor. There is evidence that such reassertion can be demonstrated with both salmeterol and formoterol in the guinea pig trachea (Fig. 2) (3). In this study, after a β_2-antagonist (sotalol) was added to the medium and washings were performed, both formoterol and salmeterol reasserted their action after the washings or after sotalol was removed. Salbutamol, an agent with a shorter side chain, was unable to reassert its action under the same conditions, whereas other agents, such as clenbuterol, which also does not have a long chain, did demonstrate this effect (11). It has also been pointed out that the chain of formoterol is probably not long enough to bind to an exosite; thus there are major doubts surrounding this theory (8).

The second proposed theory is the microkinetic diffusion model of Anderson et al. (8). This theory proposes that the property of lipid solubility is more important and suggests that salmeterol, with its very high degree of lipid solubility, associates predominantly into the lipid bilayer of the cell membrane. From here it diffuses towards the β_2-receptor, where it exerts its action. Because of its structure, salmeterol persists in the lipid bilayer. This would explain the slow onset of action and the prolonged duration of action of this agent. Formoterol, which is not as lipid-soluble as salmeterol but does have a very high affinity for the β_2-receptor, would be able to bind to the receptor and also associate into the lipid layer. It would therefore act rapidly and have a prolonged duration of action (Fig. 3). At present, this seems the more attractive theory, but further research is still required. Such a theory would explain the finding in the clinical setting

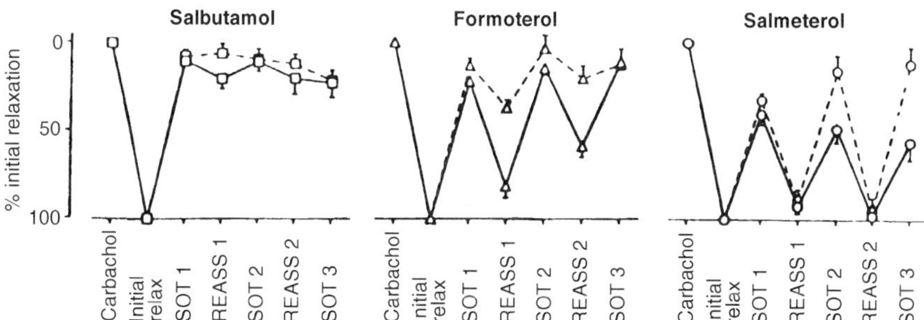

Figure 2 Reassertion of relevant effects after β_2-receptor blockade followed by washout for formoterol, salmeterol, and salbutamol. The guinea pig trachea was precontracted with 0.2 μm carbachol. The data are presented as mean (SEM) percentage of the initial relaxation caused by the β_2-agonist before β-receptor blockade with 10 μm sotalol. (From Ref. 3.)

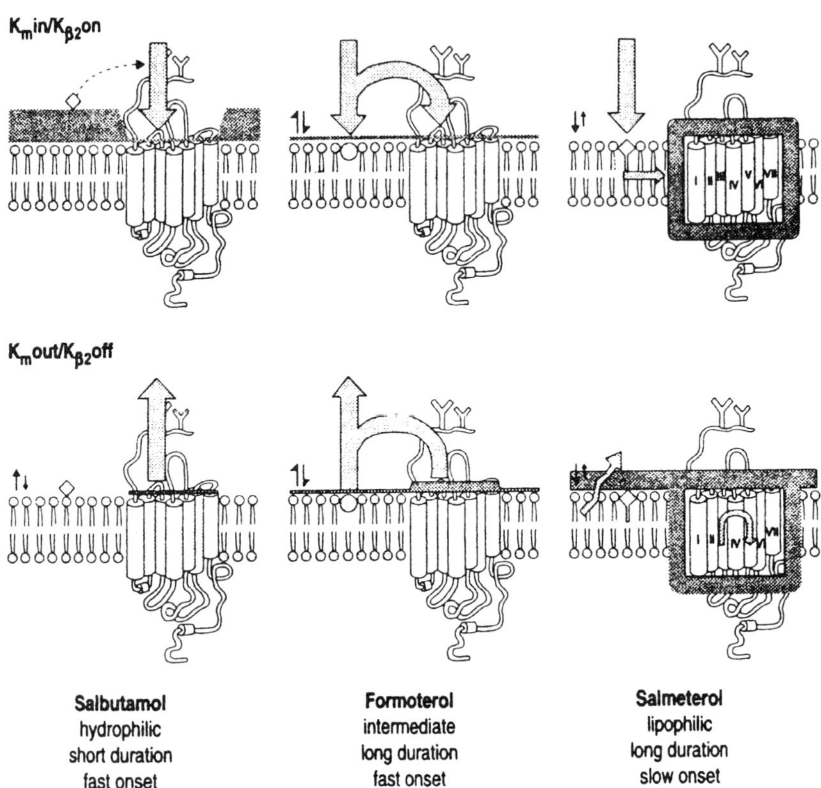

Figure 3 The microkinetic diffusion model. Top panel: During drug association with the receptor, the interaction of salbutamol with the membrane lipid is energetically unfavorable (shaded barrier) and salbutamol associates with the receptor directly, exhibiting a rapid onset, but it diffuses from tissues rapidly. The association of formoterol with both receptor and lipid is thermodynamically favorable, allowing fast onset. It is also retained in the lipid layer, allowing continual activation of the receptor. Salmeterol associates predominantly with lipid, and this interaction will cause a slow onset of action. Bottom panel: Dissociation of salbutamol and formoterol is not impeded, but formoterol has a high affinity for the receptor and is also retained with moderate affinity by lipid. Salmeterol is avidly retained by lipid accounting for its long duration of action (From Ref. 8.)

that formoterol acts more rapidly than salmeterol but that there is no difference in the duration of bronchodilation between the two drugs.

D. Pharmacokinetics

The pharmacokinetics of formoterol and salmeterol after inhalation have not been adequately studied, probably due to the small amount of drug that would get into the plasma. Both drugs are highly active by inhalation; swallowed portions of each are metabolized in the liver with a high degree of first-pass metabolism. Salmeterol is approximately 95% protein-bound, whereas formoterol shows approximately 50% protein binding. Only some 5% of salmeterol is excreted unchanged in the urine, and approximately 10% of an oral dose of formoterol is found unchanged in human urine (12).

III. Clinical Studies

A. Short-Term Use

Bronchodilation

When inhaled in the recommended therapeutic doses [12 μg formoterol, 50 μg salmeterol via a metered-dose inhaler (MDI)], both agents cause bronchodilation that persists for more than 12 hr, with the duration dependent on the dose administered. Indeed, in some studies, bronchodilation has been observed for at least 24 hr (13), although the phase and amplitude of the circadian variation in forced expiratory volume in 1 s (FEV_1) were not affected (Fig. 4) (13).

The main difference in the bronchodilator properties of these long-acting agents relates to the speed of their onset of action. When inhaled, formoterol has a rapid onset of action, with bronchodilation observed within a few minutes and a maximum effect within 60–120 min, whereas salmeterol causes a slower onset of action with a maximum bronchodilation occurring after 2–4 hr (Fig. 5) (14,15).

Protection Against Bronchoconstrictor Stimuli

The long-acting β_2-agonist drugs protect against a wide variety of bronchoconstrictor stimuli, including methacholine (13), histamine (16,17), adenosine 5′-monophosphate (AMP) (18,19), hyperventilation (20), exercise (21,22) and allergen (23). This protection is primarily due to functional antagonism of the airway smooth muscle contraction, although inhibition of mast-cell mediator release is also important in protecting against some stimuli such as AMP, hyperventilation, exercise, and the immediate response to allergen. Studies that have examined the time course of this protection have observed that in the case of both formoterol and salmeterol, its duration may last up to 24 hr, although the phase and amplitude of the circadian variation in airway hyperresponsiveness were not affected (13).

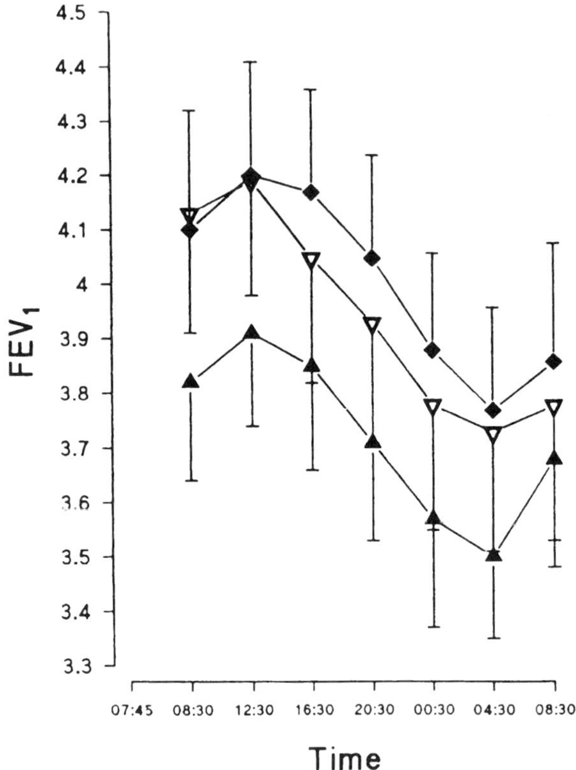

Figure 4 The bronchodilator effect of salmeterol and formoterol throughout a 24-hr period. The mean values and standard errors of mean of FEV_1 (in liters) over 24 hr after inhaling placebo (▲), formoterol (12 μg) (△), and salmeterol (50 μg) (◆) are shown. Although formoterol and salmeterol caused bronchoconstriction that persisted for at least 24 hr, these agents influenced neither the phase nor the amplitude of the circadian variation in FEV_1. (From Ref. 13.)

B. Long-Term Use

Comparison with Short-Acting β_2-Agonists

Numerous large controlled clinical trials have shown that the regular twice-daily use of salmeterol and formoterol by both children and adults produces greater improvement in symptoms, quality of life, and lung function (morning and evening peak flow) and reduces the need for rescue bronchodilators than does the use of short-acting β_2-agonists, such as salbutamol or terbutaline, when taken four times a day (24–29). The magnitude of this subjective and objective im-

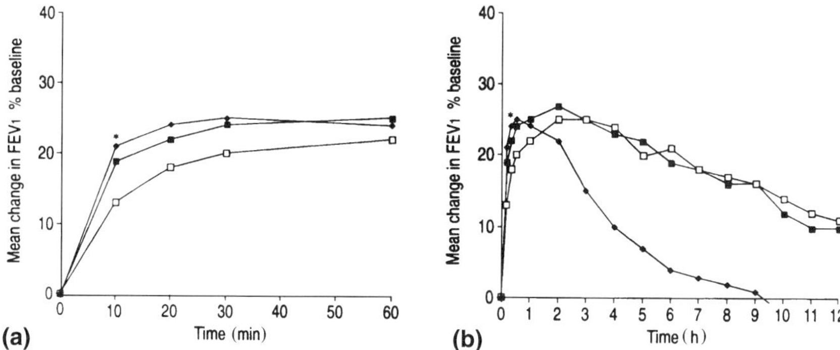

Figure 5 The time course of the bronchodilator response to inhalation of formoterol (24 μg)(■), salmeterol (50 μg)(□), and salbutamol (200 μg)(◆). The mean changes in FEV_1 (% baseline) are shown for (a) the first 60 min after inhalation; (b) the first 12 hr after inhalation. * denotes significant difference ($p < 0.05$) between salmeterol and formoterol at 10 min. (From Ref. 14.)

provement is of clinical significance and may relate in part to the administration of salmeterol and formoterol in relatively higher doses than the short-acting β_2-agonists when their greater potency is taken into consideration (30). Both the control of asthma symptoms and improvements in lung function have been shown to be maintained for at least 1 to 2 years (31,32).

One of the consistent features of these controlled clinical studies has been that despite a marked improvement in symptoms and lung function, there has been no associated reduction in the frequency of severe or ''life-threatening'' exacerbations, whether measured as a requirement for a hospital admission or emergency visits to medical care. However, this interpretation is limited by insufficient power to determine whether small yet clinically significant differences may exist. This problem was overcome by the Salmeterol Surveillance Study, undertaken specifically to investigate whether salmeterol increases the risk of a severe or life-threatening attack of asthma (33). In this study 25,180 asthmatic patients considered to require regular treatment with bronchodilators were randomly allocated to receive either salbutamol (200 μg four times a day) or salmeterol (50 μg twice daily) for a 12-week period, with major adverse events recorded to determine whether the regular use of salmeterol led to a worsening of asthma control. The study demonstrated that salmeterol did not influence the frequency of severe asthma attacks leading to hospital admission (relative risk 0.95; $p = 0.7$).

These findings could be interpreted in two ways. First, it can be concluded that the long-term use of salmeterol is not associated with deteriorating asthma control, leading to severe attacks that require admission to hospital. Conversely, despite marked symptomatic and lung function improvement, there is no associated reduction in the frequency or magnitude of severe attacks of asthma. This is perhaps not surprising, as a severe attack of asthma can be defined in terms of a lack of response to β_2-agonist therapy due to the dominant role of airways inflammation, including mucous plugging in its pathogenesis. It does, however, serve to caution medical practitioners and patients that despite marked symptomatic improvement, a concomitant amelioration in the rate of severe exacerbations requiring hospital admission cannot be expected, and that this would need to be achieved through alternative drug therapy, such as inhaled corticosteroids.

Responders and Nonresponders

Another feature of these studies is that not all subjects respond to the long-acting β_2-agonist drugs in terms of greater efficacy than to the regular use of short-acting β_2-agonists. For example, in one study, the addition of salmeterol resulted in a greater than 5% increase in morning peak expiratory flow (PEF) in only half of the symptomatic asthmatics studied after 21 weeks of treatment (34).

Furthermore, there are reports of asthmatic patients who show a striking difference in bronchodilator response to formoterol or salmeterol. For example, Ulrik et al. reported an asthmatic patient in whom formoterol was more effective than salmeterol both in immediate response and during long-term treatment (35). The clinical implication of their observations is that a poor response in an individual patient to one of the long-acting β_2-agonists should not preclude a trial with the other. Further studies are required comparing the clinical efficacy of formoterol and salmeterol; these will need to address the issue of responders and nonresponders to both drugs.

Formoterol Versus Salmeterol

At the time of this review, there has only been one published clinical study in which the long-term efficacy of formoterol and salmeterol had been compared (36). In this study, adult asthmatic patients received either formoterol 12 μg bid or salmeterol 50 μg bid, both through dry-powder delivery systems. Throughout the 6-month treatment period, there was no difference in the respiratory symptom scores, the morning prebronchodilator PEF (the primary outcome variable), or the use of rescue medication. Formoterol was superior in terms of evening prebronchodilator PEF, the clinical significance of this difference being uncertain. The authors concluded that salmeterol and formoterol had similar long-term efficacy (36).

Comparison with Inhaled Corticosteroid Therapy

Consideration of the potential role of these agents in the long-term treatment of asthma has led to their comparison with inhaled corticosteroid therapy.

Comparison as Sole Therapy

The issue of the comparative efficacy of treatment with inhaled corticosteroids or a long-acting β_2-agonist as sole therapy in asthma has been addressed in few studies. One of the major studies in children compared the efficacy of inhaled beclomethasone dipropionate (BDP) 200 μg twice daily with salmeterol 50 μg twice daily (administered by dry-powder devices) in children with mild to moderate persistent asthma who had not been treated with inhaled corticosteroids in the previous 6 months (37). During the 12-month treatment period, inhaled salbutamol was allowed as rescue medication and, if necessary, a course of oral prednisone was administered to those with severe exacerbations. The study results showed that BDP produced a significantly greater absolute increase in pre- and postbronchodilator FEV_1 than salmeterol (Fig. 6a). Airway hyperresponsiveness gradually decreased in the BDP group in contrast to the salmeterol group, in which airway hyperresponsiveness increased (2.02 versus −0.73 doubling doses of methacholine PD_{20}, respectively) (Fig. 6b). For both FEV_1 and PD_{20}, the worsening with salmeterol became more pronounced during the 2-week follow-up period at the end of the 1 year of treatment. Symptom scores improved in both treatment groups, but to a greater extent with BDP, and the number of exacerbations requiring oral prednisone was greater with salmeterol (21 versus 3, respectively). The authors concluded that monotherapy with a long-acting β_2-agonist may carry a risk of masking the severity of the disease, and that their findings supported the recommendation that long-acting β_2-agonists should not be used as sole therapy in asthma.

Comparable findings have been published in a similar study in which children received either salmeterol (50 μg bid), BDP (200 μg bid), or placebo (via a Diskhaler device) (38). The primary endpoint of airway hyperresponsiveness was significantly reduced with BDP as compared with salmeterol or placebo throughout the 12-month treatment period. Compared with placebo, both BDP and salmeterol significantly improved the FEV_1, but only BDP significantly reduced symptoms and the need for additional bronchodilator medication. In contrast to the studies in children, in a preliminary report of a 6-week study in adults, no significant differences in clinical efficacy were observed between salmeterol 50 μg bid, fluticasone 250 μg bid, or the combination (39). Interpretation of this study is difficult due to the small number of patients included and the short duration of treatment.

Addition to Existing Inhaled Corticosteroid Therapy

Studies in both children and adults have shown that when compared with placebo or regular use of short-acting β_2-agonists, the addition of salmeterol or formoterol to existing corticosteroid therapy results in a greater improvement of asthma symptoms and lung function (24–29,40,41). These findings relate to subjects with unstable asthma despite treatment with BDP or budesonide in doses up to 3200

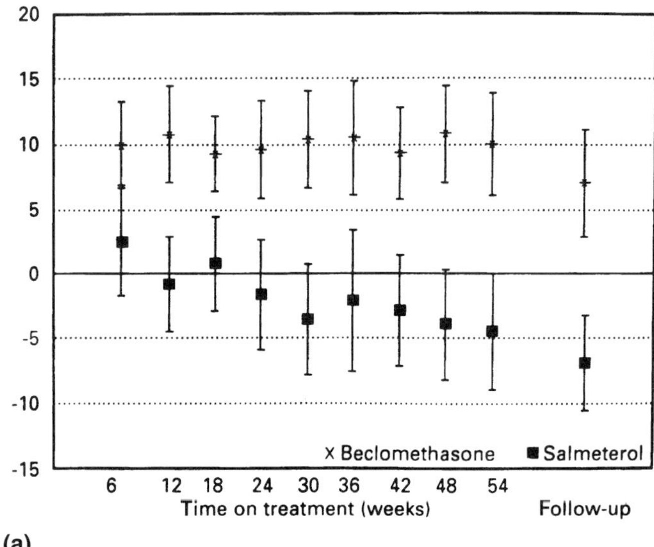

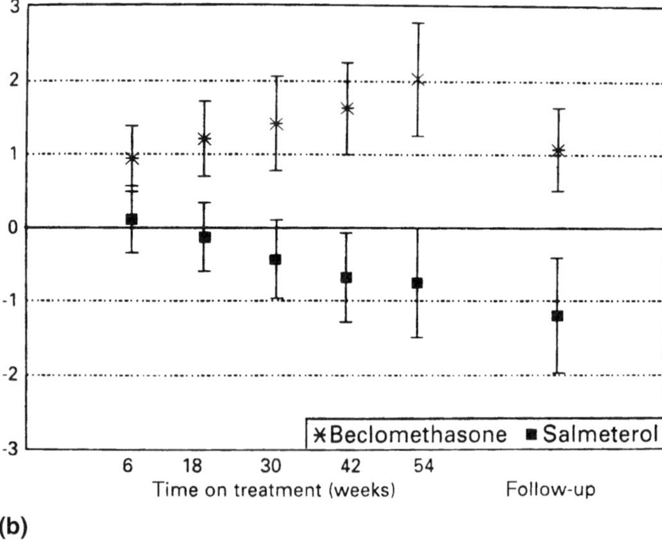

Figure 6 Comparison of the efficacy of salmeterol (■) 50 μg twice a day with beclomethasone 200 μg twice a day in children with mild to moderate persistent asthma, showing (a) changes in FEV_1% predicted (mean ±95% CI) from baseline; (b) changes in airway responsiveness (PD_{20} methacholine) in doubling doses (mean ±95% CI). (From Ref. 37.)

μg daily, with the degree of improvement apparently independent of the dose of the inhaled corticosteroid.

The issue as to whether the addition of a long-acting β_2-agonist may allow significant reduction in the dose of inhaled corticosteroids has also been studied (40). Compared with placebo, salmeterol treatment was associated with a mean 17% reduction in inhaled corticosteroid use without influencing the exacerbation rate. However, this reduction should not be interpreted as the maximum steroid-sparing effect of salmeterol, as subjects had limited freedom to reduce their inhaled corticosteroid dose according to predetermined criteria. For secondary endpoints, salmeterol was associated with higher morning and evening peak flow and a reduction in symptoms and bronchodilator use. The effect of salmeterol was maintained over 6 months with no evidence of tolerance to any clinical endpoint, including bronchodilator responsiveness to salbutamol. These findings are relevant to the use of salmeterol in clinical practice, providing reassurance that if salmeterol is introduced, a subsequent reduction in the dose of inhaled corticosteroids is unlikely to have a detrimental effect in patients who follow an appropriate management plan.

Comparison with Increasing the Dose of Inhaled Corticosteroids

Comparison of the efficacy of adding salmeterol or formoterol with that of increasing the dose of inhaled corticosteroids in patients with asthma who are symptomatic despite treatment with regular inhaled corticosteroids and short-acting β_2-agonist drugs has also been studied. In patients with severe persistent asthma who were symptomatic despite maintenance treatment with 400 μg of BDP daily, Greening et al. reported that the addition of twice-daily salmeterol was superior to increasing the dose of BDP to 1000 μg per day in terms of reducing daytime and nighttime symptoms and improving lung function (34).

Comparable findings were observed in a subsequent study of similar design in which patients with severe asthma received either 2000 μg of BDP daily or 1000 μg of BDP daily plus salmeterol at either 50 or 100 μg twice daily (42). There were improvements in symptoms and pulmonary function in both the group treated with an increase in inhaled corticosteroids and the groups treated with salmeterol, although treatment with salmeterol was more effective. There was no difference in efficacy between the two doses of salmeterol and there was no evidence of an adverse effect of salmeterol on airway hyperresponsiveness. As with the previous study (34), the greater subjective and objective improvement with salmeterol was not associated with a greater reduction in the severe exacerbation rate.

The major equivalent study with formoterol examined the efficacy of adding formoterol 12 μg twice daily to low (200 μg daily) and high (800 μg daily) doses of inhaled budesonide over the period of 1 year (43). The primary outcome measure was severe exacerbations (defined as the requirement for treatment with oral steroids or a decrease in peak flow of $>30\%$ below baseline on 2 consecutive

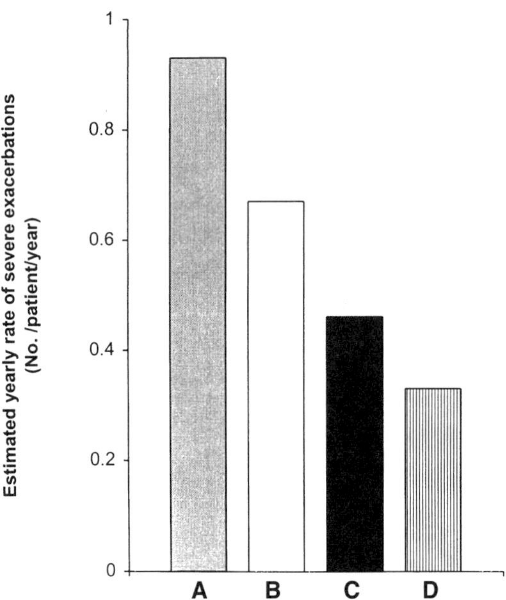

Figure 7 Frequency of severe exacerbations of asthma in patients treated with low-dose budesonide (200 μg daily) (A); low-dose budesonide (200 μg daily) plus formoterol (12 μg twice daily) (B); high-dose budesonide (800 μg daily) (C); or high-dose budesonide (800 μg daily) plus formoterol (12 μg twice daily) (D). The reduction in severe exacerbations was greater with increased doses of inhaled corticosteroids than with the addition of formoterol, while the greatest reduction was observed with the combination regimen. (From Ref. 43.)

days), which were reduced by 26, 49, and 63% with the addition of formoterol, increasing the dose of budesonide, and the combination therapeutic regimen, respectively (Fig. 7). In contrast, there was a greater improvement in symptoms of asthma and lung function with the addition of formoterol rather than the increase in inhaled corticosteroid dose; the combination was superior to either therapy alone. If prevention of severe exacerbations is considered the primary objective in the treatment of patients with severe persistent asthma, the results of this study would suggest that increasing the dose of inhaled corticosteroids is preferable to adding a long-acting β_2-agonist such as formoterol and that the combination is better than either therapeutic intervention alone.

Comparison with Other Therapy

Published clinical trials comparing long-acting β_2-agonist drugs with other drugs used in the treatment of asthma have shown salmeterol and/or formoterol to be more effective than oral theophylline (44), inhaled sodium cromoglycate or nedocromil sodium (45,46), and ketotifen (47) in terms of control of symptoms and lung function and the need for rescue medication in both adult and adolescent patients with asthma.

IV. Airway Inflammation

Since asthma is recognized as a chronic inflammatory disorder of the airway mucosa—involving a number of cell types including mast cells, eosinophils, macrophages, T lymphocytes, epithelial cells, endothelial cells, and myelofibroblasts (48)—another issue to consider is whether long-acting β_2-agonists may have clinically significant anti-inflammatory effects. β_2-receptors are present on a number of these cells and β_2-agonists have been shown to modify the function of many of these cell types in different in vitro and in vivo models (49). The evidence as to whether long-acting β_2-agonists exert a clinically significant anti-inflammatory effect is conflicting and subject to debate (50), although a number of observations can be made.

One model of allergic inflammation in asthma is the airway response to inhaled or locally instilled allergen in asthmatic subjects, where an immediate bronchoconstrictor response occurring within 10 min after challenge is followed by a late asthmatic response occurring 3–7 hr after challenge. The immediate response is primarily due to the release of mediators such as histamine, prostaglandin D_2, and leukotriene C_4 from activated mast cells, whereas the late asthmatic response involves the recruitment and activation of eosinophils and other inflammatory cells with release of various cytokines and pro-inflammatory mediators and is associated with increased airway responsiveness. Both formoterol and salmeterol have been shown to inhibit the early and late bronchoconstrictor response to allergen challenge as well as the associated enhanced airway responsiveness (Fig. 8) (13,23,51).

It is likely that these effects are due to functional antagonism of the bronchoconstrictor stimuli, inhibition of the mast cell–mediated immediate bronchoconstriction, and to some degree inhibition of the eosinophil accumulation and activation within the airways during the late response. Evidence for this latter effect comes from a study in which inhaled salmeterol given 1 hr prior to local endobronchial allergen challenge and every 12 hr thereafter reduced the increment in ECP but not eosinophil numbers in bronchoalveolar lavage (BAL) 24 hr after challenge (52). In this study there was also a decrease in allergen-related increase in IL-4 and IL-5 levels in the BAL, which is consistent with an inhibitory effect on cell activation. This cytokine regulation would be expected to reduce eosinophil recruitment, which would be consistent with the observation that sal-

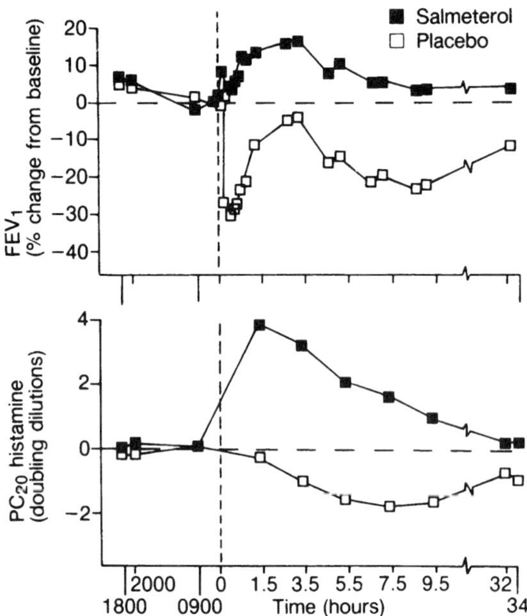

Figure 8 The inhibitory effect of inhaled salmeterol on the immediate and late phases of allergen-induced bronchoconstriction and associated allergen-induced airway hyperresponsiveness. Salmeterol (50 μg)(■) or placebo (□) was administered 10 min before allergen. The FEV_1 (% change from baseline) and histamine responsiveness (cumulative concentration of histamine to produce a greater than 20% decrease in FEV_1–PC_{20}) were measured at intervals up to 34 hr after allergen challenge in eight asthmatic subjects. (From Ref. 51.)

meterol pretreatment inhibits the increase in BAL eosinophils at the later 48-hr time point following local endobronchial allergen challenge (53).

In contrast with the findings in relation to acute allergen-induced inflammation, studies examining the long-term effects of salmeterol have been unable to identify any significant anti-inflammatory effects. In four placebo-controlled studies, treatment with salmeterol for 6 to 8 weeks had no effect on BAL differential cell counts, mediator levels (histamine, tryptase, ECP), T-lymphocyte activation status, or large airway cell populations (mast cells, eosinophils, T lymphocytes) despite reducing symptoms, improving lung function, and reducing airway hyperresponsiveness (54–57).

In summary, these findings would suggest that there are differences in the effects of long-acting β_2-agonist drugs with respect to acute and chronic airway inflammation. Treatment with a long-acting β_2-agonist may modify aspects of cell activation and recruitment following acute allergen exposure. However, long-term treatment in chronic asthma has not been shown to produce a significant effect on underlying airway inflammatory processes, despite symptomatic and physiological improvement. The difference between these findings probably relates to the differing mechanisms, with the acute response predominantly mast cell–dependent, whereas several cell populations—including eosinophils, epithelial cells, and T lymphocytes, in addition to mast cells—have a role in the chronic disease process. These other inflammatory cell types are less susceptible than mast cells to the inhibitory effects of β_2-agonist drugs. Alternatively, desensitization to the inhibitory effects of β_2-agonist therapy with long-term use may contribute to differing findings in relation to acute and long-term effects.

V. Safety

Concerns about the safety of β_2-agonist drugs relate primarily to the short-term side effects after administration, whether their regular use increases chronic asthma severity, and whether long-term use may increase the risk of death.

A. Acute Side Effects

As in the case of the short-acting β_2-agonist drugs, the use of salmeterol and formoterol is associated with extrapulmonary effects such as tremor, hypokalemia and cardiovascular effects including tachycardia, QTc prolongation, and inotropy (24,26–28,40,58). These effects are dose-related and generally attenuated within 2 weeks of commencing therapy due to the development of tolerance.

These studies have examined the side-effect profiles of salmeterol and formoterol when taken according to the recommended dosage regime. However, it is well recognized that asthmatic patients may self-administer very high doses of their β_2-agonists during a severe asthma exacerbation, doses well in excess of those recommended by the manufacturers or the patients' physicians. For example, in a study of the drug use by asthmatic patients during a severe attack, about 30% of the patients had taken more than 45 puffs of their β_2-agonist inhaler during the 24 hr prior to hospital admission (59). As a result, it is necessary to examine the extrapulmonary effects of both salmeterol and formoterol when taken repeatedly in excess of their recommended doses. This particularly applies to formoterol, in view of the regulatory approval in some countries for it to be used for the treatment of bronchoconstriction in addition to regularly scheduled use (60).

Comparison has been made of the extrapulmonary adverse effects of repeated inhalation of formoterol with those of salbutamol, fenoterol, and placebo (61). In this study, subjects inhaled either formoterol (24 μg), salbutamol (400 μg), fenoterol (400 μg), or placebo at 30-min intervals for five doses in an attempt to simulate the use of β_2-agonist drugs in the situation of severe exacerbations of asthma. With repeated inhalations, the inotropic, chronotropic, and electrophysiological effects of formoterol were less than those of fenoterol despite equivalent systemic β_2-receptor effects (Fig. 9). Formoterol behaved like salbutamol with regard to its speed of onset and magnitude of effect on the cardiovascular system, and, as expected, these effects were of greater duration. This high degree of in vivo β_2-selectivity of formoterol is consistent with the in vitro studies (3,4). These findings are reassuring in that they suggest that the adverse side-effect profile of formoterol is similar to that of salbutamol and less in terms of improved β_2-selectivity and lesser magnitude of effects than fenoterol.

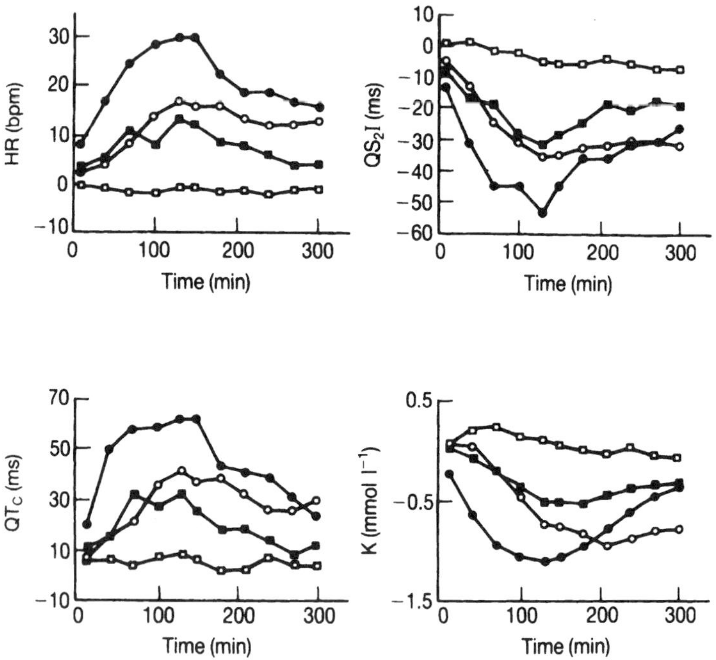

Figure 9 The extrapulmonary side effects of repeated inhalations of formoterol (24 μg per dose)(○), fenoterol (400 μg per dose)(●), salbutamol (400 μg per dose)(■), and placebo (□). The mean change in heart rate (HR), electromechanical systole (QS_21), potassium (K^+), and QTc interval are shown. Each drug was administered at 0, 30, 60, 90, and 120 min. The inotropic, chronotropic, and electrophysiological effects of formoterol were less than those of fenoterol, despite equivalent systemic β_2-receptor effects. (From Ref. 61.)

In a similar study with salmeterol, patients with mild persistent asthma inhaled at hourly intervals placebo; salmeterol 25, 50, 100 and 200 μg; or salbutamol 100, 500, 1000, and 1000 μg (62). Salmeterol and salbutamol caused a mean maximum increase in FEV_1 following the first dose; as a result, the dose equivalence for the airway effects could not be estimated. Heart rate increased and plasma potassium concentration and diastolic blood pressure decreased in a dose-dependent manner following salmeterol and salbutamol, with median dose equivalence for salmeterol compared with salbutamol of 17.7, 7.8, and 7.6 respectively. The magnitude of the responses to this cumulative dose regimen was similar to that observed when salmeterol was given as a single dose. The mean increase in heart rate (16 beats per minute) and mean fall in plasma potassium concentration (0.45 mmol/L) following inhalation of a single 400-μg dose of salmeterol (63) were similar to those observed with the cumulative dose of 375 μg administered in the former study (15 beats per minute; 0.52 mmol/L) (62).

In the clinical studies in which tolerability has been examined, no significant differences in the incidence and type of adverse events have been noted between either salmeterol or formoterol and regular salbutamol regimens (24–29,64,65). These studies, together with large monitoring surveys of prescription events, have shown that in adolescents and adults, headache and tremor are the most common reasons for cessation of treatment (66).

B. Morbidity

Since the introduction of long-acting β_2-agonist drugs, there have been concerns that their use may lead to worsening asthma control and tolerance to their bronchodilator effects, potentially leading to more severe exacerbations. These concerns have been extensively studied, although the clinical relevance of the findings remains uncertain.

Tolerance to Bronchodilator Effects

It has been established that regular administration of long-acting inhaled β_2-agonist therapy leads to the development of tolerance to their nonbronchodilator effects, including tremor, tachycardia, electrophysiological effects (QTc interval prolongation), hyperglycemia, hypokalaemia, and lymphocyte responses (67,68). In contrast, the evidence for tolerance to the bronchodilator effects of long-acting β_2-agonist drugs when taken regularly is less clear, with conflicting results from studies addressing this issue (24,26,68–75).

The difficulties with the interpretation of these studies relate primarily to differences in design and methods of analysis. In a number of the studies that did not show tolerance, there was no placebo control group, and no run-in period without β_2-agonist treatment to control for receptor desensitization before the study. When such a design is used, including a 2-week run-in period during which no β_2-agonists were given, a modest degree of bronchodilator subsensitivity to salbutamol has been demonstrated following 4 weeks of twice-daily administration of salmeterol despite persistent improvement in peak flow rates (72). It was calculated that the tolerance was equivalent to a 2.5- to 4.0-fold greater dose of salbutamol required to produce a similar improvement in FEV_1 and peak expiratory flow rate (PEFR), respectively. However, when these data were reanalyzed with absolute FEV_1 values rather than with the change in FEV_1 from baseline, no subsensitivity to salbutamol could be demonstrated (73,74). This interpretation is supported by a recent placebo-controlled study with a 2-week run-in period in which β_2-agonists were withheld, showing no tolerance to the bronchodilator response to salbutamol after chronic dosing with salmeterol (69). In contrast to these findings with salmeterol, statistically significant declines in the peak level and duration of bronchodilator effect occurred in response to formoterol after 4 weeks of twice-daily treatment, even though the regular use of formoterol was associated with a significant improvement in lung function (68,71). Perhaps the best illustration of the time course and magnitude of this effect is the FACET study (43), in which the initial improvement in morning peak flow in response to formoterol was attenuated by about 50% within days of its use. Importantly, this tolerance did not progress following this period and was not associated with an increased frequency of severe exacerbations of asthma.

Taken together, these studies suggest that some tolerance to the bronchodilator effect of long-acting β_2-agonists may occur with long-term treatment, with desensitization more likely to occur with formoterol than with salmeterol.

When tolerance does occur, it is rapidly reversed by treatment with systemic corticosteroids, with the bronchodilator response restored within 60 min of a single intravenous injection of hydrocortisone (75). This effect of steroids is associated with an upregulation of lymphocyte β_2-receptor function. The mechanism may involve an increase in the rate of synthesis of the β_2-receptors through a process of increased β_2-receptor gene transcription (76) or a reversal or inhibition of internalization of receptors from the cell surface (77). Corticosteroids are also thought to promote the formation of the coupled high-affinity state of the β_2-receptor, which, in turn, increases receptor function (77).

These observations suggest that during a severe exacerbation of asthma, systemic corticosteroids should be administered as soon as possible in order to restore normal airway β_2-receptor sensitivity, particularly in patients receiving long-acting β_2-agonist therapy. In addition, they imply that patients may need to use higher than usual doses of short-acting β_2-agonists to relieve bronchoconstriction in a severe attack of asthma.

There is considerable interindividual variability in the propensity for tolerance to the bronchodilator effects of long-acting β_2-agonist drugs, with evidence suggesting that this may be determined by genetic polymorphisms of the β_2-

receptor. In a recent study in patients with moderate to severe persistent asthma, a significantly greater degree of bronchodilator desensitization was noted after 4 weeks treatment with formoterol in patients homozygous for Gly16 as compared with those who were homozygous for Arg16 (78). An almost 50% reduction in the maximum FEV_1 response to cumulative doses of formoterol was observed in homozygous Gly16 asthmatics, as compared with no change in the maximum bronchodilator response in the homozygous Arg16 asthmatics (Fig. 10). These findings suggest that the Gly16 receptor may not only lead to a reduced efficacy of β_2-agonists when taken during a severe exacerbations of asthma but also a reduction in the bronchoprotective effects of β_2-agonists, as discussed below.

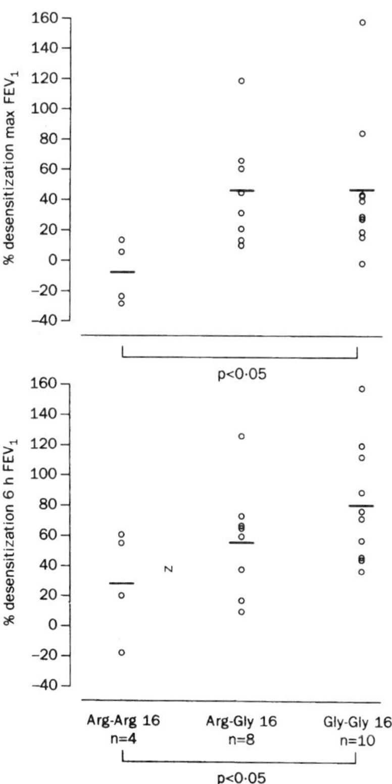

Figure 10 The degree of bronchodilator desensitization after regular formoterol therapy (24 μg twice a day) for 4 weeks. The maximum FEV_1 and 6-hr FEV_1 responses are shown. Values are divided into groups according to homozygous Arg 16, heterozygous Arg 16/ Gly 16, and homozygous Gly 16 polymorphisms of the β_2-adrenoceptor. Mean values for each group are indicated by horizontal lines. (From Ref. 78.)

Loss of Protection Against Bronchoconstrictor Stimuli

Regular administration of long-acting β_2-agonists leads to a partial loss of protection against a wide range of bronchoconstrictor stimuli, including methacholine, histamine, AMP, exercise, cold air, and allergen (18,79–84). One of the comprehensive studies to examine this phenomenon is that of Cheung et al. (80). In this study, a 10-fold increase in methacholine PC_{20} after the first dose of salmeterol was reduced to only a twofold increase after 4 weeks of salmeterol therapy (Fig. 11). This reduced bronchoprotection remained unchanged after a further 4 weeks of therapy. Despite this loss of protection, there was no associated tachyphylaxis to the bronchodilator effects of salmeterol or a change in underlying airway responsiveness.

It is likely that this effect is due to changes in the regulation of β_2-receptors, either by rapid desensitization with uncoupling of the receptors from the intracellular secondary messengers or sequestration of receptors or by a more gradual

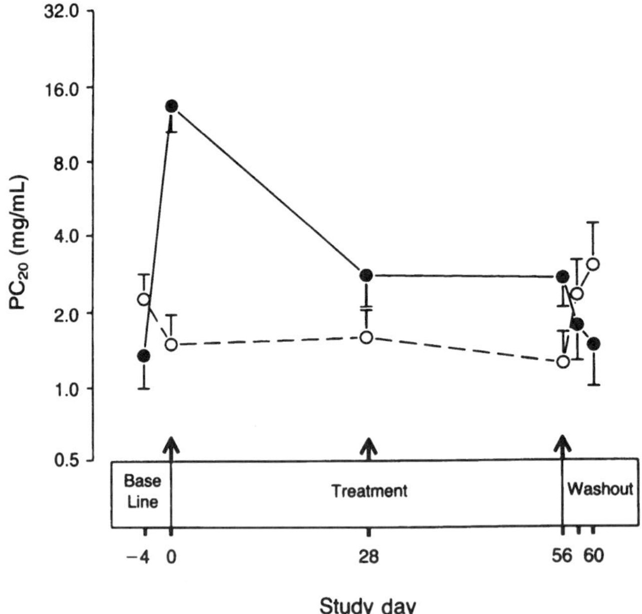

Figure 11 The airway responsiveness to methacholine at baseline, 1 hr after inhalation (arrows) of salmeterol (●) or placebo (○) on days 0, 28, and 56 during regular treatment with salmeterol (50 μg twice daily). The mean (±SEM) PC_{20} values are shown. There was a significant reduction in the protective effect of salmeterol on methacholine-induced bronchoconstriction after 4 and 8 weeks of treatment ($p < 0.001$). (From Ref. 80.)

downregulation of receptors. The development of greater tolerance to the bronchoprotective rather than the bronchodilator effects of long-acting β_2-agonists suggests a difference in receptor reserve for these two activities. This interpretation would be consistent with in vitro findings demonstrating a decline in β_2-agonist potency and efficacy as a bronchoconstrictor stimulus increases (85,86).

Tolerance to the acute bronchoprotective effects may occur after the first two doses, with a progressive increase in the magnitude of this effect over 3 to 4 days (84). This time course is consistent with the in vitro induction of β_2-receptor downregulation within 24 hr (87). In contrast to the tolerance observed when the challenge occurs within 1 hr of the last dose, there may be no loss of the bronchoprotective effects of long-acting β_2-agonists when the provoking challenge occurs 10–14 hr after the last dose of a long-acting β_2-agonist (88,89), although not all studies have confirmed this (90).

Such tolerance, which is not prevented by the coadministration of inhaled corticosteroids (83), is likely to result in a reduced bronchodilator efficacy of inhaled β_2-agonist therapy when taken prior to or in the situation of bronchoconstriction due to provoking stimuli.

Airway Hyperresponsiveness

Discontinuation of regularly administered long-acting β_2-agonists has not been shown to increase the level of airway responsiveness to stimuli such as methacholine (80,81,89,91); this contrasts with the increase in airway hyperresponsiveness observed after the discontinuation of short-acting β_2-agonist therapy (92–94). The reason for this difference between short- and long-acting β_2-agonists is unclear. It does not seem to relate to timing of the bronchial challenge tests, for these have been undertaken at different intervals up to 2 weeks after regular treatment has ended. One possibility is that regular treatment with long-acting β_2-agonists has not been continued for a sufficiently long period prior to discontinuation of therapy. This would be supported by the observation that the ''negative'' studies have generally involved 8–12 weeks of therapy, whereas a 12-month study observed a 1.86-fold doubling dose decrease in PD_{20} to methacholine with regular salmeterol (37). However, enhanced airway hyperresponsiveness was not observed after 12 months treatment with formoterol (95), and rebound increases in airway responsiveness with short-acting β_2-agonists have been observed after as little as 2 weeks of therapy (92–94). Consequently, a rebound increase in airway hyperresponsiveness after cessation of β_2-agonist treatment may be a property of short-acting rather than long-acting β_2-agonist drug therapy, although this remains to be definitely confirmed.

Severe Exacerbations

One way to assess the clinical relevance of the long-term effects of the long-acting β_2-agonist drugs is to determine whether their use influences the frequency or severity of exacerbations of asthma. In the case of salmeterol, it has been shown that its use does not influence the severe exacerbation rate. As discussed above, this evidence comes primarily from the Salmeterol Surveillance Study (33), in which the risk of admission to a hospital or intensive care unit (ICU) due to acute exacerbations of asthma was similar in patients taking salmeterol and in those taking regular salbutamol. More recently, a case-control study from the United Kingdom has found that the use of salmeterol does not increase the risk of a life-threatening attack of asthma resulting in an ICU admission (96). However, salmeterol has been shown to reduce the frequency of severe exacerbations (defined by reductions in peak flow of 60% and requirement for emergency medical assessment) not necessarily requiring hospital admission (97).

With respect to formoterol, it has recently been reported that its regular use is associated with fewer severe exacerbations (defined by a reduction in peak flow of 30% or a course of oral steroids) over a 12-month period, although there were too few subjects to determine its effect on the frequency of acute exacerbations severe enough to warrant hospital admission (43). These studies are reassuring to the extent that they indicate that potential problems relating to tolerance to bronchodilator and bronchoprotective effects are not associated with an increased frequency of severe exacerbations. However, this does not exclude these problems being of clinical relevance to individual patients in certain situations.

Compliance and Related Issues

It is not surprising that there have been reports of patients who stop taking inhaled corticosteroids after starting a long-acting β_2-agonist, presumably due in part to the symptomatic improvement they obtained (98). Such patients have been observed to develop worsening asthma, which improved again after the reintroduction of inhaled corticosteroids. However, whether poor compliance for inhaled corticosteroid therapy is more likely to occur with a long-acting as compared with a short-acting β_2-agonist drug has not been studied as yet.

Another feature that has been reported in those patients who are poorly compliant with their inhaled corticosteroid therapy is that although they may have normal lung function and few symptoms while taking a long-acting β_2-agonist regularly, they may experience a severe asthma attack when it is stopped (98). This phenomenon indicates that effective bronchodilation through regular use of long-acting β_2-agonist therapy may mask a worsening of the disease.

A recent study that has specifically addressed this issue has reported that regular inhalation of salmeterol can lead to a delay in the recognition of worsening asthma (99). In this study, a model of a stepwise reduction of inhaled corticosteroids was used to allow asthma control to gradually worsen. The subjects in the salmeterol arm of the study had a twofold greater level of sputum eosinophils in the week before a clinically recognizable exacerbation of asthma than did those in the placebo arm. It was suggested that salmeterol allowed the subjects to tolerate a degree of airway inflammation that would otherwise have led to symptoms and decreased lung function. This phenomenon was termed "masking," in that the regular use of salmeterol has the potential to "mask" a worsening of airway inflammation and thereby delay awareness of an exacerbation of asthma, since symptoms and lung function during treatment remained well controlled until the eosinophilic inflammation became more significantly advanced.

C. Mortality

Concerns that the overuse of β_2-agonists during severe exacerbations of asthma may increase the risk of mortality are based on the evidence that two specific β_2-agonist drugs, isoprenaline and fenoterol, were the major factors contributing to asthma mortality epidemics in six countries in the 1960s and later in New Zealand in the 1970s and 1980s (100–104). The role of isoprenaline forte in these asthma deaths was primarily based on analyses of time trends and case series (101,102,105–107), whereas that of fenoterol was based on a series of case-control studies. These studies showed that inhaled fenoterol was associated with an increased risk of death as compared with the most commonly used β_2-agonist drug, salbutamol (108–111), and that this association could not be explained by confounding by the severity of asthma (112–114). Therefore, it is important to address the question of whether long-acting β_2-agonist drugs may also increase the risk of death from asthma.

The major study that has investigated whether the use of salmeterol may influence the risk of mortality is the Salmeterol Nationwide Surveillance Project (33). Although this study involved 25,180 asthmatic patients, it had insufficient power to investigate the relative risk of death associated with salmeterol, as there were only 14 deaths in total throughout the study period. As a result, it was not possible to interpret the finding of a "non-statistically significant" ($p = 0.105$) threefold increased risk of death associated with the use of salmeterol. The reassurance offered by the authors that the number of deaths associated with salmeterol was no greater than one would expect in such a group of asthmatics was not entirely convincing and negated the purpose of undertaking a study with an appropriate control group; an alternative interpretation was that it was the inadequate power of the study (and the resulting imprecision in the effect estimates) that prevented the threefold increased risk of death with salmeterol from reaching statistical significance.

Likewise, the results of the subsequent monitoring study of prescription events were inconclusive (66). In this cohort study of over 15,000 patients prescribed salmeterol, there were 39 deaths due to asthma. Although the authors concluded that there was no evidence that salmeterol contributed to death in any of the patients examined, no definite clinical criteria were provided (or indeed exist) as to what evidence would indicate such an association, particularly when applied to a group of patients with severe persistent asthma with an increased risk of both morbidity and mortality. As a result of this lack of a control group, matched in terms of chronic asthma severity, the authors were unable to determine whether the use of salmeterol was causally associated with the deaths observed. Similarly, the circumstantial case reports linking patients dying from asthma with salmeterol use are unable to determine whether the drug therapy contributed to the fatal outcome (115,116).

More recently, a case-control study has been undertaken in which it was demonstrated that the use of salmeterol by patients with severe persistent asthma did not increase the risk of a near-fatal attack (96). If a near-fatal attack is considered to be an intermediate step in a process by which a severe attack of asthma may become fatal (117), these findings would suggest that salmeterol is unlikely to be associated with a significantly increased risk of death, at least by this mechanism.

Support for this interpretation is obtained when the findings of this study are compared with those of similar case-control studies investigating the role of the β_2-agonist fenoterol in the epidemic of asthma deaths in New Zealand which employed similar methodology (109–111,118). In these studies, the risk of asthma death or near-fatal attack associated with fenoterol increased when the analysis was restricted to the subgroups with greater severity of asthma. For example, in the case-control studies of a near-fatal attack, the relative risk associated with fenoterol increased from 2.0 to 2.6 in the severe subgroup, defined by patients with a recent hospital admission (118), compared with the risk with salmeterol which decreased from 2.3 to 1.4 (Fig. 12) (96). These contrasting results indicate that the increased baseline risk of a near-fatal attack associated with salmeterol, but not with fenoterol, was due to confounding by severity of disease, which is consistent with other evidence that salmeterol was preferentially prescribed to patients with more severe asthma. When confounding by severity was controlled for in the analysis, there was no significant risk of a near-fatal attack with salmeterol, in contrast with fenoterol, for which the risk increased.

Likewise, the first-time prescription of salmeterol, in comparison with ipratropium bromide or theophylline, was not associated with an increase in respiratory mortality in a recent cohort study based on the United Kingdom General Practice Research Database (119). However, this study included only 28 respiratory deaths, 19 of which occurred in patients who had chronic obstructive pulmonary diseases (COPD) or emphysema in addition to diagnosed asthma, whereas the findings were reported only for respiratory deaths in general rather than specifically for asthma. Thus, the numbers are too small to draw conclusions about respiratory deaths in general and are certainly too small to draw any conclusions about the risk of asthma death in patients prescribed salmeterol.

In conclusion, although available evidence suggests that the use of salmeterol is probably not associated with an increased risk of asthma death, this is

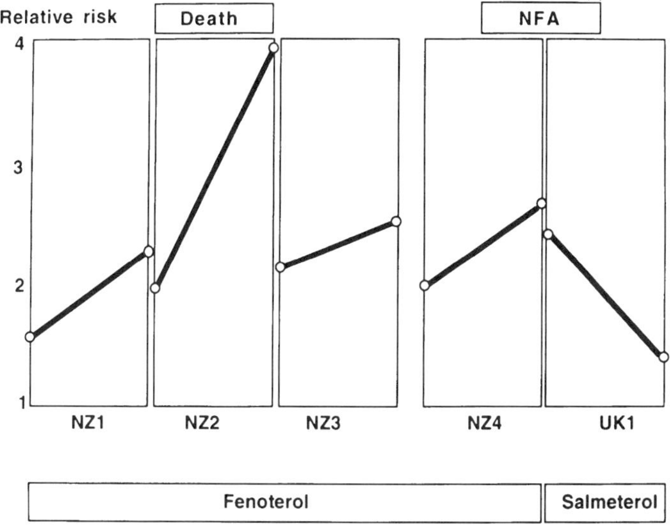

Figure 12 Comparison of the salmeterol findings with those relating to fenoterol from the similar New Zealand case-control studies of near-fatal asthma (NFA) [NZ4] (118) and deaths from asthma [NZ1, NZ2, NZ3] (109–111). For each study, the left-hand axis shows the overall relative risk of death or NFA for those prescribed fenoterol/salmeterol; the right-hand axis represents the same analysis in the subgroup of those patients with a hospital admission in the previous 12 months (the most valid marker of chronic asthma severity). These contrasting patterns indicate that when confounding by severity is controlled for in the analysis, there is no significant increased risk of a near-fatal attack with salmeterol, in contrast to fenoterol, for which the risk increased. (From Ref. 96.)

by no means certain, and it is still necessary to investigate this formally through case-control studies of asthma mortality. With respect to formoterol, there have been no studies that have specifically addressed the risk of mortality associated with its use. In view of the greater intrinsic activity of formoterol compared with salmeterol and a greater potential for formoterol to be used repeatedly during a severe attack of asthma (owing to its rapid onset of action and the recommendations of its manufacturer), it will be important to undertake case-control studies to examine the risk of mortality associated with its use in countries where it gains a significant market share.

VI. Recommended Use

The studies mentioned above have led to the recommended use of salmeterol and formoterol in patients with severe persistent asthma who are symptomatic despite the regular use of inhaled corticosteroids in combination with short-acting β_2-agonist drugs ''as needed.'' In international guidelines for the management of asthma, it is recommended that salmeterol or formoterol be introduced when patients are symptomatic despite inhaled corticosteroids in a dose of at least 800 μg BDP or budesonide daily, with provision for their introduction at an earlier level—corresponding with a daily dose of inhaled corticosteroids of 500 μg BDP or equivalent—in certain circumstances (120,121). With the addition of a long-acting β_2-agonists, short-acting β_2-agonist drugs such as salbutamol or terbutaline are still used ''as needed'' for the relief of symptoms. It is not recommended that long-acting β_2-agonists be used as sole therapy for the treatment of asthma.

A number of regulatory authorities have also approved the use of inhaled formoterol as rescue medication and as prophylaxis against exercise and allergen-induced bronchoconstriction. This approval has the restriction that a total daily dose of 72 μg should not be exceeded (60). It should be acknowledged that although self-administration by patients of formoterol according to both regularly scheduled twice-daily and ''as needed'' use may prove to be an appropriate regimen, its efficacy and safety has not been established; hence, such a regimen cannot be recommended at this time.

For both children over 4 years of age and adults, the recommended therapeutic dose of salmeterol via the MDI is 50 μg twice daily. Higher doses do not result in significantly improved efficacy yet are associated with greater side effects (41,122,123) The equivalent bronchodilator dose of formoterol is 9 μg (15), which has led to the recommended use of formoterol from the MDI in the dose of 12 μg twice daily.

References

1. Jeppson A, Löfdahl C-G, Waldeck B, Widmark E. On the predictive value of in vitro experiments in the evaluation of the effect duration of bronchodilator drugs for local administration. Pulm Pharmacol 1989; 2:81–85.
2. Naline E, Zhang Y, Qian Y, Mairon N, Anderson G, Grandordy B, Advenier C. Relaxant effects and durations of action of formoterol and salmeterol on the isolated human bronchus. Eur Respir J 1994; 7:914–920.
3. Lindén A, Bergendal A, Ullman A, Skoogh B-E, Löfdahl C-G. Long and short acting beta-2 agonists in the isolated guinea pig trachea—efficacy, potency and functional antagonism. Eur Respir J 1991; 4:199s.
4. Lindén A, Bergendal A, Ullman A, Skoogh B-E, Löfdahl C-G. Salmeterol, formoterol and salbutamol in the isolated guinea pig trachea: differences in maximum relaxant effect and potency but not in functional antagonism. Thorax 1993; 48: 547–553.
5. Roux F, Grandordy B, Douglas J. Functional and binding characteristics of long-acting beta-2 agonists in lung and heart. Am J Respir Crit Care Med 1996; 153: 1489–1495.

6. Decker N, Quennedey M, Rouot B, Schwartz J, Velly J. Effects of N-aralkyl substitution of beta agonists on alpha and beta adrenoceptor sub-types: pharmacological studies and binding assays. J Pharmacol 1982; 34:107–112.
7. Johnson M. The pre-clinical pharmacology of salmeterol: bronchodilator effects. Eur Respir Rev 1991; 1:253–256.
8. Anderson G, Lindén A, Rabe K. Why are long-acting beta adrenoceptor agonists long acting? Eur Respir J 1994; 7:569–578.
9. Nials A, Coleman R, Johnston M, Magnussen H, Rabe K, Vardey C. Effects of beta adrenoceptor agonists in human bronchial smooth muscle. Br J Pharmacol 1993; 110:1112–1116.
10. Brittain R. Approaches to a long-acting selective beta-2 adrenoceptor stimulant. Lung 1990; 168(suppl):142–153.
11. O'Donnell S. Selectivity of clenbuterol (NAB 365) in guinea pig isolated tissues containing beta adrenoceptors. Arch Int Pharmacodyn Ther 1976; 224:190–198.
12. Nyberg L. Pharmacokinetics of beta-2 adrenoceptor stimulating drugs. In: Pauwels R, O'Byrne P, eds. Beta-2 Agonists in Asthma Treatment. New York: Marcel Dekker, 1997:87–130.
13. Rabe KF, Jorres R, Nowak D, Behr N, Magnussen H. Comparison of the effects of salmeterol and formoterol on airway tone and responsiveness over 24 hours in bronchial asthma. Am Rev Respir Dis 1993; 147:1436–1441.
14. van Noord JA, Smeets JJ, Raaijmakers JAM, Bommer AM, Maesen FPV. Salmeterol versus formoterol in patients with moderately severe asthma: onset and duration of action. Eur Respir J 1996; 9:1684–1688.
15. Palmqvist M, Persson G, Lazer L, Rosenborg J, Larsson P, Lotvall J. Inhaled dry-powder formoterol and salmeterol in asthmatic patients: onset of action, duration of effect and potency. Eur Respir J 1997; 10:2484–2489.
16. von Berg A, Schmitt-Grohe S, Berdel D. Protective effect of formoterol in asthmatic children. Am Rev Respir Dis 1990; 141:A208.
17. Sovijarvi AR, Reinikainen K, Freudenthal Y, Andersson P, Riska H. Preventive effects of inhaled formoterol and salbutamol on histamine-induced bronchoconstriction—a placebo-controlled study. Respiration 1992; 59:279–282.
18. Taylor DA, Jensen MW, Aikman SL, Harris JG, Barnes PJ, O'Connor BJ. Comparison of salmeterol and albuterol-induced bronchoprotection against adenosine monophosphate and histamine in mild asthma. Am J Respir Crit Care Med 1997; 156: 1731–1737.
19. Soler M, Joos L, Bolliger CT, Elsasser S, Perruchoud AP. Bronchoprotection by salmeterol: cell stabilization or functional antagonism? Comparative effects on histamine- and AMP-induced bronchoconstriction. Eur Respir J 1994; 7:1973–1977.
20. Malo JL, Cartier A, Trudeau C, Ghezzo H, Gontovnick L. Formoterol, a new inhaled beta-2 adrenergic agonist, has a longer blocking effect than albuterol on hyperventilation-induced bronchoconstriction. Am Rev Respir Dis 1990; 142: 1147–1152.
21. Anderson SD, Todwell LJ, DuToit J. Duration of protection by inhaled salmeterol in exercise-induced asthma. Chest 1991; 100:1254–1260.
22. Henriksen JM, Agertoft L, Pedersen S. Protective effect and duration of action of

inhaled formoterol and salbutamol on exercise-induced asthma in children. J Allergy Clin Immunol 1992; 89:1176–1182.
23. Palmqvist M, Balder B, Löwhagen O, Melander E, Svedmyr N, Wahlander L. Late asthmatic reaction decreased after pretreatment with salbutamol and formoterol, a new long-acting beta$_2$-agonist. J Allergy Clin Immunol 1992; 89:844–849.
24. Pearlman DS, Chervinsky P, LaForce C, Seltzer JM, Southern DL, Kemp JP, Dockhorn RJ, Grossman J, Liddle RF, Yancey SW, Cocchetto DM, Alexander WJ, van As A. A comparison of salmeterol with albuterol in the treatment of mild-to-moderate asthma. N Engl J Med 1992; 327:1420–1425.
25. Leblanc P, Knight A, Kreisman H, Borkhoff CM, Johnston PR. A placebo-controlled, crossover comparison of salmeterol and salbutamol in patients with asthma. Am J Respir Crit Care Med 1996; 154:324–328.
26. D'Alonzo GE, Nathan RA, Henochowicz S, Morris RJ, Ratner P, Rennard SI. Salmeterol xinafoate as maintenance therapy compared with albuterol in patients with asthma. JAMA 1994; 271:1412–1416.
27. Kesten S, Chapman KR, Broder I, Cartier A, Hyland RH, Knight A, Malo JL, Mazza JA, Moote DW, Small P. A 3 month comparison of twice daily inhaled formoterol vs four times daily inhaled albuterol in the management of stable asthma. Am Rev Respir Dis 1991; 144:622–625.
28. Steffensen I, Faurschou P, Riska H, Rostrup J, Wegener T. Inhaled formoterol dry powder in the treatment of patients with reversible obstructive airway disease. Allergy 1995; 50:657–663.
29. Farschou P, Steffensen I, Jacques L. Effect of addition of inhaled salmeterol to the treatment of moderate-to-severe asthmatics uncontrolled on high-dose inhaled steroids. Eur Respir J 1996; 9:1885–1890.
30. Smyth ET, Pavord JD, Wong CS, Wisniewski AFZ, Williams J, Tattersfield AE. Interaction and dose equivalence of salbutamol and salmeterol in patients with asthma. Br Med J 1993; 306:543–545.
31. Maesen BLP, Smeets SJ, Costongs R, Costongs MAL, Maesen FPV. Long term effects of the beta-2-adrenoceptor agonist formoterol for two years on lung function of stable asthmatic patients. Chest 1993; 103(suppl):286S.
32. Britton MG, Earnshaw JS, Palmer JBD. A twelve month comparison of salmeterol with salbutamol in asthmatic patients. Eur Respir J 1992; 5:1062–1067.
33. Castle W, Fuller R, Hall J, Palmer J. Serevent nationwide surveillance study: comparison of salmeterol with salbutamol in asthmatic patients who require regular bronchodilator treatment. Br Med J 1993; 306:1034–1037.
34. Greening AP, Ind PW, Northfield M, Shaw G. Added salmeterol versus higher dose corticosteroid in asthma patients with symptoms on existing inhaled corticosteroid: Allen & Hanburys Limited UK Study Group. Lancet 1994; 344:219–224.
35. Ulrik CS, Kok-Jensen A. Different bronchodilating effect of salmeterol and formoterol in an adult asthmatic. Eur Respir J 1994; 7:1003–1005.
36. Vervloet D, Ekstrom T, Pela R, Duce Gracia F, Kopp C, Silvert BD, Quebe-Fehling E, Della Cioppa G, Di Benedetto G. A 6 month comparison between formoterol and salmeterol in patients with reversible obstructive airways disease. Respir Med 1998; 92:836–842.
37. Verberne AAPH, Frost C, Roorda RJ, van der Laag H, Kerrebijn KF. One year

treatment with salmeterol compared with beclomethasone in children with asthma. Am J Respir Crit Care Med 1997; 156:688–695.
38. Simons FER and the Canadian Beclomethasone Dipropionate-Salmeterol Xinafoate Study Group. A comparison of beclomethasone, salmeterol, and placebo in children with asthma. N Engl J Med 1997; 337:1657–1665.
39. Weersink EJM, Douma WR, Koëter G, Postma DS. Is there a synergistic effect between salmeterol and fluticasone in asthmatics with nocturnal airway obstruction? (abstr) Am J Respir Crit Care Med 1995; 151:A268.
40. Wilding P, Clark M, Coon JT, Lewis S, Rushton L, Bennett J, Oborne J, Cooper S, Tattersfield AE. Effect of long term treatment with salmeterol on asthma control: a double blind, randomised crossover study. Br Med J 1997; 314:1441–1446.
41. van der Molen T, Postma DS, Turner MO, Jong BM, Malo JL, Chapman K, Grossman R, de Graaff CS, Riemersma RA, Sears MR. Effects of the long acting beta agonist formoterol on asthma control in asthmatic patients using inhaled corticosteroids. Thorax 1997; 52:535–539.
42. Woolcock A, Lundback B, Ringdal N, Jacques LA. Comparison of addition of salmeterol to inhaled steroids with doubling of the dose of inhaled steroids. Am J Respir Crit Care Med 1996; 153:1481–1488.
43. Pauwels RA, Löfdahl C-G, Postma DS, Tattersfield AE, O'Byrne P, Barnes PJ, Ullman A. Effect of inhaled formoterol and budesonide on exacerbations of asthma. N Engl J Med 1997; 337:1405–1411.
44. Fjellbirkeland L, Gulsvik A, Palmer JBD. The efficacy and tolerability of inhaled salmeterol and individually dose-titrated sustained-release theophylline in patients with reversible airways disease. Respir Med 1994; 88:599–607.
45. Bousquet J, Aubert B, Bons J. Comparison of salmeterol with disodium cromoglycate in the treatment of adult asthma. Ann Allergy Asthma Immunol 1996; 76: 189–194.
46. Johnson ME, UK Study Group. A multicentre study to compare the efficacy and safety of salmeterol xinafoate and nedocromil sodium via metered-dose inhalers in adults with mild-to-moderate asthma. Eur J Clin Res 1994; 5:75–85.
47. Muir JF, Bertin L, Georges D. French Multicentre Study Group. Salmeterol versus slow-release theophylline combined with ketotifen in nocturnal asthma: a multicentre trial. Eur Respir J 1992; 5:1197–1200.
48. Djukanovic R, Roche WR, Wilson JW, Beasley CR, Twentyman OP, Howarth RH, Holgate ST. Mucosal inflammation in asthma: state of the art. Am Rev Respir Dis 1990; 142:434–457.
49. Barnes PJ. Beta-adrenergic receptors and their regulation: State of the Art. Am J Respir Crit Care Med 1995; 152:838–860.
50. Howarth P. Effects of beta$_2$-agonists on airway inflammation. In: Pauwels R, O'Byrne PM, eds. Beta$_2$-Agonists in Asthma Treatment. New York: Marcel Dekker, 1997:67–86.
51. Twentyman OP, Finnerty JP, Harris A, Palmer J, Holgate ST. Protection against allergen-induced asthma by salmeterol. Lancet 1990; 336:1338–1342.
52. Murray JJ, Hagermara DD, Dworksi R, Steller JR. Effect of salmeterol and beclomethasone on the late phase response to sequential antigen challenge in man. In:

Johnson M, ed. Acute and Chronic Inflammation in the Respiratory Tract. London: Colwood House, 1995:64.

53. Calhoun WJ, Hinton KL, Brick JJ, Vuchinich T. Effects of salmeterol on eosinophil recruitment to the airway following segmental antigen challenge in atopic asthmatics. In: Johnson M, ed. Acute and Chronic Inflammation in the Respiratory Tract. London: Colwood House, 1995:62.
54. Boulet LP, Turcotte H, Boulet M, Dube J, Gagnon MA, Lavidette M. Effects of salmeterol on chronic and allergen-induced airway inflammation in mild allergic asthma. In: Johnson M, ed. Acute and Chronic Inflammation in the Respiratory Tract. London: Colwood House 1995:66.
55. Kraft M, Bettinger CM, Pak J, et al. Salmeterol decreases nocturnal symptoms and β_2-agonist use in nocturnal asthma without altering airway inflammation. In: Johnson M, ed. Acute and Chronic Inflammation in the Respiratory Tract. London: Colwood House, 1995:68.
56. Howarth PH, Roberts JA, Bradding P, Walls AE, Holgate ST. The influence of β_2-agonists on airway inflammation in asthma. In: Costello JF, Mann RD, eds. Beta-agonists in the Treatment of Asthma. Carnforth, UK: Parthenon, 1992:69–77.
57. Gardiner PV, Ward C, Booth H, Allison A, Hendrick DJ, Walters EH. Effect of eight weeks of treatment with salmeterol on bronchoalveolar lavage inflammatory indices in asthmatics. Am J Respir Crit Care Med 1994; 150:1006–1011.
58. Tranfa CME, Pelaia G, Grembiale RD, Naty S, Durante S, Borrello G. Short-term cardiovascular effects of salmeterol. Chest 1998; 113:1272–1276.
59. Windom HH, Burgess CD, Crane J, Pearce N, Kwong T, Beasley R. The self-administration of inhaled beta agonist drugs during severe asthma. NZ Med J 1990; 103:205–207.
60. Adis International. New Ethicals. May 1998:172–173.
61. Bremner P, Woodman K, Burgess C, Crane J, Purdie G, Pearce N, Beasley R. A comparison of the cardiovascular and metabolic effects of formoterol, salbutamol and fenoterol. Eur Respir J 1993; 6:204–210.
62. Bennett JA, Smyth ET, Pavord ID, Wilding PJ, Tattersfield AE. Systemic effects of salbutamol and salmeterol in patients with asthma. Thorax 1994; 49:771–774.
63. Maconochie JG, Forster JK. Dose response study with high-dose inhaled salmeterol in healthy subjects. Br J Clin Pharmacol 1992; 33:342–345.
64. Stålenheim G, Wegener T, Grettve L, Lundback B, Melander B, Osterman K, Piitulainen E, Zetterstrom O. Efficacy and tolerance of a 12-week treatment with inhaled formoterol in patients with reversible obstructive lung disease. Respiration 1994; 61:305–309.
65. Dahl R. Comparative studies of inhaled salmeterol with other bronchodilators. Eur Respir Rev 1995; 5:138–141.
66. Mann RD, Kubota K, Pearce G, Wilton L. Salmeterol: a study by prescription event monitoring in a UK cohort of 15,407 patients. J Clin Epidemiol 1996; 49:247–250.
67. Maconochie JG, Minton NA, Chilton JE, Keene ON. Does tachyphylaxis occur to the non-pulmonary effects of salmeterol? Br J Clin Pharmacol 1994; 37:199–204.

68. Newnham DM, Grove A, McDevitt DG, Lipworth BJ. Subsensitivity of bronchodilator and systemic β_2-adrenoceptor responses after regular twice daily treatment with eformoterol dry powder in asthmatic patients. Thorax 1995; 50:497–504.
69. Langley SJ, Masterton CM, Batty EP, Woodcock A. Bronchodilator response to salbutamol after chronic dosing with salmeterol or placebo. Eur Respir J 1998; 11: 1081–1085.
70. Ullman A, Hedner J, Svedmyr N. Inhaled salmeterol and salbutamol in asthmatic patients: an evaluation of asthma symptoms and the possible development of tachyphylaxis. Am Rev Respir Dis 1990; 142:571–575.
71. Newnham DM, McDevitt DG, Lipworth BJ. Bronchodilator subsensitivity after chronic dosing with eformoterol in patients with asthma. Am J Med 1994; 97:29–37.
72. Grove A, Lipworth BJ. Bronchodilator subsensitivity to salbutamol after twice daily salmeterol in asthmatic patients. Lancet 1995; 346:201–206.
73. Barnes N. Bronchodilation subsensitivity to salbutamol following salmeterol (letter). Lancet 1995; 346:968.
74. Weinberger M. Bronchodilation subsensitivity to salbutamol after salmeterol (letter). Lancet 1995; 346:968.
75. Tan KS, Grove A, McLean A, Gnosspelius Y, Hall IP, Lipworth BJ. Systemic corticosteroid rapidly reverses bronchodilator subsensitivity induced by formoterol in asthmatic patients. Am J Respir Crit Care Med 1997; 156:28–35.
76. Mak JCW, Nishikawa M, Barnes PJ. Glucocorticosteroids increase β_2 adrenergic receptor transcription in human lung. Am J Physiol 1995; 12:L41–L46.
77. Davies AO, Lefkowitz RJ. Regulation of beta-adrenergic receptors by steroid hormones. Am Rev Physiol 1984; 46:119–130.
78. Tan S, Hall IP, Dewar J, Dow E, Lipworth B. Association between β_2-adrenoceptor polymorphism and susceptibility to bronchodilator desensitisation in moderately severe stable asthmatics. Lancet 1997; 350:995–999.
79. Giannini D, Carletti A, Dente FL, Bacci E, Di Franco A, Vagaggini B, Paggiaro PL. Tolerance to the protective effect of salmeterol on allergen challenge. Chest 1996; 110:1452–1457.
80. Cheung D, Timmers MC, Zwinderman AH, Bei EH, Dijkman JH, Sterk PJ. Long-term effects of a long-acting β_2-adrenoceptor agonist, salmeterol, on airway hyperresponsiveness in patients with mild asthma. N Engl J Med 1992; 327:1198–1203.
81. Yates DH, Sussman HS, Shaw MJ, Barnes PJ, Chung KF. Regular formoterol treatment in mild asthma: effect on bronchial responsiveness during and after treatment. Am J Respir Crit Care Med 1995; 152:1170–1174.
82. Ramage L, Lipworth BJ, Ingram CG, Cree A, Dhillon DP. Reduced protection against exercise induced bronchoconstriction after chronic dosing with salmeterol. Respir Med 1994; 88:363–368.
83. Yates DH, Kharitonov SA, Barnes PJ. An inhaled glucocorticoid does not prevent tolerance to the bronchoprotective effect of a long-acting inhaled β_2-agonist. Am J Respir Crit Care Med 1996; 154:1603–1607.
84. Bhagat R, Kalra S, Swystun A and Cockcoft DW. Rapid onset of tolerance to the bronchoprotective effect of salmeterol. Chest. 1995; 108:1235–1239.

85. Lemoine H, Overlack C, Kohl A, Worth H, Reinhardt D. Formoterol, fenoterol and salbutamol as partial agonists for relaxation of maximally contracted guinea-pig tracheae: comparison of relaxation with receptor binding. Lung 1992; 170:163–180.
86. Lemoine H, Overlack C. Highly potent beta$_2$ sympathomimetic convert to less potent partial agonists as relaxants of guinea pig trachea maximally contracted by carbachol: comparison of relaxation with receptor binding and adenylate cyclase stimulation. J Pharmacol Exp Ther 1992; 261:258–270.
87. Clark RB, Allal C, Friedman J, Johnson M, Barber R. Stable activation and desensitization of β_2-adrenergic receptor stimulation of adenylyl cyclase by salmeterol: evidence for quasi-irreversible binding to an exosite. Mol Pharmacol 1996; 49: 182–189.
88. Kemp J, Kalberg C, Anderson W, Emmett A, Rickard K. Effect of 24-week salmeterol therapy on airway hyperresponsiveness (abstr). Am J Respir Crit Care Med 1997; 155:A344.
89. Booth H, Fishwick K, Harkawat R, Devereaux G, Hendrick DJ, Walters EH. Changes in methacholine induced bronchoconstriction with the long acting β_2 agonist salmeterol in mild to moderate asthmatic patients. Thorax 1993; 48:1121–1124.
90. Yates DH, Wordsell M, Barnes PJ. Effect of regular salmeterol treatment on albuterol-induced bronchoprotection in mild asthma. Am J Respir Crit Care Med 1997; 156:988–991.
91. Beach JR, Young CL, Harkawat R, Gardiner PV, Avery AJ, Coward GA, Walters EH, Hendrick DJ. Effect on airway responsiveness of six weeks treatment with salmeterol. Pulm Pharmacol 1993; 6:155–157.
92. Wahedna I, Wong CS, Wisniewski AF, Pavord ID, Tattersfield AE. Asthma control during and after cessation of regular β_2-agonist treatment. Am Rev Respir Dis 1993; 148:707–712.
93. Vathenen AS, Knox AJ, Higgins BG, Britton JR, Tattersfield AE. Rebound increase in bronchial responsiveness after treatment with inhaled terbutaline. Lancet 1988; 1:554–558.
94. Kerrebijn KF, van Essen-Zandvliet EEM, Neijens HJ. Effect of long-term treatment with inhaled corticosteroids and beta-agonists on the bronchial responsiveness in children with asthma. J Allergy Clin Immunol 1987; 79:653–659.
95. Becker AB, Simons FER. Formoterol, a new long-acting selective beta$_2$-agonist, decreases airway responsiveness in children with asthma. Lung 1990; 168(suppl): 99–102.
96. Williams C, Crossland L, Finnerty J, Crane J, Holgate ST, Pearce N, Beasley R. A case-control study of salmeterol and near fatal attacks of asthma. Thorax 1998; 53:7–13.
97. Taylor DR, Town GI, Herbison GP, Boothman-Burrell D, Flannery EM, Hancox B, Harré E, Laubscher K, Linscott V, Ramsay CM, Richards G. Asthma control during long term treatment with regular inhaled salbutamol and salmeterol. Thorax 1998; 53:744–752.
98. Arvidsson P, Larsson S, Löfdahl C-G, Melander B, Svedmyr N, Wåhlander L.

Inhaled formoterol during one year in asthma: a comparison with salbutamol. Eur Respir J 1991; 4:1168–1173.
99. McIvor RA, Pizzichini E, Turner MO, Hussack P, Hargreave FE, Sears MR. Potential masking effects of salmeterol on airway inflammation in asthma. Am J Respir Crit Care Med 1998; 158:924–930.
100. Pearce N, Crane J, Burgess C, Jackson R, Beasley R. Beta agonists and asthma mortality: Deja-vu. Clin Exp Allergy 1991; 21:401–410.
101. Stolley PD. Why the United States was spared an epidemic of deaths due to asthma. Am Rev Respir Dis 1972; 105:883–890.
102. Stolley PD, Schinnar R. Association between asthma mortality and isoproterenol aerosols: a review. Prev Med 1978; 7:319–338.
103. Pearce N, Beasley R, Crane J, Burgess C. Epidemiology of asthma mortality. In: Busse WW, Holgate ST, eds. Asthma and Rhinitis. Oxford: Blackwell, 1995:58–69.
104. Jackson R. A century of asthma mortality. In: Beasley R, Pearce NE, eds. The Role of Beta Agonist Therapy in Asthma Mortality. New York: CRC Press, 1993:29–47.
105. Speizer FE, Doll R, Heaf P. Observations on recent increases in mortality from asthma. Br Med J 1968; 1:335–339.
106. Inman MHW, Adelstein AM. Rise and fall of asthma mortality in England and Wales in relation to use of pressurised aerosols. Lancet 1969; 2:279–285.
107. Fraser PM, Speizer FE, Waters SD, Doll R, Mann NM. The circumstances preceding death from asthma in young people in 1968 to 1969. Br J Dis Chest 1971; 65: 71–84.
108. Spitzer WO, Suissa S, Ernst P, Horowitz RI, Habbick B, Cockcroft D, Boivin JF, McNutt M, Buist AS, Rebuck AS. The use of beta agonists and the risk of death and near death from asthma. N Engl J Med 1992; 326:501–506.
109. Crane J, Pearce N, Flatt A, Burgess C, Jackson R, Kwong T, Ball M, Beasley R. Prescribed fenoterol and death from asthma in New Zealand, 1981–83: case-control study. Lancet 1989; 1:917–922.
110. Pearce N, Grainger J, Atkinson M, Crane J, Burgess C, Culling C, Windom H, Beasley R. Case-control study of prescribed fenoterol and death from asthma in New Zealand, 1977–1981. Thorax 1990; 45:170–175.
111. Grainger J, Woodman K, Pearce N, Crane J, Burgess C, Keane A, Beasley R. Prescribed fenoterol and death from asthma in New Zealand, 1981–1987: a further case-control study. Thorax 1991; 46:105–111.
112. Beasley R, Burgess C, Pearce N, Grainger J, Crane J. Confounding by severity does not explain the association between fenoterol and asthma death. Clin Exp Allergy 1994; 24:660–668.
113. Sackett DL, Shannon HS, Browman GW. Fenoterol and fatal asthma (letter). Lancet 1990; 1:46.
114. Pearce N, Beasley R, Crane J, Burgess C. Confounding by indication and channelling over time: the risks of β_2-agonists (letter). Am J Epidemiol 1997; 146:885–886.
115. Finkelstein FN. Risks of salmeterol (letter). N Engl J Med 1994; 331:1314.

116. Palmer JBD, Rickard KA, Thompson JR. Risks of salmeterol (letter). N Engl J Med 1994; 331:1314.
117. Beasley R, Pearce N, Crane J. Use of near-fatal asthma for investigating asthma deaths. Thorax 1993; 48:1093–1094.
118. Burgess C, Pearce N, Thiruchelvam R, Wilkinson R, Linaker C, Woodman K, Crane J, Beasley R. Prescribed drug therapy and near-fatal asthma attacks. Eur Respir J 1994; 7:498–503.
119. Meier CR, Jick H. Drug use and pulmonary death rates in increasingly symptomatic asthma patients in the UK. Thorax 1997; 52:612–617.
120. Lenfant C. International Consensus Report on Diagnosis and Management of Asthma. Bethesda, MD: National Heart, Lung and Blood Institute, National Institute of Health, U.S. Department of Health and Human Services, 1992.
121. Global Initiative for Asthma. Global strategy for asthma management and prevention NHLBI/WHO Workshop Report. Bethesda, MD: National Institutes of Health, National Heart, Lung and Blood Institute, 1996.
122. Palmer JBD, Stuart AM, Shepherd GL, Viskum K. Inhaled salmeterol in the treatment of patients with moderate-to-severe reversible obstructive airways disease: a 3 month comparison of the efficacy and safety of twice daily salmeterol (100 μg) with salmeterol (50 μg). Respir Med 1992; 86:409–417.
123. Faurschou P. Chronic dose-ranging studies with salmeterol. Eur Respir Rev 1991; 1:282–287.

6

Inhaled Glucocorticoids, Established and New

JOSEPH D. SPAHN and STANLEY J. SZEFLER

University of Colorado Health Sciences Center
and National Jewish Medical and Research Center
Denver, Colorado

I. Introduction

Glucocorticoids (GC) are the most potent and effective class of medications used in the treatment of both the acute and chronic manifestations of asthma (1,2). They have been used in the treatment of asthma for nearly 50 years, long before a rationale was developed to explain their actions (3–5). Unfortunately, much of the early enthusiasm regarding oral GC therapy was dampened with the realization that long-term use resulted in the development of a number of debilitating adverse effects. Thus, research was quickly directed toward reducing the side-effect profile by delivering GC directly into the airway. The development of potent GCs and metered-dose inhalers (MDIs), which can effectively deliver these agents into the lower airways, have revolutionized the way we care for asthma patients. No other asthma medication available today can improve asthma symptoms and baseline pulmonary function while also reducing bronchial hyperresponsiveness (BHR) to the same extent as inhaled GC therapy. In addition, by virtue of the fact that small quantities of GC are delivered topically, the incidence of adverse effects is greatly diminished as compared with chronically administered oral GC therapy. This chapter provides a brief history of the development of inhaled GC therapy, the mechanisms of inhaled glucocorticoid action and an overview of their clinical efficacy; this is followed by a discussion of their potential for causing adverse effects. The last section provides an overview of fluticasone, the most recently released inhaled GC.

II. History

The first attempt to administer GC by the inhaled route came in 1951 when Gelfand reported improvement in four of five asthma patients treated with aerosolized cortisone suspended in saline (6). Of note, the effect was likely due to systemic absorption of the drug, since very large doses (50 mg) were used. In contrast, a subsequent double-blind placebo-controlled study evaluating aerosolized hydrocortisone hemisuccinate at a much lower dose (15 mg/day) as compared with placebo failed to show significant improvement in asthma symptoms (7). Other studies evaluating hydrocortisone and prednisolone in the late 1950s and early 1960s showed variable effects, but the general consensus was that these drugs were not effective, either because of insufficient potency of the GC used, inefficient delivery of the drug to the lower airway, or rapid clearance of the GC from the bronchial tree (8).

The decade of the 1960s heralded the development of both the "modern" pressurized MDI and dexamethasone, a much more potent GC than either prednisolone or hydrocortisone. Shortly after the release of the Decadron Respihaler®, several studies were published demonstrating its oral GC-tapering effects in steroid-dependent asthma and its ability to improve asthma symptoms (9–12). Of significance, not all patients demonstrated improvement in asthma control and/or oral GC dose reduction. Children and adolescents appeared to respond more favorably than adults, along with those with a shorter duration of asthma.

The recognition that inhaled dexamethasone therapy resulted in significant adverse effects came soon after its introduction. In fact, many of the initial studies demonstrating dexamethasone's efficacy found it to significantly suppress the HPA axis. An important observation made by Dennis and Itkin (12) was the persistence of cushingoid features in many steroid-dependent asthma patients treated with inhaled dexamethasone even after they were tapered off oral GC therapy. These investigators were also the first to describe oral and laryngeal candidiasis as complications of inhaled GC therapy. In retrospect, these findings are not surprising, given that the amount of inhaled dexamethasone required for clinical efficacy was similar in magnitude to the dexamethasone equivalent of the oral GC that many of these patients were on. Thus, although it was effective, inhaled dexamethasone did not offer significant advantages over oral GC in terms providing superior topical-to-systemic potency (13).

The first inhaled steroid to offer superior topical-to-systemic potency was beclomethasone dipropionate (BDP). BDP was initially developed as a topical GC for use in atopic dermatitis, but by the early 1970s, a pressurized MDI delivering BDP (50 μg per actuation) was developed. In 1972, two open-label studies found inhaled BDP to have potent oral GC-sparing effects in patients with steroid-dependent asthma (14,15). Associated with significant reductions in oral GC dose were improvements in pulmonary function, decreased diurnal variability in peak expiratory flow rates, and less need for supplemental bronchodilator use. Of importance, BDP therapy did not result in suppression of the HPA axis. Furthermore, many steroid-dependent asthma patients treated with BDP developed steroid withdrawal syndrome as their oral steroid dose was tapered and eventually discontinued. Patients also reported exacerbations of their eczema and/or allergic rhinitis as their oral steroid dose was discontinued; in some cases, the cushingoid stigmata disappeared. These observations strengthened the concept that BDP's efficacy came mainly from its topical effects.

Controlled studies that supported the above findings soon followed (16–19). A classic study from the Medical Research Council published in 1974 (16) found BDP (400 and 800 μg/day) to be superior to placebo in terms of oral GC reduction and asthma symptoms in a large number of steroid-dependent asthma patients. This study was among the first to demonstrate dose-dependent effects of inhaled GC therapy, both in terms of clinical efficacy and adverse effects, with a greater percentage of patients tapered off oral GC therapy and a greater incidence of oral candidiasis in those treated with high-dose BDP as opposed to those treated with low-dose BDP. Another large double-blind, placebo-controlled study evaluated the long-term effects of either inhaled BDP or betamethasone valerate as compared with prednisone (17) and found the inhaled GCs to be as effective as prednisone in the management of severe asthma. In addition, a daily dose of 400 μg/day of BDP was equivalent to 7.5 mg/day of prednisone but without the adverse effects.

These studies helped to develop the foundation for the acceptability and widespread use of inhaled GC therapy for individuals with chronic asthma. Over the ensuing 20–25 years, several other potent topical steroids such as flunisolide, triamcinolone acetonide, budesonide, and fluticasone propionate were developed for use in asthma. The widespread use of spacer devices also contributed to the optimization of topical effects while minimizing the potential for systemic effects. We have learned a great deal regarding the clinical effects and the potential for adverse effects of inhaled GC therapy in asthma. Great strides have also been made in our understanding of the mechanism(s) of GC action at both the molecular and cellular levels. The following text briefly discusses the progress that has been made regarding each of these issues.

III. Mechanisms of Action

A. Effects at the Molecular Level

Given their lipid composition, GCs easily diffuse across the cell membrane and bind with high affinity to a specific cytoplasmic receptor termed the *glucocorticoid receptor* (GCR). Upon ligand binding, the GC-GCR complex is translocated to the nucleus (20), dimerizes (21), and eventually binds to specific DNA sites termed *glucocorticoid response elements* (GRE) upstream from the promoter regions of steroid-responsive genes (22). GC-GCR binding to the GRE results in either up or downregulation of gene products (23–25). It has been estimated that there are between 10 and 100 genes that have GRE sites and hence can be directly influenced by GCs (26).

Of note, many of the genes encoding for proinflammatory cytokines lack GREs. Thus, GC must also act indirectly in suppressing inflammation. Glucocorticoids accomplish this by interfering with nuclear transcription factors such as AP-1 and NF-κB, which are involved in the transcription of several proinflammatory cytokine genes (27–29). GCs can also interfere with transcription factor binding by induction of proteins such as IκBα, which can effectively neutralize specific transcription factors (30,31). Last, GC can also influence posttranscriptional events such as RNA translation, protein synthesis, and protein secretion. In particular, GCs have been shown to decrease the stability of interferon-gamma (INF-γ) mRNA by activation of a ribonuclease that degrades the AU-rich sequences in the untranslated region of this gene (32).

B. Effects at the Cellular Level

The mucosal inflammatory response seen in asthma has been shown to be associated with the production of cytokines, the upregulation of adhesion molecules on both leukocytes and vascular endothelium, the influx of inflammatory cells, and the production of mediators of inflammation including histamine, leukotrienes, prostaglandins, PAF, and the eosinophil-derived basic proteins (33). GCs display profound inhibitory effects on the inflammatory response associated with asthma. The anti-inflammatory effects of GCs come mainly from their ability to inhibit the transcription of multiple cytokines and hence to inhibit inflammatory cell activation. Multiple in vitro studies have shown GC to inhibit the production of cytokines such as interleukin-1 (IL-1) (34), IL-2 (35), IL-3 (36), IL-4 (37,38), IL-5 (39,40), IL-6, (41), IL-13, granulocyte-macrophage colony-stimulating factor (GM-CSF) (42,43), and tumor necrosis factor-alpha (TNF-α) (43). Many if not all of these cytokines are thought to be involved in airway inflammation either directly or indirectly.

Studies evaluating the effect of inhaled GC therapy on allergic inflammation in asthma patients have only recently been completed. These studies have employed bronchoscopy with bronchoalveolar lavage (BAL) and/or endobronchial biopsy prior to and following a course of inhaled GC therapy. One of the first controlled studies evaluated the effect of budesonide (1200 μg/day) or terbutaline for 3 months on airway inflammation in 14 adult asthma patients (44). Budesonide therapy was associated with an increase in the number of ciliated epithelial cells and a reduction in the number of eosinophils within the airway epithelium. Reductions in the number of eosinophils and activated T lymphocytes (CD25-positive) obtained from the BAL fluid of asthma patients treated with high-dose BDP have also been noted (45). A recent study from Trigg et al. (46) also evaluated the effect of high-dose BDP therapy (1000 μg/day) or placebo in a group of 25 patients with mild asthma. In contrast to the above studies, these investigators failed to see reductions in numbers of T-helper and activated T cells following a 4-month course of BDP, but they did find significant reductions in the number of tissue eosinophils and activated eosinophils (EG2-positive). Of significance, BDP was found to reduce the epithelial expression of GM-CSF and to reduce the thickness of the lamina reticularis, whereas no effect on either parameter was noted with placebo. Exhaled nitric oxide (NO) has been noted to be elevated in asthma patients and may serve as a useful noninvasive marker of allergic inflammation. A recent study evaluated the effect of budesonide (1600 μg/day) on exhaled NO levels (47). Following a 3-week course of budesonide therapy, NO levels fell significantly from 203 to 120 ppb, whereas there was no change following placebo administration. Although inhaled GC therapy can reduce the degree of inflammation, it cannot completely abolish the infiltration of inflammatory cells into the airways. This point was nicely demonstrated by Sont et al. (48), who performed bronchoscopy with biopsies in a group of 26 adults with mild to moderate asthma on chronic inhaled GC therapy (BDP or budesonide, mean dose of 654 μg/day). Despite the fact that all patients were on inhaled GC therapy, significant numbers of eosinophils, T lymphocytes, and mast cells were found within the lamina propria. Of interest, correlations were noted between the inflammatory cells and bronchial hyperresponsiveness but not with symptom scores, pulmonary function measures, or supplemental β-agonist use.

In summary, therapy with inhaled GC results in reductions in inflammatory cell infiltration into the lamina propria and epithelium, and it has been suggested that inhaled GCs can reduce the thickness of the lamina reticularis. These data support the hypothesis that inhaled GCs act topically by suppressing allergic inflammation and may also modulate airway remodeling.

IV. Efficacy

A vast body of literature has accumulated over the past 25 years that support the clinical efficacy of inhaled GC therapy in both children and adults. This section provides a general overview of clinical efficacy, highlighting important articles that demonstrate the effectiveness of inhaled GC therapy.

Increased bronchial responsiveness, or bronchial hyperresponsiveness (BHR), is a sentinel feature of asthma that has been shown to correlate with disease severity, frequency of symptoms, and need for treatment (49). Although the precise relationship remains elusive, airway inflammation is thought to contribute to BHR (50,51); however, the two conditions are not necessarily directly linked (52). Studies evaluating the effect of inhaled GC therapy in asthma have consistently demonstrated a favorable effect on BHR in both adults and children with asthma (53–63). Decreases in BHR from two- to sevenfold have been reported within 6 weeks of instituting inhaled GC therapy, with a plateau effect usually reached by 8 weeks. Although few studies have attempted to compare the effects of oral therapy with those of inhaled GC therapy on reductions in BHR, at least one study suggests that inhaled GC therapy may, in fact, be superior to oral GC therapy (64).

Van Essen-Zandvliet et al. (62), in one of the largest controlled studies evaluating inhaled GC therapy in children, studied 116 children assigned either to salbutamol and budesonide (600 μg/day) or salbutamol only over a 22-month period. The children on budesonide displayed a 3-fold reduction in BHR at 4 months of therapy, which became even greater by the study's end. Of even greater significance, a plateau effect had not been seen even after 22 months of budesonide therapy. Associated with the decrease in BHR were significant improvements in lung function and asthma symptoms. The children randomized to budesonide had an 11% improvement in their prebronchodilator FEV_1 as compared with the children on placebo, and this improved lung function was maintained throughout the study. The children on placebo therapy fared poorly, with over 40% requiring withdrawal from the study secondary to poor asthma control and nearly 50 requiring at least one oral GC burst during the study secondary to an asthma exacerbation. In marked contrast, only 14% of the patients on budesonide required supplemental courses of prednisone. Finally, three children required hospitalization during the study, and all three were in the placebo group.

Similar results have been noted in adult asthma patients. Haahtela et al. (61) studied the effect of budesonide (1200 μg/day) or terbutaline in 103 newly diagnosed adult asthma patients over a 96-week period and found one doubling dose reduction in BHR in those treated with budesonide. Unlike the case in the pediatric study, a plateau effect was reached by 8 weeks, and this was sustained throughout the study. Associated with the reduction in BHR were significant improvements in symptom scores, PEF rates, and a decreased need for supplemental β_2-agonist use. A greater number of patients randomized to the placebo group (n = 10) were withdrawn from the study secondary to poor asthma control as compared with those randomized to budesonide (n = 1). In summary, studies evaluating inhaled steroid therapy have consistently reported significant reductions in BHR, fewer asthma symptoms, improved pulmonary function (PEF and FEV_1), less need for supplemental β-agonist use, and fewer exacerbations requiring courses of oral GCs.

Inhaled GCs were initially reserved for use in patients with moderate to severe asthma (65); but as our understanding of this disease has advanced, inhaled GCs are now recommended for individuals with mild persistent asthma (66). The newly updated guidelines now from the National Heart, Lung and Blood Institute (NHLBI) recommend low-dose inhaled GC therapy (or cromolyn/nedocromil for children) as first-line therapy for mild persistent asthma (66). Inhaled GCs are also recommended in increasing doses for those with moderate and severe asthma. Whether inhaled GC therapy should be first-line therapy in children with mild asthma remains a topic of debate (67). Those who favor the use of inhaled GC therapy in mild asthma argue that since this medication reduces airway inflammation, BHR and the need for supplemental β-agonist therapy, it should be used in all patients with mild persistent asthma or asthma of greater severity. Given that inhaled GC therapy is not without the potential for adverse effects and that adequate long-term studies evaluating bone demineralization and growth delay have yet to be completed, others argue that its use be reserved for those with more frequent symptoms—i.e., patients with moderate to severe persistent asthma.

Two recent studies, one in children the other in adults, evaluated the efficacy and adverse effects of long-term budesonide therapy in mild asthma (68,69). Of no surprise, both found budesonide to be an effective asthma therapy, with few adverse effects noted. Of significance, both made the intriguing observation that the longer an individual had asthma prior to instituting inhaled GC therapy, the less improvement in pulmonary function was noted following institution of budesonide therapy. The results from these studies suggest that the longer the time from the initiation of symptoms and subsequent treatment with inhaled GC, the less effective this form of therapy may be.

V. Adverse Effects

Although the topical-to-systemic potency of inhaled GCs make the likelihood of GC-associated adverse effects much less than that associated with oral GCs, the potential for systemic absorption and hence systemic effects remains. In general, the development of adverse effects from inhaled GC therapy is in large part dependent on the dose and the frequency with which the inhaled GC is given (70). High doses (1000 μg/day in children) administered frequently (four times daily) are most likely to result in an increase in both local and systemic adverse effects.

A. Local Adverse Effects

The most commonly encountered adverse effects from inhaled GC therapy are local and consist of oral candidiasis and dysphonia. As is the case for systemic complications, these effects are dose-dependent and are most common in individuals on high-dose inhaled and oral GC therapy (71,72). Thrush is thought to occur as a result of local immunosuppression, while dysphonia occurs as a result of vocal cord muscle myopathy (73). The incidence of these local effects can be greatly minimized by using a spacer device, which reduces the oropharyngeal deposition of the drug (74,75). In addition, mouth rinsing using a ''swish and spit'' technique following inhaled GC inhalation leaves less drug in the oropharynx and reduces absorption of the drug from the GI tract.

B. Systemic Adverse Effects

Even though the risk of developing systemic adverse effects is much smaller for inhaled than for oral GC therapy, the potential for toxicity remains. The systemic effects of inhaled GCs are dependent on the dose delivered, the pharmacokinetic profile of the GC (i.e., degree of first-pass hepatic metabolism), the method of delivery of the GC, and individual differences in steroid sensitivity among patients (71). Several systemic effects have been reported and include suppression of the hypothalamic-pituitary-adrenal axis, growth suppression, effects on bone metabolism, dermal thinning, cataracts/glaucoma, hypoglycemia, weight gain, psychosis, and opportunistic infection.

Adrenal Suppression

Inhaled GC therapy can result in suppression of the hypothalamic-pituitary-adrenal axis. The degree of suppression is largely dependent on the dose and frequency of the inhaled GC delivered, duration of treatment, route of administration, and time of day the drug is administered (76). There are two major methods of assessing HPA axis function (77). The first method measures basal adrenal activity. Examples of this method include single morning cortisol determinations (the least sensitive method), serial serum cortisol concentrations over a fixed period of time (very sensitive), or 24-hr urinary cortisol excretion (also very sensitive). The other method measures response to stimulation (ACTH or metyrapone) or stress (insulin-induced hypoglycemia). There have been a large number of studies evaluating HPA function in asthma patients; most have measured basal cortisol activity with single morning serum cortisol determinations (78–80) or 24-hr urinary cortisol excretion (81–83), while others have measured response to stimulation (84,85). The preponderance of data would suggest that doses of 400 μg/day or less are not associated with changes in the HPA axis but that, as the inhaled dose is increased to above 1000 μg/day, HPA axis suppression clearly occurs. High-dose fluticasone propionate (FP) therapy appears to have a much greater effect on the HPA axis suppression than does therapy with the other inhaled GCs, as discussed below (86,87). Whether or not modest reductions in the HPA axis are of clinical relevance remains to be determined. Even though it is extremely unlikely that an asthma patient on less than 1000 μg/day would develop an addisonian crisis due to adrenal suppression, the fact that measurable changes in the HPA axis are present indicates systemic absorption; thus HPA axis suppression could serve as a marker for other systemic effects.

Growth Suppression

Growth suppression is the steroid-associated adverse effect that causes the most concern for clinicians caring for children (88). Whether clinically significant growth suppression can occur with chronic inhaled GC therapy remains controversial, with some studies suggesting that doses of as little as 400 mg/day of beclomethasone dipropionate can result in suppression of linear growth. Unfortunately, almost all of the studies that have attempted to determine the effect of inhaled GCs on growth have been limited. Many studies have evaluated growth over short periods of time utilizing knemometry (89,90). Of significance, reductions in the lower leg growth rate noted in short-term knemometry studies cannot be used to predict an adverse effect on long-term statural growth (91). Other studies evaluating growth over longer periods of time have not been placebo-controlled, and some studies have studied too heterogeneous a patient population in terms of scatter of ages among the children enrolled. The following discussion attempts to summarize the data, given the above limitations.

Before one can address the effect of inhaled GC therapy on growth, one must first take into account the observation that asthma, especially poorly controlled asthma, can affect growth adversely (92,93). Ninan and Russell, in one of the few studies that took this variable into account, evaluated the growth of 58 children with asthma over a 5-year period (94). All children were prepubescent at entry (mean age 3.5 years for males, 4.4 years for females); they were followed for nearly 2 years before receiving inhaled GC therapy. In addition, each child's asthma was classified as being under good, moderate, or poor control according to asthma symptoms prior to beginning inhaled GC therapy. These investigators found that the study group as a whole had diminished growth velocity at the start of the study with a mean height velocity standard deviation (HVSD) score of −0.51. The children whose asthma was in good control had the least evidence of growth suppression prior to the institution of inhaled GC therapy and continued to grow at the same rate while on therapy (HVSD score −0.01 before versus −0.07 during iGC treatment). In contrast, the subjects whose asthma was poorly controlled grew poorly regardless of whether or not they were receiving inhaled GC (HVSD score −1.50 before versus −1.55 during). Of interest, those with moderately controlled asthma actually demonstrated improved growth velocity while on inhaled GC therapy, with the HVSD score increasing from −0.83 to −0.49. These investigators concluded that poor asthma control significantly affected growth more than inhaled GC therapy.

There have now been three controlled studies demonstrating growth suppression using moderate doses of beclomethasone over a period of 7–12 months (95–97). In the first study, Tinkelman et al. (95) compared BDP 84 μg administered four times daily (336 μg/day) with theophylline in 195 children 6–16 years old with mild to moderate asthma over a 12-month period. Suppression of growth velocity was noted in the group treated with BPD, with the males being most affected. Doull et al. (96) studied the effect of 400 μg/day BDP or placebo in 94 children with mild asthma (7–9 years old) for 7 months followed by a 4-month washout period. Following 7 months of either BDP or placebo, the children randomized to BDP had grown significantly less than the children on placebo (2.66 versus 3.66 cm) with no significant catch-up growth noted during the 4 month washout period. Of note, the growth suppression occurred in the absence of suppression of the HPA axis, a finding also noted by Tinkelman et al. (95). The third study evaluated the effect of 1 year of therapy with BDP (400 μg/day) versus salmeterol in 67 children (mean age 10.5 years, range 6–16 years) with mild to moderate asthma (96). BDP was found to be superior to salmeterol in terms of efficacy (improved pulmonary function, reduced BHR, and decreased need for oral GC use). However, the average annual growth was significantly reduced, with a reduction in linear growth of 1.4 cm resulting in −0.28 SDS.

Complicating the issue further is the observation that asthma can delay the onset of puberty (97,98). Studies utilizing inhaled GC therapy in older children and in children in whom a reduction in growth velocity is noted may actually be demonstrating an exaggerated decline in growth velocity seen immediately prior to the onset of puberty (99). A study by Merkus et al. (100) evaluated the long-term (22 months) effect of either budesonide (600 μg/day) or placebo on the growth rates of 40 asthmatic teenagers (mean age 12.8 years) compared with the growth rates of 80 age-matched, nonasthmatic controls. Growth rates among the male asthmatic children were found to be significantly decreased compared to age-matched non-asthmatic controls, but when the growth rates between those treated with placebo versus those given budesonide were compared, those treated with budesonide had better growth rates (−0.44 cm/year for budesonide versus −0.70 cm/year for placebo). Thus, the growth delay noted among the asthmatic adolescents was most likely due to a delay in puberty and not to the long-term budesonide therapy.

Although inhaled GC therapy can suppress short-term linear growth, long-term studies have not shown differences in growth (68) or attainment of adult height as compared with asthmatic patients not on inhaled GC and nonasthmatic controls (98,101). Unfortunately, none of these studies were ideal in that they were either retrospective or lacking adequate controls. A large 5-year randomized, multicenter study sponsored by the National Institutes of Health, called the Childhood Asthma Management Program (CAMP), is an ongoing study designed to answer many of the questions we have regarding inhaled GC use in childhood asthma. This study, in which >1000 children have been randomized to receive either placebo, nedocromil, or budesonide over a 5-year period, is designed to measure the natural history of childhood asthma in addition to the efficacy and adverse effects of the two study medications. Of particular interest is whether 5 years of budesonide therapy will adversely affect growth in addition to other potential adverse effects, including changes in bone metabolism or osteoporosis.

Osteoporosis

Osteoporosis, is a significant and common adverse effect in asthmatic patients dependent on chronic oral GC therapy. All patients who have been on >7.5 mg prednisone (or equivalent) daily for at least 6 months are at risk for developing osteoporosis (102). Despite the fact that osteoporosis is a potentially debilitating complication of GC therapy, there have been, until recently, a paucity of studies evaluating the effect of inhaled GC on bone metabolism and even fewer studies evaluating the effect of inhaled GC on bone mineral density. GCs exert negative effects on bone formation by inhibiting osteoblast function in addition to increasing bone resorption. There are several markers available for use in analyzing the effects of GC on bone metabolism (103). The carboxypeptide of type I procollagen (PICP), osteocalcin, and alkaline phosphatase are serum markers of osteoblast function, while urinary hydroxyproline, pyridinolone, and serum tartrate resistant acid phosphatase (TRAP) and type I collagen carboxy terminal propeptide (ICTP) are markers of bone resorption. Short-term studies have demonstrated dose-dependent suppression of serum osteocalcin levels with both beclomethasone dipropionate (104,105) and budesonide (106). A study designed to assess the long-term effects of inhaled GC on bone metabolism evaluated serum PICP and ICTP levels in 70 patients randomized to receive beclomethasone dipropionate (800 μg/day) compared with those in 85 patients randomized to receive bronchodilator therapy alone over a 2.5-year period (107). Of some surprise, although decreases in serum osteocalcin levels were noted shortly after treatment (4 weeks), there were no differences in markers of bone resorption or bone formation between the two groups upon completion of the 2.5-year study. The authors concluded that long-term changes in bone turnover during inhaled GC treatment should not be deduced from short-term studies with single serum parameters of bone function. They also stated that long-term studies utilizing bone densitometry need to be performed to adequately determine the potential for detrimental effects on bone metabolism.

To assess the clinical relevance of inhaled GC therapy on bone metabolism, studies utilizing bone densitometry should be performed. Bone densitometry is the most sensitive way to assess for the presence of osteoporosis (108,109). The detection and quantitation of the degree of osteoporosis is important; as the degree of osteoporosis increases, so too does the risk of fracture (110). There have been a number of studies utilizing bone densitometry in asthma patients on inhaled GC therapy. Most studies have been cross-sectional while a few have been prospective, controlled studies. Two recently published cross-sectional studies highlight the discrepancies in results that characterize many of the studies evaluating adverse effects with inhaled GC therapy. Hanania et al. (111) studied 36 asthma patients—18 treated with BDP (mean dose 1323 μg/day; median duration 24 months) and 18 treated with bronchodilator alone. Biochemical markers of bone metabolism as well as bone mineral density were measured in all subjects. The investigators found significant reductions in osteocalcin levels in the group on BDP compared with those on bronchodilator therapy. In addition, those on BDP had significantly decreased bone mineral density of the femoral neck compared with age-matched controls. Of note, significant inverse correlations were found between bone mineral density and the dose duration (product of the average daily dose of inhaled GC in grams and the duration of therapy in months) of inhaled GC therapy.

Whereas Hanania et al. (111) found inhaled GC therapy to result in a dose-dependent reduction in bone density, Luengo et al. (112), found no difference in bone mineral density among 48 asthmatic patients on inhaled GC (BDP or budesonide; mean dose 662 ± 278 μg/day for 10.6 years) compared with 48 age- and sex-matched nonasthmatic controls at baseline or after 2 years of observation. Similar results were noted by Konig et al. (113) in a cross-sectional study performed in children. These investigators studied the effect of 300–600 μg/day of BDP on biochemical markers of bone metabolism and bone mineral density for 24 months compared with age- and sex-matched controls and children with asthma not on inhaled GC therapy. BDP in doses up to 800 μg/day had no effect on osteocalcin levels or bone mineral density, but the asthmatic patients had lower osteocalcin levels than their age-matched, nonasthmatic peers.

Given the discrepancy in results among the above studies, Toogood et al. performed bone density studies in 69 adult patients with asthma in an attempt to differentiate between the effect of inhaled GC and the potential effect of other variables such as past or current oral GC use, age, physical activity level, and postmenopausal state on bone density (114). They found inhaled GC therapy to result in a dose-dependent reduction of bone mineral density with a decrease of approximately 0.5 standard deviations for each increment of inhaled GC dose of 1 mg/day. Of some surprise, a larger lifetime exposure to inhaled GC was associated with a more normal lumbar bone density. Toogood and colleagues speculated that this "protective effect" was due to reconstitution of bone mineral density following conversion from oral to inhaled GC therapy. Last, postmenopausal women on estrogen replacement therapy were likely to have normal bone density. In conclusion, the daily dose but not the duration of therapy adversely affects bone density, and estrogen therapy may offset inhaled GC effects on bone demineralization in postmenopausal women (114).

Cataracts/Glaucoma

Cataracts and glaucoma are known ophthalmological complications of chronic systemic GC therapy (115–117). Two recent reports have suggested that chronic inhaled GC therapy is also associated with the development of these complications (118,119). Both studies have received substantial coverage in the lay press and both are large epidemiological studies that found weak but statistically significant associations between inhaled GC therapy and either cataracts or glaucoma. It should be noted that in both studies elderly individuals were evaluated, with the mean age in the cataract study being 66 years, while only subjects 65 years of age and above were evaluated in the glaucoma study. In the study by Garbe et al. (119), individuals on high-dose inhaled GC therapy (≥1500 μg/day) for prolonged periods (≥3 months) were at greatest risk for the development of glaucoma, with an odds ratio of 1.44. Cummings et al. also found an increased risk for the development of subcapsular cataracts with higher cumulative lifetime doses of inhaled GC therapy, the highest prevalence being found in subjects whose lifetime dose was >2000 mg (118). Whether the results of these studies apply to inhaled GC in children remains to be determined, although smaller studies have not found associations between inhaled GC and cataract formation (95,120).

Other Adverse Effects

There have been a number of other adverse effects associated with inhaled GC therapy, including hypoglycemia (121), the development of cushingoid features (122), opportunistic infections (123–125), dermal thinning (126,127), and psychosis (128). Most of these adverse effects have been reported as case reports, with few controlled studies performed to objectively evaluate the potential for and significance of these complications.

In summary, while this area remains controversial, most would agree that high-dose (>1000 μg/day for children, 2000 μg/day for adults) therapy for extended periods is most likely to be associated with greatest risk of adverse effects. The adverse effects of greatest concern include suppression of the HPA axis, growth suppression, and the insidious development of osteoporosis. At present many questions remain regarding the clinical significance of these adverse effects. Studies designed to address these concerns are in progress (e.g., the CAMP study); until a clear consensus emerges, it is prudent to use the lowest tolerated inhaled GC dose and to keep in mind that systemic effects can occur in those patients who require high-dose therapy for long periods to ensure adequate asthma control.

VI. Fluticasone Propionate: The Newest Inhaled GC

Four inhaled GC preparations are on the market in the United States: beclomethasone dipropionate (Vanceril, Beclovent), triamcinolone acetonide (Azmacort), flunisolide (Aerobid), and fluticasone propionate (Flovent). A fifth inhaled GC, budesonide (Pulmicort), although widely studied and used throughout the world, has only recently received FDA approval. Despite the widespread use of GCs over several years, questions persist regarding whether one steroid preparation is more potent and hence superior to another. In attempting to address this question, one must consider potency in terms of both clinical efficacy and systemic effects or potential for adverse effects of the drug in question. To date, there has yet to be a clinical study that has compared, head to head, the clinical efficacy and systemic effects of all the available inhaled steroids, thus making it difficult to determine whether one drug is any ‘‘better’’ than another. With that said, McCubbin et al. (129)—using partial suppression of the immediate asthmatic response to inhaled allergen as a measure of topical potency and 24-hr urinary free cortisol output as a measure of systemic potency—found beclomethasone dipropionate, triamcinolone, and flunisolide to have equivalent potencies for both topical and systemic effects. Since the release of fluticasone propionate (FP) in August 1996, there has been much discussion regarding whether this drug distinguishes itself from the other inhaled GCs.

A. Distinguishing Features of Fluticasone Propionate: Efficacy

Although newly introduced, FP has been widely studied, and it is from this body of research that several unique features of FP have emerged. First, because FP binds to the glucocorticoid receptor with very high affinity (130) and possesses a prolonged GC receptor binding time (131), it is among the most potent in terms of topical anti-inflammatory effects. In addition, it undergoes extensive first-pass hepatic metabolism, rendering >95% of the swallowed portion inactive once it passes the liver (132,133). It should be noted that any inhaled GC delivered to the lung is available to the systemic circulation; in the case of FP, this is the sole source of systemic absorption (134). These two features, high topical anti-inflammatory effects and extensive first-pass metabolism, give this compound a high topical-to-systemic potency ratio, which is the basis for its clinical efficacy.

Second, FP is available in three MDI dosage strengths: low (44 μg per puff), medium (110 μg per puff), and high (220 μg per puff). This allows one to treat all degrees of asthma severity while keeping the puffs required per day within an acceptable number. Third, studies in both adults and children have consistently demonstrated FP to be more effective than beclomethasone dipropionate and budesonide on a microgram-per-microgram basis. Studies comparing FP to beclomethasone dipropionate have shown FP to be approximately twice as potent in terms of improving PEFR (135,136). It should be noted that equal improvement in efficacy parameters while patients are receiving different doses of inhaled GCs (e.g., *X* μg/day of GC A versus 2*X* μg/day of GC B) do not necessarily "prove" that GC A is twice as potent as GC B (137). In an attempt to better quantify whether differences in the clinical efficacy and systemic effects of budesonide and FP exist, Agertoft and Pedersen published a study designed to compare the minimum effective dose of budesonide Turbuhaler to the fluticasone propionate Diskhaler (138). These investigators found both drugs to be equally effective on a microgram-per-microgram basis, but since the budesonide Turbuhaler is thought to deliver a greater quantity of drug to the lower airways than the fluticasone Diskhaler, the authors concluded that FP is likely to be more potent than budesonide (138).

Fourth, high-dose FP has been shown to have profound oral steroid-sparing effects in patients with steroid-dependent asthma (139). In this randomized, placebo-controlled, multicenter study, over 80% of the patients on high-dose FP therapy (2000 μg/day) were able to be completely tapered off oral GC therapy. In addition, the mean FEV_1 actually increased in this group despite the significant reduction in oral steroid dose. This degree of steroid-sparing effect has not been noted in other studies in which steroid-dependent asthma patients could be tapered off their oral GC utilizing the other available inhaled GC (140). Fifth, high-dose FP therapy has recently been shown to be as effective as prednisolone for the treatment of mild to moderate acute asthma exacerbations (141). In this study over 400 adult asthma patients with acute asthma exacerbations were enrolled in a randomized, double-blind, double-dummy parallel study that compared the efficacy of FP 2000 μg/day or a tapering dose of prednisolone over a 16-day period. The investigators found both treatments to be equally effective in the treatment of mild to moderate asthma exacerbations not requiring admission to the hospital. This is an intriguing article, which suggests that oral GC may not be required for mild-to-moderate asthma exacerbations. Although high-dose FP therapy is associated with systemic effects (see below), they would be expected to be less significant than those of oral glucocorticoid therapy.

Last, FP therapy has been shown to result in significant reductions in airway inflammatory cells/mediators of inflammation from both BAL fluid and airway tissue of adults with asthma (142,143). As discussed above, studies using other inhaled GCs have shown similar effects, so this finding is not unique to FP. Of importance, even short-term (3-week) low-dose FP (500 μg/day) therapy results in reduced airway inflammation (39). Associated with the decreased airway inflammation was a reduction in the thickness of the lamina propria, suggesting that FP can modulate the intensity of airway remodeling. BDP has also been demonstrated to decrease the thickness of the lamina propria, but at twice the dose (1000 μg/day) given over a longer period of time (4 months) (46).

B. Distinguishing Features of Fluticasone Propionate: Adverse Effects

Several studies in both adults and children have evaluated the effect of FP on suppression of the HPA axis. The majority have shown FP to have comparable systemic effects to either beclomethasone dipropionate or budesonide, especially at the doses of FP recommended for the treatment of mild and moderate asthma (176–440 μg/day) (135,136,144,145). The same cannot be said regarding high-dose fluticasone propionate (i.e., dose ≥1000 μg/day). A number of studies have demonstrated significantly greater effects on suppression of the HPA axis than equivalent doses of budesonide (86,87,146). These studies found FP to have a greater ability to suppress plasma cortisol, urinary cortisol, and ACTH levels, with the greatest degree of suppression noted at doses of ≥1000 μg/day. Specifically, Clark et al. (86) studied 12 adult asthma patients in a double-blind, placebo-controlled, crossover design comparing single doses of either inhaled budesonide (400, 1000, 1600, or 2000 μg) or FP (500, 1000, 1500, or 2000 μg) administered at 2200 hr, and found FP to exhibit at least a twofold greater degree of adrenal suppression than budesonide on a microgram-per-microgram basis. The interpretations from this study are limited by its design—i.e., a single-dose study with the drug administered at 2200 hr (maximizing potential adrenal suppression).

A subsequent study from the same group (146) studied the effect of chronic dosing of either fluticasone propionate or budesonide administered twice daily over 4 days; it found fluticasone propionate to have a more profound suppressive effect on both morning cortisol levels and overnight urinary cortisol/creatine ratios compared to budesonide, with a 3.5-fold difference in potency between the two drugs. Similar results were reported by Boorsma et al. (87), who compared the relative systemic potency of FP and budesonide in non-asthmatic adults administered twice daily over 4 days. These investigators found fluticasone to have a 3.7- to 5.2-fold greater systemic potency ratio than budesonide. Of note, high-dose FP (2000 μg/day) resulted in a reduction of over 80% in the average cortisol level, and 89% suppression of the morning level, compared with 27% and 11% suppression for 2000 μg/day of budesonide respectively.

From these three studies, FP at doses of ≥1000 μg/day can be expected to result in clinically significant adrenal suppression. This is an important and possibly unique observation for FP. Thus, one should use high-dose FP only in patients with severe, poorly controlled asthma or in those with steroid-dependent asthma. Once the patient's asthma is better controlled or the oral steroid dose has been significantly tapered, attempts should be made to titrate the FP dose downward. Since FP comes in three different dosage strengths, a simple approach would be to have the patient stop taking the inhaler providing 220 μg per puff and begin using the MDI providing 110 μg/puff at the same number of puffs.

Whether long-term high-dose FP therapy will be associated with other significant systemic adverse effects remains unknown at the present time. In one of the few studies that evaluated the effect of fluticasone propionate on bone metabolism, Bootsma et al. (147) compared the effect of fluticasone propionate 750 μg/day with that of beclomethasone 1500 μg/day in a randomized, double-blind, crossover study over 6 weeks with evaluation of serum cortisol, osteocalcin, PICP, ICTP, and deoxypyridinoline cross-links before and after treatment. Neither treatment affected morning cortisol levels, but significant decreases in osteocalcin and PICP, markers of bone formation, were noted following beclomethasone dipropionate and not fluticasone propionate therapy. Neither drug had any effect on the markers of bone resorption studied (ICTP and deoxypyridinoline cross-links).

Of concern to clinicians caring for children was a recent report of growth suppression associated with high-dose FP therapy (148). Six children with severe, symptomatic asthma despite being on ≥800 μg/day of either beclomethasone dipropionate or budesonide were placed on high-dose FP (≥1000 μg/day) in an attempt to improve their asthma control. Following institution of high-dose fluticasone therapy, all of the children displayed improved asthma control, but associated with this were decreases in their growth velocity. Of no surprise, significant adrenal suppression was also noted. There are several limitations to this study in that it was neither prospective nor controlled in any way. It does make the important observation that high-dose FP therapy may be associated with clinically significant adverse effects. Again, it is important to stress that the higher the dose of any inhaled GC, the greater the chance of developing systemic adverse effects (72). Although high-dose fluticasone therapy may be associated with growth suppression, a recently published study evaluating the short-term effects of low-dose (200, and 400 μg/day) FP and budesonide showed no effect on lower leg growth with either GC at 200 μg/day and a slight but statistically significant reduction in lower leg growth with budesonide at 400 μg/day, but not with FP at the same dose (149).

In summary, FP is a newly released inhaled GC displaying several unique features that may distinguish it from the other currently available inhaled GCs. It is an effective and safe inhaled GC preparation when given at the recommended doses. Of note, high-dose therapy (≥1000 μg/day) may be associated with a greater degree of adrenal suppression than therapy with the other inhaled GCs; thus FP should be reserved for use in severe, poorly controlled, or steroid-dependent asthma. The safety of FP should be measured in terms of its efficacy;

i.e., at equal doses, FP is likely to have greater systemic effects than other inhaled GCs, but it will also display greater clinical efficacy. Thus, for equal degrees of efficacy, a smaller amount of FP should suffice.

References

1. Szefler SJ. Glucocorticoid therapy for asthma: Clinical pharmacology. J Allergy Clin Immunol 1991; 88:147–164.
2. Spahn JD, Leung DYM. The role of glucocorticoids in the management of asthma. Allergy Asthma Proc 1996; 17:341–350.
3. Randolph TG, Rollins JP. The effect of cortisone on bronchial asthma. J Allergy 1950; 21:288–295.
4. Carryer HM, Koelsche GA, Prickman LE, Maytum CK, Lake C, Williams HL. The effect of cortisone on bronchial asthma and hay fever occurring in subjects sensitive to ragweed pollen. J Allergy 1950; 21:282–287.
5. Feinberg SM, Dannenberg TB, Malkiel S. ACTH and cortisone in allergic manifestations: Therapeutic results and studies on immunological and tissue reactivity. J Allergy 1951; 22:195–210.
6. Gelfand ML. Administration of cortisone by the aerosol method in the treatment of bronchial asthma. N Engl J Med 1951; 245:293–294.
7. Brockbank W, Brebner H, Pengelly CDR. Chronic asthma treated with aerosol hydrocortisone. Lancet 1956; 2:807.
8. Reed CE. Aerosol glucocorticoid treatment of asthma: Adults. Am Rev Respir Dis 1990; 141:S82–S88.
9. Crepea SB. Inhalation corticosteroid (dexamethasone PO_4) management of chronically asthmatic children. J Allergy 1963; 34:119–126.
10. Arbesman CE, Bonstein HS, Reisman RE. Dexamethasone aerosol therapy for bronchial asthma. J Allergy 1963; 34:354–361.
11. Snider GL, Frank MI, Aaronson AL, Radner DB, Kaplan MA, Mosko MM. The effect of dexamethasone aerosol on airway obstruction in bronchial asthma. Dis Chest 1963; 44:408–415.
12. Dennis M, Itkin IH. Effectiveness and complications of aerosol dexamethasone phosphate in severe asthma. J Allergy 1964; 35:70–76.
13. Toogood JH, Lefcoe NM. Dexamethasone aerosol for the treatment of ''steroid dependent'' chronic bronchial asthmatic patients. J Allergy 1965; 36:321–332.
14. Brown HM, Storey G, George WHS. Beclomethasone dipropionate: A new steroid aerosol for the treatment of allergic asthma. Br Med J 1972; 1:585–590.
15. Clark TJH. Effect of beclomethasone dipropionate delivered by aerosol in patients with asthma. Lancet 1972; 1:1361–1364.
16. Brompton Hospital/Medical Research Council Collaborative Trial. Double-blind trial comparing two dosage schedules of beclomethasone dipropionate aerosol in the treatment of chronic asthma. Lancet 1974; 2:303–307.
17. British Thoracic and Tuberculosis Association. Inhaled corticosteroids compared

with oral prednisone in patients starting long-term corticosteroid therapy for asthma. Lancet 1975; 2:469–473.
18. Godfrey S, Konig P. Beclomethasone aerosol in childhood asthma. Arch Dis Child 1973; 48:665–670.
19. British Thoracic and Tuberculosis Association. A controlled trial of corticosteroids in patients receiving prednisone tablets for asthma. Br J Dis Chest 1976; 70:95–103.
20. Picard D, Yamomoto KR. Two signals mediate hormone dependent nuclear localization of the glucocorticoid receptor. EMBO J 1987; 6:3333–3340.
21. Tsai SY, Carlstedt-Duke J, Weigel NL, Dahlman K, Gustafsson JA, Tsai MJ, O'Malley BW. Molecular interactions of steroid hormone receptor with its enhancer element: evidence for receptor dimer formation. Cell 1988; 55:361–369.
22. Luisi BF, Xu WX, Otwinowski Z, Freedman LP, Yamamoto KR, Siegler PB. Crystallographic analysis of the interaction of the glucocorticoid receptor with DNA. Nature 1991; 352:497–505.
23. Sakai DD, Helms S, Carlstedt-Duke J, Gustafsson JA, Rottman FM, Yamamoto KR. Hormone-mediated repression of transcription: A negative glucocorticoid response element from the bovine prolactin gene. Genes Dev 1988; 2:1144–1154.
24. Diamond MI, Miner JN, Yoshinaga SK, Yamamoto KR. Transcription factor interactions: Selectors of positive or negative regulation from a single DNA element. Science 1990; 249:1266–1272.
25. Yang-Yen H-F, Chambard J-C, Sun Y-L, Smeal T, Schmidt TJ, Drouin J, Karin M. Transcriptional interference between c-Jun and the glucocorticoid receptor: Mutual inhibition of DNA binding due to direct protein-protein interaction. Cell 1990; 62: 1205–1215.
26. Barnes PJ, Greening AP, Crompton GK. Glucocorticoid resistance in asthma. Am J Respir Crit Care Med 1995; 152:S125–S142.
27. Schule R, Rangarajan P, Kliewer S, Ransone LJ, Bolado J, Yang N, Verma IM, Evans R. Functional antagonism between oncoprotein c-Jun and the glucocorticoid receptor. Cell 1990; 62:1217–1226.
28. Adcock IM, Brown CR, Gelder CM, Shirasaki H, Peters MJ, Barnes PJ. The effects of glucocorticoids on transcription factor activation in human peripheral blood mononuclear cells. Am J Physiol 1995; 37:C331–C338.
29. Ray A, Prefontaine KE. Physical association and functional antagonism between the p65 subunit of transcription factor NF-kappa B and the glucocorticoid receptor. Proc Natl Acad Sci USA 1994; 91:752–756.
30. Scheinman RI, Cogswell PC, Lofquist AK, Baldwin AS. Role of transcriptional activation of IκBα in mediation of immunosuppression by glucocorticoids. Science 1995; 270:283–286.
31. Auphan N, DiDonato JA, Rosette C, Helmberg A, Karin M. Immunosuppression by glucocorticoids: inhibition of NF-κB activity through induction of IkB synthesis. Science 1995; 270:286–290.
32. Peppel K, Vinci JM, Baglioni C. The AU-rich sequences in the 3′ untranslated region mediate the increased turnover of interferon mRNA induced by glucocorticoids. J Exp Med 1991; 173:349–355.
33. Hegele RG, Hogg JC. The Pathology of asthma: An inflammatory disorder. In

Szefler SJ, Leung DYM, eds. Severe Asthma: Pathogenesis and Clinical Management. New York: Marcel Dekker, 1996:61–76.
34. Borish L, Mascali JJ, Dishuck J, Beam WR, Martin RJ, Rosenwasser LJ. Detection of alveolar macrophage-derived IL-1β in asthma: inhibition with corticosteroids. J Immunol 1992; 149:3078–3082.
35. Boumpas DT, Older SA, Anastassiou ED, Tsokos GC, Nelson D, Balow JE. Dexamethasone inhibits human IL-2 but not IL-2R gene expression in vitro at the level of nuclear transcription. J Clin Invest 1991; 87:1739–1747.
36. Culpepper JA, Lee F. Regulation of IL-3 expression by glucocorticoids in cloned murine T lymphocytes. J Immunol 1985; 135:3191–3197.
37. Wu CY, Fargeas C, Nakajima T, Delespesse G. Glucocorticoids suppress the production of interleukin 4 by human lymphocytes. Eur J Immunol 1991; 21:2645–2647.
38. Byron KA, Varigos G, Wooton A. Hydrocortisone inhibition of human interleukin-4. Immunology 1992; 77:624–626.
39. Rolfe FG, Hughes JM, Armour CL, Sewell WA. Inhibition of interleukin-5 gene expression by dexamethasone. Immunology 1992; 77:494–499.
40. Robinson D, Hamid Q, Ying S, Bentley A, Assoufi B, Durham, Kay AB. Prednisolone treatment in asthma is associated with modulation of bronchoalveolar lavage cell interleukin-4, interleukin-5, and interferon-γ cytokine gene expression. Am Rev Respir Dis 1993; 148:401–406.
41. Tobler A, Meier R, Seitz M, Dewald B, Baggiolini M, Fey MF. Glucocorticoids downregulate gene expression of GM-CSF, NAP-1, IL-8, IL-6, but not M-CSF in human fibroblasts. Blood 1992; 79:45–51.
42. Kato M, Schleimer RP. Antiinflammatory steroids inhibit granulocyte/macrophage colony stimulating factor production by human lung tissue. Lung 1994; 172:113–124.
43. Waage A, Bakke O. Glucocorticoids suppress the production of tumor necrosis factor by lipopolysaccharide-stimulated human monocytes. Immunology 1988; 63: 299–302.
44. Laitinen LA, Laitinen A, Haahtela T. A comparative study of the effects of an inhaled corticosteroid, budesonide, and a β2-agonist, terbutaline, on airway inflammation in newly diagnosed asthma. J Allergy Clin Immunol 1992; 90:32–42.
45. Wilson JW, Djukanovic R, Howarth PH, Holgate ST. Inhaled beclomethasone dipropionate downregulates airway lymphocyte activation in atopic asthma. Am J Respir Crit Care Med 1994; 149:86–90.
46. Trigg CJ, Manolitsas ND, Wang J, Calderon MA, McAulay A, Jordan SE, Herdman MJ, Jhalli N, Duddle JM, Hamilton SA, Devalia JL, Davies RJ. Placebo-controlled immunopathologic study of four months of inhaled corticosteroids in asthma. Am J Respir Crit Care Med 1994; 150:17–22.
47. Kharitonov SA, Yates DH, Barnes PJ. Inhaled glucocorticoids decrease nitric oxide in exhaled air of asthmatic patients. Am J Respir Crit Care Med 1996; 153:454–457.
48. Sont JK, Van Krieken JHJM, Evertse CE, Hooijer R, Willems LNA, Sterk PJ. Relationship between the inflammatory infiltrate in bronchial biopsy specimens and clinical severity of asthma in patients treated with inhaled steroids. Thorax 1996; 51:496–502.

49. Hargreave FE, Ryan G, Thomson NC, Ryan G, Thomson NC, O'Byrne PM, Latimer K, Juniper EF, Dolovich J. Bronchial responsiveness to histamine or methacholine in asthma: measurement and clinical significance. J Allergy Clin Immunol 1981; 68:347–355.
50. Barnes PJ. New concepts in the pathogenesis of bronchial hyperresponsiveness and asthma. J Allergy Clin Immunol 1989; 83:1013–1026.
51. Chung KF. Role played by inflammation in the hyperreactivity of the airways in asthma. Thorax 1986; 41:657–662.
52. Power C, Sreenan S, Hurson B, Burke C, Poulter LW. Distribution of immunocompetent cells in the bronchial wall of clinically healthy subjects showing bronchial hyperresponsiveness. Thorax 1993; 48:1125–1129.
53. Kraan J, Koeter GH, VD Mark TW, Sluiter HJ, De Vries K. Changes in bronchial hyperreactivity induced by 4 weeks of treatment with antiasthmatic drugs in patients with allergic asthma: a comparison between budesonide and terbutaline. J Allergy Clin Immunol 1985; 76:628–636.
54. Ryan G, Latimer KM, Juniper EF, Roberts RS, Tech M, Hargreave FE. Effect of beclomethasone dipropionate on bronchial hyperresponsiveness to histamine in controlled non-steroid dependent asthma. J Allergy Clin Immunol 1985; 75:25–30.
55. Dutoit JI, Salome CM, Woolcock AJ. Inhaled corticosteroids reduce the severity of bronchial hyperresponsiveness in asthma but oral theophylline does not. Am Rev Respir Dis 1987; 136:1174–1178.
56. Svendsen UG, Frolund L, Madsen F, Nielson NH, Holstein-Rathlou N-H, Weeke B. A comparison of the effects of sodium cromylglycate and beclomethasone dipropionate on pulmonary function and bronchial hyperreactivity in subjects with asthma. J Allergy Clin Immunol 1987; 80:68–74.
57. Kerrebijn KF, Van Essen-Zandvliet EEM, Neijens HJ. Effect of long-term treatment with inhaled corticosteroids and beta-agonists on the bronchial hyperresponsiveness in children with asthma. J Allergy Clin Immunol 1987; 79:653–659.
58. Kraan J, Koeter GH, Van Der Mark TW, Boorsma MM, Kukler J, Sluiter HJ, De Vries K. Dosage and time effects of inhaled budesonide on bronchial hyperreactivity. Am J Respir Dis 1988; 137:44–48.
59. Juniper EF, Kline PA, Vanzieleghem MA, Ramsdale EH, O'Byrne PM, Hargreave FE. Effect of long-term treatment with an inhaled corticosteroid (budesonide) on airway hyperresponsiveness and clinical asthma in non-steroid-dependent asthmatics. Am Rev Respir Dis 1990; 142:832–836.
60. Waalkens HJ, Gerristen J, Koeter GH, Krouwels FH, Van Aalderen WMC, Knol K. Budesonide and terbutaline or terbutaline alone in children with mild asthma: effects on bronchial hyperresponsiveness and diurnal variation in peak flow. Thorax 1991; 46:499–503.
61. Haahtela T, Jarvinen M, Kava T, Kiviranta K, Koskinen S, Lehtonen K, Nikander K, Persson T, Reinikainen K, Selroos O, Sovijarvi A, Stenius-Aarniala B, Svahn T, Tammivaara R, Laitinen LA. Comparison of a β_2-agonist, terbutaline, with an inhaled corticosteroid, budesonide, in newly diagnosed asthma. N Engl J Med 1991; 325:388–392.
62. Van Essen-Zandvliet EE, Hughes MD, Waalkens HJ, Duiverman EJ, Pocock SJ,

Kerrebijn KF. Effects of 22 months of treatment with inhaled corticosteroids and/or beta-2-agonists on lung function, airway responsiveness, and symptoms in children with asthma. Am J Respir Dis 1992; 146:547–554.

63. Djukanovic R, Wilson JW, Britten KM, Wilson SJ, Walls AF, Roche WR, Howarth PH, Holgate ST. Effect of an inhaled corticosteroid on airway inflammation and symptoms in asthma. Am Rev Respir Dis 1992; 145:669–674.
64. Jenkins CR, Woolcock AJ. Effect of prednisone and beclomethasone dipropionate on airway responsiveness in asthma: a comparative study. Thorax 1988; 43:378–384.
65. Expert Panel Report: Guidelines for the Diagnosis and Management of Asthma. National Institutes of Health, National Heart, Lung and Blood Institute. NIH publication Na 91-3042, 1991.
66. Expert Panel Report 2: Guidelines for the Diagnosis and Management of Asthma. NIH publication No. 97-4051, Bethesda, MD: National Institutes of Health, National Heart, Lung and Blood Institute, 1997.
67. Drazen JM, Israel E. Treating mild asthma—when are inhaled steroids indicated? (editorial) N Engl J Med 1994; 331:737–739.
68. Agertoft L, Pedersen S. Effects of long-term treatment with an inhaled corticosteroid on growth and pulmonary function in asthmatic children. Respir Med 1994; 88:373–381.
70. Haahtela T, Jarvinen M, Kava T, Kiviranta K, Koskinen S, Lehtonen K, Nikander K, Persson T, Selroos O, Sovijarvi A, Stenius-Aarniala B, Svahn T, Tammivaara R, Laitinen LA. Effects of reducing or discontinuing inhaled budesonide in patients with mild asthma. N Engl J Med 1994; 331:700–705.
71. Toogood JH. Complications of topical steroid therapy for asthma. Am Rev Respir Dis 1990; 141:S89–S96.
72. Toogood JH. High-dose inhaled steroid therapy for asthma. J Allergy Clin Immunol 1989; 528–536.
73. Williams AJ, Baghat MS, Stableforth DE, Cayton RM, Shenoi PM, Skinner C. Dysphonia caused by inhaled steroids: recognition of a characteristic laryngeal abnormality. Thorax 1983; 38:813–821.
74. Toogood JH, Baskerville J, Jennings B, Lefcoe NM, Johansson S-A. Use of spacers to facilitate inhaled corticosteroid treatment of asthma. Am Rev Respir Dis 1984; 129:723–729.
75. Toogood JH, Jennings B, Baskerville J, Lefcoe N, Newhouse M. Assessment of a device for reducing oropharyngeal complications during beclomethasone treatment of asthma. Am Rev Respir Dis 1981; 123:113.
76. Meltzer EO, Kemp JP, Welch MJ, Orgel HA. Effect of dosing schedule on efficacy of beclomethasone dipropionate aerosol in chronic asthma. Am Rev Respir Dis 1985; 131:732–736.
77. Pedersen SE. Efficacy and safety of inhaled corticosteroids in children. In: Schleimer RP, Busse WW, O'Byrne PM, eds. Inhaled Glucocorticoids in Asthma. New York: Marcel Dekker, 1997:551–606.
78. Johansson SA, Andersson KE, Brattsand R. Topical and systemic potencies of budesonide, beclomethasone dipropionate, and prednisone in man. Eur J Respir Dis 1982; 63(suppl 122):74–84.

79. Ebden P, Jenkins A, Houston G. Comparison of two high dose corticosteroid aerosol treatments, beclomethasone dipropionate (1500 μg/d) and budesonide (1600 μg/d), for chronic asthma. Thorax 1986; 41:869–874.
80. Springer C, Avital A, Maayan CH. Comparison of budesonide and beclomethasone dipropionate for treatment of asthma. Arch Dis Child 1987; 62:815–819.
81. Warner J, Nikolaizik W, Marchant J. The systemic effects of inhaled corticosteroids. J Allergy Clin Immunol 1989; 83:220–225.
82. Brown PH, Blundell G, Greening AP, Crompton GK. Hypothalamo-pituitary-adrenal axis suppression in asthmatics inhaling high dose corticosteroids. Respir Med 1991; 85:501–510.
83. Pedersen S, Fuglsang G. Urinary cortisol excretion in children treated with high doses of inhaled corticosteroids: a comparison of budesonide and beclomethasone. Eur Respir J 1988; 1:433–435.
84. Baran D. A comparison of inhaled budesonide and beclomethasone dipropionate in childhood asthma. Br J Dis Chest 1987; 81:170–175.
85. Prahl P, Jenson T, Bjorregaard-Anderson H. Adrenocortical function in children on high dose aerosol therapy. Allergy 1987; 42:541–544.
86. Clark DJ, Grove A, Cargill RI, Lipworth BJ. Comparative adrenal suppression with inhaled budesonide and fluticasone propionate in adult asthmatic patients. Thorax 1996; 51:262–266.
87. Boorsma M, Andersson N, Larsson P, Ullman A. Assessment of relative systemic potency of inhaled fluticasone and budesonide. Eur Respir J 1996; 9:1427–1432.
88. Ellis EF. Adverse effects of corticosteroid therapy (editorial). J Allergy Clin Immunol 1987; 80:515–517.
89. Wolthers OD, Pedersen S. Controlled study of linear growth in children during treatment with inhaled glucorticosteroids. Pediatrics 1992; 89:839–842.
90. Wolthers OD, Pedersen S. Growth of asthmatic children during treatment with budesonide: a double blind trial. Br Med J 1991; 303:163–165.
91. Pedersen S, Agertoft L. Relationship between short-term lower leg growth and long-term statural growth in asthmatic children treated with budesonide. Am J Respir Crit Care Med 1995; 56:13.
92. Reimer LG, Morris HG, Ellis FE. Growth of asthmatic children during treatment with alternate-day steroids. J Allergy Clin Immunol 1975; 55:224–231.
93. Russell G. Asthma and growth. Arch Dis Child 1993; 69:695–698.
94. Ninan TK, Russell G. Asthma, inhaled corticosteroid treatment, and growth. Arch Dis Child 1992; 67:703–705.
95. Tinkelman DG, Reed CE, Nelson HS, Offord KP. Aerosol beclomethasone dipropi onate compared with theophylline as primary treatment of chronic, mild to moderately severe asthma in children. Pediatrics 1993; 92:64–77.
96. Doull IJM, Freezer NJ, Holgate ST. Growth of prepubertal children with mild asthma treated with inhaled beclomethasone dipropionate. Am J Respir Crit Care Med 1995; 151:1715–1719.
97. Verberne AAPH, Frost C, Jan Roorda RJ, Van Der Laag H, Kerrebijn KJ. One year treatment with salmeterol compared with beclomethasone in children with asthma. Am J Respir Crit Care Med 1997; 156:688–695.

98. Martin AJ, Landau LI, Phelan PD. The effect on growth of childhood asthma. Acta Pediatr Scand 1981; 70:683–688.
99. Balfour-Lynn L. Childhood Asthma and puberty. Arch Dis Child 1985; 60:231–235.
100. Lemanske RF, Allen DB. Choosing a long-term controller medication in childhood asthma: the proverbial two-edged sword (editorial). Am J Respir Crit Care Med 1997; 156:685–687.
101. Merkus PJFM, Van Essen-Zandvliet EEM, Duiverman EJ, Van Houwelingen HC, Kerrebijn KF, Quanjer PH. Long-term effect of inhaled corticosteroids on growth rate in adolescents with asthma. Pediatrics 1993; 91:1121–1126.
102. Silverstein MD, Yunginger JW, Reed, CE, Petterson T, Zimmerman D, Li JCL, O'Fallon WM. Attained adult height after childhood asthma: effect of glucocorticoid therapy. J Allergy Clin Immunol 1997; 99:466–474.
103. Lukert BP, Raisz LG. Glucocorticoid-induced osteoporosis: pathogenesis and management. Ann Intern Med 1990; 112:352–364.
104. Toogood JH. Effects of inhaled steroid therapy for asthma on skeletal metabolism. In: Schleimer RP, Busse WW, O'Byrne PM, eds. Inhaled Glucocorticoids in Asthma. New York: Marcel Dekker, 1997:607–626.
105. Teelucksingh S, Padfield PL, Tibi L, Gough KJ, Holt PR. Inhaled corticosteroids, bone formation, and osteocalcin. Lancet 1991; 338:60–61.
106. Pouw EM, Prummel MF, Oosting H, Roos CM, Endert E. Beclomethasone inhalation decreases serum osteocalcin concentrations. Br Med J 1991; 302:627–628.
107. Wolthers OD, Riis BJ, Pedersen S. Bone turnover in asthmatic children treated with oral prednisone or inhaled budesonide. Pediatr Pulmonol 1993; 16:341–346.
108. Kerstjens HAM, Postma DS, Van Doormaal JJ, Van Zanten AK, Brand PLP, Dekhuijzen PNR, Koeter GH. Effects of short term and long term treatment with inhaled corticosteroids on bone metabolism in patients with airways obstruction. Thorax 1994; 49:652–656.
109. Johnston CC, Slemenda CW, Melton LJ. Clinical use of bone densitometry. N Engl J Med 1991; 324:1105–1109.
110. Seeman E, Wagner HW, Offord Kp, Kumar R, Johnson WJ, Riggs BL. Differential effects of endocrine dysfunction on the axial and appendicular skeleton. J Clin Invest 1982; 69:1302–1309.
111. Cummings SR, Black DM, Nevitt M, Browner W, Cauley J, Ensrud K, Genant HK, Palermo L, Scott J. Bone density at various sites for prediction of hip fracture. Lancet 1993; 341:72–75.
112. Hanania NA, Chapman KR, Sturtridge WC, Szalai JP, Kestin S. Dose-related decreases in bone density among asthmatic patients treated with inhaled corticosteroids. J Allergy Clin Immunol 1995; 96:571–579.
113. Luengo M, Del Rio L, Pons F, Picado C. Bone mineral density in asthmatic patients treated with inhaled corticosteroids: A case control study. Eur Respir J 1997; 10: 2110–2113.
114. Konig P, Hillman L, Cervantes C, Levine C, Maloney C, Douglas B, Johnson L, Allen S. Bone metabolism in children with asthma treated with inhaled beclomethasone dipropionate. J Pediatr 1993; 122:219–226.

115. Toogood JH, Baskerville JC, Markov AE, Hodsmon AB, Fraher LJ, Jennings B, Haddod RG, Drost D. Bone mineral density and the risk of fracture in patients receiving long-term inhaled steroid therapy for asthma. J Allergy Clin Immunol 1995; 96:157–166.
116. Rooklin AR, Lampert SI, Jaeger EA, McGeady SJ, Mansmann HC. Posterior subcapsular cataracts in steroid-requiring asthmatic children. J Allergy Clin Immunol 1979; 63:383–386.
117. Toogood JH, Markov AE, Baskerville J, Dyson C. Association of ocular cataracts with inhaled and oral steroid therapy during long-term treatment of asthma. J Allergy Clin Immunol 1993; 91:571–579.
118. Skuta GL, Morgan RK. Corticosteroid-induced glaucoma. In: Ritch R, Shields MB, Krupin T, eds. The Glaucomas. St Louis: Mosby–Year Book, 1996:1177–1188.
119. Cumming RG, Mitchell P, Leeder SR. Use of inhaled corticosteroids and the risk of cataracts. N Engl J Med 1997; 337:8–14.
120. Garbe E, LeLorier J, Boivin J-F, Suissa S. Inhaled and nasal glucocorticoids and the risks of ocular hypertension or open-angle glaucoma. JAMA 1997; 277:722–727.
121. Simons FER, Persaud MP, Gillespie CA, Cheang M, Shuckett EP. Absence of posterior subcapsular cataracts in young patients treated with inhaled glucocorticoids. Lancet 1993; 342:776–778.
122. Carrel AL, Somers S, Lemanske RF, Allen DB. Hypoglycemia and cortisol deficiency with low-dose corticosteroid therapy for asthma. Pediatrics 1996; 97:921–924.
123. Hollman GA, Allen DB. Overt glucocorticoid excess due to inhaled corticosteroid therapy. Pediatrics 1988; 81:452–455.
124. Shaikh WA. Pulmonary tuberculosis in patients treated with inhaled beclomethasone. Allergy 1992; 47:327–330.
125. Abzug MJ, Cotton MF. Severe chickenpox after intranasal use of corticosteroids. J Pediatr 1993; 123:577–579.
126. Sy MLT, Chin TW, Nussbaum E. Pneumocystis carinii pneumonia associated with inhaled corticosteroids in an immunocompetent child with asthma. J Pediatr 1995; 127:1000–1002.
127. Capewell S, Reynolds S, Shuttleworth D, Edwards C, Finlay AY. Purpura and dermal thinning associated with high dose inhaled corticosteroids. Br Med J 1990; 300:1548–1551.
128. Autio P, Karjalainen Risteli L, Risteli J, Kiistala, Oikarinen A. Effects of an inhaled steroid (budesonide) on skin collagen synthesis of asthma patients in vivo. Am J Respir Crit Care Med 1996; 153:1172–1175.
129. Lewis LD, Cochrane GM. Psychosis in a child inhaling budesonide. Lancet 1983; 2:634.
130. McCubbin MM, Milavetz G, Grandgeorge S, Weinberger M, Ahrens R, Sargent C, Vaughan LM. A bioassay for topical and systemic effect of three inhaled corticosteroids. Clin Pharmacol Ther 1995; 57:455–460.
131. English AF, Neate MS, Quint DJ, Sareen M. Biological activities of some corticosteroids used in asthma. Am J Respir Crit Care Med 1994; 149(suppl):A212.

132. Hogger P, Rohdewald P. Binding kinetics of fluticasone propionate to the human glucocorticoid receptor. Steroids 1994; 59:597–602.
133. Phillips GH. Structure-activity relationships of topically active steroids: the selection of fluticasone propionate. Respir Med 1990; 84(suppl A):19–23.
134. Harding SM. The human pharmacology of fluticasone propionate. Respir Med 1990; 84(suppl A):25–29.
135. Lipworth BJ. New perspectives on inhaled drug delivery and systemic bioactivity. Thorax 1995; 50:105–110.
136. Dahl R, Lundback B, Malo JL, Mazza JA, Nieminen MM, Saarelainen P, Barnacle H. A dose-ranging study of fluticasone propionate in adult patients with moderate asthma. Chest 1993; 104:1352–1358.
137. Gustafsson P, Tsanakas J, Gold M, Primhak R, Radford M, Gillies E. Comparison of the efficacy and safety of inhaled fluticasone propionate 200 μg/day with inhaled beclomethasone dipropionate 400 μg/day in mild and moderate asthma. Arch Dis Child 1993; 69:206–211.
138. Kamada AK, Szefler SJ. How should inhaled glucocorticoids be compared? J Allergy Clin Immunol 1997; 99:735–737.
139. Agertoft L, Pedersen S. A randomized, double-blind dose reduction study to compare the minimal effective dose of budesonide Turbuhaler and fluticasone propionate Diskhaler. J Allergy Clin Immunol 1997; 99:773–780.
140. Noonan M, Chervinsky P, Busse WW, Weisberg SC, Pinnas J, DeBoisblanc BP, Boltomsky H, Pearlman D, Repsher L, Kellerman D. Fluticasone propionate reduces oral prednisone use while it improves asthma control and quality of life. Am J Respir Crit Care Med 1995; 152:1467–1473.
141. Hummel S, Lehtonen L. Comparison of oral-steroid sparing by high-dose and low-dose inhaled steroid in maintenance treatment of severe asthma. Lancet 1992; 340: 1483–1487.
142. Levy ML, Stevenson C, Maslen T. Comparison of short courses of oral prednisolone and fluticasone propionate in the treatment of adults with acute exacerbations of asthma in primary care. Thorax 1996; 51:1087–1092.
143. Booth H, Richmond I, Ward C, Gardiner PV, Harkawat R, Walters EH. Effect of high dose inhaled fluticasone propionate on airway inflammation in asthma. Am J Respir Crit Care Med 1995; 152:45–52.
144. Olivieri D, Chetta A, Del Donno M, Bertorelli G, Casalini A, Pesci A, Testi R, Foresi A. Effect of short-term treatment with low-dose inhaled fluticasone propionate on airway inflammation and remodeling in mild asthma: a placebo-controlled study. Am J Respir Crit Care Med 1997; 155:1864–1871.
145. Lipworth BJ, Clark DJ, McFarlane LC. Adrenocortical activity with repeated twice daily dosing of fluticasone propionate and budesonide given via a large volume spacer to asthmatic children. Thorax 1997; 52:686–689.
146. Hoekx JCM, Hedlin G, Pedersen W, Sorva R, Hollingworth K, Efthimiou J. Fluticasone propionate compared with budesonide: a double blind trial in asthmatic children using powder devices at a dosage of 400 μg/day. Eur Respir J 1996; 9:2263–2272.
147. Clark DJ, Lipworth BJ. Adrenal suppression with chronic dosing of fluticasone

propionate compared with budesonide in adult asthmatic patients. Thorax 1997; 52:55–58.

148. Bootsma GB, Dekhuijzen R, Festin J, Mulder PGH, Swinkles LMJW, Van Herwaarden CLA. Fluticasone propionate does not influence bone metabolism in contrast to beclomethasone dipropionate. Am J Respir Crit Care Med 1996; 153:924–930.
149. Todd G, Dunlop K, McNaboe J, Ryan MF, Carson D, Shields MD. Growth and adrenal suppression in asthmatic children treated with high-dose fluticasone propionate. Lancet 1996; 348:27–29.
150. Agertoft L, Pedersen S. Short-term knemometry and urine cortisol excretion in children treated with fluticasone propionate and budesonide: a dose response study. Eur Respir J 1997; 10:1507–1512.

7

Platelet-Activating Factor Antagonists in Bronchial Asthma

DEVENDRA K. AGRAWAL and ROBERT G. TOWNLEY

Creighton University School of Medicine
Omaha, Nebraska

I. Introduction

Platelet-activating factor (PAF) is a potent mediator of inflammation. The biological response elicited by this mediator was initially reported in 1966 by Barbaro and Zvaifler (1), who observed histamine release following specific antigen challenge from a mixture of rabbit platelets and stimulated leukocytes. Subsequently, Henson reported that a factor released from sensitized leukocytes activated platelets and released vasoactive amines (2). In 1972, Benveniste and colleagues further demonstrated that the stimulation of IgE-sensitized rabbit basophils released a soluble factor that activated platelets (3). Because of its first recognized physiological effect on platelets and lack of molecular identity, it was termed the mediator, or *platelet-activating factor*. In 1979, the molecular structure was elucidated independently by two separate groups. Benveniste and colleagues (4) and Demopoulos et al. (5) identified this mediator to be mixture of 1-O-alkyl-2-acetyl-sn-glycero-3-phosphocholines (AGEPC), called the *PAF-acether*. At the same time, another laboratory named this substance *antihypertensive polar renomedullary lipid* (APRL), because its substance was isolated from the renal medulla and had a very potent hypotensive activity (6). Later on, it was found to be identical with PAF-acether.

PAF-acether is a phospholipid and is rapidly generated by the enzyme acyltransferase from its inactive precursor, lyso-PAF. PAF is newly formed mediator, which is synthesized and released from various cells in response to a stimulus. In this chapter, we discuss the relationship between PAF and bronchial asthma.

A. Bronchial Asthma and PAF

The allergic response in bronchial asthma can be classified mainly into two phases: (1) an early acute reaction that occurs 10 to 25 min following allergen challenge and (2) a delayed response, which, in about 40–50% subjects, occurs 3 to 8 hr after allergen challenge. A post–late phase (subacute/chronic inflammatory phase) has also been reported. Nonspecific airway hyperresponsiveness, which is an almost universal feature of asthma, is more pronounced in subjects undergoing a late-onset response. Therefore, the induction of airway hyperresponsiveness has been considered to be partly a consequence of the mechanisms that underlie the late-onset response.

Airway hyperresponsiveness has been characterized by an exaggerated bronchoconstriction to a variety of endogenously released mediators. The early asthmatic response occurring shortly after allergen challenge is most likely secondary to the action of both preformed and newly synthesized bronchoconstrictor molecules (e.g., histamine, cytokines, PAF, sulfidopeptide leukotrienes, and cyclooxygenase products) released by human lung mast cells as a consequence of IgE-mediated degranulation. This leads to an influx of inflammatory cells and release of mediators, corresponding to the late asthmatic phase occurring several hours after allergen challenge. Effects of PAF mimic several of the features of asthma, such as microvascular leakage, mucus secretion, bronchoconstriction, and possibly increased responsiveness (7). PAF has potent activity as a chemotactic agent and as an activator of eosinophils, which are prominent cells in asthmatic airways (8,9). Eosinophilic inflammation characterizes asthma and airway hyperresponsiveness. Thus, the interaction between PAF and eosinophils may be crucial in the pathogenesis of bronchial hyperresponsiveness in asthma. Since PAF plays a crucial role in the inflammatory cascades, this evoked interest in the development of selective and specific antagonists of PAF receptors.

The ability of PAF receptor antagonists to inhibit various aspects of the allergic response has been demonstrated in a number of animal models. Since, in experimental animals, PAF and allergen-induced eosinophil infiltration were considered to be dependent upon platelet activation (10), it was suggested that platelet activation might be an important component of the allergic process.

B. PAF in Serum or Lavage Fluid

Attempts have been made to measure PAF in serum or bronchoalveolar lavage (BAL) fluid in symptomatic or asymptomatic asthmatic subjects. In general, results are variable. Horii and colleagues (11) detected PAF equivalent to about 1.4 pmol of 1-O-hexadecyl-2-acetyl-sn-glycero-3-phosphocholine in BAL fluids from an asthmatic infant during an asthmatic attack. In contrast to the asthmatic patient, there was no detectable PAF in BAL exudates from patients with laryngeal stenosis or with respiratory distress syndrome. However, a wide variation in the amount of lysoPAF was present in individual asthmatic patients, suggesting that the level of lysoPAF cannot be taken as an indicator for the presence of PAF.

PAF was undetectable in bronchoalveolar lavage fluid in 11 atopic patients with mild asymptomatic bronchial asthma (12).

In asthma patients, PAF was present in the BAL fluid, and the presence of PAF in BAL supernatant was significantly associated with a combination of low neutrophil and high lymphocyte counts and with macrophage metabolic activity as assessed by lucigenin chemiluminescence (13).

Schauer and colleagues (14) reported that granulocytes from the symptomatic asthmatic patients showed a significantly higher PAF generation as compared with those from asymptomatic asthmatic patients or controls. However, LTC_4 generation was increased in both asymptomatic and symptomatic patients. These results suggest a regulatory role of PAF in the exacerbation of asthma.

Chang-Yeung and colleagues (15) observed a significant increase in plasma histamine and PAF levels in patients with mild seasonal asthma after allergen-induced bronchoconstriction but not in patients with asthma after bronchoconstriction induced by methacholine. There was a significant correlation between the baseline plasma PAF levels and the degree of bronchial hyperresponsiveness to methacholine.

Intracellular Versus Extracellular PAF

PAF was originally discovered as a lipid-phase mediator, which is released from several cells after synthesis. However, most of the newly synthesized PAF in endothelial cells (16), polymorphonuclear leukocytes (17,18), and other cells (19,20) is apparently retained within the cell of origin. The amount of secreted versus intracellularly retained PAF depends on the conditions used and varies dramatically in different cells. The findings that much of the PAF synthesized in many cell systems remains associated with the cells suggest its role as an intracellular messenger and direct activator of target cells. Indeed, evidence for the presence of intracellular PAF receptors has been reported (21).

The release of PAF from cells is influenced by the presence of albumin in the extracellular medium (22), pH (23), Ca^{2+} ions (24), removal of medium by a dynamic flow system (25), and cell density (23). It was also observed that the level of PAF in blood was controlled by PAF-acetylhydrolase (26), and PAF might be released extracellularly from human polymorphonuclear leukocytes stimulated in PAF-acetylhydrolase–deficient serum—i.e., under conditions close to those existing in vivo. Interestingly, Miwa and colleagues (27) discovered a specific protein that is different from albumin, binds newly synthesized PAF, and appears to facilitate its secretion. Other investigators have also reported the existence of a transport protein that is selective for PAF (28,29).

Thus, depending upon the conditions, PAF could be present both intra- and extracellulary. However, the exact mechanism of PAF secretion and the regulatory role of intracellular PAF in cell signaling are still unclear and warrant further attention.

C. PAF and Release of Mediators from Human Cells

PAF is a very potent mediator to activate various inflammatory cells and release their contents (10). There are several reports on the in vivo and in vitro effects of PAF.

PAF released superoxide radicals from highly purified human blood eosinophils, and this effect was sensitive to several antiasthmatic drugs, including salbutamol, salmeterol, theophylline, and azelastine (30).

PAF is very potent in producing eosinophil chemotaxis, and this effect was attenuated by apafant (WEB 2086 BS), a platelet-activating factor antagonist (31). However, in another report, WEB 2086 affected neither the eosinophil nor IL-5 release when administered once a day for 10 days (10–100 mg/kg/day) in mice (32). In addition, this drug never affected the IL-5 release but significantly suppressed eosinophil infiltration even when administered twice a day for 10 days (30–200 mg/kg/day). In contrast, another long-acting PAF receptor antagonist, Y-24180, when administered orally once a day for 10 days (0.3–3 mg/kg), suppressed eosinophil infiltration in a dose-dependent manner and suppressed IL-5 release at the highest dosage (32).

D. PAF Receptors in Human Blood Eosinophils

PAF receptors have been characterized by both functional and radioligand binding techniques. Characterization of PAF receptors has been made possible with the development and the availability of compounds selective for PAF receptors. To date there are several molecules synthesized by various pharmaceutical industries, and these compounds have been shown to antagonize the functional effect of PAF in various cells and tissues selectively (10,20). In general, the PAF receptor antagonists can be classified mainly into two groups: PAF-related structures and PAF-unrelated structures. PAF-unrelated antagonists have been further classified into natural PAF receptor antagonists and the synthetic compounds (33).

Specific receptors have been described in many cells and tissues in which PAF elicits effects. In general, PAF receptor belongs to the seven-transmembrane-domain group of receptor families. PAF receptor has been cloned both in animals and humans (34–36). The human receptor gene encodes a 342–amino acid protein of 39 kDa with greater than 80% homology with the guinea pig receptor. Computer analysis of the protein sequence revealed limited sequence homology with other G protein–linked receptors. The highest degree of identity, 29%, was observed with the *N*-formyl Met-Leu-Phe peptide receptor.

In human blood eosinophils, we observed a high affinity (K_D 1.2–2.4 nM) with a density of 100,000 to 166,400 receptors per cell (10). Kishimoto and colleagues (37) observed that the levels of PAF receptor mRNA in eosinophils from atopic asthmatic patients were significantly higher than those in normal subjects. This suggests that the increased expression of PAF receptor in eosinophils may be relevant to the pathogenesis of atopic asthma.

Burgers et al. (38) observed a decrease of 14% in PAF receptors immediately after allergen challenge. Interestingly, the level of PAF receptors returned to control values after about 4 hr, followed by a transient increase of 9% at 7 hr after allergen challenge. These data suggest that PAF, which is secreted in the circulation during allergic-asthmatic reaction, triggered transient sequestration of platelets, possibly in the lung.

Recently, Nagase and colleagues (39) observed airway hyperresponsiveness in transgenic mice overexpressing PAF receptors. PAF-induced bronchoconstriction in the transgenic mice was significantly reduced by a thromboxane synthesis inhibitor (indomethachin or ozagrel), an inhibitor of 5-lipoxygenase-activating protein (MK-886), or a cysteinyl leukotriene antagonist (pranulukast). This suggested that both thromboxane A_2 and cysteinyl leukotrienes (LTC_4, LTD_4, and LTE_4) were involved in the bronchial responses to PAF in mice. We have also reported that a novel thromboxane synthetase inhibitor, DP-1904, inhibited PAF-induced degranulation of human blood eosinophils (40).

E. PAF Acetylhydrolase in Human BAL

PAF is a mediator produced in human airways during acute and chronic inflammatory lung diseases. The levels of PAF are regulated by acetylhydrolase, the enzyme that converts lyso-PAF to PAF or vice versa. Triggiani and colleagues (41) reported the presence of extracellular acetylhydrolase activity mainly secreted by alveolar macrophages in human BAL fluid. Acetylhydrolase, which is highly sensitive to oxygen radical–induced damage, inactivated PAF released in the airways. These investigators concluded that the secretion and inactivation of BAL-acetylhydrolase might influence the levels of this enzyme in BAL fluid during acute and chronic inflammatory lung diseases and, ultimately, regulate the proinflammatory activities of PAF in patients with acute and chronic inflammatory lung diseases.

Tsukioka and colleagues (42) observed a higher level of plasma PAF and markedly lower level of PAF acetylhydrolase activity in asthmatic patients, both in remission and at the time of asthmatic attack, than in healthy subjects. The plasma PAF level was more closely associated with asthma both in remission and at the time of asthmatic attack than with pulmonary tuberculosis, whereas there was no significant difference in serum PAF acetylhydrolase activity between the two diseases. These authors concluded that the low serum PAF acetylhydrolase activity in asthmatic patients might have been due to saturation as a result of continuous reaction to the increased plasma PAF level in those patients.

The production of PAF by inflammatory cells is regulated by lyso-PAF acetyltransferase, and the activity of this enzyme is increased in neutrophils of stable asthmatic patients. Misso and colleagues (43) observed a decrease in lyso-PAF acetyltransferase activity together with a reduction in the enzymatic affinity constant during acute asthma. Interestingly, the affinity and maximum activity increased to levels higher than in normal control subjects after recovery. These data suggested that alterations in the affinity of acetyltransferase for acetylcoenzyme A (CoA) and in the regulation of enzyme activity might be occurring during acute asthma.

F. PAF Challenges in Humans

Various studies of the effects of PAF on human and animal airways would probably support a putative role for this lipid mediator in asthma.

The effect of cetirizine, a potent and specific H_1 receptor antagonist, was examined on PAF-induced bronchoconstriction in 10 patients with mild asthma (44). Airway responses were assessed by measuring specific airway conductance (sGaw). This study concluded that PAF-induced bronchoconstriction in humans was not mediated by histamine release, suggesting that H_1 receptor antagonists do not modify PAF-induced bronchoconstriction. This could also be supported by a finding of Louis and colleagues (45), where inhaled PAF-induced airway obstruction and neutropenia in asthma patients without any significant change of plasma histamine level. This suggests that lung mast cells or basophils do not degranulate during PAF-induced bronchoconstriction.

Our group at Creighton had investigated the protective effect of oral terfenadine, a H1 antagonist, on the dermal and pulmonary response, and changes of circulating white blood cells (WBCs) in response to injected and inhaled PAF (46). In this double-blind crossover study, nine men with mild asthma participated using 120 mg of terfenadine or placebo. Pulmonary function was measured 3 hr after administration of study drug and a PAF challenge was performed, showing a significant improvement on terfenadine. Terfenadine significantly inhibited the wheal-and-flare response to histamine and the flare response to injected PAF. Terfenadine did not have an effect on the number of circulating WBCs or the response of pulmonary function to inhaled PAF (46). These results suggested a limited role of endogenous histamine in the effects of PAF.

In our initial study, we sought to elucidate the role of PAF in airway hyperreactivity by comparing the effect of PAF on methacholine-induced airway responsiveness in six nonasthmatic subjects (47). Nonspecific airway responsiveness was not significantly increased following PAF inhalation at 6 hr, nor was it increased at 1, 2, 7, or 14 days. Thus, we were unable to confirm the finding of Cuss and colleagues (48) and Smith et al. (49) of a PAF-induced increased response to methacholine. In another study, we further examined the role of PAF in airway hyperreactivity by comparing the effect of inhaled PAF on methacholine and isoproterenol airway responsiveness in six nonasthmatic and six asthmatic subjects (50). The rationale for this study was based partly on our studies done in guinea pigs, showing that PAF increased bronchial sensitivity to methacholine and decreased the bronchial response to isoproterenol and prostaglandin E_1 (51). In this study in humans, neither nonspecific airway reactivity nor isoproterenol responsiveness was changed following PAF inhalation in the nonasthmatic subjects in the 6 days following aerosolized PAF. Asthmatic subjects had increased airway responsiveness to methacholine at 2 hr post-PAF, which did not persist. Responsiveness to isoproterenol did not change in the asthmatic subjects (50). Similar results were reported by Chung and Barnes (52).

Asthmatic subjects, as compared with normal subjects, developed an exaggerated acute airway obstruction in response to PAF, although no correlation was found between log PC_{20} methacholine and log fall in FEV_1 after PAF (53). The same group in later studies (54) examined the effects of inhaled PAF on methacholine bronchial responsiveness, circulating leukocyte counts, and ex vivo TNF-α and IL-1 production from blood monocytes in eight allergic asthma patients. Inhalation of PAF, as compared with lyso-PAF and saline, resulted in a significant decrease in PC_{20} over a period of 1 week. There was no significant difference in spontaneous TNF-α and IL-1 production or circulating neutrophil counts after PAF, lyso-PAF, or saline. Interestingly, inhaled PAF caused a significant protracted augmentation in circulating eosinophil counts.

Kaye and Smith (55) also examined the effects of inhaled leukotriene D4 and platelet-activating factor on airway reactivity in normal subjects. In this study, after inhaling PAF, 6 of the 8 subjects developed increased airway reactivity, which was maximal at 1 day and persisted for 14 days in 3 subjects. After inhaling LTD_4, 6 of the 8 subjects also developed increased airway reactivity, which was maximal at 7 days and persisted for 14 days in 2 of the subjects.

In another study, six normal subjects without bronchial hyperresponsiveness inhaled 400 μg of PAF in 10 divided cumulative doses (56). All subjects felt a hot flush and slight tracheal irritation after the inhalation of PAF. However, PAF administration did not induce bronchial hyperresponsiveness, as determined by a reduction of 20% of FEV_1 or by more sensitive indicators of ventilatory obstruction, such as $FEV_{25-75\%}$ and $FEF_{75\%}$. In another study by Lai and colleagues (57) there was no effect of PAF on bronchial hyperresponsiveness or mucosal inflammation, as determined by the immunocytochemistry for tryptase and eosinophil cationic protein, in atopic nonasthmatic subjects.

Since theophylline may possess anti-inflammatory actions that underlie its antiasthma properties, Chung and colleagues (58) sought to determine whether theophylline could inhibit the bronchoconstriction and the bronchial hyperresponsiveness induced by inhaled PAF in eight nonasthmatic subjects. PAF caused a significant decrease in PC_{40} (the concentration of methacholine needed to cause 40% fall in baseline Vp_{30}). However, theophylline had no significant effect on PAF-induced bronchoconstriction.

A therapeutic dose of salbutamol caused partial inhibition of PAF-induced bronchoconstriction and had a minimal effect on the increased bronchial responsiveness following PAF (59).

Circulating PAF increased markedly during acute asthmatic attacks, and the enhanced in vivo and in vitro production of PAF decreased to normal after successful immunotherapy (60). These data suggest that PAF might be involved in the pathogenesis of bronchial asthma.

Yamamoto and colleagues (61) observed an increased level of β-thromboglobulin and platelet factor 4 in subjects with symptomatic and asymptomatic chronic asthma, and there was a statistically significant correlation between the initial level of PAF and that of β-thromboglobulin and platelet factor 4. These results suggest that platelet activation in the circulation is sometimes provoked in asthma, but plasma level of alpha granule–derived proteins does not reflect the intensity or severity of asthma.

Louis and Radermecker (62) compared the variations in the specific conductance (sGaw) and forced expiratory volume in 1 sec (FEV_1) in 12 asthma patients and 12 normal subjects after inhalation of doubling doses of PAF (15–120 μg) and methacholine (18 to at least 144 μg). When the PD_{35} sGaw values were compared, PAF was found on a molar basis to be 33-fold more potent than methacholine in the normal subjects but only 5-fold more potent in the asthma patients. The percentage fall in FEV_1 (calculated by interpolation) or a 35% fall in sGaw was greater in asthma patients than in normal subjects for both methacholine and PAF. These results demonstrated a tachyphylaxis after inhalation of PAF in normal subjects and asthma patients and showed that the latter developed a greater bronchial obstruction than normal subjects even if methacholine was more sensitive than PAF at discriminating between the two groups.

Hozawa and colleagues (63)—in a randomized double-blind placebo-controlled two-phase crossover study—examined the effect of Y-24180, a potent, specific, orally active PAF receptor antagonist, on bronchial hyperresponsiveness to methacholine in 13 patients with extrinsic stable asthma. In this study, Y-24180 significantly improved the PC_{20}-FEV_1 value without carryover effect compared with placebo as well as period effect by analysis of variance. These results suggest that PAF is an important mediator involved in the bronchial hyperresponsiveness of bronchial asthma in humans. It has also been reported that the arterial blood-gas abnormalities shown during exacerbations of bronchial asthma could be due to endogenous release of PAF (64).

The blood PAF levels of bronchial asthmatic patients with the active symptoms were significantly higher than those of normal healthy control subjects, suggesting that PAF may play a role in bronchial asthma (65). Asthmatic individuals are more sensitive to the acute inflammatory effects of ozone than nonasthmatic individuals (66). In this study, however, there was no significant changes in leukotriene B_4 or PAF in nasal lavage fluid.

G. Leukotriene and PAF

Leukotrienes (LTs) play a significant role in the pathogenesis of bronchial asthma; this is attested to by the finding that two leukotriene receptor antagonists—zafirlukast (Accolate) and montelukast (Singulair)—as well as the leukotriene synthesis inhibitor zileuton (Zyflo) are now in clinical use in the United States. All three of these agents show significant increase in pulmonary function, which is separate from the effect of β-agonists, and protect against exercise- and allergen-induced asthma. Leukotrienes and PAF share a number of common characteristics. Both are lipid mediators produced through the arachidonic acid pathway, and both PAF and leukotrienes are synthesized and released from mast cells and basophils following allergen challenge. The cysteinyl leukotrienes as well as PAF are produced by eosinophils, whereas leukotriene B_4 and PAF are produced by neutrophils. Furthermore, both are very potent in producing microvascular leakage and both have been reported, at least in some studies, to induce airway hyperresponsiveness. The interrelationship between leukotrienes and PAF is further supported by the observation that both cause bronchoconstriction, increased secretion of mucus, microvascular leak, and edema.

Both PAF and leukotriene B_4 are associated with neutrophil chemotaxis and induction of transitory leukopenia, particularly neutropenia and a rebound leukocytosis, in both healthy subjects and patients with asthma. From these observations, it has been suggested that some of the pulmonary effects of PAF could be potentiated by the secondary release of leukotrienes. PAF can mediate production of leukotriene C_4 by human eosinophils in vitro (67). PAF inhalation results in an increase in urinary LTE_4, which is the major metabolizer of both leukotriene C_4 and D_4 (68). The PAF receptor antagonist UK 74505 has been reported to attenuate the increase in urinary LTE_4 (69). We have reported that bronchial challenge with PAF induces leukopenia, which is most marked at 5 min after inhalation, followed by a rebound leukocytosis at 15 min after challenge (47). These effects of inhaled PAF cause peripheral blood neutropenia due to neutrophil sequestration in the pulmonary circulation and are associated with marked disturbances in pulmonary gas exchange in both normal individuals and patients with mild asthma (64,70,71). Since both LTB_4 and PAF cause neutropenia, whereas LTC_4 and LTD_4 do not, Gomez and colleagues were prompted to study the effect of a 5-LO inhibitor (zileuton) on PAF-induced pulmonary abnormalities in mild asthma (72). Two different studies using two different leukotriene-receptor antagonists found attenuation of PAF-induced bronchoconstriction but not neutropenia in normal individuals (73,74). The orally active 5-LO inhibitor zileuton is effective in inhibiting bronchoconstriction in patients challenged with hyperventilation of cold air (75) or aspirin (76) and resulted in marked inhibition of calcium ionophore–stimulated blood production of LTB_4 ex vivo after a single dose of 800 mg (77). For these reasons, Gomez and colleagues (72) determined the effect of the 5-LO inhibitor zileuton in preventing PAF-induced systemic, neutropenic, pulmonary, and respiratory gas-exchange responses in patients with mild asthma.

These investigators studied subjects with mild asthma before and after PAF inhalation in a randomized double-blind placebo-controlled crossover fashion. Compared with placebo, zileuton reduced both PAF-induced neutropenia at 5 min by 43% and the subsequent rebound neutrophilia at 15 min by 50%. Furthermore, zileuton attenuated the increase in respiratory resistance by 39% and the alveolar-arterial oxygen pressure difference [P $(A\text{-}a)_{O_2}$] by 40%; it also decreased Pa_{O_2} by 27%. These findings caused the authors to conclude that PAF-induced systemic and pulmonary effects in patients with asthma are effectively mediated by the ongoing release of leukotrienes. Since only a single dose of zileuton was used, it is not possible to deduce whether all of these effects of PAF are mediated by 5-LO products. The fact that zileuton, in contrast to the leukotriene receptor antagonists (73,74), reduced both the neutropenic and rebound neutrophilic effects induced by PAF, whereas zileuton and the leukotriene receptor antagonists both attenuated the bronchoconstrictor response to inhaled PAF, points to the role of leukotriene B_4 biosynthesis in contributing to neutropenia. LTB_4 is a potent chemotactic agent for neutrophils, and inhaled LTB_4 induces transitory neutropenia and rebound neutrophilia (78). These changes with inhaled LTB_4 are very similar to those seen with PAF inhalation. Although these changes are consistent with the PAF-induced neutropenia being mediated by LTB_4 they do not prove cause and effect.

Gomez and colleagues (72) were the first to show that a single dose of a selective 5-LO inhibitor provides moderate protection against PAF-induced arterial blood gas abnormalities and ventilation-perfusion imbalance. These authors have demonstrated that the PAF-induced hypoxemic effect is not due to bronchoconstriction alone, as the administration of ipratropium bromide with its bronchodilating effect had a protective effect on airway tone but not on the systemic and neutropenic effects or pulmonary gas exchange responses provoked by PAF challenge. In contrast, salbutamol clearly inhibited all PAF-induced effects (71). These authors postulated that the pulmonary gas-exchange abnormalities caused by inhalation of PAF are a result of increased microvascular leakage (64,70,71).

Inhalation challenges with PAF are somewhat different from other bronchoconstrictive substances in that rapid tachyphylaxis occurs and the response to PAF is not marked (52,79). It is best determined using sensitive measurements of changes in airway function, such as sGaw or $V_{30}P$. In performing PAF challenges, human serum albumin may be added to minimize adherence of the material to the nebulizer or other glass surfaces. Starting concentrations vary from 0.1–2 mg/mL. It has been observed that the inhalation of PAF is associated with flushing and a sense of warmth as well as an increase in the heart rate. Bronchoconstriction occurs within 2 to 3 min and is relatively short-lived, with decreased airway caliber lasting 15–45 min (79). It has been stated that asthmatic subjects do not have a marked degree of airway responsiveness to PAF as compared with normal, nonasthmatic subjects. However, this could also be attributed to the need to use pulmonary function parameters such as sGaw and $V_{30}P$, which avoid deep inspiration and thus avoid the bronchodilating effect, which might be important in the limited bronchoconstrictor response to PAF. Thus even methacholine, when challenged in normal subjects, will induce significant changes in the sGaw and $V_{30}P$, which are not significantly different from those in asthmatic subjects. However, when a deep inspiration maneuver is used in the spirometric techniques involving forced vital capacity, there is a marked protection against methacholine in normal subjects, which is either diminished or absent in asthmatic subjects. Nevertheless, early studies in humans reported that the PAF was 100 times more potent than methacholine in a eliciting a 40% fall in the $V_{40}P$ (48) and similarly up to several hundred times more potent in eliciting a 35% fall in sGaw (48,79). Although, the mechanism of PAF-induced bronchoconstriction is not entirely known, there is evidence that it may involve leukotriene production. Leukotriene release was reported after treatment of perfused rat lungs with PAF (80). In a separate study, inhalation of 2 mg/mL of PAF in normal subjects elicited a 38% fall in sGaw and led to a 10-fold rise in urinary LTE_4 excretion (81).

In conclusion, there is considerable evidence that many of the pulmonary effects of PAF are at least in part mediated by leukotrienes.

H. Studies with PAF-Receptor Antagonists in Humans

The interaction of PAF with airway smooth muscle and the attenuation of allergic bronchoconstriction by selective PAF-receptor antagonists have raised the possibility that PAF might be involved in the underlying pathophysiology of allergic airway hyperresponsiveness. Consequently, PAF-receptor antagonists may be useful in the treatment of human asthma.

Wilkens and colleagues (82) investigated the effect of BN 52063, a specific PAF-receptor antagonist, on the early asthmatic response to exercise in six patients with exercise-induced asthma. After a treatment period of 2 days, an exercise challenge on the third day was preceded by administration of either placebo or BN 52063 240 mg PO 3 hr before challenge or 5 mg by inhalation 30 min before challenge. After the oral intake of 240 mg BN 52063, there was no effect on the initial exercise-induced bronchoconstriction, but the prolonged reduction of PEF was significantly attenuated. Additionally, intake of BN 52063 significantly diminished the rise in plasma concentrations of PF4 and β-thromboglobulin after the exercise challenge. These results suggests that platelet activation after exercise-induced asthma was markedly inhibited by BN 52063, indicating a role of PAF as a mediator in exercise-induced asthma.

Hsieh (83) examined the effect of aerosolized BN 52021, a PAF-receptor antagonist, on the bronchoconstriction induced by PAF, methacholine, or specific allergen in 21 asthmatic children and compared them with a group of healthy children. The results of the study showed that 6 of 7 asthmatic children and 1 of 7 normal subjects gave a positive bronchial provocation with PAF. Further, in asthmatics, prior inhalation of BN 52021 inhibited the bronchoconstriction induced by PAF and allergen but not by methacholine. Finally, prior inhalation of BN 52021 inhibited a marked decrease of peripheral blood eosinophils and neutrophils in normal subjects but not in asthma patients. These findings were encouraging in supporting the role of a PAF receptor antagonist in the prevention and treatment of bronchial asthma.

In healthy volunteers, premedication with WEB-2086 (40 mg) completely prevented any increase in airway resistance after PAF inhalation as well as development of most of the cardiovascular and side effects induced by PAF (84). In symptomatic atopic asthma patients, in a double-blind randomized placebo-controlled parallel group study, Spence and colleagues (85) examined the effect of the orally active PAF antagonist WEB 2086, to see whether it reduced the need for inhaled corticosteroid. There was no significant difference between the WEB 2086–and placebo-treated groups. Similar results were reported by Freitag and colleagues (86), where 1 week of treatment with an orally administered WEB 2086 did not attenuate allergen-induced early or late responses or airway hyperresponsiveness (87).

The effect of UK-74,505—a specific PAF antagonist—on early and late asthmatic response to inhaled allergen was studied (88). It was found that UK-74,505 did not affect either the early or the late asthmatic response to inhaled allergen or bronchial responsiveness, despite its potency and long duration of action. Later on, modipafant (UK-80,067) which is the (+)-enantiomer of UK-74,505, was developed as a potent and specific PAF antagonist. Kuitert and colleagues (89) assessed the effect of modipafant over 28 days in adult subjects with moderately severe asthma in a placebo-controlled parallel-group study. There was no significant difference between placebo and modipafant in diurnal variation in peak expiratory flow, clinic FEV_1, rescue bronchodilator usage, symptom score, or airway responsiveness. This suggests that PAF is not a major mediator in asthma.

Hozawa and colleagues (90) reported the effects of a potent and orally active PAF receptor antagonist, Y-24180, on bronchial hyperresponsiveness to methacholine in patients with extrinsic stable asthma. Compared with the placebo, Y-24180 significantly improved the PC_{20}-FEV_1 value without carryover or period effect. Later on this drug was shown to suppress allergic pulmonary eosinophilia in mice by attenuating the release of IL-5 (32).

In our laboratory, we examined the safety and efficacy of a 240-mg oral dose of RP-59227 in attenuating the early- and late-phase antigen challenge in asthmatics; we used a double-blind, placebo-controlled crossover design (91). RP-59227 attenuated the release of neutrophil and eosinophil chemotactic activity after antigen challenge and reduced the effect of exogenously added PAF in inducing eosinophil chemotaxis. However, RP-59227 did not protect against the antigen-induced early- or late-phase response.

SR27417A is a novel PAF antagonist with increased potency compared with previously tested compounds. In a double-blind crossover study, treatment with SR27417A significantly attenuated the late asthmatic response [area under the curve (AUC) late allergic reaction (LAR) 4–10 hr: 107 ± 24 after placebo, 79 ± 17 after SR27417A] (92). In this study, the mean percent fall in FEV_1 LAR following SR27417A treatment was significantly smaller than that after placebo. There were no effects on early asthmatic responses, allergen-induced airway responsiveness, or baseline lung measurements. These data suggested that SR27417A had a modest inhibitory effect on the late asthmatic response, suggesting that PAF may play a small role in allergic inflammation.

II. Concluding Remarks

PAF is an important phospholipid mediator that plays a regulatory role in the function of inflammatory, epithelial, endothelial, and smooth muscle cells. It is a potent bronchoconstricting agent and produces intense inflammation and edema. However, based on the studies described, the clinical trials of PAF antagonists in the treatment of bronchial asthma were not encouraging. In fact, the response to the conventional antiasthma drugs is superior than that by PAF antagonists. However, it is possible that a combination of PAF antagonist with other specific antagonist might elicit a synergistic response. In this regard, the Schering-Plough company synthesized a compound, Sch 37370, which was an orally active antagonist of PAF and histamine H_1 receptors with potential therapeutic use in the treatment of asthma (93). A single dose (5 mg/kg) of Sch 37370 antagonized both PAF and histamine, with plasma antihistamine activity lasting longer than plasma anti-PAF activity. These studies need to be explored further.

References

1. Barbaro JF, Zvaifler NJ. Antigen-induced histamine release from platelets of rabbits producing homologous PCA antibody. Proc Soc Exp Biol Med 1966; 122:1245–1250.
2. Henson PM. Role of complement and leukocytes in immunologic release of vasoactive amines from platelets. Fed Proc 1968; 18:1721–1725.
3. Benveniste J, Henson PM, Cochrane CG. Leukocyte-dependent histamine release from rabbit platelets: the role of IgE-basophils and platelet-activating factor. J Exp Med 1972; 136:1356–1360.
4. Benveniste J, Tence M, Varenne P, Bidault J, Boullet C, Polonsky J. Semisynthese et structure proposee du facteur activant les plaquettes (PAF): PAF-acether, un alkyl ether analogue de la lysophosphatidylcholine. CR Acad Sci Ser D 1979; 289:1037–1042.
5. Demopoulus CA, Pinckard RN, Hanahan DJ. Platelet-activating factor. Evidence for 1-O-alkyl-2-acetyl-sn-glycerol-3-phosphoryl-choline as the active component (a new class of lipid mediators). J Biol Chem 1979; 254:9355–9360.
6. Blank ML, Snyder F, Byers LW, Brooks B, Muirhead EE. Antihypertensive activity of an alkyl ether analog of phsophatidylcholine. Biophys Biochem Res Commun 1979; 90:1194–1200.
7. Agrawal DK, Fugate MJ, Townley RG. Platelet-activating factor-acether-induced microvascular permeability in mice. In: Handley DA, Saunders RN, Houlihan WJ, Tomesch JC, eds. Platelet-Activating Factor in Endotoxin and Immune Diseases. New York: Marcel Dekker, 1990:177–188.
8. Tamura N, Agrawal DK, Suliaman FA and Townley RG. Effects of platelet-activating factor on the chemotaxis of normodense eosinophils from normal subjects. Biochem Biophys Res Commun 1987; 142:638–644.
9. Tamura N, Agrawal DK, and Townley RG. Leukotriene C_4 production from human eosinophils in vitro: role of eosinophil chemotactic factors on eosinophil activation. J Immunol 1998; 141:4291–4297.
10. Agrawal, DK. Platelet-activating factor receptors in the airways. In: Agrawal, DK, Townley RG, eds. Inflammatory cells and mediators in bronchial Asthma. Boca Raton, FL: CRC Press, 1991:171–206.
11. Horii T, Okazaki H, Kino M, Kobayashi Y, Satouchi K, Saito K. Platelet-activating factor detected in bronchoalveolar lavage fluids from an asthmatic patient. Lipids 1991; 26:1292–1296.
12. Crea AE, Nakhosteen JA, Lee TH. Mediator concentrations in bronchoalveolar lavage fluid of patients with mild asymptomatic bronchial asthma. Eur Respir J 1992; 5:190–195.
13. Stenton SC, Court EN, Kingston WP, Goadby P, Kelly CA, Duddridge M, Ward C, Hendrick DJ, Walters EH. Platelet-activating factor in bronchoalveolar lavage fluid from asthmatic subjects. Eur Respir J 1990; 3:408–413.
14. Schauer U, Koch B, Michl U, Jager R, Rieger CH. Enhanced production of platelet-activating factor by peripheral granulocytes from children with asthma. Allergy 1992; 47:143–149.
15. Chang-Yeung M, Lam S, Chan H, Tse KS, Salari H. The release of platelet-activat-

ing factor into plasma during allergen-induced bronchoconstriction. J Allergy Clin Immunol 1991; 87:667–673.
16. McIntyre TM, Zimmerman GA, Satoh K, and Prescott SM. Cultured endothelial cells synthesize both platelet-activating factor and prostacyclin in response to histamine, bradykinin, and adenosine triphosphate. J Clin Invest 1985; 76:271–280.
17. Oda M, Satouchi K, Yasunaga K, Saito K. Molecular species of platelet-activating factor generated by human neutrophils challenged with ionophore A23187. J Immunol 1985; 134:1090–1095.
18. Sisson JH, Prescott SM, McIntyure TM, Zimmerman GA. Production of platelet-activating factor by stimulated human polymorphonuclear leukocytes: correlation of synthesis with release, functional events, and leukotriene B4 metabolism. J Immunol 1987; 138:3918–3923.
19. Henson PM. Extracellular and intracellular activities of PAF. In: Snyder F, ed: Platelet-Activating Factor and Related Lipid Mediators. New York: Plenum Press, 1987; 255–272.
20. Venable ME, Zimmerman GA, McIntyre TM, Prescott SM. Platelet-activating factor: a phospholipid autacoid with diverse actions. J Lipid Res 1993; 34:691–702.
21. Shukla SD. Platelet activating factor receptor and signal transduction mechanisms. FASEB J 1990; 6:2296–2301.
22. Ludwig JC, Hoppens CL, McManus LM, Mott GE, Pinckard RN. Modulation of platelet-activating factor (PAF) synthesis and release from human polymorphonuclear leukocytes (PMN): role of extracellular albumin. Arch Biochem Biophys 1985; 241:337–342.
23. Leyravaud S, Benveniste J. Regulation of cellular retention of PAF-acether by extracellular pH and cell concentration. Biochim Biophys Acta 1989; 1005:192–198.
24. Ludwig JC, McManus LM, Clark PO, Hanahan DJ, Pinckard RN. Modulation of platelet-activating factor (PAF) synthesis and release from human polymorphonuclear leukocytes (PMN): role of extracellular Ca^{2+}. Arch Biochem Biophys 1984; 232:102–110.
25. Cluzel M, Undem BJ, Chilton FH. Release of platelet-activating factor and the metabolism of leukotriene B4 by the human neutrophil when studied in a cell superfusion model. J Immunol 1989; 143:3659–3665.
26. Alam I, Smith JB, Silver MJ. Metabolism of platelet-activating factor by blood platelets and plasma. Lipids 1983; 18:534–542.
27. Miwa M, Sugatani J, Ikemura T, Okamoto Y, Ino M, Saito K, Suzuki Y, Matsumoto M. Release of newly synthesized platelet-activating factor (PAF) from human polymorphonuclear leukocytes under in vivo conditions: contribution of PAF-releasing factor in serum. J Immunol 1992; 148:872–880.
28. Banks JB, Wykle RL, O'Flaherty JT, Lumb RH. Evidence for protein-catalyzed transfer of platelet activating factor by macrophage cytosol. Biochim Biophys Acta 1988; 961:48–52.
29. Lumb RH, Record M, Ribbes G, Pool GL, Terce F, Chap H. PAF-acether transfer activity in HL-60 cells is induced during differentiation. Biochem Biophys Res Commun 1990; 171:548–554.
30. Ezeamuzie CI, Al-Hage M. Effects of some anti-asthma drugs on human eosinophil

superoxide anions release and degranulation. Int Arch Allergy Immunol 1998; 115: 162–168.
31. Nabe T, Yamamura H, Kohno S. Eosinophil chemotaxis induced by several biologically active substances and the effects of apafant on it in vitro. Arzneimittelforschung 1997; 47:1112–1116.
32. Yamaguchi S, Kagoshima M, Kohge S, Terasawa M. Suppressive effects of Y-24180, a long-acting antagonist for platelet-activating factor, on allergic pulmonary eosinophilia in mice. Jpn J Pharmacol 1997; 75:129–134.
33. Koltai M, Hosford D, Braquet PG. Platelet-activating factor and its antagonists in allergic and inflammatory disorders. In: Townley RG, Agrawal DK, eds. Immunopharmacology of Allergic Diseases. New York:Marcel Dekker, 1991:463–489.
34. Honda Z, Nakamura M, Miki I, Minami M, Watanabe T, Seyama Y, Okado H, Toh H, Ito K, Miyamoto T, Shimizu T. Cloning by functional expression of platelet-activating factor receptor from guinea pig lung. Nature 1991; 349:342–346.
35. Nakamura M, Honda Z, Izumi T, Sakanaka C, Mutoh H, Minami M, Bito H, Seyama Y, Matsumoto T, Noma M, Shimizu T. Molecular cloning and expression of platelet-activating factor receptor from human leukocytes. J Biol Chem 1991; 266:20400–20405.
36. Ye RD, Prossnitz ER, Zou A, Cochrane CG. Characterization of a human cDNA that encodes a functional receptor for platelet-activating factor. Biochem Biophys Res Commun 1991; 180:105–111.
37. Kishimoto S, Shimadzu W, Izumi T, Shimizu T, Sagara H, Fukuda T, Makino S, Waku K. Comparison of platelet-activating factor receptor mRNA levels in peripheral blood eosinophils from normal subjects and atopic asthmatic patients. Int Arch Allergy Immunol 1997; 114 (suppl 1):60–63.
38. Burgers JA, Bruynzeel PL, Mengelers HJ, Kreukniet J, Akkerman JW. Occupancy of platelet receptors for platelet-activating factor in asthmatic patients during an allergen-induced bronchoconstrictive reaction. J Lipid Mediat 1993; 7:135–149.
39. Nagase T, Ishii S, Katayama H, Fukuchi Y, Ouchi Y, Shimizu T. Airway responsiveness in transgenic mice overexpressing platelet-activating factor receptor: roles of thromboxanes and leukotrienes. Am J Respir Crit Care Med 1997; 156:1621–1627.
40. Agrawal DK, Takami M, Ono S. A novel thromboxane synthetase inhibitor, DP-1904, inhibits human blood eosinophil degranulation. Inflammation 1997; 21:1–8.
41. Triggiani M, De-Marino V, Sofia M, Faraone S, Ambrosio G, Carratu L, Marone G. Characterization of platelet-activating factor acetylhydrolase in human bronchoalveolar lavage. Am J Respir Crit Care Med 1997; 156:94–100.
42. Tsukioka K, Matsuzaki M, Nakamata M, Kayahara H, Nakagawa T. Increased plasma level of platelet-activating factor (PAF) and decreased serum PAF acetylhydrolase (PAFAH) activity in adults with bronchial asthma. J Invest Allergol Clin Immunol 1996; 6:22–29.
43. Misso NL, Gillon RL, Stewart GA, Thompson PJ. Lyso-PAF acetyltransferase activity in neutrophils of patients during acute asthma and after recovery. Eur Respir J 1996; 9:2243–2249.
44. Ghosh SK, Rafferty P, DeVos C, Patel KR. Effect of cetirizine, a potent H1 antago-

nist, on platelet-activating factor induced bronchoconstriction in asthma. Clin Exp Allergy 1993; 23:524–527.
45. Louis R, Bury T, Corhay JL, Radermecker M. No increase in plasma histamine during PAF-induced airway obstruction in allergic asthmatics. Chest 1993; 104:806–810.
46. Hopp RJ, Townley RG, Agrawal DK, Bewtra AK. Terfenadine effect on the bronchoconstriction, dermal response, and leukopenia induced by platelet-activating factor. Chest 1991; 100:994–998.
47. Hopp RJ, Bewtra AK, Agrawal DK, Townley RG. Effect of platelet-activating factor inhalation on nonspecific bronchial reactivity in man. Chest 1989; 96:1070–1072.
48. Cuss FM, Dixon CMS, Barnes PJ. Effects of inhaled platelet activating factor on pulmonary function and bronchial responsiveness in man. Lancet 1986; 2:189–192.
49. Smith LJ, Rubin AE, Patterson R. Mechanism of platelet activating factor-induced bronchoconstriction in humans. Am Rev Respir Dis 1988; 137:1015–1021.
50. Hopp RJ, Bewtra AK, Nabe M, Agrawal DK, Townley RG. Effect of PAF-acether inhalation on nonspecific bronchial reactivity and adrenergic response in normal and asthmatic subjects. Chest 1990; 98:936–941.
51. Agrawal DK, Bergren DR, Byorth PJ and Townley RG. Platelet-activating factor induces non-specific desensitization to bronchodilators in guinea pigs. J Pharmacol Exp Ther 1991; 259:1–7.
52. Chung KF, Barnes PJ. Effects of platelet activating factor on airway calibre, airway responsiveness, and circulating cells in asthmatic subjects. Thorax 1989; 44:108–115.
53. Louis R, Bury T, Corhay JL, Radermecker MF. Acute bronchial and hematologic effects following inhalation of a single dose of PAF: comparison between asthmatics and normal subjects. Chest 1994; 106:1094–1099.
54. Louis R, Degroote D, Bury T, Corhay JL, Kayembe JM, Franchimont P, Radermecker MF. Changes in bronchial responsiveness, circulating leukocytes and ex vivo cytokine production by blood monocytes after PAF inhalation in allergic asthmatics. Eur Respir J 1995; 8:611–618.
55. Kaye MG, Smith LJ. Effects of inhaled leukotriene D4 and platelet-activating factor on airway reactivity in normal subjects. Am Rev Respir Dis 1990; 141:993–997.
56. Gebremichael I, Leuenberger P. Platelet-activating factor does not induce bronchial hyperreactivity in nonasthmatic subjects. Respiration 1992; 59:193–196.
57. Lai CK, Djukanovic R, Wilson JW, Wilson SJ, Britten KM, Howarth PH, Holgate ST. Effect of inhaled platelet-activating factor on bronchial inflammation in atopic non-asthmatic subjects. Int Arch Allergy Immunol 1992; 99:84–90.
58. Chung KF, Lammers JW, McCusker M, Roberts NM, Nichol GM, Barnes PJ. Effect of theophylline on airway responses to inhaled platelet-activating factors in man. Eur Respir J 1989; 2:763–768.
59. Chung KF, Dent G, Barnes PJ. Effects of salbutamol on bronchoconstriction, bronchial hyperresponsiveness, and leukocyte responses induced by platelet activating factor in man. Thorax 1989; 44:102–107.
60. Hsieh KH, Ng CK. Increased plasma platelet-activating factor in children with acute asthmatic attacks and decreased in vivo and in vitro production of platelet-activating factor after immunotherapy. J Allergy Clin Immunol 1993; 91:650–657.

61. Yamamoto H, Nagata M, Tabe K, Kimura I, Kiuchi H, Sakamoto Y, Yamamoto K, Dohi Y. The evidence of platelet activation in bronchial asthma. J Allergy Clin Immunol 1993; 91:79–87.
62. Louis RE, Radermecker MF. Acute bronchial obstruction following inhalation of PAF in asthmatic and normal subjects: comparison with methacholine. Eur Respir J 1996; 9:414–420.
63. Hozawa S, Haruta Y, Ishioka S, Yamakido M. Effects of a PAF antagonist, Y-24180, on bronchial hyperresponsiveness in patients with asthma. Am J Respir Crit Care Med 1995; 152:1198–1202.
64. Felez MA, Roca J, Barbera JA, Santos C, Rotger M, Chung KF, Rodriguez-Roisin R. Inhaled platelet-activating factor worsens gas exchange in mild asthma. Am J Respir Crit Care Med 1994; 150:369–373.
65. Kurosawa M, Yamashita T, Kurimoto F. Increased levels of blood platelet-activating factor in bronchial asthmatic patients with active symptoms. Allergy 1994; 49:60–63.
66. McBride DE, Koenig JQ, Luchtel DL, Williams PV, Henderson WR Jr. Infammatory effects of ozone in the upper airways of subjects with asthma. Am J Respir Crit Care Med 1994; 149:1192–1197.
67. Bruynzeel PL, Koenderman BL, Kok PTM, Hameling ML, Verhangen J. Platelet-activating factor induced leukotriene C_4 formation and luminol dependent chemiluminiscence by human eosinophils. Pharmacol Res Commun 1986; 18(suppl):61–69.
68. Taylor IK, Ward PS, Taylor GW, Dollery CT, Fuller RW. Inhaled PAF stimulates leukotriene and thromboxane A_2 production in humans. J Appl Physiol 1991; 71: 1396–1402.
69. O'Connor BJ, Uden S, Carty TJ, Eskra JD, Barnes PJ, Chung KF. Inhibitory effect of UK 74505, a potent and specific oral platelet activating factor (PAF) receptor anatgonists on airway and systemic responses to inhaled PAF in humans. Am J Respir Crit Care 1994; 150:35–40.
70. Rodriguez-Roisin R, Felez MA, Chung KF, Barbera JA, Wagner PD, Cobos A, Barnes PJ, Roca J. Platelet-activating factor causes ventilation-perfusion mismatch in man. J Clin Invest 1994; 93:188–194.
71. Diaz O, Barbera JA, Marrades R, Chung KF, Roca J, Rodriguez-Roisin R. Inhibition of PAF-induced gas exchange defects by beta-adrenergic agonists in mild asthma is not due to bronchodilation. Am J Respir Crit Care Med 1997; 156:17–22.
72. Gomez FP, Iglesia R, Roca J, Barbera JA, Chung KF, Rodriguez-Roisin R. The effects of 5-lipoxygenase inhibition by zileuton and platelet-activating-factor-induced pulmonary abnormalities in mild asthma. Am J Respir Crit Care Med 1998; 157:1559–1564.
73. Spencer DA, Evans JM, Green SE, Piper PJ, Costello JF. Participation of the cysteinyl leukotrienes in the acute bronchoconstriction response to inhaled platelet activating factor in man. Thorax 1991; 46:441–445.
74. Kidney JC, Ridge SM, Chung KF, Barnes PJ. Inhibition of platelet-activating factor-induced bronchoconstriction by the leukotriene D4 receptor antagonist ICI 204219. Am Rev Respir Dis 1993; 147:215–217.
75. Israel E, Dermarkarian R, Rosenberg M, Sperling R, Taylor G, Rubin P, Drazen

JM. The effects of 5-lipoxygenase inhibitor on asthma induced by cold, dry air. N Engl J Med 1990; 323:1740–1744.
76. Israel E, Fischer AR, Rosenberg MA, Lilly CM, Callery JC, Shapiro J, Cohn J, Rubin P, Drazen JM. The pivotal role of 5-lipoxygenase products in the reaction of aspirin-sensitive asthmatics to aspirin. Am Rev Respir Dis 1993; 148:1447–1451.
77. Hui KP, Taylor IK, Taylor GW, Rubin P, Kesterson J, Barnes NC, Barnes PJ. Effect of a 5-lipoxygenase inhibitor on leukotriene generation and airway responses after allergen challenge in asthmatic patients. Thorax 1991; 46:184–189.
78. Sampson SE, Costello JF, Sampson AP. The effect of inhaled leukotriene B4 in normal and asthmatic subjects. Am J Respir Crit Care Med 1997; 155:1789–1792.
79. Rubin AHE, Smith LJ, Patterson R. The bronchoconstrictor properties of platelet-activating factor in humans. Am Rev Respir Div 1987; 136:1145–1151.
80. Voelkel NF, Worthen S, Reves JT, Henson PM, Murphy RC. Nonimmunological production of leukotrienes induced by platelet-activating factor. Science 1982; 218: 286–288.
81. Taylor IK, Ward PS, Taylor GW, Dollery CT, Fuller RW. Inhaled PAF stimulates leukotriene and thromboxane A2 production in humans. J Appl Physiol 1991; 71: 1396–1402.
82. Wilkens H, Wilkens JH, Uffmann J, Bovers J, Frohlich JC, Fabel H. Effects of the platelet-activating factor antagonist BN 52063 on exertional asthma. Pneumologie 1990; 44(suppl 1):347–348.
83. Hsieh KH. Effects of PAF antagonist, BN52021, on the PAF, methacholine, and allergen-induced bronchoconstriction in asthmatic children. Chest 1991; 99:877–882.
84. Adamus WS, Heuer HO, Meade CJ, Schilling JG. Inhibitory effects of the new PAF acether antagonist WEB 2086 on pharmacologic changes induced by PAF inhalation in human beings. Clin Pharmacol Ther 1990; 47:456–462.
85. Spence DP, Johnston SL, Calverley PM, Dhillon P, Higgins C, Ramhamadany E, Turner S, Winning A, Winter J, Holgate ST. The effect of the orally active platelet-activating factor antagonist WEB 2086 in the treatment of asthma. Am J Respir Crit Care Med 1994; 149:1142–1148.
86. Freitag A, Watson RM, Matsos G, Eastwood C, O'Byrne PM. Effects of platelet-activating factor antagonist, WEB 2086, on allergen-induced asthmatic responses. Thorax 1993; 48:594–598.
87. Tamura G, Takishima T, Mue S, Makino S, Itoh K, Miyamoto T, Shida T, Nakajima S. Effect of a potent platelet-activating factor antagonist, WEB 2086, on asthma: a multicenter, double-blind placebo-controlled study in Japan. Adv Exp Med Biol 1996; 416:371–380.
88. Kuitcrt LM, Hui KP, Uthayarkumar S, Burke W, Newland AC, Uden S, Barnes NC. Effect of the platelet-activating factor antagonist UK-74,505 on the early and late response to allergen. Am Rev Respir Dis 1993; 147:82–86.
89. Kuitert LM, Angus RM, Barnes NC, Barnes PJ, Bone MF, Chung KF, Fairfax AJ, Higenbotham TW, O'Connor BJ, Piotrowska B. Effect of a novel potent platelet-activating factor antagonist, modipafant, in clinical asthma. Am J Respir Crit Care Med 1995; 151:1331–1335.
90. Hozawa S, Haruta Y, Ishioka S, Yamakido M. Effects of a PAF antagonist, Y-24180,

on bronchial hyperresponsiveness in patients with asthma. Am J Respir Crit Care Med 1995; 152:1198–1202.
91. Townley RG, Eda R, Hopp RJ, Bewtra AK, Gillen MS. The effect of RP 59227, a platelet-activating factor antagonist, against antigen challenge and eosinophil and neutrophil chemotaxis in asthmatics. J Lipid Mediat Cell Signal 1994; 10:345–353.
92. Evans DJ, Barnes PJ, Cluzel M, O'Connor BJ. Effects of a potent platelet-activating factor antagonist, SR27417A, on allergen-induced asthmatic responses. Am J Respir Crit Care Med 1997; 156:11–16.
93. Billah MM, Gilchrest HG, Eckel SP, Granzow CA, Lawton PJ, Radwanski E, Brannan MD, Affrime MB, Christopher JD, Richards W. Differential plasma duration of antiplatelet-activating factor and antihistamine activities of oral Sch 37370 in humans. Clin Pharmacol Ther 1992; 52:151–159.

8

Tachykinin Receptor Antagonists

GUY F. JOOS

University Hospital Ghent
Ghent, Belgium

CHARLES ADVENIER

Faculty of Medicine Paris West
University Paris V
Paris, France

I. Introduction

Nonadrenergic, noncholinergic (NANC) neural mechanisms are implicated in the pathophysiology of asthma. While inhibitory NANC (i-NANC) effects are bronchodilatory through the activity of vasoactive intestinal peptide (VIP) and nitric oxide (NO) from cholinergic nerves, excitatory NANC (e-NANC) effects are bronchoconstrictors and mediated by sensory neuropeptides (1–4). Sensory neuropeptides include calcitonin gene–related peptide (CGRP) and the tachykinins. Five different tachykinin peptides have now been identified in mammalian nervous tissues: substance P (SP), neurokinin A (NKA), neuropeptide K (NPK), neuropeptide γ (NP γ), and neurokinin B (NKB) (2). SP and NKA are the best-studied members of the tachykinin peptide family. These neuropeptides are synthesized by sensory neurons and subsequently stored in the terminal parts of the axon collaterals. Activation of these noncholinergic excitatory nerves by mechanical and chemical stimuli generates antidromic impulses and a local axon reflex, which leads to bronchoconstriction and neurogenic inflammation (1,3–5).

SP and NKA have various effects that could contribute to the changes observed in asthmatic airways, including smooth muscle contraction, submucosal gland secretion, vasodilatation, increase in vascular permeability, stimulation of cholinergic nerves, stimulation of mast cells, stimulation of B and T lymphocytes, stimulation of macrophages, chemoattraction of eosinophils and neutrophils, and vascular adhesion of neutrophils. In view of their potential airway effects, sensory neuropeptides have been implicated in the pathogenesis of asthma. Various review articles on this topic have been published in the past few years (1,3–9).

Most of the biological actions of tachykinins are mediated via activation of one of the three tachykinin receptors, denoted neurokinin receptors 1–3 (NK_1, NK_2, and NK_3) (Table 1). The NK_1, NK_2, and NK_3 neurokinin receptors have the highest affinity for SP, NKA, and NKB, respectively (Table 1). The physiological

Table 1 Receptor Subtypes Involved in the Pharmacological Effects of Tachykinins (Substance P, Neurokinin A, and Neurokinin B) in the Airways

Effect		Receptor Subtypes		
		NK_1	NK_2	NK_3
Nerve activation	Increase in ganglionic transmission	+	+	+++
Airway smooth muscle	Contraction of ferret trachea	+	+++	
	Contraction of hamster trachea		+++(NK_{2B})	
	Contraction of guinea pig trachea	++	+++	
	Contraction of guinea pig bronchus	+	+++(NK_{2A})	
	Contraction of human bronchus	+	+++	
	Relaxation of rat trachea[a]	++		
Vascular permeability	Plasma protein extravasation	+++	+/++	
Recruitment and activation of inflammatory cells	Chemotaxis (guinea pig, human)	++		
	Lymphocyte proliferation (human)	++	+	
	Increase in neutrophils motility	++	+	
	Monocyte/macrophage stimulation	+++	+++	
	Mast cell activation[b]	?	?	
Stimulation of secretion	Mucus in guinea pig trachea	+++	±	
	Mucus in ferret trachea	+++	±	
	Mucus in human bronchus	+++	±	
	Chloride secretion from epithelial cells	+++	±	

[a]Contractile effect has also been reported.
[b]A nonreceptor effect has been suggested
Key: NK, neurokinin; Ach, acetylcholine.
Receptor subtypes involvement: $^{+++}$ very strong; $^{++}$ strong; $^{+}$ moderate; ± doubtful; ? questionable.

activity of both exogenously administered and endogenously released neuropeptides is modulated through enzymatic cleavage and inactivation by peptidases (10). In human airways, two major peptidases are neutral endopeptidase (NEP, also called enkephalinase, E.C.3.4.24.11), which is predominantly present in airway epithelium, and angiotensin-converting enzyme (ACE, E.C.3.14.5.1), present within the pulmonary endothelium (10). NEP mRNA and NEP-immunoreactive material have been identified in human airways (11). In a recent biopsy study, Sont and colleagues have shown increased expression of NEP in the airway epithelium of asthmatic patients using inhaled corticosteroids (12).

In experimental models, the effect of sensory neuropeptides can be inhibited in various ways: (1) by depleting the neuropeptides from the nerves (e.g., by the neurotoxin capsaicin); (2) by inhibiting the release of sensory neuropeptides from the nerves (e.g., by stimulation of presynaptic β_2-receptors or opioid receptors); or (3) by blocking the tachykinin receptors (by tachykinin receptor antagonists). A series of specific tachykinin receptor antagonists have been developed (Fig. 1, Table 2) (13). The first tachykinin receptor antagonists had a peptidic structure, low potency and specificity, and demonstrated partial agonist activity. Several highly selective nonpeptide tachykinin receptor antagonists have also been described, some of which are currently under clinical investigation. The following nonpeptide tachykinin receptor antagonists have been studied in airways: CP-96,345, CP-99,994, RP 67580, and SR 140333 as NK_1 receptor antagonists; SR 48968 and GR 159897 as NK_2 receptor antagonists; and SR 142801 as a NK_3 receptor antagonist (Fig. 1).

In this chapter we describe the pharmacological properties of the tachykinin receptor antagonists, reviewing their contribution to tachykinin receptor classification. Apart from animal data, we focus on their effects on human airways both in vitro and in vivo. In addition, the first clinical studies with some of these compounds are discussed.

II. Sensory Neuropeptides in Human Airways

SP and NKA are found in the human lung. Measurements by radioimmunoassay (RIA) have shown an SP content of approximately 3 pmol/g tissue in human segmental bronchi, being of a similar magnitude as in the corresponding parts of guinea pig airways (14). In contrast, a lower content of NKA was found, being approximately 0.3 pmol/g tissue (15). Nerve fibers containing SP-like immunoreactivity (SP-li-IR) have been described beneath and within the airway epithelium, around blood vessels and submucosal glands, within the airway smooth muscle layer, and around local tracheobronchial ganglion cells. These nerve fibers are also found in and around bronchi, bronchioles, and more distal airways, occasionaly extending into the alveoli (14). In a more recent study, the presence of SP

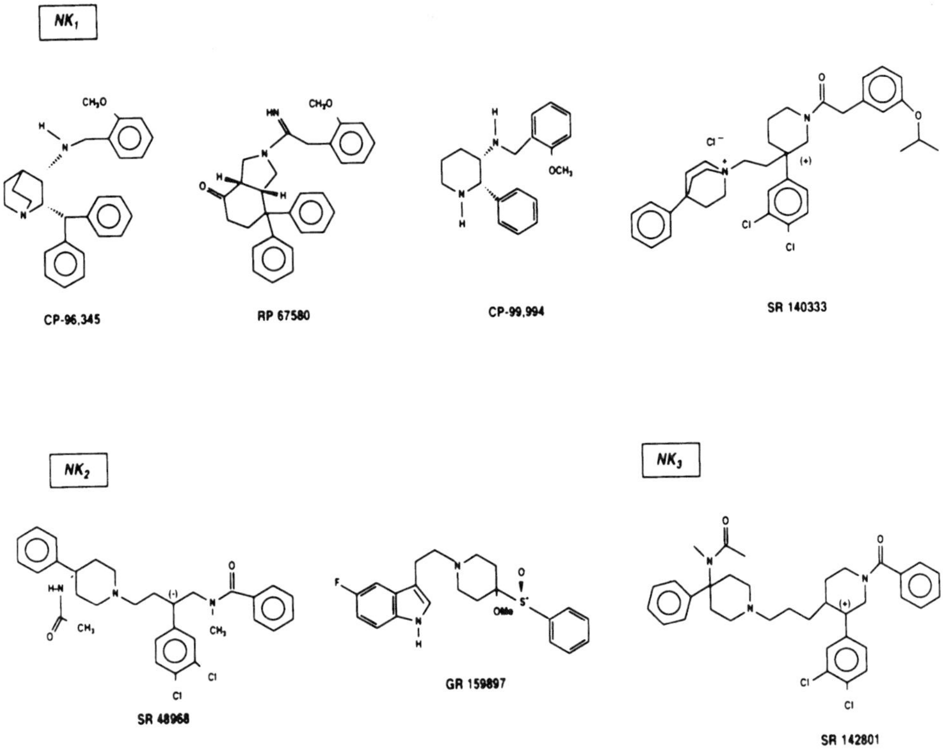

NK_1

CP-96,345 RP 67580 CP-99,994 SR 140333

NK_2

SR 48968 GR 159897

NK_3

SR 142801

Figure 1 Chemical structure of nonpeptide tachykinin antagonists.

CP-96,345:	[2S,3S)-cis-2(diphenylmethyl)-N-[2-methoxyphenyl)-methyl]-1-azabicyclo [2.2.2.] octane-3-amine
CP-99,994:	(+)-(2S,3S)-3-(2-methoxy-benzylamino)-2-phenylpiperidine
RP 67580:	(3aR, 7aR)-7,7-diphenyl-2-[1-imino-2-(2-methoxyphenyl)-ethyl] perhydroisoindol-4-one
SR 140333:	(S)-1-[2-[3-(3,4-Dichlorophenyl)-1-(3-isopropoxyphenylacetyl) piperidin-3-yl]ethyl]-4-phenyl-1-azoniabicyclo [2.2.2]octane
SR 48968:	(S)-N-methyl-N[4-acetylamino-4-phenylpiperidino)-2-(3,4-dichlorophenyl)butyl]-benzamide
GR 159897:	(R)-1-[2-(5-fluoro-1 H-indol-3-yl)ethyl]-4-methoxy-4-[(phenylsulfinyl)methyl]-piperidine
SR 142801:	(R)-(N)-(1-(3-(1-benzoyl-3-(3,4-dichlorophenyl)piperidin-3-yl)propyl)-4-phenylpiperidin-4-yl)-N-methylacetamide

Table 2 Selective Tachykinin Receptor Agonists and Antagonists

	NK_1 Receptors	NK_2 Receptors	NK_3 Receptors
Selective agonists			
Endogenous	Substance P	Neurokinin A Neuropeptide γ	Neurokinin B
Synthetic analogues	[Sar^9,$Met(O_2)^{11}$]SP Septide	[βAla^8]NKA(4–10) [Nle^{10}]NKA(4–10) [Lys^5,$MeLeu^9$, Nle^{10}]NKA(4–10)	[$MePhe^7$]NKB Senktide
Stable peptide antagonists	FK 888	MEN 10,376	
	MEN 11,149	MEN 10,627 MEN 11,42 (Nepadutant)	
Nonpeptide antagonists	CP-96,345 CP-99,994 CP-122,721 SR 140333 (Nolpitantium) RP 67580 RPR 100893 L 709210 L 732138 LY 303870 (Lanepitant) GR 203040	SR 48968 (Saredutant) SR 140190 GR 159897	SR 142801 (Onasetant) SB 223412 PD 157652 GR 138676

nerve fibers in normal larynx, trachea, and bronchi was confirmed. The authors found relatively few SP-containing nerve fibers compared to nerve fibers containing peptides such as vasoactive intestinal peptide (VIP). Moreover, according to their observations, the respiratory epithelium was lacking SP-containing nerve fibers (16). NKA and probably other related peptides are also present in human airway nerves. Using an antiserum raised against the nonmammalian tachykinin kassinin, Martling et al. demonstrated tachykinin-like immunoreactivity in human bronchi (15). Characterization of the immunoreactive material by high-performance liquid chromatography (HPLC) revealed that the tachykinin-like immunoreactivity was heterogenous and consisted of NKA, NPK, and a compound resembling the nonmammalian tachykinin eledoisin. No immunoreactive material corresponding to NKB was found (15).

Asthmatic lung tissue may contain more SP as compared with healthy lungs. In tissue obtained at autopsy, after lobectomy, and at bronchoscopy, both the number and the length of SP-immunoreactive (SP-IR) nerve fibers were increased in the airways of asthmatic subjects as compared with those of nonasthmatic controls (17). However, these findings need confirmation, since in another study, SP-IR nerves were not invariably found in bronchial biopsies from patients with mild persistent asthma (18). Moreover, in a recent study, substance P-like immunoreactivity (SP-li-IR) was measured in HPLC-purified tissue extracts from airways of both asthmatic subjects and healthy controls. Less SP-li-IR was detected in tracheal tissue from asthmatic as compared with nonasthmatic subjects, whereas parenchymal SP-li-IR content was similar in both groups. This may reflect augmented SP release in asthma (19). These findings are in accordance with a report on increased plasma levels of SP in patients with acute asthma (SP-li-IR 4.6 ± 0.4 pmol/L in 25 asthmatics compared with 2.2 ± 0.2 pmol/L in 21 healthy controls, respectively) (20).

SP has also been measured in the bronchoalveolar lavage (BAL) fluid. Increased SP levels have been measured in BAL from healthy subjects after ozone exposure (21). Nieber et al. (22) examined six atopic subjects with grass pollen allergy and six nonallergic, healthy controls. A significantly larger amount of SP was found in the BAL of atopic subjects at baseline as compared with the nonallergic controls, with a further increase following allergen challenge (22). A similar release of SP has also been demonstrated in the nasal lavage (NAL) from patients with allergic rhinitis (23).

SP has also been determined in sputum induced by inhalation of hypertonic saline. The level of SP was significantly higher in the sputum of patients with asthma (mean ± SEM: 17.7 ± 2.4 fmol/L) and of patients with chronic bronchitis (mean ± SEM: 25.6 ± 5.5 fmol/L) as compared with healthy controls (mean ± SEM: 1.1 ± 0.4 fmol/L). Moreover, in the asthmatic patients, the SP concentration was significantly related to the eosinophil count in the sputum. In all subjects the SP concentration in the hypertonic saline-induced sputum was found to correlate with FEV_1/FVC (24).

The content of SP and CGRP in human lung tissue has been shown to decrease with age and after denervation (25,26). In a comparative study of autopsy tissue from infants (0–3.5 years of age), children (8–11 years of age), and adults (17–24 years of age), relatively fewer SP- and CGRP-containing nerve fibers were found in the adult bronchioli, suggesting that, in human lung tissue, the content of both neuropeptides may decrease with age (25). In a study in transplanted human respiratory tracts removed at retransplantation, the content of neuropeptide-immunoreactive nerves was found to be lower than in the control lungs. Some immunoreactivity for SP and CGRP persisted, although the nerve fibers were more sparse as compared with nontransplanted tissue, suggesting that no reinnervation occurred (26).

Finally, recent studies have documented possible changes in neurokinin receptor expression in asthma, providing evidence for an increase in mRNA transcripts for NK_1 (27) and NK_2 (28) receptors in asthma. A new notion is that tachykinins are also present in inflammatory cells such as macrophages, eosinophils, and dendritic cells (29). Eosinophils have been shown to synthesize immunoreactive SP (30) and to express preprotachykinin-I (PPT-I) mRNA (31). Recently, we demonstrated that alveolar macrophages obtained from induced sputum of healthy volunteers contain SP and NK_1 receptors (32). As in the rat, the expression of SP by macrophages is upregulated by lipopolysaccharide (LPS) (33).

III. Bronchoconstrictor Effect of Sensory Neuropeptides

A. In Vitro Bronchoconstrictor Effect of SP and NKA

The in vitro contractile effects of SP and NKA have been studied extensively. SP contracts human bronchi and bronchioli (34,35), being less potent than histamine or acetylcholine (36,37). NKA is a more potent constrictor of human bronchi than SP and was reported to be two to three orders of magnitude more potent than histamine or acetylcholine on molar base (37,38) (Fig. 2). In contrast with guinea pigs, NKB had no contractile effect on human airways (37,38).

Noncholinergic pathways have been thought to be more important in the smaller airways. Indeed, SP was found to contract small airways to a larger extent and at lower concentrations compared with large airways (39). This effect on small airways was mediated via the release of prostanoids, specifically thromboxane A_2, and through activation of NK_1 receptors (39). In contrast, SP has been

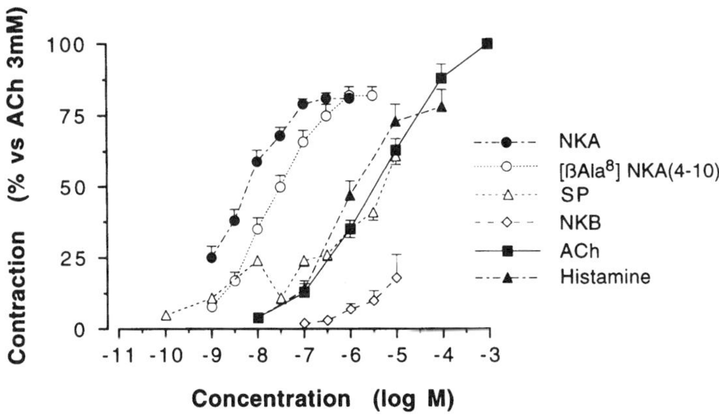

Figure 2 Concentration-response curve for neurokinin A (NKA), [βAla[8]] NKA(4-10) (a selective NK_2 receptor agonist), substance P (SP), neurokinin B (NKB), acetylcholine (ACh) and histamine on the human isolated bronchus. Values are mean ± SEM for 5 to 12 experiments.

shown to contract large bronchi through activation of NK_2 receptors (Fig. 2) (38,40).

The effect of passive sensitization on the in vitro contractile effect of SP and NKA has been studied in human bronchi (41). Human bronchi incubated overnight with serum from asthmatic patients atopic to *Dermatophagoides pteronyssinus* showed an enhanced sensitivity and an enhanced maximal contractile response to SP and NKA. This effect was independent of changes in the activity of NEP (41). Similarly, incubation of small human bronchi with interleukin-1β (IL-1β) induced an increased bronchoconstrictor response to SP (42).

It is important to stress that all the studies mentioned above have been performed in isolated airways obtained at thoracotomy, mostly from current smokers or ex-smokers with lung cancer. To our knowledge, no studies so far have reported the effect of tachykinins on isolated bronchi from asthmatic patients. Conversely, studies with adenosine 5′ monophosphate (AMP) have revealed important differences between isolated bronchi from healthy and asthmatic subjects both with regard to the potency of the agonist and its mechanism of action (43).

B. In Vivo Bronchoconstrictor Effect of SP and NKA

The in vivo bronchoconstrictor effect of SP and NKA, administered by inhalation or intravenous infusion, has been investigated by several groups. In these studies NKA was found to be a more potent bronchoconstrictor than SP, and patients with asthma appeared to be hyperresponsive to both SP and NKA (44–52).

We have studied the effect of inhaled SP and NKA on the airway caliber in both nonasthmatic and asthmatic subjects (46,47). Inhalation of SP and NKA by six healthy, nonsmoking subjects did not cause a significant change in specific airways conductance (sGaw). In asthmatic patients, inhalation of SP up to 10^{-6} mol/mL caused no change in sGaw, whereas inhalation of NKA resulted in a concentration-dependent bronchoconstriction. The bronchoconstriction occurred rapidly and sGaw returned to the baseline within 30 min in most patients. All patients reported chest tightness. No cough and no change in heart rate or blood pressure were noted (46). In another study in 19 asthmatic patients, we found a weak, though insignificant correlation between airway responsiveness to methacholine and NKA, suggesting that different mechanisms are involved in the bronchoconstrictor activity of these two agents (47). Recently, we have demonstrated that the airway response to NKA is reproducible when measured with an interval of 1 week (48).

The in vivo bronchoconstrictor effect of inhaled sensory neuropeptides in humans has been confirmed and extended by other groups. In patients with more severe asthma, Crimi et al. demonstrated that inhaled SP is also capable of causing bronchoconstriction (49). Apart from a significant decrease in forced expiratory volume in 1 sec (FEV_1), high doses of inhaled SP (up to 8 mg/mL)* also caused a significant fall in blood pressure and an increase in heart rate in asthma (50). Inhaled SP also produced bronchoconstriction in children with asthma, depending on the severity of disease (51). Using a highly efficient jet nebulizer in combination with a sensitive measure of airway caliber, Cheung et al. showed that NKA caused bronchoconstriction not only in asthmatic patients but also in healthy subjects, the asthmatic patients being more sensitive to NKA than the healthy controls (52,53).

Only few studies have investigated tachykinin effects on airway responsiveness in humans. In one study, inhaled SP has been shown to enhance the maximal airway narrowing to methacholine in asthmatic patients 24 hr after inhalation (50).

C. Mechanisms Involved in the Bronchoconstrictor Effects of Tachykinins

In guinea pig airways and isolated large human airways, the constrictor effect of the tachykinins was reported to be direct, as antihistamines and muscarinic receptor antagonists did not affect the reaction (34). However, in rabbit airways, the bronchoconstrictor activity of SP was partially inhibited by pretreatment with atropine. In Fisher 344 rats, tachykinins caused bronchoconstriction mainly by indirect mechanisms, through activation of cholinergic nerves and mast cells (54,55).

To investigate the mechanism of tachykinin-induced bronchoconstriction in asthma, the effects of nedocromil sodium, a potent mast-cell stabilizer, and the anticholinergic agents oxitropium bromide and ipratropium bromide on NKA- and SP-induced bronchoconstriction have been studied in patients with mild persistent asthma. Nedocromil sodium prevented the bronchoconstriction caused by NKA (56) and SP (49). Oxitropium bromide offered a partial protection against the bronchoconstrictor effect of NKA, which was evident in 4 out of 11 asthmatic patients (57). Ipratropium bromide caused a modest but significant rightward shift in the dose-response curve to SP in 7 patients with moderate persistent asthma (58). These findings indicate that in asthma, SP and NKA exert their bronchoconstrictor effects, at least partially, by indirect mechanisms, such as inflammatory cells (e.g., mast cells) and/or nerves.

In experimental animals, tachykinins have been shown to release acetylcholine from postganglionic cholinergic airway nerve endings (59,60). In isolated human airways, NKA but not SP potentiated the contractile response to cholinergic neural stimulation in the presence of K^+ channel blockade with 4-aminopyridine (4-AP). Because neither 4-AP per se nor the combination of 4-AP and NKA

---

*10^{-6} moles SP per milliliter equals approximately 1 mg SP per milliliter.

potentiated the postjunctional effects of acetylcholine, it was suggested that the potentiation of the neural response by NKA was occurring at the level of the postganglionic nerve terminal (61).

Substance P has been shown to cause dose-dependent release of histamine and serotonin (5-HT) from rat peritoneal and pleural mast cells. This is a rapid phenomenon, occurring within 15 sec, more than 90% of the response occurring within 1 min (62). SP-induced histamine release has also been documented in rat lung in vitro (63). Similarly, Joos et al. demonstrated tachykinin-induced contraction of rat trachea by secondary release of 5-HT from mast cells. This effect was mediated by NK_1 receptors (64). Furthermore, the protective effect of nedocromil sodium against SP- and NKA-induced bronchoconstriction in asthma suggests a possible involvement of mast cells in human airway response to tachykinins (49,56). Indeed, SP has been shown to release histamine from mast cells recovered from BAL fluid of asthmatic patients (65). In this study, mast cell counts significantly correlated with SP-induced histamine release (65). According to recent observations, SP elevated the histamine content in cultures of human nasal mucosa. In this study, it was shown by histomorphometry that SP increased the percentage of degranulated mast cells (66). Conversely, the lack of effect of pretreatment with astemizole and terfenadine, two potent and specific H_1-antagonists, on NKA-induced bronchoconstriction in asthmatic subjects suggests that histamine does not play a major role in NKA-induced bronchoconstriction in humans (58,67).

In the last decade, direct evidence has been provided for a close contact between mast cells and nerves. A large number of intestinal mucosal mast cells from healthy and nematode-infected rats have been shown to be in direct contact with nerve profiles, some of which contained SP or CGRP (68). A similar association has been found in rat lung (69).

IV. Classification of Tachykinin Receptor Antagonists

The tachykinin receptor antagonists are classified according to their specificity for the NK_1, NK_2, or NK_3 receptor, respectively. They have also been classified according to their chemical structure into three generations of tachykinin receptor antagonists (Fig. 1) (13).

The first generation of tachykinin receptor antagonists was developed in the beginning of the 1980s, based on insertion of multiple D-Trp residues on the backbone of SP. These compounds have been useful tools to study tachykinin receptors, although they had a number of drawbacks—such as low potency, poor selectivity, and not negligible intrinsic activity. Furthermore, due to limitations linked to their peptide nature, these compounds have not been considered as serious candidates for human use. The second generation of tachykinin receptor antagonists includes peptidic substances with a markedly improved potency and specificity. Some of them have a long duration of action (e.g., MEN 10,627; MEN 11,420) due to their cyclic structure with conformational constraints, increasing the resistance to degradation by peptidases. The third generation of these antagonists arose from the discovery of potent nonpeptide ligands that were highly selective for NK_1, NK_2, and NK_3 receptors (Fig. 1, Table 2) (9,13,70–80). Owing to their nonpeptide nature in combination with a favorable pharmacokinetic profile and relatively few adverse effects, these compounds seemed to be the most obvious candidates to be applied in humans in vivo.

The specificity of these compounds has been established by binding studies on human tachykinin receptors cloned and expressed in Chinese hamster ovary (CHO) cells and on classic in vitro bioassays (13). The most frequently used preparations in studies of tachykinin receptor pharmacology include the following: (1) for the NK_1 receptor, rabbit pulmonary artery (endothelium-dependent relaxation), the guinea pig ileum, the rat urinary bladder; (2) for the NK_2 receptor, rabbit pulmonary artery (endothelium-denuded) and vena cava, guinea-pig and human airways, and isolated rat vas deferens; (3) for the NK_3 receptor, rat portal vein and guinea pig ileum. Receptor specific agonists have been derived from SP, NKA, and NKB by modification of the peptide structure. The principal NK_1 receptor agonists are SP-OMe, and [Sar^9, $Met(O_2)^{11}$] SP. [Nle^{10}]NKA(4-10), [βAla^8]NKA(4-10) and [Lys^5, $MeLeu^9$, Nle^{10}]NKA (4-10) are NK_2 receptor agonists. $MePhe^7$ NKB and senktide are agonists specific for the NK_3 receptor (Table 2) (13).

There is evidence for pharmacological differences in tachykinin receptors among species. Based on differences in affinity for the nonpeptide NK_1 receptor antagonists CP-96,345 and RP 67580, the NK_1 receptor can be divided in two major categories: (1) the NK_1 receptor found in humans, bovine animals, guinea pigs, hamsters and rabbits, for which CP-96,345 is more potent, and (2) the NK_1 receptor found in rats, mice and chickens, for which RP 67580 is more potent. A similar species-dependent heterogeneity has been demonstrated for the NK_2 receptor. Based on differences in rank order of potency of the NK_2 receptor antagonists, Maggi et al. introduced the $NK_{2A/B}$ classification to distinguish the pharmacological characteristics of the NK_2 receptor found in humans, bovine animals, guinea pigs, and rabbits (NK_{2A} receptor) versus the pharmacological characteristics of this receptor found in hamsters and rats (NK_{2B} receptor) (80). Antagonists with a high affinity for the NK_{2A} receptor include SR 48968, MEN 10,207, and MEN 10,376, whereas substances with specificity for the NK_{2B} receptor are R 396, L 659,877, MEN 10,573, MEN 10,612, and MEN 10,627. Species heterogeneity (rat versus human and guinea pig) has also been reported for the NK_3 receptor (76,81). Recently still another subtype of NK_1 receptors has been proposed: an NK_1 receptor sensitive to septide [($pGlu^6$, Pro^9) SP (6–11)] has been identified in isolated guinea pig bronchi. However, since NK_1 receptor antagonists are more effective against septide than against SP, and because no distinct receptor molecule for septide has been cloned so far, it is possible that septide may not act on a receptor subtype but on a site of the NK_1 receptor molecule with lower affinity (82–85). Further research is needed to clarify this phenomenon.

Analysis of the binding sites of the tachykinin receptor antagonists has revealed interesting findings. A recent study has demonstrated that the binding sites for the nonpeptide ligands CP-96,345 and SR 48968 on the NK_1 and the NK_2 receptor, respectively, are distinct from those of SP or NKA. Furthermore, it has been suggested that CP-96,345 and SR 48968 act through epitopes located around the outer part of the transmembrane segments VI on their respective receptors (13,86,87). This may account for the slowly reversible antagonism exerted by SR 48968 in some studies (86,88).

V. Effects of Tachykinin Receptor Antagonists on Airways

A. Bronchoconstriction

Animal Studies

In guinea pig isolated airways, electrical field stimulation produces a typical biphasic response. The first component of this response is atropine-sensitive and hence clearly related to stimulation of cholinergic fibers, while the second, slowly raising noncholinergic excitation component, is largely mediated by endogenous tachykinins released from capsaicin-sensitive nerve afferents. SR 48968 potently abolished this NANC response (89–91), confirming previous reports with peptide NK_2 receptor antagonists (92). SR 48968 has been used to demonstrate the involvement of tachykinins through NK_2 receptor stimulation in the effects provoked by several agents in guinea pig airways, including capsaicin (91,93–95), resiniferatoxin (95,96), citric acid (97), serotonin (after blockade of 5-HT_2 receptors) (98), sodium metabisulfite (99), and diethylether (100), or in hyperpnea-induced bronchoconstriction (101).

In guinea pigs in vivo, SR 48968 provided at least partial inhibition of bronchoconstriction induced by NK_2 receptor stimulation directly through the NK_2 receptor agonist, [Nle^{10}]NKA(4-10), or indirectly by irritants such as capsaicin, resiniferatoxin, or citric acid (91,93,96,97,102,103).

Joos et al. have compared the effects of the tachykinins SP and NKA with those of the specific NK_1 and NK_2 receptor agonists in the airways of Fisher 344 and BDE rats. In addition, they studied the effect of potent nonpeptide NK_1 and NK_2 receptor antagonists on the SP- and NKA-induced airway effects (104). In these in vivo experiments, the tachykinins have been shown to cause bronchoconstriction in the Fisher 344 rats both by direct and indirect mechanisms, involving stimulation of the NK_1 receptors and mast-cell activation, whereas in BDE rats bronchoconstriction was induced exclusively by a direct effect—i.e., through activation of the NK_2 receptors (104). Moreover, they found that SP and NKA contract isolated trachea from Fisher 344 rats mainly by interaction with the NK_1 receptor (105). Thus, these genetically different inbred rat strains differ with regard to the airway sensitivity to tachykinins and the mechanisms involved in the airway response (104,105).

FK 224 is a cyclopeptide tachykinin receptor antagonist that inhibits NK_1 and NK_2 receptor-mediated airway responses in the guinea pig (106). In a study of Fisher 344 rats, this compound blocked both the NKA-induced bronchoconstriction and the airway mast-cell activation (107).

Human In Vitro Studies

In isolated human bronchi, SR 48968 displayed competitive antagonism for contraction induced by the specific NK_2 receptor agonist [Nle^{10}]NKA(4-10) with a pA_2 of 9.40 (40,108). SR 48968 also inhibited contraction of isolated human airway smooth muscle induced by neuropeptide gamma, with a similar pA_2 (108,109), but it did not affect responses to capsaicin (108). Under similar conditions, GR 159897, another nonpeptide NK_2 receptor antagonist, exhibited a pA_2 of 8.6 when tested against [Nle^{10}]NKA(4-10) (110). However, no effect was found on bronchoconstriction induced by acetylcholine, histamine, KCl or prostaglandin $F_{2\alpha}$ (40), or bradykinin (111). SR 48968 caused a rightward shift in the dose-response curve to SP (40). Since the specific NK_1 receptor antagonist CP-96,345 did not affect this response, these findings suggest that SP-induced contraction of the large airways of nonasthmatic subjects in vitro is mediated mainly through the stimulation of NK_2 receptors (40). Similar observations have been made for NKA (40,112,113). Recently, evidence has been provided that NK_1 receptors are also partially involved in the contractile response of human small airways (see also Sec. III.A) (39).

B. Effects on Inflammatory Responses

Allergic Bronchoconstriction

In guinea pigs sensitized with ovalbumin (OVA), SR 48968 markedly reduced the bronchoconstrictor response to low doses of OVA and completely blocked this response when combined with the nonpeptide NK_1 receptor antagonist CP-96,345 (114). After high doses of OVA, the combination of both NK_1 and NK_2 receptor antagonists markedly attenuated the late bronchoconstrictor response occurring after 10–20 min (114). Similar results were obtained with the long-acting peptide NK_2 receptor antagonist MEN 10,627, showing that tachykinins are involved in allergen-induced bronchoconstriction, at least in guinea pigs (115).

Using NEP inhibition by thiorphan in humans in vivo, the involvement of tachykinins could not be demonstrated in allergen-induced bronchoconstriction

(116). However, these findings have not yet been confirmed by application of specific tachykinin receptor antagonists in allergen challenge.

Plasma Protein Leakage

Both pharmacological and immunohistochemical studies provided evidence that NK_1 receptors are involved in the neurogenic inflammation within the central airways of guinea pigs and rats (117,118). The nonpeptide NK_1 receptor antagonists CP-96,345 and CP-99,994 inhibited the microvascular leakage induced by SP, bradykinin (119,120), hypertonic saline (121), and allergen in guinea pig airways (122). Although NKA is a considerably less potent inducer of microvascular leakage than SP, the NK_2 receptor antagonist SR 48968 inhibited the NKA-induced microvascular leakage in guinea pig airways (120). Similarly, Toussignant and co-workers demonstrated that neurogenic inflammation in peripheral guinea pig airways is partially mediated by NK_2 receptors (123). Using the specific NK_2 receptor agonist, [β-Ala^8]NKA(4-10) in combination with the specific NK_2 receptor antagonist SR 48968, they demonstrated that microvascular leakage induced by NK_2 receptor stimulation is found only in secondary bronchi and intraparenchymal airways (123). In lower airways of guinea pigs, SR 48968 also partially inhibited the plasma extravasation induced by electrical vagal stimulation (124).

Boichot et al. showed that, apart from its direct effect, aerosolized SP potentiates histamine-induced microvascular leakage in the airways of phosphoramidon-pretreated guinea pigs 24 hr after inhalation, whereas no increase in microvascular leakage was noted without exposure to SP (125). Accordingly, the NK_1 receptor antagonist SR 140333 markedly reduced the SP-induced potentiation of the microvascular leakage, whereas the NK_2 receptor antagonist SR 48968 had no inhibiting effects, strengthening the role of the NK_1 receptor in the microvascular leakage following tachykinin stimulation (125). In addition, similar protective effects against histamine-induced microvascular leakage were obtained by SR 140333 applied in guinea pigs exposed to aerosolized citric acid (126).

Mucus Secretion

Currently, it has been established that the in vitro secretion of a variety of mucus markers in the lower airways of various species—including humans, guinea pigs, ferrets, and cats—is mediated by NK_1 receptor stimulation. This was first demonstrated by investigating the rank order of potency of natural tachykinins and, more recently, by application of the tachykinin NK_1 receptor antagonist FK 888 (127,128).

Inflammatory Cells

Tachykinins exert several effects on inflammatory cells. It has been demonstrated that SP is capable of inducing the release of peroxidase from guinea pig eosinophils (129). SP is also known to stimulate the chemotaxis of human monocytes (130) and rabbit neutrophils (131). In addition, a moderate SP-induced chemotactic activity has been observed on neutrophils from both healthy and asthmatic subjects (132). Interestingly, SP or IL-1–induced polymorphonuclear leukocyte accumulation was prevented by an NK_1 receptor antagonist but not by an NK_2 receptor antagonist (133). Furthermore, administration of IL-1 has been shown to induce the release of endogenous tachykinins, possibly SP (139).

Apart from chemoattractant activity, tachykinins may also act as growth factors in vitro, stimulating the proliferation of human T and B lymphocytes and pulmonary fibroblasts (134–137). Tachykinins may also modulate inflammatory cell activation through the secondary release of various cytokines. Lotz et al. reported SP-induced release of IL-1, IL-6, and tumor necrosis factor alpha (TNF-α) from human monocytes (138). In another study, SP released IL-8 from human polymorphonuclear leukocytes and potentiated the release of IL-8 induced by substances such as *N*-formyl-methionyl-leucyl-penhylalamine (fMLP) (139). Finally, in association with human T-lymphocyte proliferation, SP has been shown to increase the expression of IL-2 messenger ribonucleic acid (mRNA) (140).

Conversely, inflammatory cells can elicit tachykinin release from sensory neurons. Eosinophils isolated from human allergic volunteers have been shown to induce SP synthesis in cultured dorsal root ganglion neurons from rats. This effect was mediated through the release of major basic protein (MBP) (141).

The hypothesis that tachykinin receptors play a role in inflammatory cell activation within the airways has recently been strengthened by observations with tachykinin receptor antagonists. In venules of the rat trachea, adhesion of leukocytes induced by SP or capsaicin was attenuated by the selective tachykinin NK_1 receptor antagonist CP-96,345 and therefore appears to be mediated by tachykinin NK_1 receptors (142). Applying the same NK_1 receptor antagonist in sensitized mice in vivo, Kaltreider et al. reported a moderate though significant reduction in the total numbers of leukocytes, lymphocytes, and granulocytes in the BAL after antigen challenge (143). Similar results were obtained in sensitized guinea pigs with the NK_1 receptor antagonist SR 140333 (144). These findings suggest that immune responses within the airways may elicit secretion of endogenous tachykinins, inducing infiltration of leukocytes into lung tissue. In contrast, in rabbits immunized to *Alternaria tenuis*, chronic treatment with capsaicin attenuated the airway hyperresponsiveness without inhibiting the recruitment of inflammatory cells—eosinophils and neutrophils—into the airways (145). Finally, in primates, dual antagonism offered by an NK_1 receptor antagonist (CP-99,994) combined with an NK_2 receptor antagonist (SR 48968) markedly reduced the allergen-induced eosinophil recruitment in BAL fluid, whereas each antagonist used alone was ineffective (146).

In guinea pigs pretreated with the NEP inhibitor phosphoramidon, airway responses to SP were not associated with recruitment of granulocytes into the airways (147). In contrast, in these guinea pigs, increases in chemiluminescence and in arachidonate release by alveolar macrophages ex vivo were observed after inhalation of SP (147,148). In another guinea pig study, SP induced the release of superoxide anions and thromboxane from alveolar macrophages in vitro (149) through stimulation of NK_2 receptors and, to a lesser extent, NK_1 receptors (150). More recently, SP has been shown to induce gelatinase production by alveolar macrophages through activation of the NK_2 receptor (151). In contrast with these observations in guinea pigs, alveolar macrophages from both healthy subjects and asthmatic patients were only poorly activated by SP in vitro, if at all (152).

Airway Hyperresponsiveness

Several lines of evidence suggest that tachykinins may be involved in the pathophysiology of airway hyperresponsiveness. Indeed, SP has been shown to potentiate bronchoconstriction (30 min or 24 hr after inhalation) induced by acetylcholine or histamine in guinea pigs (153–155), and NKA increased airway responsiveness to methacholine in monkeys for as long as 4 weeks (156). Similarly, inhibitors of tachykinin metabolism, such as thiorphan or phosphoramidon, potentiated toluene diisocyanate hyperresponsiveness in guinea pigs (157). In asthmatic subjects, Cheung et al. observed a significant increase in airway responsiveness to methacholine 24 hr after inhalation of SP (50). Conversely, depleting tachykinins from NANC nerve endings of guinea pigs by chronic treatment with high doses of intraperitoneal capsaicin reduced the airway hyperresponsiveness to carbachol, methacholine, or histamine induced by acute capsaicin (158), ovalbumin (159,160), toluene diisocyanate (157), endotoxin (161), PAF (162), or ozone (163). Similar findings were obtained in mice (164,165) (regarding airway hyperresponsiveness induced by dinitrofluorobenzene or toluene diisocyanate) and in rabbits (with regard to airway hyperresponsiveness induced by *A. tenuis*) (166).

In addition, Ellis and Undem have shown that ovalbumin challenge potentiated the e-NANC response to electrical field stimulation in isolated guinea pig main bronchi, probably through the release of histamine, again suggesting a link between tachykinins and allergic airway inflammation (167).

Boichot et al. have investigated the effects of the tachykinin receptor antagonists SR 48968 and SR 140333 on ovalbumin-induced airway hyperresponsiveness in sensitized guinea pigs. Ovalbumin caused increased airway responsiveness to acetylcholine 48 hr after challenge, which was prevented by intraperitoneal pretreatment with the NK_2 receptor antagonist SR 48968 but not by SR 140333, an NK_1 receptor antagonist (168). However, in another study in sensitized guinea pigs, SR 140333 has been shown to protect both against the allergen-induced airway hyperresponsiveness to histamine and the allergen-induced airway inflammation (144). Furthermore, SR 48968 also inhibited airway hyperresponsiveness induced by citric acid (169), substance P (170), IL-5 (171), and the potentiation by cold air of antigen-induced bronchoconstriction(172). In another guinea pig study by Perretti et al., the peptide NK_2 receptor antagonist, MEN 10,627, reduced the PAF-induced airway hyperresponsiveness to histamine (173). Finally, Tocker et al. found that vagal stimulation potentiated pulmonary anaphylaxis in the sensitized, perfused guinea pig lung. This potentiation was abolished by NK_2 receptor blockade; conversely, NKA but not SP could mimic the effects of vagal stimulation (174).

The findings with tachykinin receptor antagonists mentioned above confirm previous observations with capsaicin or exogenous tachykinins, suggesting that tachykinins are involved in the pathophysiology of airway hyperresponsiveness. Furthermore, pharmacological evidence has been provided that NK_2 and perhaps also NK_1 receptor stimulation may play a role in this phenomenon in guinea pig airways. In mice, on the other hand, tracheal hyperreactivity induced by toluene diisocyanate has been completely blocked by the NK_1 receptor antagonist RP 67580, suggesting a more prominent role for the NK_1 receptor in this model (165).

This raises the question of the site of action of the tachykinins (and tachykinin receptor antagonists). We suggest that tachykinin receptor antagonists act either locally on the efferent regulation of tissue responses (i.e., on target cells involved in bronchoconstriction and inflammation) or on nerve transmission. Interestingly, a recent study in OVA-sensitized guinea pigs shows a four- to fivefold increase in the neuropeptide level in the lung tissue as well as an increase in the percentage of SP/NKA-immunoreactive neurons in the nodose ganglion from 25% to a maximum of 48% 24 hr after allergen challenge (175). Furthermore, in nodose ganglia removed from OVA-immunized guinea pigs and exposed to the sensitizing antigen, SP depolarized 83% of the neurons. In contrast, SP produced no discernible changes in membrane electrophysiological properties in control ganglia (176). This SP effect was blocked by the NK_2 receptor antagonist SR 48968 and mimicked by the specific NK_2 receptor agonist [β-Ala^8) NKA (4–10), thus showing that it was mediated through NK_2 receptor stimulation (176). Similarly, the percentage of neurons expressing preprotachykinin A (PPT A)-mRNA was increased in vagal sensory ganglia of sensitized guinea pigs 12–24 hr after allergen challenge (175). Finally, it may be suggested that tachykinin receptor antagonists might act on the hyperalgesia associated with airway hyperresponsiveness—i.e., on the threshold of stimulation of sensory nerves. Indeed based on their animal experiments, Adcock and Garland suggested that tachykinins might decrease the threshold for stimulation of sensory nerve endings in the lung in a similar manner as in inflammed tissues, where they are clearly involved in hyperalgesia (177).

C. Cough

The cough reflex is usually considered to be mediated by rapidly adapting pulmonary stretch receptors (irritant receptors), with myelinated afferents and by stimulation of C-fiber endings through the release of tachykinins (178). Inhalation of capsaicin or an aqueous solution of citric acid causes cough in humans and in guinea pigs (179). In guinea pigs, this response seems to involve sensory mechanisms, since it can be prevented by pretreatment with a high concentration of capsaicin, causing depletion of neuropeptides through degeneration of the sensory nerves (180). The NK_2 receptor antagonist SR 48968 has been shown to reduce dose-dependently the cough induced by inhalation of an aqueous solution of citric acid in unanesthetized guinea pigs, suggesting that NK_2 receptor stimulation may play an important role in the pathophysiology of cough (181–183). In a comparative study in guinea pigs, SR 48968 was approximately 150 times more potent than codeine; in contrast to the latter, the effects of SR 48968 were not inhibited by naloxone (181). Similar results have been obtained by Robineau et al. with SR 48968 on capsaicin-induced cough in guinea pigs (184) and by Evangelista et al., who demonstrated that MEN 10,627, a peptide NK_2 receptor antagonist, inhibits antigen-induced bronchoconstriction and cough in sensitized guinea pigs (115).

Based on conflicting data from animal studies, the antitussive effect of tachykinin NK_1 receptor antagonists remain still under debate. In two studies in unanesthetized guinea pigs, neither CP-99,994 nor SR 140333, two potent nonpeptide NK_1 receptor antagonists, was able to protect against citric acid–induced cough (182,185). However in the same animal model, FK 888, another peptide NK_1 receptor antagonist, has been shown to inhibit cough induced by various irritants, including tobacco smoke, substance P, citric acid, and phosphoramidon (183,186). Moreover, Bolser et al. observed that CP-99,994 and SR 48968 inhibit cough in experimental animals by acting on the central nervous system (CNS) (187). Similarly, SR 140333 has been reported to potentiate the antitussive activity of an NK_2 receptor antagonist (SR 48968) on citric acid–induced cough in guinea pigs (182). In the same model, FK 888 and SR 48968 had small additive effects (183).

VI. Clinical Studies with Tachykinin Receptor Antagonists in Asthma

Presently, only four tachykinin receptor antagonists have been applied in clinical trials in asthma, including FK 224, a cyclic peptide tachykinin antagonist for NK_1 and NK_2 receptors; CP-99,994, a nonpeptide NK_1 receptor antagonist; FK 888, an NK_1 receptor antagonist; and SR 48968, a nonpeptide NK_2 receptor antagonist. Most of these trials have examined the protective effect of the tachykinin receptor antagonists against various challenges, whereas only very few long-term studies have been conducted investigating their effects on the disease outcome parameters.

FK 224 delivered at 4 mg by a metered-dose aerosol, has been shown to inhibit the bradykinin-induced bronchoconstriction and cough in nine asthmatic patients (188). Using a similar dose, Joos et al. studied the effect of inhaled FK 224 on NKA-induced bronchoconstriction in 10 patients with mild persistent asthma (48). In this group of asthmatic patients, FK 224 neither affected baseline FEV_1 nor provided protection against NKA-induced bronchoconstriction (48). In a long-term placebo-controlled trial in patients with mild to moderate persistent asthma, Lunde et al. evaluated the effects of 4 weeks of treatment with this compound (4 mg q.i.d. via metered-dose inhaler) on the disease parameters (189). In this study, FK 224 neither improved symptom scores nor lung function parameters (189). However, as FK 224 was not able to antagonize the airway effects of NKA in asthmatics, the study by Lunde et al. (189) does not reject a possible role for sensory neuropeptides in asthma.

In another study in 14 asthmatic males, the effect of pretreatment with the nonpeptide NK_1 receptor antagonist CP-99,994 (250 μg/kg iv) was investigated on the airway response to hypertonic saline (190). In these asthmatic patients, CP-99,994 failed to affect both the hypertonic saline-induced bronchoconstriction and cough (190). However, it remains to be demonstrated whether this compound at the given dose and route of administration, is able to block the airway responses to inhaled SP or NKA.

The peptide NK_1 receptor antagonist FK 888 has been studied in nine subjects with exercise-induced asthma (191). Pretreatment with a single dose (2.5 mg) of inhaled FK 888 did not affect baseline lung function. Although no protection could be shown against the exercise-induced maximal fall in lung function, FK 888 significantly reduced the time to recovery after exercise-induced bronchoconstriction (191). The observations from this study suggest that NK_1 receptor–mediated mechanisms may be involved in exercise-induced airway narrowing, at least during the recovery phase.

The effect of the nonpeptide tachykinin NK_2 receptor antagonist SR 48968 (saredutant) on neurokinin A–induced bronchoconstriction was studied in 12 asthmatic subjects (192). Pretreatment with SR 48968 (100 mg orally) significantly inhibited NKA-induced bronchoconstriction, causing a mean threefold rightward shift of the dose-response curve.

VII. Conclusions

1. Tachykinins are present in neurons and inflammatory cells within the airways. They may be released from the airways by stimuli such as ozone and allergen.

2. Tachykinins cause contraction of human airway smooth muscle both in vitro and in vivo. NKA and SP induce bronchoconstriction in humans, asthmatic patients being more sensitive than normal subjects. The bronchoconstrictor effect

Table 3 Proposed Models to Evaluate the Activity of Tachykinin Receptor Antagonists in Asthma

Experimental models	Airway effects of inhaled tachykinins, e.g., NKA or SP
Clinical models	Exercise-induced bronchoconstriction
(acute effects)	Hypertonic saline-induced bronchoconstriction
	Hyperventilation-induced bronchoconstriction
	Cold air challenge
	Allergen-induced bronchoconstriction
Chronic disease	As monotherapy (mild disease)
(long-term effects)	Steroid-sparing effect in moderate disease
	Cotherapy in severe disease

of these neuropeptides is in part indirect. The exact mechanism by which they cause bronchoconstriction is still unknown. Tachykinin NK_2 receptors are present on smooth muscle of both large and small airways. They mediate a major part of the bronchoconstrictor effect of tachykinins. Tachykinin NK_1 receptors are localized in smooth muscle of small airways and are responsible for a transient, low-intensity contraction subject to rapid desensitization.

3. NK_2 receptor antagonists protect against tachykinin-induced bronchoconstriction.

4. The effect of tachykinins is, however, not limited to airway smooth muscle contraction, which is only one component of airway obstruction. Tachykinins are involved, at least in animal models, in neurogenic inflammation (vasodilatation, plasma extravasation), as well as in airway hypersecretion, regulation of neural transmission, and attraction and activation of inflammatory cells. Many of these effects are mediated through the NK_1 receptor.

5. Thus the potential therapeutic effect of tachykinin receptor antagonists may not be restricted to inhibition of tachykinin-induced bronchoconstriction, and, conversely, inhibition of bronchoconstriction may not be predictive of the overall beneficial effect of tachykinin receptor antagonists in asthma. Obviously, more clinical studies are needed to evaluate the possible therapeutic role of this new class of compounds (Table 3).

Acknowledgments

We gratefully thank Mrs. C. Vandeven for typing the manuscript.

References

1. Lundberg JM, Saria A. Polypeptide-containing neurons in airway smooth muscle. Annu Rev Physiol 1987; 49:557–572.

2. Helke CJ, Krause JE, Mantyh PW, Couture R, Bannon MJ. Diversity in mammalian tachykinin peptidergic neurons: multiple peptides, receptors, and regulatory mechanisms. FASEB J 1990; 4:1606–1615.
3. Barnes PJ, Baraniuk JN, Belvisi MG. Neuropeptides in the respiratory tract: Part I. Am Rev Respir Dis 1991; 144:1187–1198.
4. Barnes PJ, Baraniuk JN, Belvisi MG. Neuropeptides in the respiratory tract: Part II. Am Rev Respir Dis 1991; 144:1391–1399.
5. Joos GF, Germonpré PR, Kips JC, Peleman RA, Pauwels RA. Sensory neuropeptides and the human lower airways: present state and future directions. Eur Respir J 1994; 7:1161–1171.
6. Ellis JL, Undem BJ. Pharmacology of non-adrenergic, non-cholinergic nerves in airway smooth muscle. Pulm Pharmacol 1994; 7:205–223.
7. Lundberg JM. Pharmacology of cotransmission in the autonomic nervous system: integrative aspects on amines, neuropeptides, adenosine triphosphate, amino acids and nitric oxide. Pharmacol Rev 1996; 48:113–178.
8. Maggi CA, Giachetti A, Dey RD, Said SI. Neuropeptides as regulators of airway function: vasoactive intestinal peptide and the tachykinins. Physiol Rev 1995; 75: 277–322.
9. Advenier C, Lagente V, Boichot E. The role of tachykinin receptor antagonists in the prevention of bronchial hyperresponsiveness, airway inflammation and cough. Eur Respir J 1997; 10:1892–1906.
10. Nadel JA. Neutral endopeptidase modulates neurogenic inflammation. Eur Respir J 1991; 4:745–754.
11. Baraniuk JN, Ohkubo K, Kwon OJ, Maj J, Ali M, Davies R, Twort C, Kaliner M, Letarte M, Barnes PJ. Localization of neutral endopeptidase (NEP) mRNA in human bronchi. Eur Respir J 1995; 8:1458–1464.
12. Sont JK, van Krieken JHJM, van Klink HCJ, Roldaan AC, Apap CR, Willems LNA, Sterk PH. Enhanced expression of neutral endopeptidase (NEP) in airway epithelium in biopsies from steroid-versus nonsteroid-treated patients with atopic asthma. Am J Respir Cell Mol Biol 1997; 16:549–556.
13. Regoli D, Bourdon A, Fauchère J-L. Receptors and antagonists for substance P and related peptides. Pharmacol Rev 1994; 46:551–599.
14. Lundberg JM, Hökfelt T, Martling C-R, Saria A, Cuello C. Substance P immunoreactive sensory nerves in the lower respiratory tract of various mammals including man. Cell Tissue Res 1984; 235:251–261.
15. Martling C-R, Theodorsson-Norheim E, Lundberg JM. Occurrence and effects of multiple tachykinins; substance P, neurokinin A and neuropeptide K in human lower airways. Life Sci 1987; 40:1633–1643.
16. Luts A, Uddman R, Alm P, Basterna J, Sundler F. Peptide-containing nerve fibers in human airways: distribution and coexistence pattern. Int Arch Allergy Immunol 1993; 101:52–60.
17. Ollerenshaw SL, Jarvis D, Sullivan CE, Woolcock AJ. Substance P immunoreactive nerves in airways from asthmatics and nonasthmatics. Eur Respir J 1991; 4: 673–682.
18. Howarth PH, Springall DR, Redington AE, Djukanovic R, Holgate ST, Polak JM. Neuropeptide-containing nerves in endobronchial biopsies from asthmatic and nonasthmatic subjects. Am J Respir Cell Mol Biol 1995; 13:288–296.

19. Lilly CM, Bai TR, Shore SA, Hall AE, Drazen JM. Neuropeptide content of lungs from asthmatic and nonasthmatic patients. Am J Respir Crit Care Med 1995; 151: 548–553.
20. Cardell LO, Uddman R, Edvinsson L. Low plasma concentrations of VIP and elevated levels of other neuropeptides during exacerbations of asthma. Eur Respir J 1994; 7:2169–2173.
21. Hazbun ME, Hamilton R, Holian A, Eschenbacher WL. Ozone-induced increases in substance P and 8-Epi-Prostaglandin $F_{2\alpha}$ in the airways of human subjects. Am J Respir Cell Mol Biol 1993; 9:568–572.
22. Nieber K, Baumgarten CR, Rathsack R, Furkert J, Oehme P, Kunkel G. Substance P and β-endorphin-like immunoreactivity in lavage fluid of subjects with and without allergic asthma. J Allergy Clin Immunol 1992; 90:646–652.
23. Mosimann BL, White MV, Hohman RJ, Goldrich MS, Kaulbach HC, Kaliner MA. Substance P, calcitonin-gene related peptide, and vasoactive intestinal peptide increase in nasal secretions after allergen challenge in atopic patients. J Allergy Clin Immunol 1993; 92:95–104.
24. Tomaki M, Ichinose M, Miura M, Hirayama Y, Yamauchi H, Nakajima N, Shirato K. Elevated substance P content in induced sputum from patients with asthma and patients with chronic bronchitis. Am J Respir Crit Care Med 1995; 151:613–617.
25. Hislop AA, Wharton J, Allen KM, Polak JM, Haworth S. Immuno-histochemical localization of peptide-containing nerves in human airways: age-related changes. Am J Respir Cell Mol Biol 1990; 3:191–198.
26. Springall DR, Polak JM, Howard L, Power RF, Krausz T, Manickam S, Banner NR, Khagani A, Rose M, Yacoub MH. Persistence of intrinsic neurones and possible phenotypic changes after extrinsic denervation of human respiratory tract by heart-lung transplantation. Am Rev Respir Dis 1990; 141:1538–1546.
27. Adcock IM, Peters M, Gelder C, Shirasaki H, Brown CR, Barnes PJ. Increased tachykinin receptor gene expression in asthmatic lung and its modulation by steroids. J Mol Endocrinol 1993; 11:1–7.
28. Bai TR, Zhou D, Weir T, Walker B, Hegele R, Hayashi S, McKay K, Bondy GP, Fong T. Substance P (NK1) and neurokinin A (NK2) receptor gene expression in inflammatory diseases. Am J Physiol 1995; 269:L309–L317.
29. Maggi CA. The effects of tachykinins on inflammatory and immune cells. Regul Peptides 1997; 70:75–90.
30. Aliakbar J, Sreedharan SP, Turck CW, Goetzl EJ. Selective localization of vasoactive intestinal peptide and substance P in human eosinophils. Biochem Biophys Res Commun 1987; 148:1440–1445.
31. Metwali A, Blum AM, Ferraris L, Klein JS, Fiocchi C, Weinstock JV. Eosinophils within the healthy or inflamed human intestine produce substance P and vasoactive intestinal peptide. J Neuroimmunol 1994; 52:69–78.
32. Germonpré PR, Joos GF, Bullock GR, Pauwels RA. Expression of substance P and its receptor by human sputum macrophages. Am J Respir Crit Care Med 1997; 155:A821.
33. Killingsworth CR, Shore SA, Alessandrini F, Dey RD, Paulauskis JD. Rat alveolar macrophages express preprotachykinin gene-I mRNA-encoding tachykinins. Am J Physiol 1997; 273:L1073–L1081.

34. Lundberg JM, Martling C-R, Saria A. Substance P and capsaicin induced contraction of human bronchi. Acta Physiol Scand 1983; 119:49–53.
35. Finney MJB, Karlsson J-A, Persson CGA. Effects of bronchoconstrictors and bronchodilators on a novel human small airway preparation. Br J Pharmacol 1985; 85: 29–36.
36. Martling C-R, Theodorsson-Norheim E, Lundberg JM. Occurrence and effects of multiple tachykinins; substance P, neurokinin A and neuropeptide K in human lower airways. Life Sci 1987; 40: 1633–1643.
37. Advenier C, Naline E, Drapeau G, Regoli D. Relative potencies of neurokinins in guinea pig trachea and human bronchus. Eur J Pharmacol 1987; 139:133–137.
38. Naline E, Devillier P, Drapeau G, Toty L, Bakdach H, Regoli D, Advenier C. Characterization of neurokinin effects and receptors in human isolated bronchi. Am Rev Respir Dis 1989; 140:679–686.
39. Naline E, Molimard M, Regoli D, Edmonds-Alt X, Advenier A. Evidence for functional tachykinin NK_1 receptors on human isolated small bronchi. Am J Physiol (Lung Cell Mol Physiol 15) 1996; 271:L763–L767.
40. Advenier C, Naline E, Toty L, Bakdach H, Edmonds-Alt X, Vilain P, Brelière J-C, Le Fur G. Effects on the isolated human bronchus of SR 48968, a potent and selective nonpeptide antagonist of the neurokinin A (NK_2) receptors. Am Rev Respir Dis 1992; 146:1171–1181.
41. Ben-Jebria A, Marthan R, Rossetti M, Savineau J-P. Effect of passive sensitization on the mechanical activity of human isolated bronchial smooth muscle induced by substance P, neurokinin A and VIP. Br J Pharmacol 1993; 109:131–136.
42. Naline E, Barchasz E, Molimard M, Moreau J, Emonds-Alt X, Advenier C. Interleukin-1β induces and hyperresponsiveness of human isolated bronchi to (Sar^9, Met $(02)^{11}$) substance P, a tachykinin NK_1 receptor agonist (abstr). Am J Respir Crit Care Med 1998; 157:A490.
43. Björck T, Gustafsson LE, Dahlen S-E. Isolated bronchi from asthmatics are hyperresponsive to adenosine, which apparently acts indirectly by liberation of leukotrienes and histamine. Am Rev Respir Dis 1992; 145:1087–1091.
44. Fuller RW, Maxwell DL, Dixon CMS, McGregor GP, Barnes VF, Bloom SR, Barnes PJ. Effect of substance P on cardiovascular and respiratory function in subjects. J Appl Physiol 1987; 62:1473–1479.
45. Evans TW, Dixon CM, Clarke B, Conradson T-B, Barnes PJ. Comparison of neurokinin A and substance P on cardiovascular and airway function in man. Br J Clin Pharmacol 1988; 25:273–275.
46. Joos G, Pauwels R, Van Der Straeten M. The effect of inhaled substance P and neurokinin A on the airways of normal and asthmatic subjects. Thorax 1987; 42: 779–783.
47. Joos GF. The role of sensory neuropeptides in the pathogenesis of asthma. Clin Exp Allergy 1989; 19 (suppl 1):9–13.
48. Joos GF, Van Schoor J, Kips JC, Pauwels RA. The effect of inhaled FK224, a tachykinin NK_1 and NK_2 receptor antagonist on neurokinin A induced bronchoconstriction in asthmatics. Am J Respir Crit Care Med 1996: 153:1781–1784.
49. Crimi N, Palermo F, Oliveri R, Palermo B, Vancheri C, Polosa R, Mistretta A.

Effect of nedocromil on bronchospasm induced by inhalation of substance P in asthmatic subjects. Clin Allergy 1988; 18:375–382.
50. Cheung D, Van Der Veen H, Den Hartigh J, Dijkman JH, Sterk PJ. Effects of inhaled substance P on airway responsiveness to methacholine in asthmatic subjects in vivo. J Appl Physiol 1994; 77:1325–1332.
51. Nakai J, Iikura Y, Akimoto K, Shiraki K. Substance P-induced cutaneous and bronchial reactions in children with bronchial asthma. Ann Allergy 1991; 66:155–161.
52. Cheung D, Bel EH, Den Hartigh J, Dijkman JH, Sterk PJ. The effect of an inhaled neutral endopeptidase inhibitor, thiorphan, on airway responses to neurokinin A in normal humans in vivo. Am Rev Respir Dis 1992; 145:1275–1280.
53. Cheung D, Timmers MC, Zwinderman AH, den Hartigh J, Dijkman JH, Sterk PJ. Neutral endopeptidase activity and airway hyperresponsiveness to neurokinin A in asthmatic subjects in vivo. Am Rev Respir Dis 1993; 148: 1467–1473.
54. Joos GF, Pauwels RA, Van Der Straeten ME. The mechanism of tachykinin-induced bronchoconstriction in the rat. Am Rev Respir Dis 1988; 137:1038–1044.
55. Joos G, Pauwels R. The in vivo effect of tachykinins on airway mast cells of the rat. Am Rev Respir Dis 1993; 148:922–926.
56. Joos G, Pauwels R, Van Der Straeten M. The effect of nedocromil sodium on the bronchoconstrictor effect of neurokinin A in asthmatics. J Allergy Clin Immunol 1989; 83:663–668.
57. Joos GF, Pauwels RA, Van Der Straeten ME. The effect of oxitropium bromide on neurokinin A–induced bronchoconstriction in asthmatics. Pulm Pharmacol 1988; 1: 41–45.
58. Crimi N, Palermo F, Oliveri R, Palermo B, Vancheri C, Polosa R, Mistretta A. Influence of antihistamine (astemizole) and anticholinergic drugs (ipratropium bromide) on bronchoconstriction induced by substance P. Ann Allergy 1990; 65:115–120.
59. Tanaka DT, Grunstein MM. Mechanisms of substance P induced contraction of rabbit airway smooth muscle. J Appl Physiol 1984; 57:1551–1557.
60. Hall AK, Barnes PJ, Meldrum LA, Maclagan J. Facilitation by tachykinins of neurotransmission in guinea-pig pulmonary parasympathetic nerves. Br J Pharmacol 1989; 97:274–280.
61. Black JL, Johnson PRA, Alouan L, Armour CL. Neurokinin A with K^+ channel blockade potentiates contraction to electrical stimulation in human bronchus. Eur J Pharmacol 1990; 180:311–317.
62. Fewtrell CMS, Foreman JC, Jordan CC, Oehme P, Renner H, Stewart JM. The effects of substance P on histamine and 5-hydroxytryptamine release in the rat. J Physiol 1982; 330:393–411.
63. Ali H, Leung KBP, Pearce FL, Hayes A, Foreman JC. Comparison of the histamine releasing action of substance P on mast cells and basophils from different species and tissues. Int Arch Allergy Appl Immunol 1983; 79:121–124.
64. Joos GF, Lefebvre RA, Bullock GR, Pauwels RA. Role of 5-hydroxytryptamine and mast cells in the tachykinin-induced contraction of rat trachea in vitro. Eur J Pharmacol 1997; 338:259–268.
65. Heaney LG, Cross LJM, Stanford CF, Ennis M. Substance P induces histamine release from human pulmonary mast cells. Clin Exp Allergy 1995; 25:179–186.

66. Schierhorn K, Brunnée T, Schultz K-D, Jahnke V, Kunkel G. Substance-P-induced histamine release from human nasal mucosa in vitro. Int Arch Allergy Immunol 1995; 107:109–114.
67. Crimi N, Oliveri R, Polosa R, Palermo F, Mistretta A. The effect of oral terfenadine on neurokinin–A induced bronchoconstriction. J Allergy Clin Immunol 1993; 91: 1096–1098.
68. Stead RH, Tomioka M, Quinonez G, Sinon GT, Felten SY, Bienenstock J. Intestinal mucosal mast cells in normal and nematode-infected rat intestines are in intimate contact with peptidergic nerves. Proc Natl Acad Sci USA 1987; 84:2975–2979.
69. Nilsson G, Alving K, Ahlstedt S, Hökfelt T, Lundberg JM. Peptidergic innervation of rat lymphoid tissue and lung: Relation to mast cells and sensitivity to capsaicin and immunization. Cell Tissue Res 1990; 282:125–133.
70. Snider RM, Constantine JQ, Lowe JA. III, Longo KP, Lebel WS, Woody HA, Drozda SE, Desai MC, Vinick FJ, Spencer RW, Hess HJ. A potent nonpeptide antagonist of the substance P (NK-1) receptors. Science (Wash DC) 1991; 251: 435–437.
71. McLean S, Ganong A, Seymour PA, Snider RM, Desai JC, Rosen T, Bryce DK, Longo KP, Reynolds LS, Robinson G, Schmidt AW, Siok C, Heym J. Pharmacology of CP 99994: a nonpeptide antagonist of the tachykinin NK-1 receptor. Regul Pept 1993; 46:120.
72. Garret C, Carruette A, Fardin V, Moussaoui S, Peyronel JF, Blanchard JC, Laduron PM. Pharmacological properties of a potent and selective nonpeptide substance P antagonist. Proc Natl Acad Sci USA 1991; 88:10208–10212.
73. Emonds-Alt X, Doutremepuich J-D, Heaulme M, Neliat G, Santucci V, Steinberg R, Vilain P, Bichon D, Ducoux J-P, Proietto V, Van Broeck D, Soubrié P, Le Fur G, Brelière J-C. In vitro and in vivo biological activities of SR140333, a novel potent non-peptide tachykinin NK_1 receptor antagonist. Eur J Pharmacol 1993; 250: 403–413.
74. Emonds-Alt X, Vilain P, Goulaouic P, Proietto V, Van Broeck D, Advenier C, Naline E, Neliat G, Brelière J-C, Le Fur G. A potent and selective non-peptide antagonist of the neurokinin A (NK_2) receptor. Life Sci 1992; 50:PL101–PL106.
75. Beresford IJM, Sheldrick RLG, Ball DI, Turpin MP, Walsh DM, Hawcock AB, Coleman RA, Hagan RM, Tyers MB. GR 159897, a potent non-peptide antagonist at tachykinin NK_2 receptors. Eur J Pharmacol 1995; 272:241–248.
76. Emonds-Alt X, Bichon D, Ducoux J-P, Heaulme M, Miloux B, Poncelet M, Proietto V, Van Broeck D, Vilain P, Neliat G, Soubrié P, Le Fur G, Brelière J-CG. SR 142801, the first potent non-peptide antagonist of the tachykinin NK_3 receptor. Life Sci 1995; 56:PL27–PL32.
77. Maggi CA, Astolfi M, Giuliani S, Goso C, Manzini S, Meini S, Patacchini R, Pavone V, Pedone C, Quartara L, Renzetti AR, Giachetti A. MEN 10,627, a novel polycyclic peptide antagonist of tachykinin NK_2 receptors. J Pharmacol Exp Ther 1994; 271:1495–1500.
73. Maggi CA, Patacchini R, Rovero P, Giachetti A. Tachykinin receptors and tachykinin receptor antagonists. J Auton Pharmacol 1993; 13:23–93.
74. Wu L-H, Vartanian MA, Oxender DL, Chung F-Z. Identification of methionine 314 and alanine 146 in the second transmembrane segment of the human tachykinin

NK_3 receptor as residues involved in species-selective binding to SR 48968. Biochem Biophys Res Commun 1994; 198:961–966.

75. Maggi CA, Patacchini R, Meini S, Giuliani S. Evidence for the presence of a septide-sensitive tachykinin receptor in the circular smooth muscle of the guinea pig ileum. Eur J Pharmacol 1993; 235:309–311.
76. Zeng X-P, Lavielle S, Burcher E. Evidence for tachykinin NK-2 receptors in guinea-pig airways from binding and functional studies, using [^{125}I]-[Lys^5,Tyr(I$_2$)^7, MeLeu^9, Nle^{10}]-NKA(4–10). Neuropeptides 1994; 26:1–9.
77. Zeng X-P, Burcher E. Use of selective antagonists for further characterization of tachykinin NK-2, NK-1 and possible ''septide-selective'' receptors in guinea pig bronchus. J Pharmacol Exp Ther 1994; 270:1295–1300.
78. Emonds-Alt X, Advenier C, Cognon C, Croci T, Daoui S, Ducoux JP, Landi M, Naline E, Neliat G, Poncelet M, Proietto V, Van Broeck D, Vilain P, Manara L, Soubrié P, Le Fur G, Maffrand JP, Brelière JC. Biochemical and pharmacological activities of SR 144190, a new potent nonpeptide tachykinin NK_2 receptor antagonist. Neuropeptides 1997; 31:449–458.
79. Catalioto R-M, Criscuoli M, Cucchi P, Giachetti A, Giannotti D, Giuliani DS, Lecci A, Lippi A, Patacchini R, Quartara L, Renzetti AR, Tramontana M, Arcamone F, Maggi CA. MEN 11420 (Nepadutant), a novel glycosylated bicyclic peptide tachykinin NK_2 receptor antagonist. Br J Pharmacol 1998; 123:81–96.
80. Maggi CA, Patacchini R, Rovero P, Giachetti A. Tachykinin receptors and tachykinin receptor antagonists. J Auton Pharmacol 1993; 13:23–93.
81. Wu L-H, Vartanian MA, Oxender DL, Chung F-Z. Identification of methionine 314 and alanine 146 in the second transmembrane segment of the human tachykinin NK3 receptor as residues involved in species-selective binding to SR 48968. Biochem Biophys Res Commun 1994; 198:961–966.
82. Maggi CA, Patacchini R, Meini S, Giuliani S. Evidence for the presence of a septide-sensitive tachykinin receptor in the circular smooth muscle of the guinea pig ileum. Eur J Pharmacol 1993; 235:309–311.
83. Zeng X-P, Lavielle S, Burcher E. Evidence for tachykinin NK-2 receptors in guinea-pigs airways from binding and functional studies, using [^{125}I]-[Lys^5, Tyr(I$_2$)^7, MeLeu^9, Nle^{10}]-NKA(4–10). Neuropeptides 1994; 26:1–9.
84. Zeng X-P, Burcher E. Use of selective antagonists for further characterization of tachykinin NK-2, NK-1 and possible ''septide-selective'' receptors in guinea pig bronchus. J. Pharmacol Exp Ther 1994; 270:1295–1300.
85. Maggi CA, Schwartz TW. The dual nature of the tachykinin NK_1 receptor. TiPS 1997; 18:351–355.
86. Gether U, Johansen TE, Snider RM, Lowe III JA, Emonds-Alt X, Yokota Y, Nakanishi S, Schwartz T. Binding epitopes for peptide and non-peptide ligands on the NK_1 (substance P) receptor. Regul Pept 1993; 49:49–58.
87. Gether U, Yokota Y, Emonds-Alt X, Brelière J-C, Lowe III, JA, Snider RM, Nakanishi S, Schwartz T. Two nonpeptide tachykinin antagonists act through epitopes on corresponding segments of the NK_1 and NK_2 receptors. Proc Natl Acad Sci USA 1993; 90:6194–6198.
88. Advenier C, Rouissi N, Nguyen QT, Emonds-Alt X, Brelière J-C, Neliat G, Naline

E, Regoli D. Neurokinin A (NK_2) receptor revisited with SR 48968, a potent nonpeptide antagonist. Biochem Bioph Res Commun 1992; 184:1418–1424.

89. Maggi CA, Astolfi M, Giuliani S, Goso C, Manzini S, Meini S, Patacchini R, Pavone V, Pedone C, Quartara L, Renzetti AR, Giachetti A. MEN 10,267, a novel polycyclic peptide antagonist of tachykinin NK_2 receptors. J Pharmacol Exp Ther 1994; 271:1489–1500.
90. Martin CAE, Naline E, Emonds-Alt X, Advenier C. Influence of (±)-CP-96,345 and SR 48968 on electrical field stimulation of the isolated guinea-pig main bronchus. Eur J Pharmacol 1992; 224:137–143.
91. Lou Y-P, Lee L-Y, Satoh H, Lundberg JM. Postjunctional inhibitory effect of the NK_2 receptor antagonist, SR 48968, on sensory NANC bronchoconstriction in the guinea-pig. Br J Pharmacol 1993; 109:765–773.
92. Maggi CA, Patacchini R, Rovero P, Santicioli P. Tachykinin receptors and noncholinergic bronchoconstriction in the guinea-pig isolated bronchi. Am Rev Respir Dis 1991; 144:363–387.
93. Bertrand C, Nadel JA, Graf PD, Geppetti G. Capsaicin increases airflow resistance in guinea pigs in vivo by activating both NK_2 and NK_1 tachykinin receptors. Am Rev Respir Dis 1993; 148:909–914.
94. Lilly CM, Besson G, Israel E, Rodger IW, Drazen JM. Capsaicin-induced airway obstruction in tracheally perfused guinea pig lung. Am J Respir Crit Care Med 1994; 49:1175–1179.
95. Ellis JL, Undem BJ. Inhibition by capsazepine of resiniferatoxin- and capsaicin-induced contractions of guinea pig trachea. J Pharmacol Exp Ther 1994; 268:85–89.
96. Foulon DM, Champion E, Masson P, Rodger IA, Jones TR. NK_1 and NK_2 receptors mediate tachykinin and resiniferatoxin-induced bronchospasm in guinea pigs. Am Rev Respir Dis 1993; 148:915–921.
97. Satoh H, Lou Y-P, Lundberg JM. Inhibitory effects of capsazepine and SR 48968 on citric acid–induced bronchoconstriction in guinea-pigs. Eur J Pharmacol 1993; 236:367–372.
98. Buckner CK, Liberati N, Dea D, Lengel D, Stinson-Fisher C, Campbell J, Miller S, Shenvi A, Krell RD. Differential blockade by tachykinin NK_1 and NK_2 receptor antagonists of bronchoconstriction induced by direct-acting agonists and the indirect-acting mimetics capsaicin, serotonin and 2-methyl-serotonin in the anesthetized guinea pig. J Pharmacol Exp Ther 1993; 267:1168–1175.
99. Sakamato T, Tsukagoshi H, Barnes PJ, Chung KF. Involvement of tachykinin receptors (NK_1 and NK_2) in sodium metabisulfite-induced airway effects. Am J Respir Crit Care Med 1994; 149:387–391.
100. Vilain P, Emonds-Alt X, Advenier C, Brelière J-C. Involvement of tachykinins in the bronchospasm induced by diethyl ether in the guinea-pig: inhibition by SR 48968 (abstr). Am J Respir Crit Care Med 1994; 149:A475.
101. Solway J, Kao BM, Jordan JE, Gitter B, Rodger IW, Howbert J, Alger LE, Necheles J, Leff AR, Garland A. Tachykinin receptor antagonists inhibit hyperpnea-induced bronchoconstriction in guinea pigs. J Clin Invest 1993; 92:315–323.
102. McKee KT, Millar L, Rodger IW, Metters KM. Identification of both NK_1 and NK_2 receptors in guinea-pig airways. Br J Pharmacol 1993; 110:693–700.

103. Maggi CA, Patacchini R, Giuliani S, Giachetti A. In vivo and in vitro pharmacology of SR 48968, a non-peptide tachykinin NK_2 receptor antagonist. Eur J Pharmacol 1993; 234:83–90.
104. Joos GF, Kips JC, Pauwels RA. In vivo characterization of the tachykinin receptors involved in the direct and indirect bronchoconstrictor effect of tachykinins in the rat. Am J Respir Crit Care Med 1994; 149:1160–1166.
105. Joos GF, Lefebvre RA, Kips JC, Pauwels RA. Tachykinins contract trachea from Fisher 344 rats by interaction with a NK_1 receptor. Eur J Pharmacol 1994; 271: 47–54.
106. Hirayama Y, Lei Y-H, Barnes PJ, Rogers DF. Effects of two novel tachykinin antagonists, FK 224 and FK 888, on neurogenic airway plasma exudation, bronchoconstriction and systemic hypotension in guinea pigs. Br J Pharmacol 1993; 108: 844–851.
107. Joos GF, Kips JC, Lefebvre R, Pauwels RA. The effect of FK 224, a NK_1 and NK_2 antagonist, on the in vivo and in vitro airway effects of neurokinin A in the rat (abstr). Eur Respir J 1993; 6:264s.
108. Ellis JL, Sham JSK, Undem BJ. Tachykinin-independent effects of capsaicin on smooth muscle in human isolated bronchi. Am J Respir Crit Care Med 1997; 155: 751–755.
109. Qian Y, Advenier C, Naline E, Bellamy JF, Emonds-Alt X. Effects of SR 48968 on the neuropeptide gamma-induced contraction of the human isolated bronchus. Fundam Clin Pharmacol 1994; 8:71–75.
110. Ball DI, Beresford IJM, Wren GPA, Pendry YD, Sheldrick RLG, Walsh DM, Turpin MP, Hagan RM, Coleman RA. In vitro and in vivo pharmacology of the non-peptide antagonist at tachykinin NK_2-receptors, GR 459897. Br J Pharmacol 1994; 112:48P.
111. Molimard M, Martin CAE, Naline E, Hirsch A, Advenier C. Contractile effects of bradykinin on the isolated human small bronchus. Am J Respir Crit Care Med 1994; 149:123–127.
112. Ellis JL, Undem BJ, Kays JS, Ghanekar SV, Barthlow HG, Buckner CK. Pharmacological examination of receptors mediating contractile responses to tachykinins in airways isolated from human, guinea pig and hamster. J Pharmacol Exp Ther 1993; 267:95–101.
113. Astolfi M, Treppiari S, Giachetti A, Merini S, Maggi CA, Manzini S. Characterization of the tachykinin NK_2 receptor in the human bronchus: influence of amastatin-sensitive metabolic pathway. Br J Pharmacol 1994; 111:570–574.
114. Bertrand C, Geppetti P, Graf PD, Foresi A, Nadel JA. Involvement of neurogenic inflammation in antigen-induced bronchoconstriction in guinea pigs. Am J Physiol 1993; 265 (Lung Cell Mol Physiol 9):L507–L511.
115. Evangelista S, Ballati J, Perretti F. MEN 10,627, a new selective NK_2 receptor antagonist, inhibits antigen-induced bronchoconstriction in sensitized guinea-pigs. Neuropeptides 1994; 26(suppl 1):39–40.
116. Diamant Z, van der Veen H, Kuijpers EAP, Bakker PF, Sterk PJ. The effect of inhaled thiorphan on allergen-induced airway responses in asthmatic subjects. Clin Exp Allergy 1996; 26:525–532.
117. Lei H-Y, Barnes PJ, Rogers DF. Inhibition of neurogenic plasma exudation in

guinea-pig airways by CP-96,345, a new non-peptide NK_1 receptor antagonist. Br J Pharmacol 1992; 105:261–262.

118. Germonpré PR, Joos GF, Everaert E, Kips JC, Pauwels RA. Characterization of neurogenic inflammation in the airways of two highly inbred rat strains. Am J Respir Crit Care Med 1995; 152:1796–1804.
119. Sakamoto T, Barnes PJ, Chung KF. Effect of CP-96,345, a non-peptide NK_1 receptor antagonist, against substance P-, bradykinin- and allergen-induced airway microvascular leakage and bronchoconstriction in the guinea pig. Eur J Pharmacol 1993; 231:31–38.
120. Qian Y, Emonds-Alt X, Advenier C. Effects of capsaicin, (±)-CP-96,345 and SR 48968 on the bradykinin-induced airways microvascular leakage in guinea-pigs. Pulm Pharmacol 1993; 6:63–67.
121. Piedimonte G, Bertrand C, Geppetti P, Snider RM, Desai MC, Nadel JA. A new NK_1 receptor antagonist (CP-99,994) prevents the increase in tracheal vascular permeability produced by hypertonic saline. J Pharmacol Exp Ther 1993; 266:270–273.
122. Bertrand C, Geppetti P, Baker J, Yamawaki I, Nadel JA. Antigen-induced vascular extravasation in guinea pig trachea. J Immunol 1993; 150:1479–1485.
123. Tousignant C, Chan C-C, Guevremont D, Brideau C, Hale JJ, MacCoss M, Rodger IW. NK_2 receptors mediate plasma extravasation in guinea-pig lower airways. Br J Pharmacol 1993; 108:383–386.
124. Savoie C, Tousignant C, Rodger IW, Chan CC. Involvement of NK_1 and NK_2 receptors in pulmonary responses elicited by non-adrenergic, non-cholinergic vagal stimulation in guinea pigs. J Pharm Pharmacol 1995; 47:914–920.
125. Boichot E, Biyah K, Germain N, Emonds-Alt X, Lagente V, Advenier C. Involvement of tachykinin NK_1 and NK_2 receptors in substance P–induced microvascular leakage hypersensitivity and airway hyperresponsiveness in guinea-pigs. Eur Respir J 1996; 9:1445–1450.
126. Biyah K, Molimard M, Emonds-Alt X, Advenier C. SR 140333 prevents potentiation by citric acid of plasma exudation induced by histamine in airways. Eur J Pharmacol 1996; 308:325–328.
127. Ramnarine SI, Rogers DF. Non-adrenergic, non-cholinergic neural control of mucus secretion in the airways. Pulm Pharmacol 1994; 7:19–33.
128. Rogers DF. Neurokinin receptors subserving airways secretion. Can J Physiol Pharmacol 1995; 73:932–939.
129. Kroegel C, Giembycz MA, Barnes PJ. Characterization of eosinophil cell activation by peptides: Differential effects of substance P, mellitin and f-met-leu-phe. J Immunol 1990; 145:2581–2587.
130. Ruff MR, Wahl SM, Pert CB. Substance P receptor-mediated chemotaxis of human monocytes. Peptides 1985; 6:107–111.
131. Marasco WA, Showell JH, Becker EL. Substance P binds to the formyl-peptide chemotaxis receptor on the rabbit neutrophil. Biochem Biophys Res Commun 1981; 99:1065–1072.
132. Rabier M, Damon M, Chanez P, Mencia-Huerta JM, Braquet P, Bousquet J, Michel FB, Godard P. Neutrophil chemotactic activity of PAF, histamine and neuromediators in bronchial asthma. J Lipid Med 1991; 4:265–275.

133. Perretti M, Ahluwalia A, Flower RJ, Manzini S. Endogenous tachykinins play a role in IL-1 induced neutrophil accumulation: Involvement of NK-1 receptors. Immunology 1993; 80:73–77.
134. Payan DG, Goetzl EJ. Substance P receptor–dependent responses of leukocytes in pulmonary inflammation. Am Rev Respir Dis 1987; 136:S39–S46.
135. Payan DG, Levine JD, Goetzl EJ. Modulation of immunity and hypersensitivity by sensory neuropeptides. J Immunol 1984; 132:1601–1604.
136. Laurenzi MA, Persson MA, Dalsgaard CJ, Ringden O. Stimulation of B-lymphocyte differentiation by the neuropeptide substance P and neurokinin A. Scand J Immunol 1989; 30:695–701.
137. Harrison NK, Dawes KF, Kwon OJ, Barnes PJ, Laurent GJ, Chung KF. Effects of neuropeptides on human lung fibroblast proliferation and chemotaxis. Am J Physiol 1995; 268:L278–L283.
138. Lotz M, Vauthan JH, Carson DA. Effect of neuropeptides on production of inflammatory cytokines by human monocytes. Science 1988; 241:1218–1221.
139. Serra MC, Calzetti F, Ceska M, Cassatella MA. Effect of substance P on superoxide anion and IL-8 production by human PMNL. Immunology 1994; 82:63–69.
140. Calvo CF, Chavanel G, Senik A. Substance P enhances IL-2 expression in activated human T-cells. J Immunol 1992; 148:3498–3504.
141. Garland A, Necheles J, White SR, Neeley SP, Leff AR, Carson SS, Alger LE, Mc Allister K, Solway J. Activated eosinophils elicit substance P release from cultured dorsal root ganglion neurons. Am J Physiol 1997; 273:L1096–L1102.
142. Baluk P, Bertrand C, Geppetti P, McDonald D, Nadel JA. NK_1 receptors mediate leukocyte adhesion in neurogenic inflammation in the rat trachea. Am J Physiol 1995; 268:L263–L269.
143. Kaltreider HB, Ichikawa S, Byrd PK, Ingram DA, Kishiyama JL, Sreedharan SP, Warnock ML, Beck JM, Goetzl E. Upregulation of neuropeptides and neuropeptide receptors in a murine model of immune inflammation in lung parenchyma. Am J Respir Cell Mol Biol 1997; 16:133–144.
144. Schuiling M, Zuidhof AB, Zaagsma J, Meurs H. Involvement of tachykinin NK_1 receptor in the development of allergen-induced airway hyperreactivity and airway inflammation in conscious unrestrained guinea pigs. Am J Respir Crit Care Med 1999; 159:423–430.
145. Herd CM, Gozzard N, Page CP. Capsaicin pretreatment prevents the development of antigen-induced airway hyperresponsiveness in neonatally immunised rabbits. Eur J Pharmacol 1995; 282:111–119.
146. Turner CR, Andresen CJ, Patterson DK, Keir RF, Obach S, Lee P, Watson JW. Dual antagonism of NK_1 and NK_2 receptors by CP 99,994 and SR 48968 prevents airway hyperresponsiveness in primates (abstr). Am J Respir Crit Care Med 1996; 153:A160.
147. Boichot E, Lagente V, Paubert-Braquet M, Frossard N. Inhaled substance P induces activation of alveolar macrophages and increases airway responses in the guinea-pig. Neuropeptides 1993; 25:307–313.
148. Boichot E, Germain N, Emonds-Alt, Lagente V, Advenier C. Effects of the tachykinin NK_1 (SR 140333) and NK_2 (SR 48968) receptor antagonists on antigen and

substance P–induced activation of guinea-pig alveolar macrophages. Am J Respir Crit Care Med 1996; 153:A417.

149. Hartung HP, Toyka KV. Activation of macrophages by substance P: induction of oxidative burst and thromboxane release. Eur J Pharmacol 1983; 89:301–305.
150. Brunelleschi S, Vanni L, Ledda F, Giotti A, Maggi CA, Fantozzi R. Tachykinins activate guinea-pig alveolar macrophages: Involvement of NK_2 and NK_1 receptors. Br J Pharmacol 1990; 100:417–420.
151. D'Ortho MP, Jarreau PH, Delacourt C, Pezet S, Lafuma C, Harf A, Macquin-Mavier I. Tachykinins induce gelatinase production by guinea-pig alveolar macrophages: involvement of NK_2 receptors. Am J Physiol 1996; 269:L631–L636.
152. Pujol JL, Bousquet J, Grenier J, Michel F, Godard P, Chanez P, De Vos C, Crastes-de-Paulet A, Michel FB. Substance P activation of bronchoalveolar macrophages from asthmatic patients and normal subjects. Clin Exp Allergy 1989; 19:625–628.
153. Omini C, Brunelli G, Hernandez A, Daffonchio L. Bradykinin and substance P potentiate acetylcholine-induced bronchospasm in guinea pig. Eur J Pharmacol 1989; 163:195–197.
154. Umeno E, Hirose T, Nishima S. Pretreatment with aerosolized capsaicin potentiates histamine-induced bronchoconstriction in guinea pigs. Am Rev Respir Dis 1992; 146:159–162.
155. Boichot E, Lagente V, Paubert-Braquet M, Frossard N. Inhaled substance P induces activation of alveolar macrophages and increases airway responses in the guinea-pig. Neuropeptides 1993; 25:307–313.
156. Tamura G, Sakai K, Taniguchi Y. Neurokinin A-induced bronchial hyperresponsiveness to methacholine in Japanese monkeys. Tohoku J Exp Med 1989; 159:69–73.
157. Sheppard D, Scypinski L. A tachykinin receptor antagonist inhibits and an inhibitor of tachykinin metabolism potentiates toluene diisocyanate-induced airway hyperresponsiveness in guinea-pigs. Am Rev Respir Dis 1988; 138:547–551.
158. Hsiue, T-R, Garland A, Ray DW, Hershenson MB, Leff AR, Solway J. Endogenous sensory neuropeptide release enhances nonspecific airway responsiveness in guinea pigs. Am Rev Respir Dis 1992; 146:148–153.
159. Matsuse T, Thomson RJ, Chen X-R, Salari H, Schellenberg RR. Capsaicin inhibits airway hyperresponsiveness but not lipoxygenase activity or eosinophilia after repeated aerosolized antigen in guinea pigs. Am Rev Respir Dis 1991; 144:366–372.
160. Ladenius AR, Nijkamp FP. Capsaicin pretreatment of guinea pigs in vivo prevents ovalbumin-induced tracheal hyperreactivity in vitro. Eur J Pharmacol 1993; 235: 127–131.
161. Jarreau P-H, D'Ortho M-P, Boyer V, Harf A, Macquin-Mavier I. Effects of capsaicin on the airway responses to inhaled endotoxin in the guinea pig. Am J Respir Crit Care Med 1994; 149:128–133.
162. Perretti F, Manzini S. Activation of capsaicin-sensitive sensory fibers modulates PAF-induced bronchial hyperresponsiveness in anesthetized guinea pigs. Am Rev Respir Dis 1993; 148:927–931.
163. Koto H, Aizawa H, Takata, S, Inoue H, Hara N. An important role of tachykinins in ozone-induced airway hyperresponsiveness. Am Rev Respir Crit Care Med 1995; 151:1763–1769.

164. Buckley TL, Nijkamp FP. Airways hyperreactivity and cellular accumulation in a delayed-type hypersensitivity reaction in the mouse: modulation by capsaicin-sensitive Nerves. Am J Respir Crit Care Med 1994; 149:400–407.
165. Scheerens H, Buckley TL, Muis T, Van Loveren H, Nijkamp FP. The involvement of sensory neuropeptides in toluene diisocyanate-induced tracheal hyperreactivity in the mouse airways. Br J Pharmacol 1996; 119:1665–1671.
166. Herd CM, Gozzard N, Page CP. Capsaicin pretreatment prevents the development of antigen-induced airway hyperresponsiveness in neonatally immunised rabbits. Eur J Pharmacol 1995; 282:111–119.
167. Ellis JL, Undem BJ. Antigen-induced enhancement of noncholinergic contractile responses to vagus nerve and electrical field stimulation in guinea pig isolated trachea. J Pharmacol Exp Ther 1992; 262:646–653.
168. Boichot E, Germain N, Lagente V, Advenier C. Prevention by the tachykinin NK_2 receptor antagonist, SR 48968, of antigen-induced airway hyperresponsiveness in sensitized guinea-pigs. Br J Pharmacol 1995; 114:259–261.
169. Girard V, Yavo JC, Emonds-Alt X, Advenier C. The tachykinin NK_2 receptor antagonist SR 48968 inhibits citric acid-induced airway hyperresponsiveness in guinea pigs. Am J Resp Crit Care Med 1996; 153:1496–1502.
170. Boichot E, Biyah K, Germain N, Emonds-Alt X, Lagente V, Advenier C. Involvement of tachykinin NK_1 and NK_2 receptors in substance P–induced microvascular leakage hypersensitivity and airway hyperresponsiveness in guinea-pigs. Eur Respir J 1996; 9:1445–1450.
171. Kraneveld AD, Nijkamp FP, Van Oosterhout AJM. Role for neurokinin-2 receptor in interleukin-5–induced airway hyperresponsiveness but not eosinophilia in guinea-pigs. Am J Respir Crit Care Med 1997; 156:367–374.
172. Yoshihara S, Geppetti P, Linden A, Hara M, Chan B, Nadel JA. Tachykinins mediate the potentiation of antigen-induced bronchoconstriction by cold air in guinea-pigs. J Allergy Clin Immunol 1996; 97:756–760.
173. Perretti F, Ballati L, Manzini S, Maggi CA, Evangelista S. Antibronchospastic activity of MEN 10,627, a novel tachykinin NK_2 receptor antagonist, in guinea-pig airways. Eur J Pharmacol 1995; 273:129–135.
174. Tocker JE, Gertner SB, Welton AF, Selig WM. Vagal stimulation augments pulmonary anaphylaxis in the guinea-pig lung. Am J Respir Crit Care Med 1995; 151: 461–469.
175. Fischer A, McGregor GP, Saria A, Philippin B, Kummer W. Induction of tachykinin gene and peptide expression in guinea pig nodose primary afferent neurons by allergic airway inflammation. J Clin Invest 1996; 98:2284–2291.
176. Weinreich D, Moore KA, Taylor GE. Allergic inflammation in isolated vagal sensory ganglia unmasks silent NK_2 tachykinin receptors. J Neurosci 1997; 17:7683–7693.
177. Adcock JJ, Garland LG. The contribution of sensory reflexes and hyperalgesia to airway hyperresponsiveness. In: Page CP, Gardiner PJ. Airway Hyperresponsiveness: Is It Really Important for Asthma? Oxford: Blackwell, 1993:234–255.
178. Widdicombe JG. Neurophysiology of the cough reflex. Eur Respir J 1995; 8:1193–1202.

179. Laude EA, Higgins KS, Morice AH. A comparative study of the effects of citric acid, capsaicin and resiniferatoxin on the cough challenge in guinea-pig and man. Pulm Pharmacol 1993; 6:171–175.
180. Forsberg K, Karlsson JA, Theodorsson E, Lundberg JP, Persson CGA. Cough and bronchoconstriction mediated by capsaicin-sensitive sensory neurons in the guinea-pig. Pulm Pharmacol 1988; 1:33–39.
181. Advenier C, Girard V, Naline E, Vilain P, Emonds-Alt X. Antitussive effect of SR 48968, a non-peptide tachykinin NK_2 receptor antagonist. Eur J Pharmacol 1993; 250:169–171.
182. Girard V, Naline E, Vilain P, Emonds-Alt X, Advenier C. Effect of the two tachykinin antagonists, SR 48968 and SR 140333, on cough induced by citric acid in the unanaesthetized guinea-pig. Eur Respir J 1995; 8:1110–1114.
183. Yasumitsu R, Hirayama Y, Imai T, Miyayasu K, Hiroi J. Effects of specific tachykinin receptor antagonists on citric acid-induced cough and bronchoconstriction in unanesthetized guinea-pigs. Eur J Pharmacol 1996; 300:215–219.
184. Robineau P, Petit C, Staczek J, Peglion J-L, Brion J-D, Canet E. NK_1 and NK_2 receptors involvement in capsaicin induced cough in guinea-pigs (abstr). Am J Respir Crit Care Med 1994; 149:A186.
185. Fox AJ, Bernareggi M, Lalloo UG, Chung KF, Barnes PJ, Belvisi MG. The effect of substance P on the cough reflex and airway sensory nerves in guinea-pigs (abstr). Am J Respir Crit Care Med 1996; 153:A161.
186. Ujiie Y, Sekizawa K, Aikawa T, Sasaki H. Evidence for substance P as an endogenous substance causing cough in guinea-pigs. Am Rev Respir Dis 1993; 148:1628–1632.
187. Bolser DC, DeGennaro FC, O'Reilly S, McLeod RL, Hey JA. Central antitussive activity of the NK_1 and NK_2 tachykinin receptor antagonists, CP-99,994 and SR 48968, in the guinea-pig and cat. Br J Pharmacol 1997; 121:165–170.
188. Ichinose M, Nakajima N, Takahashi T, Yamauchi H, Inoue H, Takishama T. Protection against bradykinin-induced bronchoconstriction in asthmatic patients by neurokinin receptor antagonist. Lancet 1992; 340:1248–1251.
189. Lunde H, Hedner J, Svedmyr N. Lack of efficacy of 4 weeks treatment with the neurokinin receptor antagonist FK 224 in mild to moderate asthma (abstr). Eur Respir J 1994; 7(suppl 18):151s.
190. Fahy JV, Wong HH, Geppetti P, Reis JM, Harris SC, Maclean DB, Nadel JA, Boushey HA. Effect of an NK-1 receptor antagonist (CP-99,994) on hypertonic saline-induced bronchoconstriction and cough in male asthmatic subjects. Am J Respir Crit Care Med 1995; 152:879–884.
191. Ichinose M, Miura M, Yamauchi H, Kageyama N, Tomaki M, Oyake T, Ohuchi Y, Hida W, Miki H, Tamura G, Shirato K. A neurokinin 1-receptor antagonist improves exercise-induced airway narrowing in asthmatic patients. Am J Respir Crit Care Med 1996; 153:936–941.
192. Van Schoor J, Joos G, Chasson B, Brouard R, Pauwels R. The effect of the oral nonpeptide NK_2 receptor antagonist SR 48968 on neurokinin A–induced bronchoconstriction in asthmatics. Eur Respir J 1998; 12:17–23.

9

Therapeutic Potential of Phosphodiesterase Type 4 Inhibitors in the Treatment of Asthma

BERNADETTE HUGHES

Pfizer Central Research
Sandwich, England

GERRY HIGGS

Celltech Therapeutics
Slough, Berkshire, England

I. Introduction

The pioneering work of Sutherland and colleagues in the 1960s established the concept of intracellular second messengers, which relay the signals from hormones acting at specific cell-surface receptors (1). Cyclic adenosine 3′,5′-monophosphate (cAMP) has become the paradigm for this concept, occupying a pivotal role in cell metabolism as well as cell functions such as secretion, muscle relaxation, ion conductance, differentiation, apoptosis, and growth. The generation, actions, and catabolism of cAMP have, therefore, been the focus of tremendous research interest among biologists and medicinal chemists hoping to understand cell processes and how to intervene with the objective of achieving a therapeutic effect.

Our understanding of the functional significance of the multiplicity of cAMP signaling components continues to grow with the identification of subtle variants in the key elements involved in the synthesis, detection, and degradation of cAMP. To date, nine forms of the cAMP-synthesizing enzyme adenylate cyclase have been detected in mammalian cells, together with up to 30 isoforms of the phosphodiesterases (PDEs), which degrade cAMP and multiple forms of the heterodimeric protein kinase A (PKA), which is responsible for transducing the cAMP signal (2). Such diversity around the processing of a single signaling species may suggest a certain amount of redundancy, but it is just as likely to be the requirement of highly discreet and specific signaling pathways. If this is the case, therein lies the opportunity for selective modulation by drugs.

In 1859, a report in the *Edinburgh Medical Journal* noted that "strong, black coffee was the most common and best remedy for attacks of asthma" (3). Similar properties were attributed to tea, and in 1888 the active principle was extracted from tea leaves and named theophylline, a methylxanthine closely related to caffeine. After nearly a century of use of theophylline as a therapy in asthma, Butcher and Sutherland (4) proposed that its bronchodilator activity is due to the inhibition of PDE activity, thereby elevating levels of intracellular cAMP in bronchial smooth muscle, leading to relaxation. This was one of the first associations between drug activity and regulation of cyclic nucleotide metabolism. The identification of multiple forms of PDEs in the early 1970s (5) led to the consideration of specific PDEs in a variety of different tissues as targets for selective inhibitors that would have therapeutic effects in a number of pathologies including hypertension, congestive heart failure, depression and dementia, metabolic disorders, respiratory diseases, chronic inflammation, and sexual dysfunction. This chapter concentrates on the investigation of the functional role of cAMP in tissues involved in asthmatic responses and reviews the evidence that selective inhibitors of the appropriate PDEs may lead to a new class of antiasthma drugs.

II. The Asthmatic Response

Bronchial asthma is characterized by episodes of acute bronchoconstriction, often initiated by exposure to allergens, followed by a late onset of wheeziness and prolonged hyperresponsiveness of the airways. There is chronic inflammation in the lungs, which is accompanied by a reduction in the dynamic compliance of the small airways. A risk factor for asthma is atopy, which is the genetic predisposition to allergy; the disease is therefore regulated by the immune system.

On exposure to allergen, cross-linking of IgE and its receptors on the surface of pulmonary mast cells leads to release of histamine, and this, together with synthesis of the cysteinyl leukotrienes by these and other cells in the airway accounts for the acute bronchoconstriction (6). The recruitment, activation, and proliferation of T lymphocytes in the airways and the subsequent generation of interleukin-5 (IL-5) leads to the selective accumulation of eosinophils in the lungs (7). Allergen-specific T lymphocytes are found in the lungs of asthmatics, and they have an upregulated capacity to produce the cytokines IL-3, IL-4, IL-5, and granulocyte-macrophage colony-stimulating factor (GM-CSF) (8).

IL-5 stimulates eosinophil differentiation and maturation in the bone marrow (9) and regulates peripheral blood eosinophilia and eosinophil infiltration of the lungs (10). Alveolar macrophages isolated from asthmatic patients release GM-CSF, which, in turn, activates eosinophils to generate the powerful bronchoconstrictor leukotriene C_4 (LTC_4) (11). The selective airway eosinophilia induced by platelet activating factor (PAF) (12) is enhanced by coadministration of GM-

CSF (13). A key factor in eosinophil recruitment is the local generation of eotaxin, a peptide from the C-C branch of the platelet factor 4 superfamily of chemotactic cytokines (14). It is now thought that IL-5 acts as a hormone to stimulate the release into the circulation of a rapidly mobilizable pool of bone marrow eosinophils and that eotaxin generated in the lungs localizes their recruitment into the small airways (15).

One of the most prominent features of the bronchial inflammation in asthma is the pronounced eosinophilia in bronchoalveolar lavage fluid and airway biopsies. A large proportion of these cells are degranulated in active disease, and high levels of eosinophil cationic protein (ECP) and major basic protein (MBP) can be detected in the tissues (16,17). These cytotoxic proteins contribute to the ongoing inflammation leading to damage to the epithelial mucosa of the airways (18) (Fig. 1).

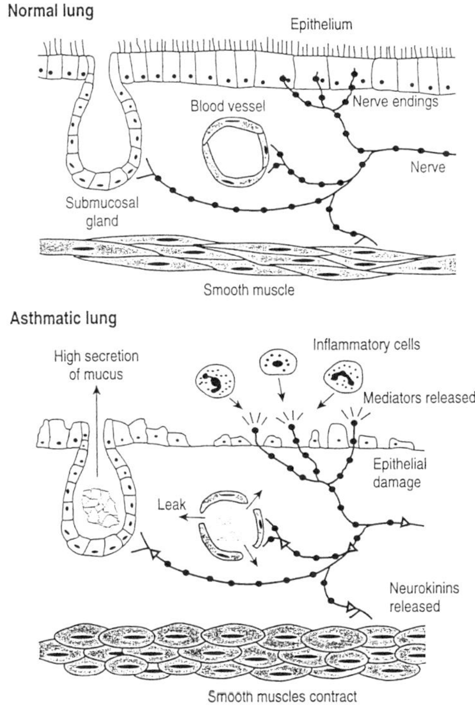

Figure 1 Resident tissues and infiltrating leukocytes involved in allergic responses in the lung. The IgE-dependent release of histamine and leukotrienes from allergen-sensitized resident tissues leads to smooth muscle constriction of the airways, vascular leakage, and edema. Infiltration of inflammatory leukocytes results in epithelial damage and exposure of sensory nerves, which triggers axon reflexes and the release of tachykinins, leading to enhancement of bronchoconstriction, inflammation, mucus secretion and hyperresponsiveness. All of these tissue responses are susceptible to regulation by cAMP. (Adapted from Ref. 19.)

Damage to the airway epithelium exposes sensory nerve endings, which release the neuropeptides substance P (SP), neurokinin A (NKA), and calcitonin gene–related peptide (CGRP). These peptides contribute to bronchoconstriction and inflammation by contracting airway smooth muscle, dilating precapillary blood vessels, and increasing postcapillary vascular permeability, thereby narrowing the small airways and enhancing tissue edema (19). It has also been suggested that the sensory neurons participate in an axon reflex mechanism in which there is a neuronal amplification of bronchoconstriction, inflammation, and mucus secretion (20).

It is evident therefore, that asthma involves a complex sequence of actions and interactions between resident tissues and infiltrating cells in the airways (Fig. 1). Several critical events in these responses are susceptible to regulation by cAMP.

III. The Regulation by cAMP of Tissue Responses in Asthma

A number of hormones act at specific cell-surface receptors linked through a guanine nucleotide binding protein (G protein) to adenylate cyclase. Binding at the receptor increases the rate at which Mg^{2+}-ATP is converted to cAMP (Fig. 2). The target enzymes for this reaction are cAMP-dependent protein kinases (e.g., PKA), which then mediate physiological responses by phosphorylating key substrates such as enzymes and ion transport systems, which regulate cell functions. The elevation of intracellular cAMP can result in suppression of cell activation. For example, responses that occur in asthma—such as mast-cell degranulation, stimulation of phospholipase A_2 (PLA_2), constriction of airway smooth muscle, activation of inflammatory leukocytes, synthesis of cytokines, and firing of sensory neurons—are all suppressed by elevation of cAMP. Endogenous regulation is mediated by catecholamines, adenosine, and eicosanoids, which signal through receptors linked to adenylate cyclase and elevate intracellular cAMP.

A. Cyclic AMP in Airway Smooth Muscle

Stimulation of a number of airway smooth muscle receptors leads to the elevation of cAMP. Circulating hormones such as epinephrine, neurotransmitters such as norepinephrine, and autocoids such as prostaglandin E_2 (PGE_2) and prostacyclin bind to receptors that activate adenylate cyclase to catalyze the conversion of ATP to cAMP (Fig. 2). The functional consequence of this is PKA-dependent muscle relaxation. Phosphorylation by PKA decreases the activity of myosin light chain kinase (MLCK) and lowers its affinity for calcium/calmodulin complex, leading to muscle relaxation. At the same time, cAMP-induced falls in cytoplasmic calcium concentrations produce a similar effect (6).

In response to stress, endogenous catecholamines induce airway relaxation and increase ventilation of the lungs by a direct, cAMP-dependent effect on air-

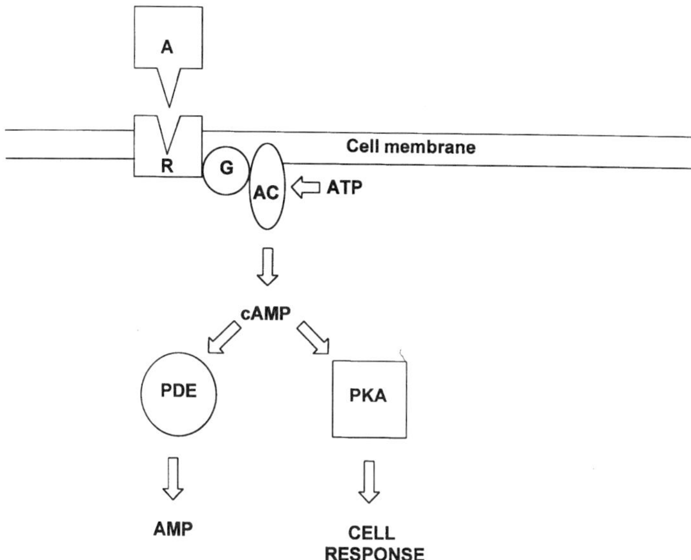

Figure 2 Schematic representation of receptor-mediated elevation of intracellular cAMP. Agonists (A) such as isoprenaline or prostaglandin E_2 bind at specific cell membrane receptors (R), which are linked to adenylate cyclase (AC) through G proteins (G). Adenylate cyclase catalyzes the conversion of ATP to cAMP, which is either broken down to AMP by phosphodiesterases (PDE) or activates protein kinase A (PKA) to phosphorylate cell proteins, which bring about a cell response.

way smooth muscle. The elevation of cAMP by β-adrenergic agonists or PDE inhibitors is thought to be the mechanism by which drugs such as salbutamol (a specific β_2-agonist) and theophylline (a nonspecific PDE inhibitor) exert their bronchodilator activity (21).

B. Cyclic AMP in Mast Cells

The nonhydrolyzable cAMP analogue dibutyryl cAMP inhibits the secretion of histamine from mast cells and basophils following cross-linking of IgE receptors. The β-adrenergic agonist isoprenaline causes a rapid monophasic increase in cAMP in human lung mast cells, and this is associated with inhibition of both IgE-induced histamine release and leukotriene synthesis (22). Similar effects are seen when intracellular cAMP is elevated by the eicosanoid PGE_2, the direct adenylate cyclase activator forskolin, or the nonspecific PDE inhibitor isobutylmethylxanthine (IBMX). In both the basophil and the human lung mast cell, agonist-induced elevation of cAMP correlates well with inhibition of mediator release (22). Paradoxically, IgE receptor cross-linking also causes a rapid rise in cAMP, which precedes histamine release (6). It is possible that stimulus-induced elevation of cAMP is a negative feedback mechanism for regulating the rate and extent of degranulation.

The combination of IBMX and forskolin inhibits antigen-induced production of both prostaglandins (PGD_2) and leukotrienes (LTC_4) by murine mast cells (23). These responses are accompanied by an abolition of increases in cytosolic calcium and the subsequent inhibition of PLA_2. The calcium-dependent activation of PLA_2 results in the liberation of arachidonic acid from phospholipids, which, in turn, leads to the synthesis of prostaglandins and leukotrienes (6). The major part of acute allergic bronchoconstriction in humans is accounted for by a combination of histamine and the cysteinyl leukotrienes (24).

C. cAMP in Inflammatory Cells

Alveolar Macrophages

Alveolar macrophages are the most numerous cells in human airways and they release inflammatory mediators following immunological challenge. Challenge with IgE immune complexes or opsonized zymosan results in the release from human alveolar macrophages of eicosanoids (thromboxane, prostaglandins, and leukotrienes), superoxide, and *N*-acetyl glucosamine (25). The generation of thromboxane and superoxide is inhibited by forskolin, indicating that cAMP partially regulates the activation of these cells. In some studies, β-adrenergic stimulation did not prevent alveolar macrophage activation, possibly because of a downregulation of the receptor (25). Other findings, however, show that salbutamol or isoprenaline elevate cAMP in alveolar macrophages from healthy volunteers but that these responses are significantly impaired in cells from asthmatics (26), which may be due to a reduction in the receptor number or impairment of signal transduction. Theophylline elevates cAMP in alveolar macrophages, and this is accompanied by inhibition of the respiratory burst (27) and cytokine synthesis (28).

Neutrophils

As in all inflammatory responses, neutrophils appear in the lungs soon after an irritant or damaging stimulus, and they continue to participate in the chronic inflammation seen in asthma. Neutrophils are a source of inflammatory eicosanoids and cytokines as well as tissue-degrading lysosomal enzymes. Release of these factors contributes to and augments the local inflammation. Elevation of cAMP in neutrophils prevents the release of lysosomal enzymes (29), the production of eicosanoids (30), and the synthesis of platelet activating factor (31). Elevation of cAMP also inhibits the oxidative burst in neutrophils (32) induced by chemoattractants (33) and cytokines (34,35). Furthermore, increased cAMP concentrations in neutrophils caused by adenylate cyclase stimulants or PDE inhibitors prevent chemotaxis (36) and adhesion to vascular endothelium (37).

Eosinophils

The infiltrate of inflammatory leukocytes into the lungs following allergen challenge is different from other acute inflammatory responses in the high proportion of eosinophils. Eosinophils are usually associated with the defense mechanisms involved in parasitic infections, and there has been some speculation that pulmonary eosinophilia in allergic asthma is a throwback to times when respiratory parasites were more prevalent. The activated eosinophil is thought to be a key cell in initiating and sustaining inflammatory damage in the lung in asthma (18).

The generation of oxygen radicals from eosinophils by opsonized zymosan is inhibited by β-agonists and inhibitors of cAMP PDEs but not by inhibitors of cGMP PDEs (38,39). Eosinophil chemotaxis induced by complement factor 5a (C5a) or PAF is inhibited by forskolin, dibutyryl-cAMP, or PDE inhibitors (40). Elevated cAMP also prevents the release of ECP, eosinophil-derived neurotoxin (41), and leukotrienes (42) from activated eosinophils. Theophylline reduces the synthesis by eosinophils of the potent bronchoconstrictor leukotriene LTC_4 (42).

Lymphocytes

Allergen-specific T-helper lymphocytes occupy a pivotal position in the development of the immune and inflammatory reactions in asthma. The IL-2 mediated clonal proliferation of these cells is inhibited by dibutyryl cyclic AMP and theophylline (43). The mitogen-driven synthesis of IL-2 in T cells is also inhibited by elevation of cAMP by either forskolin or PGE_2 (44). Similarly, allergen-induced synthesis of IL-2, IL-4, and IL-5 by peripheral blood lymphocytes taken from atopic asthmatic patients is inhibited by dibutyryl cAMP, forskolin, PGE_2, or a PDE inhibitor (45).

D. Cyclic AMP in Vascular Tissue

Vascular Smooth Muscle

In common with airway smooth muscle, elevation of cAMP in vascular smooth muscle results in relaxation. This is the basis of catecholamine- or prostaglandin-induced vasodilatation. In inflammation, dilatation of precapillary arterioles in the microcirculation results in greater perfusion of the tissues and, in combination with increased vascular permeability of the postcapillary venules, there is an augmentation of tissue edema. Cardiovascular side effects of β-agonists and PDE inhibitors used to treat asthma are a real problem. The predominant β-receptor in the airways is β_2; therefore some selectivity for the airways can be achieved with specific β_2-agonists such as salbutamol. Nonetheless, this type of drug is used mainly in asthma only by inhalation for reasons of safety and toleration. Theophylline is a nonspecific inhibitor of PDEs and, as a result, elevates cAMP in a wide range of tissues (46). The cardiovascular side effects of theophylline, which is effective only by the oral route, are a serious limitation to the use of the drug. Inhibition of PDEs in cardiac and vascular tissue leads to tachycardia, and elevation of cAMP in the central nervous system causes sleeplessness, nausea, and in some cases convulsions. The discovery of tissue-specific isoforms of cAMP PDEs holds out the prospect of more selective and better-tolerated inhibitors (46); this is discussed in the following sections in relation to the treatment of asthma.

Vascular Endothelial Cells

Aortic endothelial cells respond to forskolin with elevations in cAMP, which can be augmented by PDE inhibitors (47). In inflammation, cytokines such as IL-1 induce the expression of adhesion molecules on the surface of vascular endothelium: this leads to leukocyte margination prior to infiltration of the tissues. It is not known if the induction of adhesion molecules is subject to regulation by cAMP.

E. Cyclic AMP in Sensory Neurons

The long-acting β_2-adrenergic agonist salmeterol has been shown to elevate cAMP in a neuronal cell line, and this effect is augmented by phosphodiesterase inhibition (48). Phosphodiesterase inhibition has also been shown to inhibit the excitatory noncholinergic neurotransmission in isolated bronchi (49), indicating that cAMP may regulate the release of bronchoconstrictor tachykinins from sensory neurons in the lung. There is evidence that cAMP augments the nonadrenergic noncholinergic (NANC) relaxation of human bronchi (50). Tachykinins released in the airways also cause vascular leakage, mucus secretion, chemotaxis, and augmentation of cholinergic transmission (51).

In summary, it can be seen that cAMP plays a key role in regulating many of the responses to allergen of resident and recruited cells in the airways. It is also clear that PDE inhibition can augment the effects of cAMP in these responses. In most cases this leads to a suppression of cellular activity, which translates to a beneficial effect in disease. The elevation of cAMP accounts for the therapeutic effects of the widely used β_2-agonists and is likely to contribute to the activity of another major group, the theophylline-like drugs. Methylxanthines like theophylline are nonselective PDE inhibitors that block all the isoforms of the enzyme in different tissues. The elucidation of classes and subclasses of PDEs (2,5) with differential tissue distribution has led to attempts to target selective inhibitors for the elevation of cAMP in specific cells.

IV. Molecular Diversity of Phosphodiesterases

A. Biochemical Classification of PDEs

Mammalian tissues contain multiple molecular forms of cyclic nucleotide PDEs (52–54). In the original characterization of these enzymes, a variety of techniques were used to determine substrate specificity (i.e., cAMP, cGMP), maximum velocities, susceptibility to cofactors (e.g., calcium/calmodulin), and inhibition by pharmacological agents. Currently there are seven clearly defined PDE subgroups (PDE1–PDE7) (2) and evidence is emerging for the existence of others.

The characterization of the PDE isoforms has been driven by the search for more potent and selective therapeutic agents that elevate cAMP in target tissues. Butcher and Sutherland's findings that drugs such as theophylline inhibit cAMP hydrolysis (4) initiated a comprehensive search for compounds with improved activity. At first, compounds were screened against homogenates of whole tissues, and this almost certainly led to the failure to recognize isoform-selective PDE inhibitors. Most tissues contain multiple forms of PDE, and so only nonselective inhibitors such as the methylxanthines were seen to produce marked inhibition of total cAMP hydrolysis. A number of reports showed that certain agents produced a maximal inhibition of up to 20% at relatively low concentrations, and these effects are now reinterpreted to indicate that the compound was a good selective inhibitor of a single PDE isoform (55).

The first report that PDEs exist in multiple molecular forms was from Thompson and Appleman (56), who identified three forms of PDE in rat brain cortex. Since then, PDE isoforms have been identified in a number of other tissues through the use of a variety of isolation methods including centrifugation, gel electrophoresis, isoelectric focusing, and anion-exchange chromatography (for review, see Ref. 57). Using these techniques, three distinct peaks of PDE activity present in cardiac tissue were eluted from a DEAE column. These enzyme activities differed in substrate specificity, kinetics, and the ability to be stimulated by calmodulin (57). This became the basis of the first classification of PDE activity as PDE I, II, and III. As a result, inhibitors could be assessed in terms of their selectivity against these three peaks of activity.

The study of selective inhibitors led to the further definition of PDE isoforms. The investigation of cAMP hydrolysis in the brain led to the discovery of rolipram (58), which was subsequently shown to be a potent inhibitor of a subfraction of PDE III. Further evaluation showed that the peak of activity that corresponded to PDE III consisted of two isoforms, one with a low Km for both cAMP and cGMP and one that was cAMP-specific. The rolipram-sensitive isoform was cAMP-specific and was designated PDE IV. The detection of a cGMP-specific PDE activity defined the PDE V and PDE VI subclasses (59). The current classification of cyclic nucleotide PDEs covers seven subgroups (PDEs 1–7), with PDE7 representing a high-affinity cAMP-specific PDE that is not sensitive to rolipram (60).

B. Molecular Cloning of PDEs

A study of behavior in mutant fruit flies (*Drosophila melanogaster*) led to an association between learning and enzymes metabolizing cAMP (61). Two groups described structural genes for cAMP PDE in *Drosophila* (62) and yeast (63). At around the same time, Beavo's group produced the first comparative N-terminal primary sequence information on PDE isoforms from bovine tissues, which strongly supported the conclusion that gene loci demonstrated in *Drosophila* and yeast encoded for cyclic nucleotide PDE genes (64). This was confirmed by cDNA cloning and expression of active enzyme (65,66). The cloning of a mammalian PDE was achieved with the construction of a rat brain cDNA library in a yeast expression vector and the subsequent isolation of a gene encoding high-affinity cAMP PDE (67). This was followed by the cloning and expression of a low-Km, rolipram-sensitive cAMP PDE from a human monocyte cDNA library (68).

The five known families of PDEs that can hydrolyze cAMP (PDEs 1, 2, 3, 4, and 7) have a central catalytic region of around 330 amino acid residues. Outside this core region there is little or no homology between the PDEs. The PDE genes appear to be highly complex, with, for example, at least 16 exons spanning the 49-kb of base pairs required for assembly of the PDE4A isoform (2). This explains the large number of alternative mRNA splice variants seen for PDE genes 1, 2, and 4.

C. Tissue Distribution of PDEs

Most tissues have a mixture of PDE activities and most PDEs—with the exception of PDE6, which is located principally in the eye—are widely distributed. This wide distribution of PDE activity explains why nonspecific PDE inhibitors have a variety of adverse as well as therapeutic effects. It is important to realize, however, that most of the information to date is based on the detection of mRNA encoding a particular PDE isoform, and this does not necessarily correlate with expression of active enzyme. Similarly, detection of protein does not necessarily signify a functional role in any particular cellular activity. For example, in airway smooth muscle, PDE1 accounts for 85% of the cAMP hydrolytic activity and PDE3 and PDE4 only 10 and 5% respectively. Nonetheless, the activity of selective PDE3 and PDE4 inhibitors clearly indicates that these isoforms are more important than PDE1 in regulating muscle tone in intact tissues (69,70). This has led to the concept of ''compartmentalization'' of cAMP signaling pathways (71).

There is some experimental evidence to support the concept of compartmentalization. Particulate and soluble forms of PDEs have been described in cardiac tissue (72), and inhibition of membrane-bound PDE3 results in an inotropic effect, whereas inhibition of soluble PDE4 has no effect. The inotropic effect induced by isoprenaline correlates closely with the activity of cAMP-dependent protein kinase, but elevation of cardiac cAMP by forskolin does not result in a proportional activation of protein kinase (73), indicating a compartmentalization of cAMP generation by different activators.

The association of PDE isoforms with particular cell functions holds out the prospect of selective effects of inhibitors. The observations that inflammatory leukocytes contain predominantly the PDE4 isoform and that cAMP elevation in leukocytes suppresses their activation has led to the proposal that PDE4 inhibitors will have therapeutic value in inflammatory diseases (74). This hypothesis is the focus of a great deal of research in the pharmaceutical industry and a number of novel compounds are currently being evaluated in humans.

D. Phosphodiesterase Type 4

There are four distinct genes that encode PDE4 enzymes: PDE4A, B, C, and D. The organization of rat and human PDE4 genes is very similar and the genomic sequences show a high conservation of the intron/exon boundaries (75) (R. Owens, personal communication, 1996). Analysis of the four rat and human amino acid sequences reveals three highly conserved regions (Fig. 3). In addition to the catalytic domain, which is common to all PDEs, the PDE4 isoforms contain two upstream conserved regions, UCR1 and UCR2 (76). The functional importance of these *N*-terminal regions is not entirely clear, although a PKA phosphorylation site has been demonstrated in UCR1 and some splice variants contain SH3 binding motifs which may be important in the cellular localization of the enzyme (2).

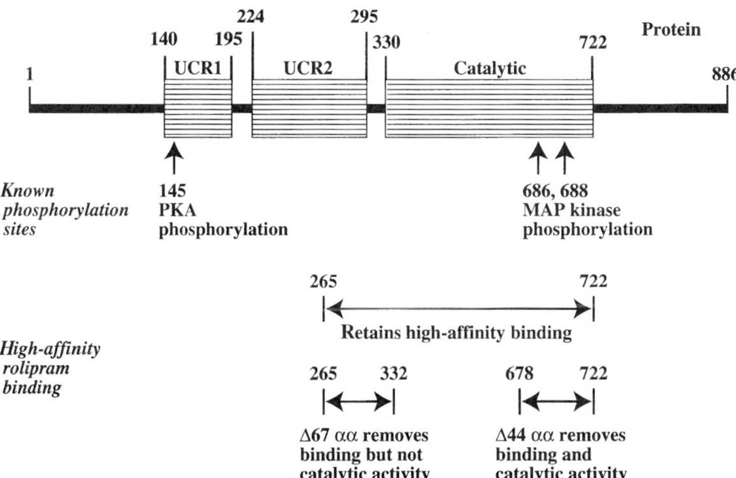

Figure 3 Schematic representation of the linear sequence of amino acids in human phosphodiesterase type 4A.

The discovery of rolipram was facilitated by its high-affinity binding in brain tissues (58). Initially there was a marked difference in the activities reported for the binding affinity of rolipram (Kd = 1–2 nM) and its potency in inhibiting the catalytic activity of the enzyme (Ki = 1 μM). This led to doubts as to whether the two activities were related. The cloning of human recombinant PDE4, however, demonstrated the coexpression of cAMP PDE activity and high-affinity rolipram binding on the same molecule (77). The disparity between Ki and Kd is probably explained by the existence of the enzyme in at least two different forms.

Truncation of PDE4A to residues 265–722 retains both catalytic activity and high-affinity binding (Fig. 3). Further truncation of the N-terminal end to residue 332 removes high-affinity binding of rolipram, but the protein remains catalytically active (78,79). Also, the C-terminal region of the catalytic region, residues 678–722, is required for both binding and catalytic activity (78). One interpretation of these observations is that the tertiary structure of the molecule in situ allows a coupling of N-terminal and C-terminal regions to form the high-affinity binding site that is not present in the uncoupled form. Both forms are capable of catalytic activity. Interestingly, the solubilization of particulate PDE4 or the treatment of membrane-bound PDE4 with vanadate-glutathione results in a tenfold increase in the potency of rolipram but not RP73401 in inhibiting cAMP hydrolysis (80), indicating that the conformation of the enzyme determines its differential susceptibility to inhibitors.

The mRNAs for all four subtypes of PDE4 are found in most tissues although, notably, PDE4C is not found in blood leukocytes (81). PDE4B is the predominant isoform found in neutrophils and PDE4D in eosinophils (81). The functional significance of these distribution patterns is not yet clear, and so far they have not shed any light on the differential effects of PDE4 inhibitors on various tissue responses.

V. The Discovery of Novel PDE Inhibitors

A. Methylxanthines

The association of theophylline with elevation of cAMP and inhibition of PDEs (4) led to the investigation of a wide range of methylxanthines and their analogues for therapeutic effects. It has been difficult, however, to optimize the benefits of xanthine therapy due to the problems of intolerance and toxicity frequently encountered in practice. Furthermore, Polson and colleagues (82) reported that at therapeutic concentrations, theophylline prevented PDE activity by only about 10%, indicating that other properties of the drug contribute to its overall effect.

Theophylline and the methylxanthines competitively antagonize the actions of adenosine at its cell surface receptors (A_1, A_2, and A_3), with varying effects on intracellular cAMP in a wide range of tissues. Stimulation of A_1 purinoceptors decreases cAMP, whereas stimulation of A_2 receptors activates adenylate cyclase and leads to an increase in cAMP (83). Thus, adenosine antagonism leads to a complex profile of responses. Adenosine is released in the lungs following antigen challenge, ischemia or hypoxia (84), and because adenosine causes bronchoconstriction in patients with asthma, adenosine antagonism has been proposed as a contributing factor in the therapeutic effects of theophylline. Certainly, downregulation of the A_1 receptor in the lungs of sensitized rabbits using a specific antisense DNA treatment results in reduced responsiveness to antigen (85).

The actions of the methylxanthines at adenosine receptors also help to explain their other therapeutic actions in, for example, acute cardiac failure as well as their adverse effects, such as central nervous system stimulation, gastric hypersecretion, gastroesophageal reflux, cardiotoxicity, and diuresis.

Despite the relative nonspecificity of the methylxanthines, a number of novel compounds in the class and some close analogues have been developed and extensively investigated in relation to their PDE inhibitory actions (Fig. 4). The elucidation of PDE isoforms enabled a more selective screening process to be employed in the discovery of more potent and specific inhibitors. Elevation of cAMP in brain tissues augments the effects of neurotransmitters such as norepinephrine, acetylcholine, and dopamine. On the basis of this, selective inhibi-

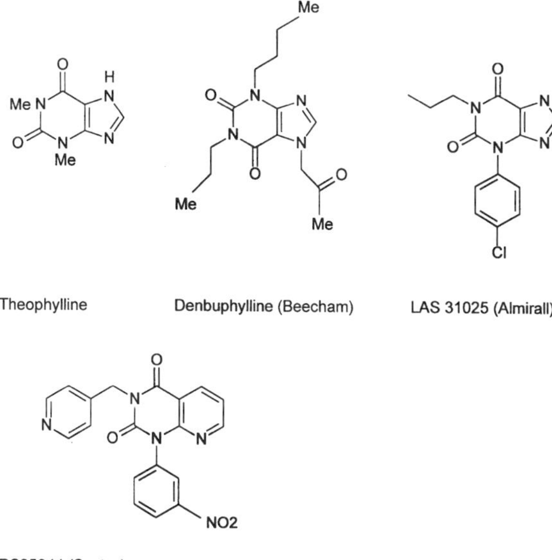

Figure 4 The methylxanthine theophylline and related selective PDE4 inhibitors.

tion of brain PDE4 has been proposed as a possible therapy for dementia (for review, see Ref. 86). The characterization of the low-Km cAMP-specific PDE4 led to the discovery of denbufylline (Fig. 4) as a selective PDE4 inhibitor, which progressed to clinical evaluation in dementia.

More recently, a novel methylxanthine (LAS 31025; Fig. 4) with selective PDE4 inhibitory activity has been evaluated in allergic airway responses (87). This compound has significant activity in preclinical models of asthma and is believed to show therapeutic effects in early clinical trials in patients. LAS 31025 is, however, a potent adenosine antagonist, and its mixed pharmacological properties will not permit a clear interpretation of its mode of action in vivo. Denbuphylline and a number of other methylxanthines have been withdrawn from clinical development because of unacceptable adverse effects, and it remains to be seen whether the latest generation of xanthines, such as LAS 31025, will offer any advantages over theophylline.

Another approach to the medicinal chemistry of PDE4 inhibitors, which is related to the xanthines, is the work on N-aryl quinazolines such as RS25344 (Fig. 4). These are among the most potent and selective PDE4 inhibitors yet described. RS25344 is relatively more potent in its activity at the high-affinity binding site on PDE4 than at the catalytic site (88). The high-affinity binding activity is thought to be related to induction of emesis and gastric side effects (89), and this is likely to be a barrier to the development of this type of compound. It has been suggested, therefore, that the target PDE4 inhibitor should be optimized at the catalytic site, with relatively less activity at the high-affinity binding site (88).

B. Nonxanthine Inhibitors

When interest developed in PDE inhibitors as putative therapies for diseases of the central nervous system, the lack of specificity of the xanthines was seen as a real obstacle to progress. The effects of xanthines and related compounds on adenosine frustrated the interpretation of the effects of PDE inhibition by these compounds in brain tissue. Theophylline and IBMX are adenosine antagonists, and other PDE inhibitors such as papaverine and dipyridamole are potent adenosine uptake inhibitors (58). Since adenosine plays a pivotal role in the control of cAMP-generating systems in the brain, any PDE inhibitor that interacts with adenosine is of limited value.

The first series of compounds in which PDE inhibitory activity could be dissociated from effects on adenosine is represented by the phenyl-2-pyrrolidone ZK 62711, later called rolipram (Fig. 5). Rolipram is a close analogue of an earlier PDE inhibitor, Ro 20-1724, which has a number of central effects including adenosine uptake inhibition and monoamine oxidase inhibition (58). Rolipram, however, is free from these activities and is 100 times more potent than

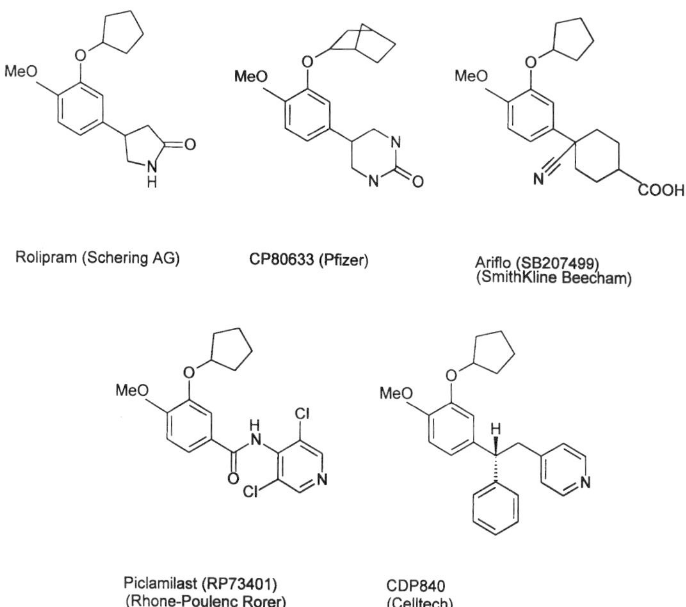

Figure 5 Nonxanthine selective PDE4 inhibitors.

Ro 20-1724 in inhibiting low-Km cAMP-specific PDE in brain tissue. Rolipram itself was developed for evaluation in clinical depression, where it showed significant antidepressant activity but appeared to be dose-limited by the onset of nausea and vomiting (90). These adverse effects may again be due to rolipram's activity at the high-affinity binding site (88,89).

The discovery of rolipram is probably most important for the chemical lead it gave to a novel series of cyclopentyloxy methoxyphenyl analogues, which have been found to be progressively more potent against PDE4 and with improved side-effect profiles (Fig. 5). Initially, these analogue programs were directed toward putative antidepressant drugs (91), but increasingly the medicinal chemistry has become targeted at antiasthmatic and anti-inflammatory activity (92–94).

Rolipram and its close analogues inhibit the cAMP hydrolytic activity of isolated PDE4 with IC_{50}s in the region of 0.1–1 μM (91). A breakthrough in terms of potency came with the discovery of the benzamide RP73401 (Fig. 5), which was shown to be up to 1000 times more potent than rolipram (80). The extended bi-aryl structure represented by RP73401 has now been further developed with the description of a series of triaryl ethanes, of which CDP840 (Fig. 5) is the prototype (95). The new nonxanthine generation of selective PDE4 inhibitors illustrated in Fig. 5 have been extensively studied in pre-clinical models of allergic and inflammatory diseases and are now under investigation in clinical trials. These compounds, which do not have activity at adenosine receptors, have a distinctly different pharmacology from the methylxanthines and in some cases have surprisingly different profiles from each other. These activities are reviewed in the following sections.

VI. The Pharmacology of PDE4 Inhibitors

A. Effects on Airway Smooth Muscle

There is substantial evidence linking cAMP and cGMP in the regulation of airway muscular tone (96,97). The β-adrenergic receptor agonists induce relaxation by elevating cAMP, and there is a correlation between inhibition of PDEs and tracheal relaxation by methylxanthines (98) or chemically unrelated PDE inhibitors (99).

In 1989, Harris and colleagues (70) published a careful and revealing study of the effects of PDE inhibitors on large airway responses in vitro and in vivo. They found that tracheal tissue contained two low-Km cAMP phosphodiesterase activities, which we now know correspond to PDE3 and PDE4. They then compared the effects of nonspecific and selective PDE inhibitors on tracheal responses induced by the spasmogens histamine, carbachol, and leukotriene D_4. The nonspecific inhibitors theophylline and papavarine caused a weak, monophasic reversal of the effects of all three spasmogens, whereas the selective PDE3 inhibitor CI-930 and the selective PDE4 inhibitor rolipram both caused biphasic relaxations of the constricted tissues (Fig. 6). The first phase of relaxant activity occurred at low concentrations (10–100 nM) of each agent, but complete relaxation was not achieved until concentrations of 0.1–1 mM were reached. If either selective inhibitor was titrated in the presence of low concentrations of the other, then marked relaxation was obtained at 0.1–1 μM, showing clear synergy between the two types of inhibitor. These experiments demonstrated that both PDE3 and PDE4 are important regulators of airway tone, and this has led to the proposal that dual inhibitors would have a value in treating allergic bronchoconstriction (71). The problem with this approach is that PDE3 is also a key regulator of cardiovascular responses. Inhibitors of PDE3 have a direct inotropic effect on the heart; by inducing relaxation in the peripheral vasculature, they also cause a reflex tachycardia (71,72). The adverse side effects of theophylline, such as tachycardia, are attributed to inhibition of PDE3.

Another important observation made by Harris et al. (70) was the relationship between high-affinity binding and tracheal relaxation. There is a highly significant correlation of activity at the high binding site with both tracheal relaxation in vitro and bronchodilation in vivo. It is possible that the PDE4 isoform

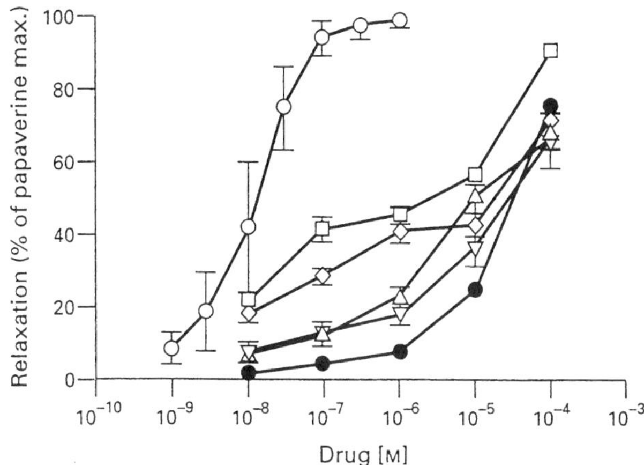

Figure 6 The relaxant effects of drugs in guinea pig isolated tracheas preconstricted with histamine. The drugs are salbutamol (open circles), rolipram (open squares), RP73401 (open diamonds), CDP840 (open triangles), CT1730 (inverted open triangles), and aminophylline (closed circles). (Data from Ref. 101.)

present in airway smooth muscle is in the high-affinity coupled conformation. If correct, the theory that high-affinity binding is also linked to the central and emetic effects of PDE4 inhibitors (88,89) may mean that direct bronchodilator activity of PDE4 inhibitors may be difficult to dissociate from adverse side effects.

With the development of more potent PDE4 inhibitors such as RP73401, there is some evidence that PDE4 inhibition could achieve a potency in bronchodilation comparable to that of the β-adrenergic agonists (100). However, in a study comparing PDE4 inhibitors with salbutamol (101), RP73401 and rolipram caused a biphasic reversal of histamine-induced tracheal constriction, confirming the findings of Harris et al. (70) and showing that PDE4 inhibitors are more than 1000 times less potent than salbutamol in producing a full reversal of the histamine response (Fig. 6).

The efficacy of PDE inhibitors in any cell system will depend upon the rate of generation of cAMP. If there is no adenylate cyclase activity, PDE inhibitors will not be able to elevate cAMP. Conversely, stimulation of receptors linked to adenylate cyclase (Fig. 2) by agonists such as isoprenaline, salbutamol, PGE_2, or adenosine results in a marked increase in the ability of PDE inhibitors to elevate intracellular cAMP. For example, rolipram exerts little effect on cAMP levels in unstimulated eosinophils; but in the presence of isoprenaline, rolipram potently increases cAMP accumulation (39). This has led to the proposal that specific PDE isoforms in airway smooth muscle are linked to adrenergic receptor–adenylate cyclase complexes (102).

In human bronchial muscle, rolipram but not the PDE3 inhibitor siguazodan potentiates the bronchodilator effects of isoprenaline (103); experiments using the β_2-agonist salbutamol indicate that the β_2-adrenergic receptor is functionally linked to PDE4 (102). In another study in guinea pig airways, however, isoprenaline potentiates the effects of both type 3 and type 4 PDE inhibitors (104). Because isoprenaline is a mixed β_1-and β_2-agonist, these results are consistent with the suggestion that β_1 is linked to PDE3 and β_2 is linked to PDE4 (102). The augmentation of β-adrenergic agonists is seen with PDE4 inhibitors such as rolipram and RP73401, which have direct bronchodilator activity themselves (100), but not with CDP840, which is not a bronchodilator (101). This again indicates that the PDE4 isoform present in airway smooth muscle adopts a conformation that is differentially sensitive to inhibitors.

B. Effects on Mast Cells

The mast cell is central to the allergic response in a number of tissues, including the skin and lungs. Mast cells release preformed and newly synthesized inflammatory mediators following exposure to allergens. Histamine and 5-hydroxytryptamine (5-HT) are stored in the basophilic granules of these cells and are released when antigens cross-link cell surface–bound IgE. This release is accompanied by secretion of proteases such as tryptase and the synthesis of eicosanoids and cytokines (105). If signaling through the high-affinity IgE receptor is prevented, none of these mediators are released (106).

The mast cell has been the target for the development of new antiallergic drugs for many years. Also, effects on mast cells have been evoked to explain the mechanism of action of drugs such as cromoglycate in asthma. Little is known about the PDE isoforms present in mast cells, although a preliminary biochemical characterization indicates that both PDE3 and PDE4 are present (107). The β_2-adrenergic agonists and the methylxanthines ''stabilize'' mast cells and basophils through the elevation of cAMP (22). Interestingly, however, selective inhibitors of PDE1, 2, 3, 4, or 5 are not as effective as the nonspecific inhibitor IBMX in preventing the degranulation of primary human lung mast cells (108). The de novo synthesis of arachidonic acid metabolites such as the cysteinyl-leukotrienes by basophils and mast cells is more sensitive to elevations in intracellular cAMP than the release of preformed mediators via the secretory process (22,108,109). A major component of acute allergic bronchoconstriction is due to leukotriene D_4, and it is possible that some PDE inhibitors have greater effects on airway function through inhibition of bronchoconstrictor mediators than through a direct relaxant effect on airway smooth muscle.

C. Effects on Inflammatory Leukocytes

Macrophages

The predominant PDE isoform in macrophages is PDE4 (107,110), and N-terminal sequence analysis has revealed the presence of PDE4A and PDE4D in human monocytes (111). Rolipram elevates cAMP in monocytes but has little or no effect on the fMLP-induced respiratory burst in human cells (110) but weakly inhibits the superoxide burst in guinea pig macrophages (112,113).

An important effect on monocytes/macrophages is the ability of PDE inhibitors to regulate cytokine synthesis. The methylxanthines were shown to inhibit endotoxin (LPS)-induced generation of tumor necrosis factor (TNF) by mononuclear cells (114), and in 1992, Molnar-Kimber and colleagues (115) demonstrated that PDE4 inhibitors are much more potent than PDE3 or nonspecific PDE inhibitors in suppressing human macrophage cytokine production. Rolipram is more effective in inhibiting TNF than IL-1β, and there is some evidence that combined inhibition of PDE3 and PDE4 is most effective (115,116).

Elevation of cAMP in human monocytes by adenylate cyclase stimulation, PDE inhibition, or addition of db-cAMP prevents the induction of TNF mRNA but actually increases IL-1β mRNA (117). This suggests that cAMP mediates TNF gene transcription and IL-1β message translation. Further investigation of the mechanism of cytokine suppression has shown that IL-10 plays a key role. Selective PDE4 inhibitors augment IL-10 production in macrophages and the inhibitory effects of rolipram or RP73401 on TNF production are reduced by anti-IL-10 monoclonal antibodies (118,119).

In peripheral blood mononuclear leukocytes from atopic patients, antigen-induced IL-5 and interferon gamma (IFN-γ) gene expression are blocked by IBMX or rolipram but not by siguazodan (120). The PDE inhibitors did not inhibit IL-4 gene expression, and it is not known if IL-5 or IFN-γ gene expression is regulated by IL-10.

Rolpiram or CP-80633 (Fig. 5) elevates plasma cAMP concentrations in mice following oral administration, and this effect is associated with reductions in LPS-induced TNF production in vivo (121). With rolipram, the effects on cAMP and TNF in vivo are dependent on release of corticosterone and epinephrine (122), but the major component of TNF inhibition by CP-80633 is independent of adrenal stimulation (121). Rolipram also elevates cAMP in alveolar macrophages and inhibits TNF synthesis in endotoxin-induced inflammation in mouse lungs (123).

There are few reports on the effects of PDE4 inhibitors on leukotriene production by macrophages. The weak PDE4 inhibitor Ro 20-1724 failed to prevent leukotriene or thromboxane synthesis in alveolar macrophages (25). Leukotriene C_4 generation by murine macrophages is blocked by rolipram or the dual PDE3/4 inhibitor zardavarine (116), but at much higher concentrations than those required to prevent TNF generation in the same cells. Furthermore, there was no synergy between the PDE inhibitors and adenylate cyclase stimulation in suppressing leukotrienes, suggesting a different mechanism of action (116).

Neutrophils

The methylxanthine IBMX inhibits a number of neutrophil functions, including degranulation (124), chemotaxis (36), superoxide production (33), and adhesion to bronchial epithelial cells (125). Xanthines also reduce arachidonic acid metabolism in neutrophils, with the consequent inhibition of leukotriene and PAF production (30,126). Functional and biochemical characterization studies indicate that PDE4 is the predominant if not the only PDE4 present in neutrophils (107,127). Selective PDE4 inhibitors (rolipram or Ro 20-1724) but not inhibitors of PDE3 or PDE5 suppress the neutrophil respiratory burst (32). Ro 20-1724 also potentiates the inhibition of neutrophil phagocytosis by an adenosine A_2 receptor agonist (128).

The recruitment of leukocytes to inflamed tissues is regulated by cAMP, which suppresses responsiveness to chemoattractants and prevents some adhesion events required for extravasation of the cells. Chemotactic peptide-induced adhesion of neutrophils to vascular endothelium is blocked by rolipram but not by the PDE3 inhibitor milrinone (37). In these experiments, fMLP induced the expression of β_2 integrins CD11a/CD18 and CD11b/CD18 on the surface of neutrophils. These molecules are required for adhesion to endothelial cells and are downregulated by rolipram. Similarly, rolipram blocks PAF-induced expression of CD11b/CD18 on neutrophils and prevents the shedding of L-selectin, another adhesion molecule involved in neutrophil migration from blood vessels (129).

Eosinophils

Eosinophils, which are characteristically involved in pulmonary inflammation in allergic responses, contain PDE4 (39), which appears to be the major PDE activity (107). The predominant PDE4 isoform in eosinophils is PDE4D (80,81). In these cells there seems to be a tight coupling between β_2-stimulation and PDE4, with marked potentiation of rolipram effects by isoprenaline (39) or salbutamol (130).

Rolipram and a number of other selective PDE4 but not PDE3 inhibitors reduce superoxide generation by eosinophils (38,39,80,130,131). Interestingly, there is some evidence that inhibition of the respiratory burst in eosinophils correlates with activity at the catalytic site rather than at the high binding site (131). This may be the basis for separating the anti-inflammatory effects from the adverse effects of PDE4 inhibitors. PDE4 inhibitors could reduce eosinophil accumulation in the lung because they block chemotaxis (40,132) and prevent shedding of the adhesion molecule L-selectin (129). They also downregulate eosinophil activation by inhibiting the release of MBP, ECP, and EPO from the eosinophilic granules (41,80,95). Studies of the metabolism of arachidonic acid by eosinophils show that PDE4 inhibitors reduce the synthesis of leukotrienes (42,133), thromboxane (134), and PAF (133).

There is, therefore, a great deal of evidence that PDE4 inhibitors potently suppress the activation of eosinophils by preventing movement, degranulation, and mediator synthesis. These effects could be of particular therapeutic value in a disease like asthma, where the eosinophil is thought to play a pivotal role in the development of pulmonary inflammation and bronchial epithelial damage (18).

Lymphocytes

Mixed lymphocyte preparations—including T and B lymphocytes as well as natural killer cells—contain a cAMP PDE activity that is sensitive to Ro 20-1724 (135). Purified preparations of T lymphocytes contain PDE3 and PDE4 in the particulate and soluble fractions respectively (136,137). $CD4^+$ and $CD8^+$ T lymphocytes contain comparable profiles of PDE activity, which is predominantly membrane-associated PDE3 and soluble PDE4 (107). A significant amount of T-cell cAMP hydrolytic activity is not sensitive to selective inhibitors of PDEs 1–5; this led to the characterization of the low-Km cAMP PDE7 in the human T-cell line HUT-78 (138).

Lymphocyte proliferation is inhibited by theophylline (43) or by elevation of intracellular cAMP induced by isoprenaline or PGE_2 (139). Elevation of cAMP is also associated with a reduction in IL-2 synthesis (44,140). Adhesion of T cells to dermal endothelial cells is blocked by IBMX (141), but it is not known if this is due to nonspecific PDE inhibition or inhibition of a single PDE subtype. The selective PDE4 inhibitor T-440 prevents allergen-induced IL-5 generation and proliferation in peripheral blood mononuclear cells from asthmatic patients (45). Rolipram but not siguazodan blocks gene expression and protein synthesis for IL-4, IL-5, and IFN-γ in both Th1 and Th2 lymphocyte clones, and there is some evidence that the Th2 phenotype is more sensitive to PDE4 inhibitors, possibly due to differential expression of PDE4 isoforms between Th1 and Th2 cells (142).

High concentrations of rolipram inhibit mitogen- or anti-CD3–induced proliferation of $CD4^+$ or $CD8^+$ T-lymphocytes, but the selective PDE3 inhibitor SK&F 95654 was inactive (143). Combinations of the PDE3 inhibitor with rolipram, however, show a marked synergy, with an increase in potency for rolipram of approximately 100-fold (143). These data indicate that both PDE3 and PDE4 are important regulators of cAMP in lymphocytes. IL-2 synthesis by murine splenocytes is suppressed by PDE4 inhibitors, and this activity correlates with inhibition of a "low-affinity" conformer of PDE4 (144).

D. The Profile of PDE4 Inhibitors in Preclinical Models of Disease

Effects on Pulmonary Dynamics

Airway Resistance and Dynamic Compliance

Harris and colleagues (70) reported that rolipram has a potent activity in reversing histamine-induced bronchoconstriction following intravenous infusions into anesthetized guinea pigs. The selective PDE4 inhibitors rolipram and denbufylline are 100–1000 times more potent than theophylline in reversing this histamine-induced bronchoconstriction (70,145). Rolipram also prevents the bronchoconstriction caused by antigen challenge in sensitized guinea pigs (109). In these studies, histamine- or LTD_4-induced bronchoconstriction was not affected by doses of rolipram that completely abolished responses to the antigen. It was suggested, therefore, that rolipram is more likely to reduce bronchoconstriction by inhibiting mast-cell degranulation than through a direct bronchodilator effect (109). Comparison of PDE-selective inhibitors demonstrates that rolipram is significantly more potent than the PDE3 inhibitor CI-930 and that the PDE5 inhibitor zaprinast is inactive against antigen-induced bronchoconstriction in vivo (146,147). Rolipram is also more potent in preventing leukotriene-dependent antigen-induced bronchoconstriction at nonbronchodilator doses, again suggesting that PDE4 regulates the synthesis or release of constrictor mediators (146). Dual inhibition of PDE3 and PDE4 produces an additive or synergistic inhibition of bronchospasm in the guinea pig (147).

To investigate the relationship between PDE4 inhibition and the effects of endogenous catecholamines, studies with adrenalectomized guinea pigs or coadministration of adrenergic receptor blockers has been carried out. Pretreatment of sensitized guinea pigs with the β-blockers propranolol or nadolol resulted in enhanced bronchial reactivity to antigen and an abolition of the inhibitory effects of rolipram on antigen-induced bronchoconstriction (148). Similarly, bilateral adrenalectomy enhanced reactivity and reduced the effects of rolipram. Rolipram did not alter circulating levels of catecholamines in normal animals, indicating that it does not stimulate the adrenals. However, circulating catecholamines are clearly important in regulating responses to antigen as well as in the efficacy of PDE4 inhibitors. When circulating catecholamines are blocked by β-blockers or lowered by adrenalectomy, there is insufficient adenylyl cyclase drive to enable PDE4 inhibitors to elevate intracellular cAMP. The authors of this study speculated that a key activity of the PDE4 inhibitors is their synergy with endogenous catecholamines in suppression of mast-cell degranulation (148).

Many of the studies of the effects of PDE inhibitors on pulmonary dynamics have been carried out in guinea pigs, and there is some concern that there is a greater involvement of endogenous catecholamines in these animals than in other species. An alternative model is the neonatal immunization of rabbits, which has been used as a way of inducing an asthma-like condition in adult animals (149,150). Gozzard and colleagues (151,152) have used this model to comprehensively evaluate the effects of PDE inhibitors on antigen responses in the airways and also to make comparisons with current treatments.

Following neonatal immunization, adult rabbits respond to aerosols of antigen with an acute bronchoconstriction and a late-phase pulmonary inflammation 24 hr after challenge. Theophylline, rolipram, or the corticosteroid budesonide have no bronchodilator properties in this model and do not affect antigen-induced increases in large airway resistance (151,152). Theophylline and rolipram also failed to prevent antigen-induced falls in the dynamic compliance of small airways, whereas budesonide inhibited small-airway changes, indicating an anti-inflammatory effect. CDP840, which is a more potent PDE4 inhibitor than rolipram, reduced antigen-induced changes in both the large and small airways and in these terms gave a therapeutic profile superior to that of budesonide (Fig. 7).

It has been suggested that the best preclinical models of asthma are those in primates where there is a naturally occurring sensitivity to antigens such as Ascaris suum in sub-groups of animals in colonies of monkeys. Exposure of these animals to antigen leads to an IgE-mediated pulmonary insufficiency which has many of the features of human asthma (153). Rolipram failed to prevent ascaris-induced increases in large airway resistance in *Macaca fascicularis* monkeys but did have some anti-inflammatory effects in the late phase (154). The most impressive effects on large airway resistance so far reported for a PDE4 inhibitor have been in ascaris-sensitive squirrel monkeys (155). Oral or intravenous administration of CDP840 to squirrel monkeys produced a marked suppression of antigen-induced acute and late phase (3–6 hr) bronchoconstriction. In this model, bronchoconstriction is largely dependent on endogenous leukotriene production (156) and this indicates that CDP840 (which is not a bronchodilator in the monkey) is working by blocking the synthesis or release of the cysteinyl leukotrienes.

Bronchial Hyperresponsiveness

Asthmatics compared with normals have an increased responsiveness to materials that can produce an increase in resistance to bronchial airflow. This has been most frequently demonstrated with the inhalation of histamine or methacholine. Normal subjects show small increases in bronchial resistance to cumulative doses of methacholine over a wide dose range, whereas asthmatic patients show a characteristic bronchial hyperresponsiveness (BHR) with a lowering in threshold sensitivity, a steepening of the dose-response curve, and an increase in the maximum response (157). In the 1960s, it was widely believed that BHR is a major risk factor for asthma and that asthmatic patients show a deficiency in the inhibitory control of the nervous system to bronchial smooth muscle (158). Although allergic inflammation in the lungs is likely to contribute to the damage associated with BHR, the evidence that BHR can precede inflammation and that removal

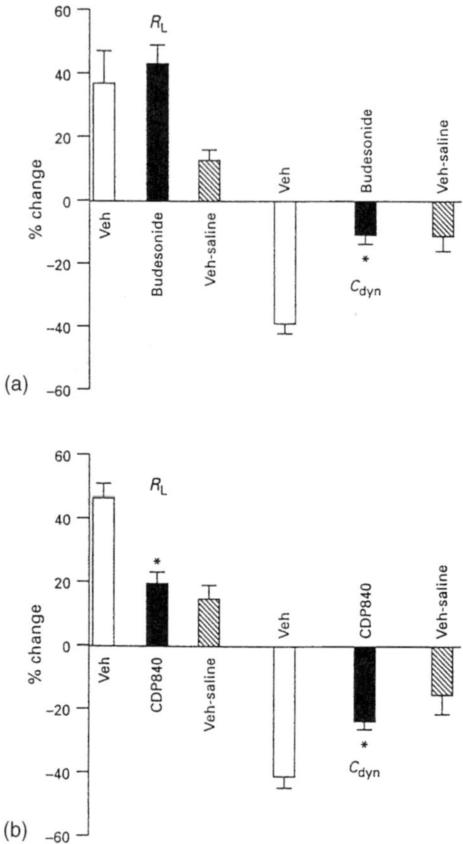

Figure 7 The effects of budesonide (a) or CDP840 (b) on antigen-induced changes in large airway resistance (R_L) and small airway compliance (C_{dyn}) in neonatally sensitized rabbits challenged with antigen. Budesonide (50 μg) was administered by inhalation and CDP840 (1 mg/kg) was given intraperitoneally. The effects of treatment were compared with vehicle controls; *indicates a statistically significant effect. (Data from Ref. 152.)

of inflammation has little effect on BHR give credibility to the theory that a neuronal lesion is a principle factor in the development of asthma (158).

The PDE inhibitors are active in a number of models of BHR. The potent PDE4 inhibitor RP73401 reduces PAF-induced BHR to bombesin in anesthetized guinea pigs (100) and theophylline, rolipram, and CDP840 prevent antigen-induced BHR to histamine in rabbits (151,152). Rolipram and CDP840 but not RP73401 or aminophylline reverse ozone-induced BHR to histamine in guinea pigs (101) (Fig. 8).

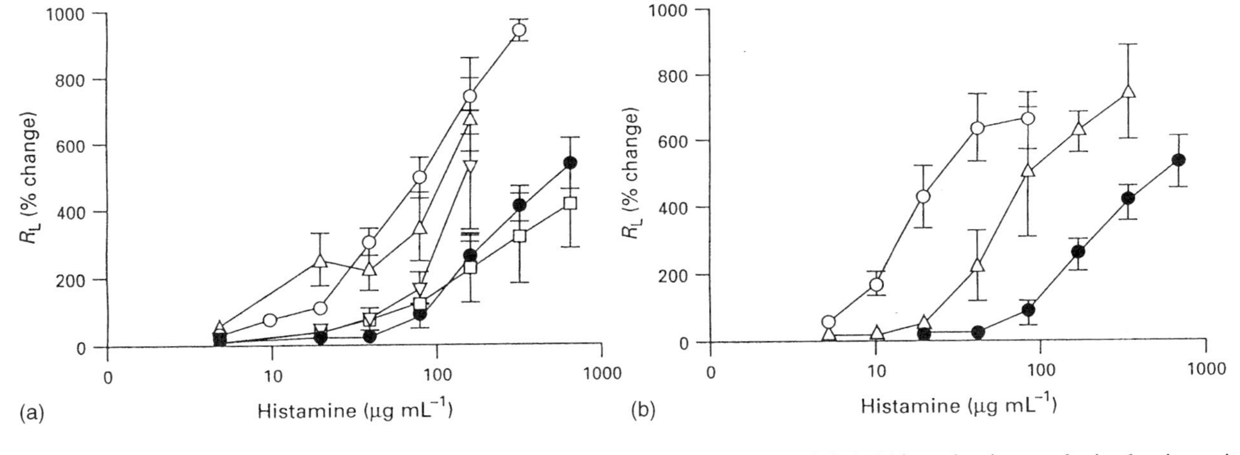

Figure 8 The effect of CDP840 on ozone-induced bronchial hyperresponsiveness to inhaled histamine in anesthetized guinea pigs. In both panels (a and b), the filled circles show the increase in lung resistance caused by histamine in normal guinea pigs; the open circles show the responses to histamine in animals exposed to ozone prior to challenge with histamine. Panel a shows the effects of CDP840 given intraperitoneally at 1 µg/kg (open triangles), 3 µg/kg (open inverted triangles), or 10 µg/kg (open squares). Panel b shows the effect of CDP840 given orally at 100 µg/kg (open triangles). (Data from Ref. 101.)

The tachykinins substance P and neurokinin A are potent bronchoconstrictors and are responsible for vagally mediated noncholinergic bronchoconstriction (51). Tachykinins are released from sensory nerve endings on stimulation, and rolipram but not the PDE3 inhibitor siguazodan or the PDE5 inhibitor zaprinast inhibits excitatory noncholinergic neurotransmission in guinea pig (49) and human (103) bronchi in vitro. Electrically induced nonadrenergic noncholinergic (NANC) contractile responses of guinea pig isolated tracheas are blocked by inhibitors of PDE3, PDE4, and PDE5 but, interestingly, the PDE4 inhibitor Ro 20-1724 failed to inhibit capsaicin-elicited responses (160). The more potent and selective PDE4 inhibitor rolipram inhibits electrically induced contractions and potentiates electrically induced relaxations of isolated trachea (50,161), indicating a regulatory role for cAMP in both excitatory and inhibitory NANC responses in airway tissue.

In anesthetized guinea pigs, CDP840 does not prevent substance P–induced bronchoconstriction but is a potent inhibitor of electrically induced, vagally mediated noncholinergic bronchoconstriction, being approximately equipotent with rolipram (101). It is possible, therefore, that PDE4 is an important regulator of cAMP levels in sensory neurons in the lungs and that this, in turn, influences the release of tachykinins. The effects of PDE4 inhibitors in suppressing noncholinergic bronchoconstriction as well as antigen- or ozone-induced BHR could be through the inhibition of tachykinin release.

Anti-inflammatory Effects

The prediction that PDE4 inhibitors should have anti-inflammatory effects (74,161) has now been substantiated by numerous reports using a variety of preclinical models of inflammatory disease. Most attention has focused on allergic inflammation in the lung, but a number of other nonpulmonary models have been investigated.

The most marked effect on inflammatory leukocytes is seen with the suppression of eosinophil recruitment in vivo. Antigen challenge of sensitized guinea pigs results in the accumulation of inflammatory cells in the lungs, with a high proportion of eosinophils. Rolipram and siguazodan reduce the number of eosinophils in guinea pig bronchial alveolar lavages, but the best effects are seen with the dual PDE3/PDE4 inhibitor zardaverine (109,147). The effects of rolipram on antigen-induced pulmonary eosinophillia in guinea pigs have been confirmed in other studies, and local administration of RP73401 (100) or oral administration of CDP840 (95) produces similar effects. Rolipram also reduces antigen-induced eosinophil accumulation in the lungs of rats (162), rabbits (151), and monkeys (154).

The effects of PDE4 inhibitors on the recruitment of other inflammatory leukocytes are not so clear. In guinea pigs (95,147) or rabbits (151,152), neutrophil and monocyte accumulation following antigen challenge is not significantly changed by rolipram or CDP840; but in rats (162) and monkeys (154) there is an inhibition of neutrophils. Characteristically, the effects of PDE inhibitors on eosinophil migration peak at around 60% inhibition, which indicates that there are some mechanisms of eosinophil accumulation that are not susceptible to regulation by cAMP. There is, however, some evidence that eosinophils that are not prevented from migration by PDE4 inhibitors are in a less activated state. The eosinophils in pleural exudates from CDP840-treated animals contain higher levels of eosinophil peroxidase than cells from control animals, suggesting that PDE4 inhibition has a stabilizing effect on eosinophil degranulation (95).

As well as having a direct effect on leukocytes, there are some reports that PDE inhibitors suppress inflammatory symptoms such as edema. Arachidonic acid–induced ear edema in mice is reduced by rolipram (163). Also, guinea pigs subjected to aerosols of endotoxin develop a pulmonary edema that is inhibited by rolipram, milrinone, or aminophylline (164). Carrageenan-induced paw edema is reduced by PDE4 inhibitors (165), but carrageenan-induced pleural exudates are only weakly inhibited by high doses of rolipram and not at all by CDP840 (95). Histamine-induced vascular leakage in the airway microvasculature is inhibited by PDE4 inhibitors (100).

Some of the effects of PDE inhibitors on inflammatory responses have been attributed to inhibition of cytokine release or action. Intratracheal administration of IL-5 in guinea pigs induces an eosinophilia that is blocked by Ro 20-1724 or theophylline but not by milrinone or zaprinast (166). IL-5-induced pleural eosinophilia in rats is inhibited by CDP840, rolipram, and RP73401 (95). In monkeys, rolipram significantly reduces IL-8 and TNF concentrations in bronchial alveolar lavage fluids following antigen challenge, and this is accompanied by reductions in eosinophil and neutrophil accumulation (154). Furthermore, the reduction by rolipram of carrageenan-induced rat paw edema is associated with suppression of TNF generation in the paw tissues (165).

There are some reports of the effects of PDE inhibitors in models of chronic inflammatory diseases. In adjuvant-induced arthritis in rats, rolipram and another selective PDE4 inhibitor, CP-77059, reduced ankle swelling and radiological evidence of joint damage (165). In collagen type II–induced arthritis in rats, rolipram delayed the onset of disease and markedly suppressed the severity of the response (167). In both of these experiments, there was evidence of TNF suppression.

The effects of rolipram have been investigated in experimental allergic encephalomyelitis (EAE) in rats and monkeys. In rats, rolipram delays the onset and suppresses the severity of the symptoms (168). In monkeys, there is a sustained reduction in clinical EAE, marked inhibition of histopathological changes, and a clear protection against this autoimmune demyelinating condition (169).

Adverse Effects

Rolipram was discovered in the search for phosphodiesterase inhibitors that would elevate cAMP in brain tissues and augment the activity of neurotransmitters (58). A number of preclinical studies indicate that rolipram has antidepressant activity, and the hypothesis was advanced that specific PDE inhibitors act at both pre- and postsynaptic sites to increase norepinephrine turnover and augment neurotransmission (170). This led to the clinical investigation of rolipram as an antidepressant and the comparison of its activity with existing drugs (90,171,172). Rolipram produced a significant antidepressant effect in these studies but was considered inferior in its therapeutic activity to imipramine (90) and amitryptyline (171). All the clinical studies reported that rolipram was well tolerated, and although an incidence of nausea in up to 20% of the patients was recorded, this did not achieve statistical significance in any of the trials. It is often assumed that rolipram was taken out of development because of its emetic properties, but it is just as likely that the lack of a clear advantage over existing therapies was the reason. In any case, emesis was identified as a characteristic of PDE4 inhibitors that would have to be ''designed out'' of any successful drug with this mechanism.

Preclinical and clinical studies have generally suggested that selective PDE4 inhibitors are free from serious adverse side effects. They do not have profound effects on the cardiovascular system in humans or laboratory animals (90,171–173); however, centrally mediated side effects could limit the utility of PDE4 inhibitors. PDE4 is abundantly distributed in the brain, mainly in association with the limbic system (174), and PDE4 inhibitors have been shown to produce behavioral and thermoregulatory effects in rodents (170) and respiratory stimulation in primates (175). It is their potential to induce emesis, however, that has received the most attention.

The xanthine bronchodilators such as theophylline cause nausea and emesis in humans, and this is one of the dose-limiting properties of these drugs (176). Using the ferret as a species susceptible to emetics, the relationship between emetic potency, adenosine antagonism, and PDE inhibition has been investigated (176). There is a close correlation between the rank order of emetic potency and PDE inhibition and no correlation with adenosine antagonism.

Despite the widely held belief that PDE4 inhibitors are emetic in laboratory animals and humans, there are few comprehensive studies addressing this activity and its mechanistic basis. At doses of less than 0.1 mg/kg iv, rolipram induced emesis, anxiety, and behavioral changes in conscious dogs and increased heart rate in anesthetized dogs not treated with a β-adrenoceptor antagonist (177). The cardiovascular effects are apparently related to activity in the central nervous system, since they are associated with a reversal of pentobarbitone-induced anesthesia. In these studies, rolipram was more emetic by the oral route of administration, suggesting an involvement of local intestinal reflexes.

The emetic response in dogs is associated with excitation of area postrema neurons, which trigger the emetic reflex following stimulation of a number of adenylate cyclase–coupled receptors (178). Theophylline, IBMX, and Ro 20-1724 augment these cAMP-dependent effects. The relationship between central and peripheral actions of PDE4 inhibitors has been probed with the use of a novel series of rolipram analogues designed to be relatively poorly taken up in the central nervous system (179). Compounds were synthesized with the objective of reducing binding at the high-affinity site, which is thought to be involved in uptake in the brain, while retaining inhibition of the PDE4 catalytic activity. Substantial reductions in high-affinity binding were accompanied by reductions in emetic potency in the ferret (179).

In a primate model of EAE, relatively high doses of rolipram induce salivation, vomiting, excessive grooming, and head twists, and these side effects are prevented by administration of the 5-HT_3 receptor antagonist ondansetron (169). Partial protection against emesis induced by PDE4 inhibitors in ferrets was also seen with ondansetron or the neurokinin receptor antagonist CP-99,994 (180). It is likely, therefore, that PDE4 inhibitors have mixed activities involving central neurokinin and peripheral 5-HT responses. There is some evidence that peripheral emetogenic activity is linked to PDE4 inhibitor-induced increased gastric acid secretion (89). Rolipram and IBMX but not siguazodan or zaprinast increase acid secretion in rabbit-isolated gastric glands.

With the discovery of multiple isoforms of PDE4 and the possibility that the enzyme adopts different conformations, it is possible that selectivity could be achieved between inhibitors of the PDE4 isoform involved in emesis and the isoforms of PDE4 that are the targets of therapeutic activity. There is, however, no definitive evidence that such selectivity explains the differentials in emetogenic and therapeutic activity already described for a number of PDE4 inhibitors. What is clear is that the new generation of PDE4 inhibitors are more potent than rolipram in inhibiting the catalytic activity of PDE4, have comparable potency to rolipram in reducing inflammatory responses, but are less emetogenic than rolipram (180–183). For example, CDP840 produces a similar anti-inflammatory effect to rolipram in the ferret but is significantly less emetogenic than rolipram in the same species (182). Also, SB 207499 (Ariflo) and rolipram have comparable effects on antigen-induced activation of inflammatory leukocytes, but SB 207499 is 100 times less potent than rolipram in inducing gastric acid secretion (183). In clinical trials with CDP840, there were no reports of nausea or vomiting (184), and recent reports suggest that SB 207499 is also well tolerated in humans (199,200). If these differential effects can be ascribed to isoform selectivity, this will enable the rational optimization of PDE4 inhibitory activity to permit the choice of compounds with the best ratio of therapeutic effects to side effects.

VII. Clinical Trials with PDE4 Inhibitors in Inflammatory Diseases

A. Asthma

A number of novel PDE4 inhibitors have been investigated in clinical asthma and some trials are currently ongoing. There is as yet, however, a lack of published data from these studies. In 1992, the compound tibenelast (LY 186655) was claimed to be a weak PDE inhibitor with putative antiasthma activity in preclinical models (185). Interestingly, this compound had already been evaluated in patients with moderately severe asthma based on its theophylline-like properties (186). Tibenelast reduced spontaneous bronchoconstriction in patients but also caused nausea (186).

The dual PDE3/PDE4 inhibitor AH 21-132 was the first isoform-selective PDE inhibitor to be investigated in humans (187). The drug was, however, given only to healthy volunteers and evaluated for its bronchodilator activity. Intravenous or inhaled administration of AH 21-132 reversed methacholine-induced bronchoconstriction with no effects on blood pressure or pulse rates and no reports of nausea (187). The effects were relatively short-lived, and it may have been considered that the activity offered no advantages over that of existing bronchodilators. There have been no reports of the drug's activity in patients with asthma. Another dual PDE3/PDE4 inhibitor, zardaverine, has been evaluated in asthmatic patients (188). In a group of 12 patients, inhalation of zardaverine produced a modest and short-lasting bronchodilatation, but some patients experienced nausea and vomiting (188).

The most recent clinical studies have been performed using selective PDE4 inhibitors. A preliminary report indicated that RP73401 does not improve pulmonary dynamics after intratracheal installation in 11 asthma patients (189). In a 6-week study in 34 patients, RP 73401 had no bronchodilator effects, did not reduce hyperresponsiveness to methacholine, and had no effects on expired nitric oxide, a measure of inflammation in the lungs (190). RP 73401 given twice a day by inhalation was, however, well tolerated.

The xanthine PDE4 inhibitor LAS 31025 is a bronchodilator (191) and, in a 6-week study, LAS 31025 improved peak flow and reduced asthma episodes when given orally in a slow-release formulation (192).

The evaluation of CDP840 is the most extensive clinical investigation of a selective PDE4 inhibitor in asthma so far published (184). CDP840 (Fig. 5) is a potent PDE4 inhibitor that is orally active in suppressing antigen-induced bronchoconstriction and pulmonary inflammation in guinea pigs, rabbits, and monkeys (95,151,152,155). In ferrets, CDP840 is significantly less emetic than rolipram (182).

A total of 54 asthma patients were recruited to three double-blind, placebo-controlled studies in which orally administered CDP840 was investigated for bronchodilator activity, its effects on histamine-induced bronchoconstriction, and its effects on early and late bronchoconstrictor responses to inhaled antigen (184). CDP840 had no bronchodilator activity or any effect on histamine-induced bronchoconstriction, thus confirming the pre-clinical findings (95). Pretreatment with 15 mg of CDP840 twice a day for 10 days prior to antigen challenge did, however, significantly reduce the late-phase bronchoconstrictor response (Fig. 9), potentially indicating anti-inflammatory activity. None of the patients in any of the studies reported nausea or emesis.

The clinical investigations of CDP840 are relatively limited, since no direct inflammatory parameters were recorded, antigen-induced hyperresponsiveness was not investigated and only one dosing regimen was evaluated. Nonetheless, the drug produced a therapeutic effect at a well-tolerated dose with no nausea. Unconfirmed reports suggest that other investigations of novel rolipram analogues in asthma have been limited by emesis at doses that had no beneficial effects. If this is true, CDP840 is the first of the new generation of selective PDE4 inhibitors to show encouraging effects in asthma. CDP840 is the prototype for a series of selective PDE4 inhibitors being developed by Celltech and Merck.

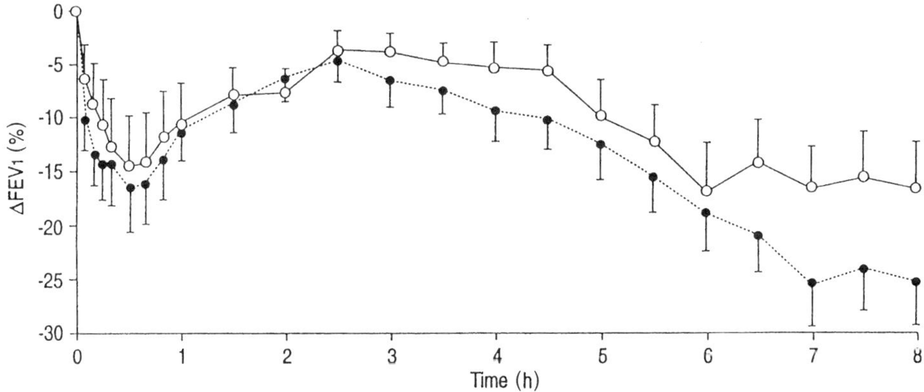

Figure 9 The effect of CDP840 on the responses of a group of 13 asthmatic patients to inhaled antigen. CDP840 was given orally (15 mg twice daily) for 9.5 days prior to antigen challenge. The results are expressed as percentage changes in forced expiratory volume in 1 sec (FEV_1). When the treated group (open circles) was compared with the placebo group (closed circles), the $AUC_{3-8\,hr}$ was 30% less for the treated group than the placebo group ($p = 0.016$). (Data from Ref. 184.)

The metabolism of CDP840 is complex (193); because of this, a backup compound with a superior metabolic profile is being sought for further development.

B. Other Inflammatory Disease

The regulatory control by cAMP on inflammatory leukocyte activation indicates that PDE inhibition is likely to have therapeutic value in other inflammatory conditions as well as asthma. The investigation of these possibilities is somewhat behind the asthma studies in both preclinical and clinical models. Nothetheless, some PDE inhibitors have been evaluated in skin diseases such as psoriasis and atopic dermatitis, and there is one preliminary report of a PDE4 inhibitor in human rheumatoid arthritis.

Papaverine cream produces an improvement in psoriatic lesions that was attributed to cAMP and cGMP PDE inhibition (194), but the selective cAMP PDE inhibitor Ro 20-1724 produces a significantly better effect (195), suggesting that inhibition of PDE4 is the mechanism of action. In these clinical trials, the PDE inhibitors were not as effective as topically applied corticosteroid cream (195); this may explain why there was no further development of Ro 20-1724 for this indication.

More recently, a selective PDE4 inhibitor has been evaluated in human atopic dermatitis (196). The production of PGE_2, IL-4, and IL-10 by peripheral blood leukocytes from patients with atopic dermatitis is greater than in normals. Furthermore, the production of these mediators is more susceptible to inhibition by PDE4 inhibitors in the atopic cells. These in vitro assays were used to evaluate the potency of a number of PDE4 inhibitors prior to the selection of one for clinical testing. Theophylline, rolipram, and Ro 20-1724 show increasing potency in inhibiting PDE activity in atopic mononuclear leukocytes, but CP 80,633 (Fig. 5) was 10–1000 times more potent. Topical application of CP 80,633 causes a significant reduction in erythema, induration, and excoriation of the inflamed skin in patients with atopic dermatitis (196).

The potent inhibition of the synthesis of TNF by some PDE4 inhibitors (115–119) has indicated that this activity may be of benefit in treating arthritic conditions in which TNF is involved (165,167). The efficacy of a TNF-neutralizing monoclonal antibody in human rheumatoid arthritis (197) has validated this target, and a preliminary evaluation of RP 73401 in rheumatoid arthritis shows promising trends to reductions in the numbers of tender joints and disease activity (198).

VIII. Conclusions

There is abundant evidence that elevation of intracellular cAMP suppresses tissue responses in asthma. It is not so clear, however, that Butcher and Sutherland's original contention that theophylline works by this mechanism (4) is correct. The methylxanthines are effective drugs that have a number of properties besides PDE inhibition, and it is difficult to ascribe their therapeutic effects to specific mechanisms with any confidence.

The hypothesis that isoform-selective PDE inhibitors will be effective drugs with advantages of selectivity and potency has yet to be proved. What is clear is that various PDE inhibitors with differing selectivities possess widely different pharmacological profiles. While it is tempting to explain this by differential inhibition of tissue-specific PDE isoforms, there is little definitive evidence to support this theory. Although there are differences in the pharmacological profiles of PDE3 and PDE4 inhibitors that can be related to their isoform selectivity, no such distinction has yet been established for selective inhibitors of the many PDE4 isoforms. While PDE4 inhibitors have therapeutic effects by inhibiting a number of airway and inflammatory responses, often the best activity is achieved only with dual inhibition of PDE3 and PDE4 (70,109,143,147). Furthermore, even the highly selective PDE4 inhibitors still retain adverse side effects; it may be that the role of cAMP is so fundamental and that the PDE isoforms are so widely distributed that the specificity required for a safe, effective drug cannot be achieved.

Lack of specificity need not, however, be a major problem in a class of drugs. The steroids, for example, are highly effective therapeutic agents that interfere with a range of cellular functions, and this broad spectrum of activity accounts for their impressive efficacy. In this regard, it has been argued that the PDE4 inhibitors are a likely alternative to the steroids because they target such pivotal mechanisms in cellular activation. They also offer the possibility of combining reversal of bronchoconstriction with anti-inflammatory activity. The current therapies do not have this combination of effects, and both bronchodilators and steroids have to be inhaled to reduce systemic side effects. An orally active prophylactic drug would be preferable.

There are also a number of encouraging results in the evaluation of PDE4 inhibitors. Compounds that have reduced activity at the high-affinity binding site on the enzyme retain inhibition of catalytic activity but are less emetic (179). Furthermore, a clear differential has been established for some PDE4 inhibitors between anti-inflammatory activity and their adverse effects on gastric acid secretion (183). These two observations offer the possibility of rational optimization of the therapeutic ratio.

As regards efficacy, it is impressive that an orally active PDE4 inhibitor suppresses both acute antigen bronchoconstriction and the late inflammatory phase in conscious monkeys at well-tolerated doses (155). Furthermore, PDE4 inhibitors are potent blockers of bronchial hyperresponsiveness (100,101, 151,152); if this activity can be achieved in patients, it may have a long-term disease-modifying effect. Finally, a therapeutic effect of a PDE4 inhibitor in human asthma has been demonstrated without adverse effects (184).

There is clearly a clinical need for improved asthma therapies, as the incidence of the disease is on the increase. It is possible that the development of well-tolerated PDE4 inhibitors in the next few years will meet that need.

Acknowledgments

We should like to acknowledge helpful discussions with our colleagues in the preparation of this chapter, in particular, Rodger Allen, Ray Owens, Martin Perry, and Graham Warrellow at Celltech and Ian Rodger and Bob Young at Merck Frosst Canada.

Note Added in Proof

Editors note: Since this chapter was written, Phase II clinical trial data with the oral PDE IV inhibitor SB 207,499 (Ariflo) in asthma and in COPD have been published in poster and abstract form (199,200). The reported encouraging effects on lung function and on symptoms suggest that further instalments in this exciting approach to novel treatments for inflammatory lung diseases can be anticipated.

References

1. Robinson GA, Butcher RW, Sutherland EW. Cyclic AMP. Annu Rev Biochem 1968; 37:149–173.
2. Houslay MD, Milligan G. Tailoring cAMP-signalling responses through isoform multiplicity. TIBS 1997; 22:217–224.
3. Salter H. On some points in the treatment and clinical history of asthma. Edinburgh Med J 1859; 4:1109–1115.
4. Butcher RW, Sutherland EW. Adenosine 3′,5′-phosphate in biological materials. J Biol Chem 1962; 237:1244–1250.
5. Thompson WJ, Terasaki WL, Epstein PN, Strada SJ. Assay of cyclic nucleotide phosphodiesterase and resolution of multiple molecular forms of the enzyme. In: Brooker G, Greengard P, Robinson GA, eds. Advances in Cyclic Nucleotide Research. Vol. 10. New York: Raven Press, 1979:69–92.
6. Dale MM, Foreman JC, Fan TD. Textbook of Immunopharmacology. 3d ed. Oxford, UK: Blackwell, 1994.
7. Corrigan CJ, Kay AB. CD4 T-lymphocyte activation in acute severe asthma—relationship to disease severity and atopic status. Am Rev Respir Dis 1990; 141: 970–977.
8. Robinson DS, Hamid Q, Ying S, Tricopo Ulos A, Barkans J, Bentley AM, Corrigan

CJ, Durham SR, Kay AB. Predominant T_{H2}-like bronchoalveolar T-lymphocyte population in atopic asthma. N Engl J Med 1992; 326:298–304.
9. Sanderson CJ, Warren DJ, Strath M. Identification of a lymphokine that stimulates eosinophil differentiation in vitro: its relationship to interleukin-3 and functional properties of eosinophils produced in cultures. J Exp Med 1985; 162:60–65.
10. Coffman RL, Seymour WP, Hudak S, Jackson J, Rennick DM. Antibody to interleukin-5 inhibits helminth-induced eosinophilia in mice. Science 1989; 245:308–310.
11. Howell CJ, Pujol J-L, Crea AEG, Davidson R, Gearing AJH, Godard PH, Lee TH. Identification of an alveolar macrophage-derived activity in bronchial asthma that enhances leukotriene C_4 generation by human eosinophils stimulated by ionophore A23187 as a granulocyte-macrophage colony-stimulating factor. Am Rev Respir Dis 1989; 140:1340–1347.
12. Lellouch-Tubiana A, Lefort J, Simon M-T, Pfister A, Vargaftig BB. Eosinophil recruitment into guinea-pig lungs after PAF-acether and allergen administration. Am Rev Respir Dis 1989; 137:948–954.
13. Sanjar S, Smith D, Kings MA, Morley J. Pretreatment with rhGM-CSF, but not rhIl-3, enhances PAF-induced eosinophil accumulation in guinea-pig airways. Br J Pharmacol 1990; 100:399–400.
14. Jose PJ, Griffiths-Johnson PA, Collins PD, Walsh DT, Moqbel R, Totty NF, Truong O, Hsuan JJ, Williams TJ. Eotaxin: a potent eosinophil chemoattractant cytokine detected in a guinea-pig model of allergic airways inflammation. J Exp Med 1994; 179:881–887.
15. Collins PD, Marleau S, Griffiths-Johnson, DA, Jose PJ, Williams, TJ. Co-operation between interleukin-5 and the chemokine eotaxin to induce eosinophil accumulation in vivo. J Exp Med 1995; 182:1169–1174.
16. Djukanovic R, Roche WR, Wilson JW, Beasley CRW, Twentyman OP, Howarth PH, Holgate ST. Mucosal inflammation in asthma. Am Rev Respir Dis 1990; 142: 434–457.
17. Adelroth E, Rosenhall L, Johannson S-A, Linden M, Venge P. Inflammatory cells and eosinophil activity in asthmatics investigated by bronchoalveolar lavage: the effects of antiasthmatic treatment with budesonide or terbutaline. Am Rev Respir Dis 1990; 142:91–99.
18. Gleich GJ. The eosinophil and bronchial asthma: Current understanding. J Allergy Clin Immunol 1990; 85:422–436.
19. Barnes PJ. Neural and inflammatory peptides: therapeutic prospects in asthma. In: Barnes PJ, ed. New Drugs for Asthma. London: IBC, 1989:149–160.
20. Barnes PJ. Asthma as an axon reflex. Lancet 1986; 1:242–245.
21. Barnes PJ. New Drugs for Asthma. London: IBC, 1989.
22. Peachell PT, MacGlashen DW Jr, Lichtenstein LM, Schleimer RP. Regulation of human basophil and lung mast cell function by cyclic adenosine monophosphate. J Immunol 1988; 140:571–579.
23. Undem BJ, Torphy TJ, Goldman D, Chilton FH. Inhibition by adenosine 3′:5′-monophosphate of eicosanoid and platelet-activating factor biosynthesis in the mouse PT-18 mast cell. J Biol Cem 1990; 265:6750–6758.
24. Roquet A, Dahlen B, Kumlin M, Ihre E, Anstren G, Binks S, Dahlen SE. Combined

antagonism of leukotrienes and histamine produces predominant inhibition of allergen-induced early and late phase airway obstruction in asthmatics. Am J Respir Crit Care Med 1997; 155:1856–1863.
25. Fuller RW, O'Malley G, Baker AJ, MacDermot J. Human alveolar macrophage activation: inhibition by forskolin but not beta-adrenoceptor stimulation or phosphodiesterase inhibition. Pulm Pharmacol 1988; 1:101–106.
26. Beusenberg FD, Van Amsterdam JG, Hoogsteden HC, Hekking PR, Brouwers JW, Schermers HP, Bonta IL. Stimulation of cyclic AMP production in human alveolar macrophages induced by inflammatory mediators and beta-sympathomimetics. Eur J Pharm 1992; 228:57–62.
27. Dent G, Giembycz MA, Rabe KF, Wolf B, Barnes PJ, Magnussen H. Theophylline supresses human alveolar macrophage respiratory burst through phosphodiesterase inhibition. Am J Respir Cell Mol Biol 1994; 10:565–572.
28. Bidani A, Wang CZ, Heming TA. Early effects of smoke inhalation on alveolar macrophage functions. Burns 1996; 22:101–106.
29. Zurier RB, Weissmann G, Hoffstein S, Kammerman S, Tai HH. Mechanisms of lyzosomal enzyme release from human leukocytes: II. Effects of cAMP and cGMP autonomic agonists and agents which effect microtubule function. J Clin Invest 1974; 53:297–309.
30. Kuehl FA Jr, Zanetti ME, Soderman DD, Miller DK, Ham EA. Cyclic AMP-dependent regulation of lipid mediators in white cells: A unifying concept for explaining the efficacy of theophylline in asthma. Am Rev Respir Dis 1987; 136: 210–213.
31. Chilton FH, Schmidt D, Torphy T, Goldman D, Undem B. cAMP inhibits platelet activating factor (PAF) biosynthesis in human neutrophils. FASEB J 1989; 3: A308.
32. Nielson CP, Vestal RE, Sturm RJ, Heaslip R. Effects of selective phosphodiesterase inhibitors on the polymorphonuclear leukocyte respiratory burst. J Allergy Clin Immunol 1990; 86:801–808.
33. Ahmed MU, Hazeki K, Hazeki O, Katada T, Ui M. Cyclic AMP-increasing agents interfere with chemoattractant-induced respiratory burst in neutrophils as a result of the inhibition of phosphatidylinositol 3-kinase rather than receptor-operated Ca^{2+} influx. J Biol Chem 1995; 270:23816–23822.
34. Ottonello L, Morone MP, Dapino P, Dallegri F. Cyclic AMP-elevating agents downregulate the oxidative burst induced by granulocyte-macrophage colony-stimulating factor (GM-CSF) in adherent neutrophils. Clin Exp Immunol 1995; 101: 502–506.
35. Ottonello L, Morone MP, Dapino P, Dallegri F. Tumour necrosis alpha-induced oxidative burst in neutrophils adherent to fibronectin: effects of cyclic AMP-elevating agents. Br J Haematol 1995; 91:566–570.
36. Harvath L, Robbins JD, Russell AA, Seamon KB. cAMP and human neutrophil chemotaxis. Elevation of cAMP differentially affects chemotactic responsiveness. J Immunol 1991; 146:224–232.
37. Derian CK, Santulli RJ, Rao PE, Solomon HF, Barrett JA. Inhibition of chemotactic peptide-induced neutrophil adhesion to vascular endothelium by cAMP modulators. J Immunol 1995; 154:308–317.

38. Dent G, Giembycz MA, Barnes PJ. Inhibition of eosinophil oxygen radical production by type IV but not type III-selective cAMP phosphodiesterase inhibitors. Br J Pharmacol 1990; 99:165P.
39. Souness JE, Carter CM, Diocee BK, Hassall GK, Wood LJ, Turner NC. Characterisation of guinea-pig eosinophil phosphodiesterase activity: assessment of its involvement in regulating superoxide generation. Biochem Pharmacol 1991; 42: 937–945.
40. Kaneko T, Alvarez R, Ueki IF, Nadel JA. Elevated intracellular cyclic AMP inhibits chemotaxis in human eosinophils. Cell Signal 1995; 7:527–534.
41. Hatzelmann A, Tenor H, Schudt C. Differential effects of non-selective phosphodiesterase inhibitors on human eosinophil functions. Br J Pharmacol 1995; 114:821–831.
42. Tenor H, Hatzelmann A, Church MK, Schudt C, Shute JK. Effects of theophylline and rolipram on leukotriene C_4 (LTC_4) synthesis and chemotaxis of human eosinophils from normal and atopic subjects. Br J Pharmacol 1996; 118:1727–1735.
43. Knudsen TE, Larsen CS, Johnsen HE. A study of cyclic nucleotides as second messengers after interleukin-2 stimulation of human T lymphocytes. Scand J Immunol 1987; 25:527–531.
44. Mary D, Aussel C, Ferrua B, Fehlmann M. Regulation of interleukin-2 synthesis by cAMP in human T cells. J Immunol 1987; 139:1179–1184.
45. Kaminuma O, Mori A, Suko M, Kikkawa H, Ikezawa K, Okudaira H. Interleukin-5 production by peripheral blood mononuclear cells of asthmatic patients is suppressed by T-440: relation to phosphodiesterase inhibition. J Pharm Exp Ther 1996; 279:240–246.
46. Krishna MT, Gristwood R, Higgs GA, Holgate ST. Phosphodiesterase inhibitors. In: Austen KF, Burakoff SJ, Rosen FS, Strom TB, eds. Therapeutic Immunology. Cambridge, MA: Blackwell, 1996:170–178.
47. Souness JE, Diocee BK, Martin W, Moodie SA. Pig aortic endothelial-cell cyclic nucleotide phophodiesterases. Biochem J 1990; 266:127–132.
48. McCrea KE, Hill SJ. Salmeterol, a long-acting β_2-adrenoceptor agonist mediating cyclic AMP accumulation in a neuronal cell line. Br J Pharmacol 1993; 110:619–626.
49. Qian Y, Girard V, Martin CAE, Molimard M, Advenier C. Rolipram but not siguazodan or zaprinast, inhibits the excitatory non-cholinergic neurotransmission in guinea-pig bronchi. Eur Respir J 1994; 7:306–310.
50. Fernandez LB, Ellis JL, Undem BJ. Potentiation of nonadrenergic noncholinergic relaxation of human isolated bronchus by selective inhibitors of phosphodiesterase isozymes. Am J Respir Crit Care Med 1994; 150:1384–1390.
51. Stretton D. Non-adrenergic non-cholinergic neural control of the airways. Clin Exp Pharmacol Physiol 1991; 18:675–684.
52. Wells JN, Hardman JG. Cyclic nucleotide phosphodiesterases. Adv Cyclic Nucl Res 1977; 8:119–143.
53. Weishaar RE, Burrows SD, Kobylarz DC, Quade DC, Evans DB. Multiple molecular forms of cyclic nucleotide phosphodiesterase in cardiac and smooth muscle and in platelets. Biochem Pharmacol 1986; 35:787–800.

54. Beavo JA. Multiple isozymes of cyclic nucleotide phosphodiesterase. Adv Second Messenger Phosphoprotein Res 1988; 22:1–38.
55. Beavo JA, Reifsnyder DH. Primary sequence of cyclic nucleotide phosphodiesterase isozymes and the design of selective inhibitors. TIPS 1990; 11:150–155.
56. Thompson WJ, Appleman MM. Characterisation of cyclic nucleotide phosphodiesterases of rat tissues. J Biol Chem 1971; 246:3145–3150.
57. Weishaar RE, Cain MH, Bristol JA. A new generation of phosphodiesterase inhibitors: Multiple molecular forms of phosphodiesterases and the potential for drug selectivity. J Med Chem 1985; 28:537–545.
58. Schwabe U, Miyake M, Ohaja Y, Daly JW. 4-(3-Cyclopentyloxy-4-methoxy)-2-pyrolidone (ZK 62711): a potent inhibitor of adenosine cyclic 3′5′-mono-phosphate phosphodiesterase in homogenates and tissue slices from rat brain. Mol Pharmacol 1976; 12:900–910.
59. Beavo JA. Phosphodiesterases. Physiol Rev 1996; 75:725–748.
60. Michaeli T, Bloom TJ, Martins T, Loughney K, Ferguson K, Riggs M, Rodgers L, Beavo JA, Wigler M. Isolation ans characterization of a previously undetected human cAMP phosphodiesterase by complementation of cAMP phosphodiesterase-deficient *Saccharomyces cerevisiae*. J Biol Chem 1993; 268:12925–12932.
61. Byers D, Davis RL, Kiger JA. Defect in cyclic AMP phosphodiesterase due to the dunce mutation of learning in *Drosophila melanogaster*. Nature 1981; 289:79–81.
62. Chen CN, Denome S, Davis RL. Molecular analysis of cDNA clones and the corresponding genomic coding sequences of the Drosophila dunce+ gene, the structural gene for cAMP phosphodiesterase. Proc Natl Acad Sci USA 1986; 83:9313–9317.
63. Sass P, Field J, Nikawa J, Toda T, Wigler M. Cloning and characterization of the high-affinity cAMP phosphodiesterase of *Saccharomyces cerevisiae*. Proc Natl Acad Sci USA 1986; 83:9303–9307.
64. Charbonneau H, Beier N, Walsh KA, Beavo JA. Identification of a conserved domain among cyclic nucleotide phosphodiesterases from diverse species. Proc Natl Acad Sci USA 1986; 83:9308–9312.
65. Qiu YH, Chen CN, Malone T, Richter L, Beckendorf SK, Davis RL. Characterization of the memory gene dunce of *Drosophila melanogaster*. J Mol Biol 1991; 222: 553–565.
66. Swinnen JV, Joseph DR, Conti M. The mRNA encoding a high-affinity cAMP phosphodiesterase is regulated by hormones and cAMP. Proc Natl Acad Sci USA 1989; 86:8197–8201.
67. Colicelli J, Birchmeier C, Michaeli T, O'Neill K, Riggs M, Wigler M. Isolation and characterization of a mammalian gene encoding a high affinity cAMP phosphodiesterase. Proc Natl Acad Sci USA 1989; 86:3599–3603.
68. Livi GP, Kmetz P, McHale MM, Cieslinski LB, Sathe GM, Taylor DP, Davis RL, Torphy TJ, Balcarek JM. Cloning and expression of cDNA for a human low-Km, rolipram-sensitive cyclic AMP phosphodiesterase. Mol Cell Biol 1990; 10:2678–2686.
69. Hall IP, Donaldson J, Hill SJ. Inhibition of histamine stimulated inositol phospholipid hydrolysis by agents which increase cAMP levels in bovine tracheal smooth muscle. Br J Pharmacol 1989; 97:603–613.

70. Harris AL, Connell MJ, Ferguson EW, Wallace AM, Gordon RJ, Pagani ED, Silver PJ. Role of low Km cAMP phosphodiesterase inhibition in tracheal relaxation and bronchodilation in the guinea-pig. J Pharmacol Exp Ther 1989; 251:199–206.
71. Nicholson CD, Challis RAJ, Shahid M. Differential modulation of tissue function and therapeutic potential of selective inhibitors of cyclic nucleotide phosphodiesterase isoenzymes. TIPS 1991; 12:19–27.
72. Weishaar RE, Kobylarz-Singer DC, Steffen RP, Kaplan HR. Subclasses of cyclic AMP-specific phosphodiesterase in left ventricular muscle and their involvement in regulating myocardial contractility. Circ Res 1987; 61:539–547.
73. England PJ, Shahid M. Effects of forskolin on contractile responses and protein phosphorylation in the isolated perfused rat heart. Biochem J 1987; 246:687–695.
74. Torphy TJ, Undem BJ. Phosphodiesterase inhibitors: new opportunities for the treatment of asthma. Thorax 1991; 46:512–523.
75. Monaco L, Vicini E, Conti M. Structure of two rat genes coding for closely related rolipram-sensitive cAMP phosphodiesterases: multiple mRNA variants originate from alternative splicing and multiple start sites. J Biol Chem 1994; 269:347–357.
76. Bolger G, Michaeli T, Martins T, St. John T, Steiner B, Rodgers L, Riggs M, Wigler M, Ferguson K. A family of human phosphodiesterases homologous to the dunce learning and memory gene product of *Drosophila melanogaster* are potential targets for antidepressant drugs. Mol Cell Biol 1993; 13:6558–6571.
77. Torphy TJ, Stadel JM, Burman M, Cielinski LB, McLaughlin MM, White JR, Livi GP. Coexpression of human cAMP-specific phosphodiesterase activity and high affinity rolipram binding in yeast. J Biol Chem 1992; 267:1798–1804.
78. Jacobitz S, Mclaughlin MM, Livi GP, Burman M, Torphy TJ. Mapping the functional domains of human recombinant phosphodiesterase 4A: structural requirements for catalytic activity and rolipram binding. Mol Pharmacol 1996; 50:891–899.
79. Owens RJ, Catterall C, Batty D, Jappy J, Russell A, Smith B, O'Connell J, Perry M. Human phosphodiesterase 4A: characterization of full-length and truncated enzymes expressed in COS cells. Biochem J 1997; 326:53–60.
80. Souness JE, Maslen C, Webber S, Foster M, Raeburn D, Palfreyman MN, Ashton MJ, Karlsson J-A. Suppression of eosinophil function by RP73401, a potent and selective inhibitor of cyclic AMP-specific phosphodiesterase: comparison with rolipram. Br J Pharmacol 1995; 115:39–46.
81. Muller T, Engels P, Fozard JR. Subtypes of the type 4 cAMP phosphodiesterases: structure, regulation and selective inhibition. TIPS 1996; 17:294–298.
82. Polson JB, Krzanowski JJ, Goldman AL, Scentivanyi A. Inhibition of human phosphodiesterase activity by therapeutic levels of theophylline. Clin Exp Pharmacol 1978; 5:536–539.
83. Finnerty JP, Holgate ST. Critical evaluation of the therapeutic efficacy of methylxanthine derivatives in asthma. In: Vane JR, Higgs GA, Marsico SA, Nistico G, eds. Asthma: Basic Mechanisms and Therapeutic Perspectives. Rome-Milan: Pythagora Press, 1989:193–222.
84. Mentzer RM, Rubio R, Berne RM. Release of adenosine by hypoxic canine lung tissue and its possible role in pulmonary circulation. Am J Physiol 1975; 229:1625–1631.

85. Nyce JW, Metzger WJ. DNA antisense therapy for asthma in an animal model. Nature 1997; 385:721–725.
86. Nicholson CD. Pharmacology of nootropics and metabolically active compounds in relation to their use in dementia. Psychopharmacology 1990; 101:147–159.
87. Bou J, Beleta J, Llupia J, Miralpeix M, Cardelus I, Domenech T, Puig J, Salcedo C, Gras J, Fernandez AG, Llenas J, Berga P, Gristwood RW, Palacios JM. Pharmacological characterisation of LAS 31025: A new type 4 selective cyclic nucleotide phosphodiesterase inhibitor with antiasthmatic potential. Third International Conference on Cyclic Nucleotide Phosphodiesterases. Glasgow, July 1996; Abstr. 84.
88. Hughes B, Owens R, Perry M, Warrellow G, Allen R. PDE4 inhibitors: the use of molecular cloning in the design and development of novel drugs. Drug Discovery Today 1997; 2:89–101.
89. Barnette MS, Grous M, Cieslinski LB, Burman M, Christensen SB, Torphy TJ. Inhibitors of phosphodiesterase IV (PDE IV) increase acid secretion in rabbit isolated gastric glands: correlation between function and interaction with a high affinity rolipram binding site. J Pharm Exp Ther 1995; 273:1396–1402.
90. Hebenstreit GF, Fellerer K, Fichte K, Fischer G, Geyer N, Meya U, Sastre-y-Hernandez M, Schony W, Schratzer M, Soukop W, Trampitsch E, Varosanec S, Zawada E, Zochling R. Rolipram in major depressive disorder: Results of a double-blind comparative study with imipramine. Pharmacopsychiatry 1989; 22:156–160.
91. Saccomano NA, Vinick FJ, Koe BK, Nielsen JA, Whalen WM, Meltz M, Phillips D, Thaidieo PF, Jung S, Chapin DS, Lebel LA, Russo LL, Helweg DA, Johnson JL, Ives JL, Williams IH. Calcium-independent phosphodiesterase inhibitors as putative antidepressants: [3-(Bicycloalkyloxy)-4-methoxyphenyl]-2-imidazolidinones. J Med Chem 1991; 34:291–298.
92. Lowe JA, Archer RL, Chapin DS, Cheng JB, Helweg D, Johnson JL, Koe BK, Lebel LA, Moore PF, Nielsen JA, Russo LL, Shirley JT. Structure-activity relationship of quinazolinedione inhibitors of calcium-independent phosphodiesterase. J Med Chem 1991; 34:624–628.
93. Ashton MJ, Cook DC, Fenton G, Karlsson J-A, Palfreyman MN, Raeburn D, Ratcliffe AJ, Souness JE, Thurairatnam S, Vicker N. Selective type IV phosphodiesterase inhibitors as antiasthmatic agents: the synthesis and biological activities of 3-(Cyclopentyloxy)-4-methoxybenzamides and analogues. J Med Chem 1994; 37:1696–1703.
94. Feldman PL, Brackeen MF, Cowan DJ, Marron BE, Schoenen FJ, Stafford JA, Suh EM, Domanico PL, Rose D, Leesnitzer MA, Brawley ES, Strickland AB, Verghese MW, Connolly KM, Bateman-Fite R, Noel LS, Sekut L, Stimpson SA. Phosphodiesterase type IV inhibition: Structure-activity relationships of 1,3-disubstituted pyrrolidines. J Med Chem 1995; 38:1505–1510.
95. Hughes B, Howat D, Lisle H, Holbrook M, James T, Gozzard N, Blease K, Hughes P, Kingaby R, Warrellow G, Alexander R, Head J, Boyd E, Eaton M, Perry M, Wales M, Smith B, Owens R, Catterall C, Lumb S, Russell A, Allen R, Merrimam M, Bloxham D, Higgs G. The inhibition of antigen-induced eosinophilia and bronchoconstriction by CDP840, a novel stereo-selective inhibitor of phosphodiesterase type 4. Br J Pharmacol 1996; 118:1183–1191.

96. Chu SS. Bronchodilators: Part I. Adrenergic drugs. Drugs Today 1984; 20:439–464.
97. Chu SS. Bronchodilators: Part II. Methylxanthines. Drugs Today 1984; 20:509–527.
98. Polson JB, Krzanowski JJ, Szentivanyi A. Inhibition of a high affinity cAMP phosphodiesterase and relaxation of canine tracheal smooth muscle. Biochem Pharmacol 1982; 31:3403–3406.
99. Newman DJ, Colella DF, Spainhour DC, Brann EG, Zabko-Potapovich B, Wardell JR. cAMP phosphodiesterase inhibitors and tracheal smooth muscle relaxation. Biochem Pharmacol 1978; 27:729–732.
100. Raeburn D, Underwood SL, Lewis SA, Woodman VR, Battram CH, Tomkinson A, Sharma S, Jordan R, Souness JE, Webber SE, Karlsson JA. Anti-inflammatory and bronchodilator properties of RP73401, a novel and selective phosphodiesterase type 4 inhibitor. Br J Pharmacol 1994; 113:1423–1431.
101. Holbrook M, Gozzard N, James T, Higgs G, Hughes B. Inhibition of bronchospasm and ozone-induced airway hyperresponsiveness in the guinea-pig by CDP840, a novel phosphodiesterase type 4 inhibitor. Br J Pharmacol 1996; 118:1192–1200.
102. Tomkinson A, Karlsson J-A, Raeburn D. Comparison of the effects of selective inhibitors of phosphodiesterase types III and IV in airway smooth muscle with differing beta-adrenoceptor subtypes. Br J Pharmacol 1993; 108:57–61.
103. Qian Y, Naline E, Karlsson J-A, Raeburn D, Advenier C. Effects of rolipram and siguazodan on the human isolated bronchus and their interaction with isoprenaline and sodium nitroprusside. Br J Pharmacol 1993; 109:774–778.
104. Planquois JM, Ruffin-Morin Y, Lagente V, Payne AN, Dahl SG. Salbutamol potentiates the relaxant effects of selective phosphodiesterase inhibitors on guinea-pig isolated trachea. Fundam Clin Pharmacol 1996; 10:356–367.
105. Stevens RL, Austen KF. Recent advances in the cellular and molecular biology of mast cells. Immunol Today 1989; 10:381–386.
106. Costello PS, Turner M, Walters AE, Cunningham CN, Bauer PH, Downward J, Tybulewicz VLJ. Critical role for the tyrosine kinase Syk in signalling through the high affinity IgE receptor of mast cells. Oncogene 1996; 13:2595–2605.
107. Tenor H, Schudt C. Analysis of PDE isoenzyme profiles in cells and tissues by pharmacological methods. In: Phosphodiesterase Inhibitors. New York: Academic Press, 1996:21–40.
108. Weston MC, Anderson N, Peachell PT. Effects of phosphodiesterase inhibitors on human lung mast cell and basophil function. Br J Pharmacol 1997; 121:287–295.
109. Underwood DC, Osborn RR, Novak LB, Matthews JK, Newsholme SJ, Undem BJ, Hand JM, Torphy TJ. Inhibition of antigen-induced bronchoconstriction and eosinophil infiltration in the guinea-pig by the cyclic AMP-specific phosphodiesterase inhibitor, rolipram. J Pharm Exp Ther 1993; 266:306–313.
110. Elliott KRF, Leonard EJ. Interactions of formylmethionyl-leucyl-phenylalanine, adenosine, and phosphodiesterase inhibitors in human monocytes. FEBS Lett 1989; 254:94–98.
111. Truong VH, Muller T. Isolation, biochemical characterization and N-terminal sequence of rolipram-sensitive cAMP phosphodiesterase from human mononuclear leukocytes. FEBS Lett 1994; 353:113–118.

112. Turner NC, Wood LJ, Burns FM, Gueremy T, Souness JE. The effect of cyclic AMP and cyclic GMP phosphodiesterase inhibitors on the superoxide burst of guinea-pig peritoneal macrophages. Br J Pharmacol 1993; 108:876–883.
113. Banner KH, Moriggi E, Da Ros B, Schioppacassi G, Semeraro C, Page CP. The effect of selective phosphodiesterase 3 and 4 isoenzyme inhibitors and established anti-asthma drugs on inflammatory cell activation. Br J Pharmacol 1996; 119: 1255–1261.
114. Endres S, Fulle H-J, Sinha B, Stoll C, Dinarello CA, Gerzer R, Weber PC. Cyclic nucleotides differentially regulate the synthesis of tumour necrosis factor-α and interleukin-1β by human mononuclear cells. Immunology 1991; 72:56–60.
115. Molnar-Kimber KL, Yonno L, Heaslip RJ, Weichman BM. Differential regulation of TNF-α and Il-1β production from stimulated human monocytes by phosphodiesterase inhibitors. Med Inflam 1992; 1:411–417.
116. Schade FU, Schudt C. The specific type III and IV phosphodiesterase inhibitor zardaverine suppresses formation of tumor necrosis factor by macrophages. Eur J Pharmacol 1993; 230:9–14.
117. Verghese MW, McConnell RT, Strickland AB, Gooding RC, Stimpson SA, Yarnall DP, Taylor JD, Furdon PJ. Differential regulation of human monocyte-derived TNFα and Il-1β by type IV cAMP-phosphodiesterase (cAMP-PDE) inhibitors. J Pharmacol Exp Ther 1995; 272:1313–1320.
118. Kambayashi T, Jacob CO, Zhou D, Mazurek N, Fong M, Strassmann G. Cyclic nucleotide phosphodiesterase type IV participates in the regulation of IL-10 and in the subsequent inhibition of TNF and IL-6 release by endotoxin-stimulated macrophages. J Immunol 1995; 155:4909–4916.
119. Allen R, Rapecki S, Higgs G. The role of Il-10 in the inhibition of LPS-mediated TNFα release from human PBMCs by phosphodiesterase 4 (PDE4) inhibitors. Inflam Res 1997; 46:S218.
120. Essayan DM, Huang SK, Kagey-Sobotka A, Lichtenstein LM. Effects of nonselective and isozyme selective cyclic nucleotide phosphodiesterase inhibitors on antigen-induced cytokine gene expression in peripheral blood mononuclear cells. Am J Respir Cell Mol Biol 1995; 13:692–702.
121. Cheng JB, Watson JW, Pazoles CJ, Eskra JD, Griffiths RJ, Cohan VL, Turner CR, Showell HJ, Pettipher ER. The phosphodiesterase type 4 (PDE4) inhibitor CP-80633 elevates plasma cyclic AMP levels and decreases tumour necrosis factor-α production in mice: effect of adrenalectomy. J Pharm Exp Ther 1997; 280:621–626.
122. Pettipher ER, Eskra JD, Labasi JM. The inhibitory effect of rolipram on TNF-α production in mouse blood ex vivo is dependent upon the release of cortisone and adrenaline. Cytokine 1997; 9:582–586.
123. de Moraes VLG, Singer M, Vargaftig BB, Chignard M. Effects of rolipram on cyclic AMP levels in alveolar macrophages and lipopolysaccharide-induced inflammation in mouse lung. Br J Pharmacol 1998; 123:631–636.
124. Nourshargh S, Hoult JRS. Inhibition of human neutrophil degranulation by forscolin in the presence of phosphodiesterase inhibitors. Eur J Pharmacol 1986; 122: 205–212.
125. Bloemen PG, van der Tweel MC, Henricks PA, Engels F, Kester MH van der Loo

PG, Blomjous FJ, Nijkamp FP. Increased cAMP levels in stimulated neutrophils inhibit their adhesion to human bronchial epithelial cells. Am J Physiol 1997; 272: L580–L587.
126. Fonteh AN, Winkler JD, Torphy TJ, Heravi J, Chilton FH. Influence of isopreterenol and phosphodiesterase inhibitors on platelet-activating factor biosynthesis in the human neutrophil. J Immunol 1993; 151:339–350.
127. Schudt C, Winder S, Forderkunz S, Hatzelmann A, Ulrich V. Influence of selective phosphodiesterase inhibitors on human neutrophil functions and levels of cAMP and Ca_i. Naunyn Schmiedebergs Arch Pharmacol 1991; 344:682–690.
128. Zalavary S, Stendahl O, Bengtsson T. The role of cAMP, calcium and filamentous actin in adenosine modulation of Fc receptor-mediated phagocytosis in human neutrophils. Biochim Biophys Acta 1994; 1222:249–256.
129. Berends C, Dijkhuizen B, deMonchy JG, Dubois AE, Gerritsen J, Kauffman HF. Inhibition of PAF-induced expression of CD11b and shedding of L-selectin on human neutrophils and eosinophils by the type IV selective PDE inhibitor rolipram. Eur Respir J 1997; 10:1000–1007.
130. Dent G, Giembycz MA, Evans PM, Rabe KF, Barnes PJ. Suppression of human eosinophil burst and cyclic AMP hydrolysis by inhibitors of type IV phosphodiesterase: interaction with the beta adrenoceptor agonist albuterol. J Pharmacol Exp Ther 1994; 271:1167–1174.
131. Barnette MS, Manning CD, Cieslinski LB, Burman M, Christensen SB, Torphy TJ. The ability of phosphodiesterase IV inhibitors to suppress superoxide production in guinea pig eosinophils is correlated with inhibition of phosphodiesterase IV catalytic activity. J Pharm Exp Ther 1995; 273:674–679.
132. Alves AC, Pires AL, Cruz HN, Serra MF, Diaz BL, Cordeiro RS, Lagente V, Martins MA. Selective inhibition of phosphodiesterase type IV suppresses the chemotactic responsiveness of rat eosinophils in vitro. Eur J Pharmacol 1996; 312:89–96.
133. Tool AT, Mul FP, Knol EF, Verhoeven AJ, Roos D. The effect of salmeterol and nimesulide on chemotaxis and synthesis of PAF and LTC_4 by human eosinophils. Eur Respir J Suppl 1996; 22:141s–145s.
134. Nicholson CD, Shahid M, Bruin J, Barron E, Spiers I, de Boer J, van Amsterdam RG, Zaagsma J, Kelly JJ, Dent L. Characterization of ORG 20241, a combined phosphodiesterase IV/III cyclic nucleotide phosphodiesterase inhibitor for asthma. J Pharmacol Exp Ther 1995; 274:678–687.
135. Epstein PM, Hachisu R. Cyclic nucleotide phosphodiesterase in normal and leukaemic human lymphocytes and lymphoblasts. Adv Cyclic Nucleotide Protein Phosphoryl Res 1984; 16:303–324.
136. Robiscek SA, Krzanowski JJ, Szentivanyi A, Polson JB. High pressure chromatography of cyclic nucleotide phosphodiesterase from purified human T lymphocytes. Biochem Biophys Res Commun 1989; 163:554–560.
137. Robiscek SA, Blanchard DK, Djeu JY, Krzanowski JJ, Szentivanyi A, Polson JB. Multiple high affinity cAMP phosphodiesterases in human T-lymphocytes. Biochem Pharmacol 1991; 42:869–877.
138. Bloom TJ, Beavo JA. Identification of type VII PDE in HUT T-lymphocyte cells. FASEB J 1994; 8:A372.

139. Van Tits LJH, Michel MC, Motulsky HJ, Maisel AS, Brodde O-E. Cyclic AMP counteracts mitogen-induced inositol phosphate generation and increases in intracellular Ca^{2+} concentrations in human lymphocytes. Br J Pharmacol 1991; 103: 1288–1294.
140. Lacour M, Arrighi J-F, Muller KM, Carlberg C, Saurat J-H, Hauser C. cAMP upregulates IL-4 and IL-5 production from activated $CD4^+$ T cells while decreasing IL-2 release and NF-AT induction. Int Immunol 1994; 6:1333–1343.
141. Bruynzeel I, van der Raaij LM, Willemze R, Stoof TJ. Pentoxyphylline inhibits human T-cell adhesion to dermal endothelial cells. Arch Derm Res 1997; 289:189–193.
142. Essayan DM, Kagey-Sobotka A, Lichtenstein LM, Huang S-K. Differential regulation of human antigen-specific Th1 and Th2 lymphocyte responses by isozyme selective cyclic nucleotide phosphodiesterase inhibitors. J Pharm Exp Ther 1997; 282:505–512.
143. Giembycz MA, Corrigan CJ, Seybold J, Newton R, Barnes PJ. Identification of cyclic AMP phosphodiesterases 3, 4 and 7 in human $CD4^+$ $CD8^+$ T-lymphocytes: role in regulating proliferation and the biosynthesis of interleukin-2. Br J Pharmacol 1996; 118:1945–1958.
144. Souness JE, Houghton C, Sardar N, Withnall MT. Evidence that cyclic AMP phosphodiesterase inhibitors suppress interleukin-2 release from murine splenocytes by interacting with a ''low-affinity'' phosphodiesterase 4 conformer. Br J Pharmacol 1997; 121:743–750.
145. Cortijo J, Bou J, Beleta I, Cardelus J, Llenas J, Morcillo E, Gristwood RW. Investigation into the role of phosphodiesterase IV in bronchorelaxation, including studies with human bronchus. Br J Pharmacol 1993; 108:562–568.
146. Howell RE, Sickels BD, Woeppel SL. Pulmonary antiallergic and bronchodilator effects of isozyme-selective phosphodiesterase inhibitors in guinea-pigs. J Pharm Exp Ther 1993; 264:609–615.
147. Underwood DC, Kotzer CJ, Bochnowicz S, Osborn RR, Luttmann MA, Hay DWP, Torphy TJ. Comparison of phosphodiesterase III, IV and dual III/IV inhibitors on bronchospasm and pulmonary eosinophil influx in guinea-pigs. J Pharmacol Exp Ther 1994; 270:250–259.
148. Underwood DC, Matthews JK, Osborn RR, Bochnowicz S, Torphy TJ. The influence of endogenous catecholamines on the inhibitory effects of rolipram against early and late phase response to antigen in the guinea-pig. J Pharmacol Exp Ther 1997; 280:210–219.
149. Larsen GL, Wilson MC, Clark ARF, Behrens BL. The inflammatory reaction in the airways of an animal model of the late asthmatic response. Fed Proc 1987; 46: 105–112.
150. Minshall EM, Riccio MM, Herd CM, Douglas GJ, Seeds EAM, McKenniff MG, Saski M, Spina D, Page CP. A novel animal model for investigating persistent airway hyperresponsiveness. J Pharmacol Toxicol Meth 1993; 30:177–188.
151. Gozzard N, Herd CM, Blake SM, Holbrook M, Hughes B, Higgs GA, Page CP. Effects of the non-selective phosphodiesterase inhibitor theophylline and a phosphodiesterase type 4 inhibitor rolipram on antigen-induced airway responses in neonatally immunised rabbits. Br J Pharmacol 1996; 117:1405–1412.

152. Gozzard N, El-Hashim A, Herd CM, Blake SM, Holbrook M, Hughes B, Higgs GA, Page CP. Effect of the glucocorticosteroid budesonide and a novel phosphodiesterase type 4 inhibitor CDP840 on antigen-induced airway responses in neonatally immunised rabbits. Br J Pharmacol 1996; 118:1201–1208.
153. Turner CR, Andresen CJ, Smith WB, Watson JW. Characterization of a primate model of asthma using anti-allergy/anti-asthma agents. Inflam Res 1996; 45:239–245.
154. Turner DR, Andresen CJ, Smith WB, Watson JW. Effects of rolipram on responses to acute and chronic antigen exposure in monkeys. Am J Respir Crit Care Med 1994; 149:1153–1159.
155. Jones TR, McAuliffe M, McFarlane C, Piechuta H, MacDonald D, Rodger IW. Effects of a selective PDE IV inhibitor (CDP840) in a leukotriene-dependent nonhuman primate model of allergic asthma. Am J Respir Crit Care Med 1996; 153: A346.
156. McFarlane CS, McAuliffe M, Piechuta H, Jones TR, Rodger IW. Effects of MK-0476, a potent and selective leukotriene D_4 receptor antagonist, on ascaris antigen-induced early and late phase airway responses in conscious squirrel monkeys. Am J Respir Crit Care Med 1994; 149:A533.
157. O'Connor G, Sparrow D, Taylor D, Segal M, Weiss S. Analysis of dose-response curves to methacholine: an approach suitable for population studies. Am Rev Respir Dis 1987; 136:1412–1417.
158. Smith H. Asthma, inflammation, eosinophils and bronchial hyperresponsiveness in asthma. Clin Exp Allergy 1992; 22:187–197.
159. Spina D, Harrison S, Page CP. Regulation by phosphodiesterase isoenzymes of non-adrenergic non-cholinergic contraction in guinea-pig isolated main bronchus. Br J Pharmacol 1995; 116:2334–2340.
160. Undem BJ, Meeker SN, Chen J. Inhibition of neurally mediated nonadrenergic, noncholinergic contractions of guinea-pig bronchus by isozyme-selective phosphodiesterase inhibitors. J Pharmacol Exp Ther 1994; 271:811–817.
161. Giembycz MA, Dent G. Prospects for selective cyclic nucleotide phosphodiesterase inhibitors in the treatment of bronchial asthma. Clin Exp Allergy 1992; 22:337–344.
162. Howell RE, Jenkins LP, Fielding LE, Grimes D. Inhibition of antigen-induced pulmonary eosinophilia and neutrophilia by selective inhibitors of phosphodiesterase types 3 or 4 in Brown Norway rats. Pulm Pharm 1995; 8:83–89.
163. Griswold DE, Webb EF, Breton J, White JR, Marshall PJ, Torphy TJ. Effect of selective phosphodiesterase type IV inhibitor, rolipram, on fluid and cellular phases of inflammatory response. Inflammation 1993; 17:333–344.
164. Howell RE, Jenkins LP, Howell DE, Inhibition of lipopolysaccharide-induced pulmonary edema by isozyme-selective phosphodiesterase inhibitors in guinea pigs. J Pharmacol Exp Ther 1995; 275:703–709.
165. Sekut L, Yarnall D, Stimpson SA, Noel LS, Bateman-Fite R, Clark RL, Brackeen MF, Menius JA, Connolly KM. Anti-inflammatory activity of PDE-IV inhibitors in acute and chronic models of inflammation. Clin Exp Immunol 1995; 100:126–132.
166. Lagente V, Pruniaux MP, Junien JL, Moodley I. Modulation of cytokine-induced eosinophil infiltration by phosphodiesterase inhibitors. Am J Respir Crit Care Med 1995; 151:1720–1724.

167. Nyman U, Mussener A, Larsson E, Lorentzen J, Klareskog L. Amelioration of collagen II-induced arthritis in rats by the type IV phosphodiesterase inhibitor rolipram. Clin Exp Immunol 1997; 108:415–419.
168. Sommer N, Loschmann P-A, Northoff GH, Weller M, Steinbrecher A, Steinbach JP, Lichtenfels R, Meyermann R, Riethmuller A, Fontana A, Dichgans J, Martin R. The antidepressant rolipram suppresses cytokine production and prevents autoimmune encephalomyelitis. Nature Med 1995; 1:244–248.
169. Genain GP, Roberts T, Davis RL, Nguyen M-H, Uccelli A, Faulds D, Li Y, Hedgpeth J, Hauser SL. Prevention of autoimmune demeyelination in non-human primates by a cAMP-specific phosphodiesterase inhibitor. Proc Natl Acad Sci USA 1995; 92:3601–3605.
170. Wachtel H. Potential antidepressant activity of rolipram and other selective cyclic adenosine 3′,5′-monophosphate phosphodiesterase inhibitors. Neuropharmacology 1984; 22:267–272.
171. Scott AIF, Perini AF, Shering PA, Whalley LJ. In-patient major depression: is rolipram as effective as amitriptyline? Eur J Clin Pharmacol 1991; 40:127–129.
172. Fleischhacker WW, Hinterhuber H, Bauer H, Pflug B, Berner P, Simhandl C, Wolk R, Gerlach W, Jaklitsch H, Sastre-y-Hernandez M, Schmeding Wiegel H, Sperner-Unterweger B, Voet B, Schbert H. A multicenter double-blind study of three different doses of the novel cAMP-phosphodiesterase inhibitor rolipram in patients with major depressive disorder. Neuropsychobiology 1992; 26:59–64.
173. Heaslip RJ, Buckley SK, Sickels BD, Grimes D. Bronchial vs cardiovascular activities of selective phosphodiesterase inhibitors in the anaesthetized beta-blocked dog. J Pharmacol Exp Ther 1991; 257:741–747.
174. Kaulen P, Bruning G, Schneider HH, Sarter M, Baumgarten HG. Autoradiographic mapping of a selective cyclic adenosine monophosphate phosphodiesterase in rat brain with the antidepressant [^{3}H] rolipram. Brain Res 1989; 503:229–245.
175. Howell LL. Comparative effects of caffeine and selective phosphodiesterase inhibitors on respiration and behavior in rhesus monkeys. J Pharm Exp Ther 1993; 266: 894–903.
176. Howell RE, Muehsam WT, Kinnier WJ. Mechanism for the emetic side effect of xanthine bronchodilators. Life Sci 1990; 46:563–568.
177. Heaslip RJ, Evans DY. Emetic, central nervous system and pulmonary activities of rolipram in the dog. Eur J Pharmacol 1995; 286:281–290.
178. Carpenter DO, Briggs DB, Knox AP, Strominger N. Excitation of area postrema neurons by transmitters, peptides and cyclic nucleotides. J Neurophysiol 1988; 59: 358–369.
179. Duplantier AJ, Biggers MS, Chambers RJ, Cheng JB, Cooper K, Damon DB, Eggler JF, Kraus KG, Marfat A, Masamune H, Pillar JS, Shirley JT, Umland JP, Watson JW. Biarycarboxylic acids and amides: Inhibition of phosphodiesterase type IV versus [^{3}H] rolipram binding activity and their relationship to emetic behavior in the ferret. J Med Chem 1996; 39:120–125.
180. Robichaud A, Tattersall FD, Choudhury I, Rodger IW. Emesis induced by inhibitors of type IV cyclic nucleotide phosphodiesterase (PDEIV). Naunyn-Schmiedeberg's Arch Pharm 1998; 358(S2):P22.11.
181. Dale TJ, Ball DI, Nials AT, Coleman RA. The anti-inflammatory and emetogenic

properties of phosphodiesterase (PDE) inhibitors in conscious ferrets. Br J Pharmacol 1995; 116:91P.

182. Dale TJ, Ball DI, Myles DD, Nials AT. The anti-inflammatory and emetogenic effects of phosphodiesterase (PDE) IV inhibitors in conscious ferrets. Third International Conference on Cyclic Nucleotide Phosphodiesterases. Glasgow, July 1996; Abstr 106.
183. Barnette MS, Christiensen SB, Essayan DM, Grous M, Prabhakar U, Rush JA, Kagey-Sobotka A, Torphy TJ. SB 207499 (Ariflo), a potent and selective second-generation phosphodiesterase 4 inhibitor: in vitro anti-inflammatory actions. J Pharmacol Exp Ther 1998; 284:420–426.
184. Harbinson PL, MacLeod D, Hawksworth R, O'Toole S, Sullivan PJ, Heath P, Kilfeather S, Page CP, Costello J, Holgate ST, Lee TH. The effect of a novel orally active selective PDE4 isozyme inhibitor (CDP840) on allergen-induced responses in asthmatic subjects. Eur Respir J 1997; 10:1008–1014.
185. Louis R, Bury T, Corhay JL, Redermecker M. LY 186655, a phosphodiesterase inhibitor, inhibits histamine release from basophils, lung and skin fragments. Int J Immunopharm 1992; 14:191–194.
186. Isreal E, Mathur PN, Tashkin D, Drazen JM. LY 186655 prevents bronchospasm in asthma of moderate severity. Chest 1988; 94(suppl):71S.
187. Foster RW, Rakshi K, Carpenter JR, Small RC. Trials of the bronchodilator activity of the isozyme-selective phophodiesterast inhibitor AH 21-132 in healthy volunteers during a methacholine challenge test. Br J Clin Pharmacol 1992; 34:527–534.
188. Brunnee T, Engelstatter R, Steinijans VW, Kunkel G. Bronchodilatory effects of inhaled zardaverine, a phosphodiesterase III and IV inhibitor, in patients with asthma. Eur Respir J 1992; 5:982–985.
189. Jonkers GJ, Tijhuis GJ, De Monchy JGR. RP 73401 (a phosphodiesterase inhibitor) does not prevent allergen induced bronchoconstriction during the early phase reaction in asthmatics. Eur J Respir 1996; 9(suppl 23):82S.
190. McGrath JL, Aikman SL, Cook RM, Kharitinov SA, O'Connor BJ. Six week treatment with inhaled RP 73401, a PDE IV inhibitor: effect on airway responsiveness and exhaled NO in mild to moderate asthma. Am J Respir Crit Care Med. 1997; 155:A660.
191. Ferrer SH, Xuan TD, Canal I, Lockhart A, Bousquet J, Luria X. Bronchodilator activity of LAS 31025, a new selective phosphodiesterase IV inhibitor. Am J Respir Crit Care Med 1997; 155:A660.
192. Luria X, Ferrer SH. A six week double blind randomised parallel placebo-controlled clinical trial to assess efficacy and safety of LAS 31025 in asthmatic patients. Am J Respir Crit Care Med 1997; 155:A203.
193. Li C, Chauret N, Trimble L, Nicoll-Griffith D, Silva J, Yergey J, Parton T, Alexander R, Warrellow G. Capillary HPLC/CF-LSIMS characterisation of a novel phase II metabolite of phosphodiesterase-IV inhibitor CDP-840. 45th ASMS Conference 1998.
194. Stawiski MA, Powell JA, Lang PG, Schork A, Duell EA, Voorhees JJ. Papavarine: its effects on cyclic AMP in vitro and psoriasis in vivo. J Invest Dermatol 1975; 64:124–127.
195. Stawiski MA, Rusin LJ, Burns TL, Weinstein GD, Voorhees JJ. Ro 20-1724: an

agent that significantly improves psoriatic lesions in double-blind clinical trials. J Invest Dermatol 1979; 73:261–263.

196. Hanifin JM, Chan SC, Cheng JB, Tofte SJ, Henderson WR, Kirby DS, Weiner ES. Type 4 phosphodiesterase inhibitors have clinical and in vitro anti-inflammatory effects in atopic dermatitis. J Invest Dermatol 1996; 107:51–56.
197. Elliott MJ, Maini RN, Feldmann M, Long-Fox A, Charles P, Bijl H, Woody JN. Repeated therapy with monoclonal antibody to tumour necrosis factor alpha (cA2) in patients with rheumatoid arthritis. Lancet 1994; 344:1125–1127.
198. Chikanza JC, Jawed SJ, Blake DR, Perot S, Menkes CJ, Barnes CG, Perry JD, Wright MG. Treatment of patients with rheumatoid arthritis with RP 73401 phosphodiesterase type IV inhibitor. Am Coll Rheum 1996; Florida: Abstr 1527.
199. Compton CH, Cedar E, Nieman RB, Amit O, Langley SJ, Sapene M. Ariflo improves lung function in patients with asthma: results of a study in patients taking inhaled corticosteroids. Am J Resp Crit Care Med 1999; 159:A624.
200. Compton CH, Gubb J, Cedar E, Nieman RB, Amit O, Brambilla C, Ayres J. The efficacy of Ariflo (SB 207499), a second-generation oral PDE4 inhibitor in patient's with COPD. Am J Resp Crit Care Med 1999; 159:A806.

10

Leukotriene Modulators

ANTHONY P. SAMPSON

Southampton General Hospital
Southampton, England

ZUZANA DIAMANT

Erasmus University Medical Centre
Rotterdam, The Netherlands

I. Introduction

It has become axiomatic over the last 15 years that human bronchial asthma consists of much more than acute episodes of bronchoconstriction causing wheeze, breathlessness, and cough triggered by a variety of otherwise trivial inhaled stimuli. Instead, this so-called nonspecific airway hyperresponsiveness (AHR; i.e., the ease with which the airways narrow after exposure to constrictor agents) is recognized as a consequence of chronic airway inflammation, even if the relationship between the two phenomena remains ill-defined (1,2). Characterization of airway inflammation in asthma has been aided by the flexible fiberoptic bronchoscope, which allows safe and convenient sampling of bronchoalveolar lavage (BAL) fluid and cells and biopsy of the bronchial wall (3). Such studies have demonstrated a Th2-lymphocyte-driven process, in which specific cytokines including interleukin (IL)-5 promote eosinophil maturation, migration, survival, and function, while others such as IL-4 and IL-13 promote IgE production by B cells (4) (Fig. 1). These cytokines may also be released by IgE-dependent activation of mast cells (5). Activated mast cells and eosinophils release final effector mediators, which cause inflammatory changes in airway smooth muscle, airway mucous glands, vascular endothelium, airway epithelium, and infiltrating and res-

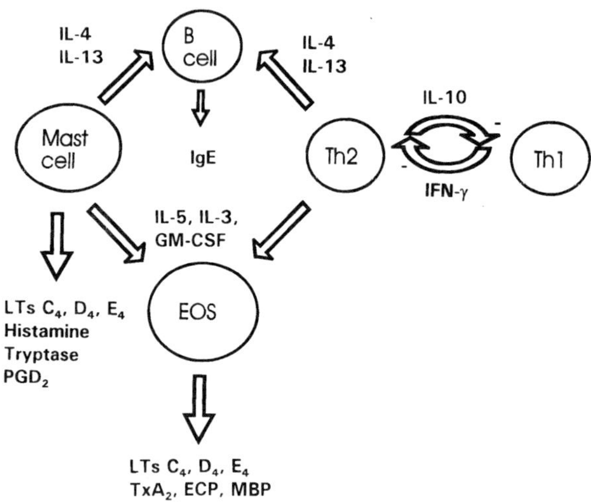

Figure 1 Cytokine networks in allergic asthma.

ident leukocytes. This inflammatory process, being the hallmark of asthma, eventually results in structural changes within the airways, so-called airway remodeling (6,7), determining the severity of the symptoms (ranging from intermittent to severe and persistent) (8).

The field of classic mediators implicated in asthma has been narrowed down within the last few years. Some mediators—such as platelet-activating factor (PAF) (9), prostanoids (10–12), and histamine (13–15)—mimic asthma symptoms and may be detected in asthma in vivo but have failed the most important of Dale's postulates (16), which require that specific pharmacological blockade should significantly alter the severity or progression of the disease. Dale's postulates have been fulfilled for only one family of mediators, cysteinyl-(or sulfidopeptide-) leukotrienes (LTs). This status is based on their extraordinary potency in constricting airway smooth muscle, stimulating mucus secretion, enhancing vascular permeability, and chemoattracting eosinophils (17). Uniquely, specific receptor antagonists and synthesis inhibitors directed against cysteinyl-LT activity have potent efficacy in experimental models of asthma and in clinical asthma (18). Cysteinyl-LTs are the principal transducers of stimulation by diverse precipitants of asthma—including allergen; exercise; cold, dry air; and aspirin-like drugs—into a final common pathway leading to acute and chronic airflow limitation. In the past few years, antileukotriene drugs entered clinical practice in many countries as the novel targeted approach to asthma therapy for decades.

This chapter reviews the remarkable success story of leukotriene research since the late 1970s, outlines the principal actions of cysteinyl-leukotrienes in the lung, and examines the evidence for their involvement in asthma. In addition, clinical studies of leukotriene modulator drugs are surveyed and potential applications of these drugs in the treatment of asthma are discussed.

II. The Generation of Leukotrienes

A. The 5-Lipoxygenase Pathway

A number of inflammatory mediators are lipid molecules, such as platelet-activating factor (PAF), a modified phospholipid, and the eicosanoids, including prostanoids (PGs) and leukotrienes (LTs), derivatives of the 20-carbon polyunsaturated fatty acid, arachidonic acid (eicosatetra-5,8,11,14-enoic acid; 20:4ω6). Arachidonic acid is a major fatty acid component of cell membranes, particularly in the nuclear envelope (19), usually esterified at the *sn*-2 position of membrane phospholipids, particularly phosphatidylcholine. Release of free arachidonate from membrane phospholipids is essential for eicosanoid synthesis, and occurs by the calcium-dependent action of phospholipase (PL)A_2 or by the sequential action of PLC and a diglyceride lipase (20,21).

Free arachidonate can be converted by cyclooxygenase-1 (COX-1) and COX-2 isoenzymes and then by a number of synthases and isomerases to PGD_2, $PGF_{2\alpha}$, PGE_2, prostacyclin (PGI_2), or thromboxane (TX)A_2, which act at specific prostanoid receptors (22) to affect the tone of bronchial and vascular smooth muscle and to enhance nociception of painful stimuli (23). Alternatively, various lipoxygenases can convert arachidonate to mono-, di-, and trihydroxylated derivatives such as the lipoxins and leukotrienes (24). LTs are not stored inside the cell but are synthesized de novo following cell activation. LT synthesis (Fig. 2) is

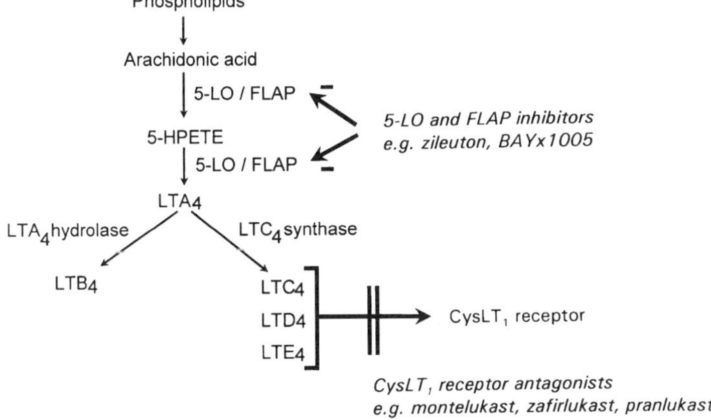

Figure 2 The 5-lipoxygenase pathway of leukotriene synthesis.

initiated by 5-lipoxygenase (5-LO), a 78-kDa hydrophilic enzyme (25,26), which synthesizes 5-hydroperoxyeicosatetraenoic acid (5-HPETE) (27). 5-HPETE may degrade nonenzymatically to the weak neutrophil chemotaxin 5-HETE or be further transformed by 5-LO to the unstable epoxide LTA_4 (28). 5-LO is suicide-inactivated by covalent binding of the LTA_4 product to the active site, but this may become rate-limiting only at very high rates of turnover (29). 5-LO is the target of one class of antileukotriene drugs, the 5-LO inhibitors, exemplified by zileuton (A-64077; Zyflo). 5-LO inhibitors compete with arachidonate at the 5-LO active site and block the synthesis of LTA_4 and of all its biologically active derivatives (30). The activity of 5-LO in intact cells requires Ca^{2+} and ATP (26) and the provision of arachidonate by a unique 18-kDa integral membrane protein termed 5-LO-activating protein (FLAP) (31–33). FLAP is located in the nuclear envelope (34). Cellular activation leads to the translocation of PLA_2 and 5-LO from the cytoplasm to the nuclear envelope (34–36), where arachidonate liberated by PLA_2 is transferred to FLAP and then donated to 5-LO (37). This process is blocked by the FLAP inhibitors, the second class of antileukotriene drugs, exemplified by MK-886, MK-0591, BAY-x1005, and BAY-y1015, which bind to FLAP and prevent it from donating arachidonate to 5-LO (38,39).

LTA_4 hydrolase is a 68- to 71-kDa cytosolic zinc-containing epoxide hydrolase with a high degree of substrate specificity (40) and with additional activity as an arginine aminopeptidase (41). It is rapidly suicide-inactivated by covalent binding of its substrate to the active site (42). The fate of LTA_4 in a particular cell type depends on the profile and activity of terminal enzymes in the leukotriene pathway. LTA_4 may be converted by LTA_4 hydrolase to the potent chemotaxin LTB_4 (5S,12R-dihydroxy-6,8,11,14-ETE) (Fig. 2). Released from the cell by a specific export carrier (43), LTB_4 is a potent chemoattractant for neutrophils and other leukocytes, acting at specific surface (BLT) receptors on target cells. The BLT receptor has been cloned in HL-60 cells and shown to be a 352–amino acid G protein–linked receptor, activation of which leads to a rise in intracellular Ca^{2+} and chemotaxis (44). LTB_4 instilled into the human airway causes neutrophil influx into BAL fluid (45), but inhaled LTB_4 does not cause bronchoconstriction or alter airway responsiveness in healthy individuals or asthmatic patients (46). A specific BLT receptor antagonist (LY293111) had no effect on the early or late responses to inhaled allergen in patients with asthma or on allergen-induced changes in airway responsiveness, although neutrophil counts were reduced in the BAL fluid (47). Overall, there is little coherent evidence that LTB_4 has a significant role in human bronchial asthma (48), and BLT receptor antagonists will not be discussed further, although they may find clinical applications in COPD (49).

Alternatively, LTA_4 may be conjugated with glutathione at the C-6 position by LTC_4 synthase, producing the first of the cysteinyl leukotrienes implicated in asthma (Fig. 2). LTC_4 synthase is a homodimeric integral membrane protein of

16.6-kDa subunits with striking sequence homologies with FLAP (50,51). It is inhibited by high concentrations of FLAP inhibitors such as MK-886 (52). LTC_4 is released from the cell by a specific export carrier (53) and may be converted by gamma glutamyl transpeptidase and dipeptidase activities in lung tissue and plasma to LTD_4 and LTE_4, respectively (54–56). Together, the three cysteinyl leukotrienes (LTC_4, LTD_4, and LTE_4) comprise the ''slow-reacting substance of anaphylaxis'' (SRS-A), first described as bronchoconstrictor activity nearly 60 years ago by Kellaway and Trethewie (57,58). Although separate receptors for LTC_4 and LTD_4 have been identified in guinea-pig lung, in human airways both leukotrienes appear to act at the same receptor (59), named $CysLT_1$ receptor. The third major group of antileukotriene drugs comprises the cysteinyl-LT receptor antagonists (cysLTRAs) (18), which specifically block the $CysLT_1$ receptor on airway smooth muscle and other lung tissues. They include zafirlukast (ICI-204,219; Accolate), montelukast (MK-0476; Singulair), and pranlukast (ONO-1078; Onon = SB205,312; Ultair). At present, only one cysLTRA (Bay u9773) also blocks the $CysLT_2$ receptor that is suspected of mediating some of the vascular actions of cysteinyl-LTs in human lung (60). Current information on human lung cysteinyl-LT receptors has been reviewed (61).

Complete degradation of the cysteinyl-LTs occurs by ω-oxidation followed by successive cycles of β-oxidation in the liver (62). However, a fixed proportion of intravenous or inhaled ^3H-LTC_4 ($\sim$5%) is excreted as LTE_4 in the urine (63), such that urinary LTE_4 concentrations are used as a marker of whole-body production of cysteinyl-LTs and hence as a measure of the bioactivity of LT synthesis inhibitors (LTSIs) in vivo.

B. Cellular Sources of Leukotrienes

The profile of leukotrienes generated in response to immunological and nonimmunological stimuli shows considerable cell-type specificity (Table 1). Intact cells can generate LTs only when they coexpress 5-LO and FLAP (33), but the subsequent synthesis of LTB_4 or of the cysteinyl LTs depends on the relative activities of LTA_4 hydrolase, and LTC_4 synthase. Some cells express both enzymes, while others predominantly or exclusively express only one. Thus, neutrophils preferentially secrete LTB_4, while eosinophils preferentially generate LTC_4 (64,65). Basophils and human lung mast cells also preferentially secrete cysteinyl LTs (66–68). Monocytes can generate both LTB_4 and smaller amounts of cysteinyl LTs (69); the capacity of monocytes to synthesize LTB_4 increases as they differentiate into alveolar macrophages (70). In contrast to myeloid cells, the capacity of lymphocytes to generate LTs is contentious. Early reports that T lymphocytes generate LTs (71) have been disputed (72). However, lymphoblastoid B-cell lines and human tonsillar B cells have low levels of 5-LO and FLAP activity (73,74). In addition, a range of lymphocyte cell lines, tonsillar B cells,

Table 1 Cellular Sources of Leukotrienes[a]

Cell Type	LTC_4	LTB_4
Mast cells	+++	+
Eosinophils	+++	0
Basophils	++	0
Neutrophils	0	++
Monocytes	+	++
Macrophages	+	+++
T lymphocytes	0	+
B lymphocytes	0	+

[a]The relative capacities of leukocyte subtypes to synthesize leukotriene (LT)C_4 or LTB_4 is indicated by the number of (+) signs, based on references discussed in Section II.B.

and peripheral T cells have LTA_4 hydrolase activity (75), suggesting that LTB_4 may be formed by T or B lymphocytes (76). Lymphocytes appear to lack LTC_4 synthase and thus do not generate cysteinyl LTs.

The synthesis of LTB_4 or LTC_4 by activated leukocytes may be rate-limited by the activity of LTA_4 hydrolase (77,78) or LTC_4 synthase. Excess LTA_4 substrate may then be released and utilized by platelets, which express LTC_4 synthase, to generate cysteinyl LTs (79), or by LTA_4 hydrolase in endothelial cells, epithelial cells, lymphocytes, erythrocytes and plasma to generate LTB_4 (76,80–83). Close apposition of leukocytes infiltrating the lung to other leukocytes or to structural elements of the airway may thus radically modulate the profile or the amounts of leukotrienes generated by leukocytes alone (84).

C. Regulation of the 5-Lipoxygenase Pathway

A plethora of studies has shown that the capacity of leukocyte subtypes to generate leukotrienes in response to an activating stimulus can be primed by cytokines implicated in asthma, including tumor necrosis factor-alpha (TNF-α), interferon gamma (IFN-γ), granulocyte-macrophage colony stimulating factor (GM-CSF), IL-8, IL-3, IL-4, IL-5, and stem-cell factor (SCF) (85). Part of the effect may be due to rapid tyrosine kinase–dependent phosphorylation or to induced expression of cytosolic PLA_2 or of other arachidonate-generating phospholipases (86–88), leading to a nonspecific upregulation in eicosanoid synthesis. However, longer-term effects may occur on gene transcription and protein expression of specific 5-LO pathway enzymes at both proximal and distal sites in the pathway.

The human gene for 5-LO has been characterized (89) and localized to chromosome 10. Its promoter contains recognition sequences for the Sp1 and

AP-2 transcription factors but lacks the TATA and CCAAT sequences expected in an inducible gene (90). The 5-LO gene promoter does contain a recognition sequence for the NF-κB transcription factor. NF-κB sites are also found in the gene promoters of a range of cytokines and adhesion molecules, suggesting that 5-LO products can be coregulated with other proinflammatory mediators. The gene for FLAP has been localized to chromosome 13 and, in contrast to 5-LO, the FLAP promoter has TATA sequences and other features characteristic of a highly inducible gene (91). The promoter also has a glucocorticoid recognition element (GRE), suggesting that FLAP expression may be regulated by anti-inflammatory corticosteroids. Curiously, in human neutrophils, dexamethasone increases expression of FLAP (92), when a reduction might have been expected. Both LTA_4 hydrolase and LTC_4 synthase cDNAs have also been cloned (51,93). Intriguingly, the LTC_4 synthase gene localizes to human chromosome 5q35 (94), close to the loci of genes coding for IL-3, IL-4, IL-5, IL-6, IL-9, IL-13, and other eosinophil- and mast cell–regulating molecules implicated in asthma.

In human neutrophils, expression of 5-LO and FLAP can be induced by GM-CSF (92,95), resulting in enhanced LTB_4 synthesis (96). Such increases in 5-LO and FLAP expression are the cause of the increased capacity to generate LTB_4 that occurs as monocytes differentiate into alveolar macrophages (97). In eosinophils, IL-5 and IL-3 promote the sequential expression of 5-LO, FLAP, and LTC_4 synthase in eosinophils differentiating from $CD34^+$ cord blood precursor cells, accompanied by increased LTC_4 synthesis (98). In mature eosinophils from human blood, IL-5 also promotes the expression of FLAP but not of 5-LO (99). In murine mast cells, IL-3 promotes the expression of 5-LO, FLAP, and LTC_4 synthase (100); in the human mast-cell line HMC-1, stem-cell factor increases 5-LO expression and activity (101). Thus, the cytokine microenvironment within the asthmatic lung may not only promote the influx of eosinophils and activation of mast cells but also divert their capacity for eicosanoid synthesis toward the cysteinyl-LT pathway.

In addition, there is some evidence that 5-LO pathway enzymes and their products may have a role as signal-transduction or nuclear transcription factors, thus regulating expression of cytokines and other genes, as well as their better-defined role as extracellular mediators. First, exogenous LTB_4 has been shown to stimulate synthesis of IL-2, IL-4, IL-5, IL-6, IL-8, and IFN-γ in human blood T cells, monocytes, and neutrophils (102–106). LTB_4 activates not only the nuclear transcription factor NF-κB (102), which regulates a number of inflammatory cytokines and adhesion molecules, but also the nuclear transcription factor PPARα, which enhances expression of the enzymes that catabolize LTB_4 and other eicosanoids (107). Second, 5-LO and FLAP inhibitors have been shown to block proliferation (thymidine uptake) and the synthesis of cytokines, including IL-2 and IL-6, by peripheral blood mononuclear cells and lymphocyte cell lines (108,109). Third, 5-LO appears to be found inside the nucleus in mature alveolar macrophages and adherent neutrophils, as compared with a cytosolic location in their blood precursors (110,111). Leukocyte activation results in rapid translocation of 5-LO from either cytosolic or intranuclear sites to the nuclear envelope to interact with FLAP (34). Perhaps this differential subcellular localization may reflect different targeting of the products of 5-LO activation for either cellular export or a nuclear transcription role. It is possible that leukotriene synthesis inhibitors may have additional anti-inflammatory benefit based on inhibition of leukotriene-induced leukocyte proliferation and cytokine synthesis.

III. Actions of Cysteinyl Leukotrienes Relevant to Asthma

A. Airway Smooth Muscle

''Slow-reacting substance of anaphylaxis (SRS-A)'' was named for its ability to cause long-lived contractions of bronchial tissue from animals. The structural elucidation in 1979–1980 of SRS-A activities from animal and human sources (112–115) and the consequent availability of synthetic cysteinyl LTs, allowed the further characterization of their diverse biological activities. In particular, several studies confirmed that the cysteinyl-LT constituents of SRS-A (LTC_4, LTD_4, and LTE_4) are potent bronchoconstrictors in non-asthmatic and asthmatic subjects, with LTC_4 and LTD_4 being more than 1000-fold more potent than histamine and producing contractions lasting 30–40 min, as compared with the 5- to 15-min contractions induced by histamine (116–121). LTD_4 is the most potent cysteinyl LT, while LTE_4 is less potent but produces the most sustained contractions. Cysteinyl LTs contract human airway smooth muscle via stimulation of the $CysLT_1$ receptors, and, according to recent albeit indirect evidence in humans, by secondary release of neuropeptides as well (122).

Inhaled LTC_4 and LTD_4 are more potent in patients with asthma than in healthy subjects, which agrees with the nonspecific AHR to various bronchoconstrictor stimuli seen generally in asthma. However, the degree of AHR is less than that seen with other agonists: asthmatic subjects respond to methacholine at a 55-fold lower concentration than healthy subjects, but they respond to LTC_4 at a quarter, and LTD_4 at an eleventh of the concentration required in healthy subjects (119,123). This could be due to significant production of endogenous cysteinyl LTs in asthmatic airways, leading to downregulation of the $CysLT_1$ receptors and thus a reduced response to exogenous cysteinyl LTs but not to other agonists (124). However, asthmatic airways appear to be uniquely hyperresponsive to LTE_4, being 14-, 15-, 6-, 9-, and 219-fold more responsive to histamine, methacholine, LTC_4, LTD_4 and LTE_4, respectively, than the airways of healthy subjects (125). These results are difficult to explain except on the basis of differential expression of the cysLT receptor subtypes in healthy subjects and patients with asthma.

B. Vascular Smooth Muscle and Endothelium

Cysteinyl LTs have potent actions on the vasculature. In human skin, cysteinyl LTs induce a wheal, caused by increased vascular permeability, with a central pallor suggesting vasoconstriction (126). Vasoconstrictor responses may limit the formation of edema in response to cysteinyl LTs alone; however, in combination with vasodilator prostanoids, cysteinyl LTs are highly effective inducers of edema (127).

The principal vascular effect of cysteinyl LTs is a direct action on the permeability of postcapillary venules (128). Cysteinyl LTs are two to three orders of magnitude more potent than histamine in causing plasma extravasation in guinea pig trachea in vivo, and this effect is blocked by the early specific cysLTRA, termed FPL-55712 (129). The increase in plasma extravasation that occurs in the trachea, bronchi, and bronchioles of guinea-pigs following antigen exposure is blocked by the cysLTRA pranlukast, showing that endogenous cysteinyl-LTs are involved in this response (130). Since airflow is proportional to the fourth power of the airway diameter, even a limited degree of edema in the bronchial wall may have a disproportionate effect on reducing airflow. Although difficult to distinguish in the acute phase from the functional effects of airway smooth muscle contraction, cysteinyl LT–dependent edema may enhance and perpetuate airflow obstruction in the medium term following allergen-dependent or other triggers of acute asthma. LTC_4 and LTD_4 also promote adhesion of PMN leukocytes to human endothelial cells in vitro, an effect that seems to be mediated by PAF released by the endothelial cells (131).

C. Mucus Secretion

Plugging of the small airways by mucus containing shed epithelial cells is a common pathological postmortem finding in the status asthmaticus lung. However, hypersecretion of mucus is also thought to occur in the airways of patients with moderate persistent asthma. Although mucus secretion is difficult to quantify, expectoration of mucus is a common experience of subjects undergoing inhalation challenge with cysteinyl LTs. In vitro, the cysteinyl LTs are 100-fold more potent than the cholinergic agonist methacholine in increasing mucus glycoprotein release by isolated human bronchi, although the effect is not stereospecific, suggesting a receptor-independent process (132). Cysteinyl LTs are also reported to slow mucociliary transport in human bronchial explants (133). In vivo, mucociliary transport in the asthmatic airway is slowed by inhaled allergen challenge; this response is reported to be inhibited by the cysLTRA FPL-55712 (134), showing that endogenous cysteinyl LTs are involved in mucus hypersecretion following allergen stimulation. The contribution of mucus hypersecretion to impaired lung function in asthma, and the role that persistent cysteinyl-LT overproduction may play in inducing mucus release, are underinvestigated areas.

D. Airway Hyperresponsiveness (AHR) and Airway Remodeling

We have seen above that asthmatic airways seem to show an anomalous degree of hyperresponsiveness to cysteinyl LTs, especially to LTE_4 (125). Cysteinyl LTs themselves cause increases in airway responsiveness to other mediators. In healthy subjects, inhalation of a single bronchoconstrictor dose of LTD_4 increases airway responsiveness to methacholine twofold, with the maximal increase at 7 days and persisting for up to 14 days (135). In asthmatic subjects, inhaled cysteinyl LTs induce a three- to fourfold AHR to histamine, with the effect of a single dose of LTE_4 lasting up to a week (136). This effect may be mediated in part by secondary release of a prostanoid (137), possibly thromboxane A_2 (138). Inhalation of LTD_4 increases subsequent airway responsiveness to inhaled PGD_2 by fourfold in healthy subjects (139); simultaneous release of cysteinyl LTs and PGD_2 from mast cells following allergen-dependent stimulation may thus have a synergistic effect. The synergistic effect of bronchoconstrictor prostanoids may be mediated by cholinergic stimulation (139), leading to elevated basal airway tone, mucus secretion, and edema.

The mechanisms underlying AHR in allergic asthma are not fully understood, but a number of factors may be involved. Evidence has been provided that AHR may be due to subthreshold airway narrowing caused by persistent overproduction of cysteinyl LTs by activated mast cells and/or eosinophils, which would increase resting airway smooth muscle tone and promote airway edema (129) and mucus plugging (134). Moreover, the resting tone of nonasthmatic human bronchi has been reduced by a specific LTSI (AA-861) and by a cysLTRA (MCI-286) but not by specific blockade of prostaglandin, thromboxane, histamine, or muscarinic cholinergic activity (140), suggesting that cysteinyl LTs do play a central role in regulating basal airway tone.

In addition, although airway smooth muscle in vitro does not appear to show increased sensitivity to spasmogens, there is an increase in total airway smooth muscle mass in the airways of patients with long-standing asthma as a result of long-term airway remodeling (7). In rats, the increase in airway responsiveness following allergen exposure is caused by an increase in airway smooth muscle mass (141). Both these increases are blocked by the cysLTRAs MK-571 and pranlukast (141,142). Alternatively, AHR may be related to disruption of the airway epithelium, allowing increased access of irritant stimuli to the bronchial mucosa and sensory nerve fibers, inducing the so-called axon reflex (143). Epithelial cell proliferation and hyperplasia are features of airway inflammation in asthma, and the cysteinyl LTs are extraordinarily potent mitogens for human airway epithelial cells in culture, with LTC_4 being active at subpicomolar concentrations (144). The effect of the 5-LO inhibitor zileuton in reducing AHR to cold, dry air in susceptible asthmatics lasts for up to 10 days after the drug is withdrawn and eliminated (145). This suggests that leukotriene-induced AHR is indeed due to structural changes in fixed elements of the airways, such as epithelium or smooth muscle. Although several studies have shown that some anti-LT drugs produced 1.5- to 5.0-fold reductions in baseline- and allergen-induced AHR (146–149), other trials do not support a significant role of cysteinylLTs in AHR (150,151). Nevertheless, in mice, targeted disruption of the 5-LO gene completely abolished the development of AHR following antigen challenge that occurs in the 5-LO wild-type mouse (152). Hence, the role of 5-LO products in AHR in humans warrants further investigation.

E. Leukocyte Chemoattraction

Chronic airway eosinophilia is a consistent finding in asthma (153). Eosinophil maturation and survival are regulated by eosinophilopoietic cytokines including IL-3, IL-5, and GM-CSF (154). IL-5 is a specific chemoattractant for eosinophils, although its effects are rather weak (155). IL-5 and IL-4 may have a greater effect on eosinophilia by upregulating eosinophil-specific adhesion mechanisms on vascular endothelium, such as VCAM-1/VLA-4 interactions (156), or by reducing eosinophil apoptosis (157). In contrast, several lipid mediators such as PAF and LTB_4 are potent chemotaxins for eosinophils but also cause nonspecific chemoattraction of other cell types, especially neutrophils (158). Eosinophils that have been specifically primed by IL-5, however, may be selectively recruited by such a chemotaxin (159).

More recently however, it has been recognized that the cysteinyl LTs are both potent and specific chemoattractants for eosinophils (17). In vitro, subnanomolar concentrations of LTD_4 cause chemotaxis of human eosinophils but not neutrophils (160). This response is blocked by the cysLTRA pobilukast (SKF-104,353). In guinea pigs, inhalation of a single dose of LTC_4 or LTD_4 (but not LTB_4) produces a dose-related eosinophil infiltration of the lung, which persists for at least 4 weeks (161,162). It is blocked by the cysLTRAs MK-571 and pranlukast and by an antibody to IL-5 (161,162). In ovalbumin-sensitized guinea pigs, antigen inhalation induces a fourfold eosinophil infiltrate of the bronchial submucosa at 12 hr postchallenge. This response is dependent on endogenous cysteinyl-LT production, as it is specifically blocked by a cysLTRA (MK-571) but not by histamine H_1 or H_2 antagonists or by a cyclooxygenase inhibitor (163). In another animal model, the cynomolgus monkey, the increases in airway responsiveness and lavage eosinophil counts induced by inhaled antigen are blocked by the specific cysLTRA ICI 198,615 (164). Similarly, the rises in BAL eosinophils and in airway responsiveness induced by antigen challenge in sheep are blocked by 5-LO inhibitor zileuton (A-64077) (165). In a mouse model, most of the rise in airway eosinophils, and all of the rise in airway responsiveness, that occurs following allergen challenge of wild-type mice is absent in 5-LO gene–disrupted mice (152). Although these studies indicate that 5-LO products are the predominant factors in allergen-induced airway eosinophilia in these animal models, with IL-5 playing a subsidiary role, it is not clear whether cysteinyl LTs and IL-5 act independently or synergistically to elicit the response.

The most valuable evidence of an eosinophilotactic role of the cysteinyl LTs comes from studies in humans in vivo. In a study in four asthmatic subjects, inhalation of a single dose of LTE_4 caused pronounced (3- to 24-fold) increases in eosinophils and smaller increases in neutrophils in the bronchial mucosa at 4 hr after inhalation (166). There were no changes in mononuclear cell counts. Similarly, inhalation of LTD_4 by asthmatic subjects has been shown to induce eosinophilia in hypertonic saline–induced sputum (167). One week of treatment with the cysLTRA zafirlukast (160 mg bid) dramatically reduced BAL fluid eosinophil and basophil counts 2 days after segmental allergen challenge in 19 subjects with mild to moderate persistent asthma (168). This suggests that cysteinyl LTs generated by allergen challenge have a role in chemoattracting or activating a wide variety of inflammatory leukocytes, including eosinophils, mast cells, basophils, and lymphocytes. Furthermore, 1 week of treatment of 12 subjects with nocturnal asthma with the 5-LO inhibitor zileuton reduced BAL eosinophil counts and even reduced peripheral blood eosinophil counts (169). Further studies of inflammatory leukocytes and their activation status in BAL fluid or bronchial biopsies during anti-LT drug treatment are required to determine the precise role of LTs in the inflammatory pathophysiology of clinical asthma.

IV. In Vivo Evidence for Cysteinyl-LT Production in Asthma

Early studies showed that SRS-A, a mixture of the three cysteinyl LTs, was released by IgE-dependent activation of animal and human lung (58,170). More recently, allergen-dependent contractions of isolated human lungs from nonasthmatic and asthmatic subjects have been shown to be due almost entirely to cysteinyl-LT release, with only a small contribution from histamine (171). In the allergen challenge model, basal levels of LTC_4 are higher in the BAL fluid of asthmatics than in healthy subjects (172). A significant rise in BAL fluid concentrations of LTC_4 occurs 5 min after allergen inhalation only in atopic asthmatics (172). The release of LTC_4 is accompanied by release of histamine, PGD_2, TXB_2, and tryptase, suggesting a mast-cell source for all five mediators (173–175).

Since a small proportion of inhaled or intravenous LTC_4 emerges as LTE_4 in the urine (176,177), urinary LTE_4 levels have been regularly used as a marker of whole-body cysteinyl-LT synthesis. Urinary LTE_4 excretion is markedly elevated following acute exacerbations in atopic asthmatic adults and children (178,179) and after allergen inhalation by atopic asthmatic patients (178,180). Exercise challenge of susceptible asthmatic children also leads to increased urinary LTE_4 excretion, although this does not correlate with exercise-induced falls in lung function (181). Furthermore, urinary LTE_4 levels are increased at night in patients with nocturnal asthma as compared with daytime values or with nighttime values in nonasthmatic subjects, and the levels correlate with the ''morning dip'' in lung function (182). Modest elevations in urinary LTE_4 are apparent even in patients with stable mild persistent asthma (183). More pronounced elevations in baseline urinary LTE_4 are seen in aspirin-sensitive asthmatics (180,184,185). Presumably, this enhanced LT synthesis may be the result of increased numbers of mast cells and eosinophils, which have been found at baseline in bronchial biopsies in patients with this type of asthma as compared with those who are aspirin-tolerant (186). Oral or inhaled aspirin challenge of aspirin-sensitive asthmatic patients causes further dramatic rises in urinary LTE_4 levels (180,184) and in BAL fluid cysteinyl LTs (187) as well as acute asthma symptoms. Apart from urine, cysteinyl LTs and/or LTB_4 have been detected in exhaled air, blood, sputum, and BAL fluid of asthmatic patients (188–195).

Overall, studies in experimental models and in clinical disease have clearly demonstrated excess production of cysteinyl LTs in vivo in a number of asthma phenotypes at baseline and with further increases during spontaneous and provocation-induced exacerbations. In addition, accumulating evidence points toward involvement of LTs in both the acute inflammatory process and the long-term structural changes within the asthmatic airways. Furthermore, inhaled cysteinyl LTs have been shown to produce symptoms of asthma. Consequently, these observations provided evidence that cysteinyl LTs play an important role in the pathophysiology of asthma, warranting the development of antileukotriene drugs.

V. Antileukotriene Drugs

A. Human Models of Asthma

When one is testing novel potential antiasthma therapies, all features of asthma should be taken into account. Only limited information can be gathered from in vitro and animal studies because of the marked incongruities between in vitro and in vivo conditions and because of additional differences between species in airway anatomy, histology, and immune response (196). Hence, it is essential to perform experimental studies in humans in vivo. For this purpose, various validated bronchoprovocation tests are being used to mimic exacerbations of asthma, including the allergen bronchoprovocation test (197), exercise and cold, dry air challenges (197), experimental viral infection (198), aspirin challenge (199,200), or withdrawal from regular antiasthma therapy (201).

In particular, allergen challenge has been shown to be an important model of asthma and can be performed in two ways: inhalation of aerosolized allergen or local instillation of allergen by bronchoscopy into a pulmonary segment.

Within 10 min of challenge, acute airway narrowing occurs in susceptible patients, the so-called early asthmatic response (EAR), which subsides within 1–3 hr and is followed by a late asthmatic response (LAR) in approximately 50% of patients (202). The LAR is an episode of airway narrowing, mostly occurring between 3–7 hr after allergen challenge, which is associated with an increase in nonspecific AHR that may last for several weeks (202). The EAR involves IgE-triggered release of mast-cell mediators predominantly causing airway smooth muscle contraction, whereas the LAR is characterized by inflammatory events within the airways, in which activated eosinophils play a pivotal role through the release of proinflammatory mediators likely to cause the subsequent AHR (203). In general, the EAR and the LAR are depicted as percent fall in FEV_1 from baseline or as areas under the curve (AUC) during the defined time spans of the respective responses (197).

Despite their advantages for intervention studies (mostly single or multiple drug doses), the asthma models are likely to reflect only the acute inflammatory events during exacerbations of asthma and fail to reproduce the chronic structural changes within the asthmatic airway. Therefore, long-term follow-up studies in patients with asthma of varying severity are essential for final evaluation of the clinical outcome of novel antiasthma drugs.

B. Leukotriene Modulation

Although various proinflammatory mediators including histamine, prostanoids, and PAF are involved in the pathophysiology of asthma (204–206), so far—with the exception of leukotriene modulators—antimediator drugs have shown disappointing results in various experimental studies in asthma. In theory, it is possible to block the metabolic pathway of arachidonic acid at various sites (Fig. 2). For instance, eicosapentaenoic acid (EPA) is an n-3 fatty acid, derived from fish oil and capable of competitive inhibition of the generation of eicosanoids from arachidonic acid (207). Therefore, it was thought that dietary supplementation with EPA could attenuate asthma symptoms. However, despite a marked protection against the late response to allergen (208), regular treatment with EPA has thus far resulted in little if any beneficial effects on the severity of symptoms in day-to-day asthma (209–211).

Inhibition of the total leukotrienes synthesis can be achieved either by blocking 5-LO or FLAP, while the leukotriene receptor ($CysLT_1$ and BLT) antagonists specifically block the effects of the respective leukotrienes at receptor sites on target tissues (Fig. 2).

C. 5-Lipoxygenase (LO) Inhibitors

Up to the present, several 5-LO inhibitors have been studied in humans in vitro and in vivo, including piriprost (U-60257), A-78773, and zileuton (A-64077;

Zyflo), followed by the second-generation 5-LO inhibitors, including ZD-2138 and ABT-761 (18,212). The in vivo pharmacological activity of 5-LO inhibitors can be measured by calcium ionophore (A-23187)–stimulated LTB_4 biosynthesis in whole blood ex vivo (213) and by urinary LTE_4 excretion (214). Many of the early compounds have been withdrawn from development because of lack of potency, an unfavorable pharmacokinetic profile, or sometimes for reasons of toxicity.

D. Effects of 5-LO Inhibitors in Human Models of Asthma

Undoubtedly the most extensively studied 5-LO inhibitor is zileuton, which has been recently registered (Zyflo) in several countries worldwide. A single oral dose of 600 mg of this first-generation 5-LO inhibitor produced a 10–15% increase in baseline FEV_1 within 30 min of ingestion in patients with stable, moderate to severe persistent asthma (215). Furthermore, pretreatment with a single oral dose (800 mg) of zileuton has been shown to protect against cold dry air–induced airway narrowing in asthmatic subjects (216). In patients with aspirin-sensitive asthma, multiple oral doses of zileuton (600 mg qid), during 6–8 days substantially reduced urinary LTE_4 excretion along with a 76% decrease in clinical symptoms, including airway obstruction and nasal, gastrointestinal, and dermal reactions after aspirin challenge (217). In addition, pretreatment with four oral daily doses of zileuton (600 mg) attenuated exercise-induced bronchoconstriction by 41% in individuals with exercise-induced asthma (218). However, despite an almost complete blockade of LTB_4 biosynthesis and a nearly 50% inhibition of urinary LTE_4 excretion, a single oral dose of zileuton (800 mg) produced only a nonsignificant trend to a reduced EAR, with no effect on the LAR or on airway responsiveness in atopic asthmatic subjects (150).

ZD-2138, a second-generation 5-LO inhibitor with a superior pharmacological profile to zileuton, dose-dependently (350 or 1000 mg orally) reduced the bronchoconstriction induced by cold, dry air in asthmatic subjects (219). In aspirin-sensitive asthma, two single oral daily doses of ZD-2138 (350 mg) provided a level of protection against aspirin-induced bronchoconstriction and related clinical symptoms similar to that provided by zileuton (220). However, despite an almost complete blockade of ex vivo LTB_4 synthesis ($>$82% inhibition) and a mean reduction in urinary LTE_4 excretion of 52%, pretreatment with one oral dose (350 mg) of this drug failed to protect against allergen-induced airway responses (221).

ABT-761 is another second-generation 5-LO inhibitor that is more potent than zileuton. In asthmatic patients, pretreatment with a single oral dose (200 mg) of this compound provided a substantial protection against exercise and adenosine challenges, reducing the airway responses by 61% and 83%, respectively (222). When a similar dose of this compound was used in another study in asthma patients, a similar reduction of the exercise-induced bronchoconstriction could be achieved (when expressed as reduction in AUC), which was accompanied by a reduction in LTB_4 biosynthesis of at least 80% and in LTE_4 urinary secretion of 55% (223).

In summary, 5-LO inhibitors have so far been shown to produce an almost complete blockade of ex vivo LTB_4 synthesis but to reduce urinary LTE_4 excretion by only 50%. This degree of leukotriene synthesis inhibition is accompanied by clinically significant protection against airway narrowing induced by adenosine, aspirin, exercise, and cold dry air. Curiously, statistically significant effects on allergen-induced airway responses have not been reported.

E. 5-Lipoxygenase Activating Protein (FLAP) Inhibitors

The FLAP inhibitors that have entered clinical trials include MK-886, MK-0591, BAY-x1005, and BAY-y1015 (18,212). As with the 5-LO inhibitors, their in vivo pharmacological activity can be measured by calcium ionophore (A-23187)–stimulated LTB_4 biosynthesis in whole blood ex vivo and by urinary LTE_4 excretion (213,214). Although all these compounds have now been withdrawn from development, they have provided valuable information on the role of leukotrienes in human models of asthma.

F. FLAP Inhibitors in Human Models of Asthma

In atopic asthma patients, two oral doses of MK-886 (500 and 250 mg) reduced LTB_4 synthesis by 54% as well as urinary LTE_4 excretion by 54% at 0–3 hr and by 80% at 3–9 hr following allergen challenge (224). This partial blockade of LT production resulted in a mean 58% inhibition of the AUC (0–3 hr) during the EAR and a 44% inhibition of the AUC (3–7 hr) during the LAR. The protection was lost by 7 hr, which is in keeping with the lack of inhibition of allergen-induced AHR 30 hr after allergen challenge (224). When combined with the findings from allergen challenge studies with the 5-LO inhibitors zileuton and ZD-2138, these results suggest that the moderate protection against allergen-induced airway responses can be at least partly explained by lack of potency of these compounds.

Pretreatment of atopic asthmatics with the structurally related but more potent FLAP inhibitor MK-0591 (3×250 mg orally) produced an almost complete inhibition of ex vivo LTB_4 synthesis (>96%) and urinary LTE_4 excretion (>84%). Although this was accompanied by a substantial inhibition (79%) of the AUC (0–3 hr) during the EAR, only a moderate reduction (39%) of the AUC (3–8 hr) during the LAR could be detected (151). The protection was lost between 8 and 12 hr after inhalation and no inhibition of allergen-induced AHR was found at 24 hr postchallenge (151).

Another FLAP inhibitor, BAY-x1005, has also been studied in the allergen challenge model. This compound has a similar in vitro potency as MK-0591, decreasing the contractile response of anti-IgE-stimulated human bronchi by 72% (225). In atopic asthmatic patients, 3.5 days of pretreatment with oral BAY-x1005 (500 mg bid) produced a mean inhibition of 87% of the AUC (0–3 hr) during the EAR and a mean inhibition of 60% of the AUC (3–7 hr) during the LAR (226). Although in this study neither ex vivo LTB_4 synthesis nor urinary LTE_4 excretion was measured, in a comparable study with 750 mg of oral BAY-x1005 before allergen challenge, a 76% inhibition of urinary LTE_4 excretion was found as compared with placebo (227). Furthermore, in a recent study in asthma, a single oral dose of BAY-x1005 (750 mg) provided substantial protection against cold dry air induced–airway narrowing (228).

Similarly, pretreatment with the FLAP inhibitor BAY-y1015 (50 or 200 mg orally before exercise) produced a dose-dependent mean inhibition of 42% of the exercise-induced maximal drop in lung function in asthmatic individuals (229).

From the pathophysiological point of view, the results with potent leukotriene synthesis inhibitors are encouraging, although almost complete blockade of leukotriene synthesis seems to be more effective against the EAR and less effective against the LAR to inhaled allergen. Several mechanisms could account for this phenomenon, including the involvement of other inflammatory mediators in the LAR as well as LTs (174,203). Furthermore, it is striking that in most studies, although 50–70% of patients respond to some extent, approximately 30–50% are nonresponders. The pathophysiological differences between responders and nonresponders remain to be clarified.

G. $CysLT_1$ Receptor Antagonists (CysLTRAs)

The first members of this category of drugs that were investigated in humans in vivo included FPL-55712, L-648051, L-649923, LY-171883 (tomelukast), LY-170680 (sulukast), RG-12525, and SKF-104353 (pobilukast) (230–236). These early compounds have been withdrawn from development due to lack of potency—i.e., causing a relatively minor rightward shift of the dose-response curve to inhaled LTD_4 (Table 2). In the past decade, more potent and/or selective cysLTRAs have been developed, of which Ultair (pranlukast; ONO-1078/SB-205312), Accolate [zafirlukast; ICI(ZD)-204219], and Singulair (montelukast; MK-0476) have recently been licensed for use in several countries worldwide (18,212) [Table 2 (237)]. These drugs are administered orally at a recommended dose of once or twice daily. Like the LTSIs, the cysLTRAs have bronchodilator properties. Both oral and intravenous administration of various cysLTRAs (e.g., zafirlukast, MK-571 and its R-enantiomer MK-0679, respectively) resulted in 5–10% increases in baseline FEV_1, which were additive to those obtained with β_2-agonists, suggesting a distinct mechanism of action (238–241). Furthermore,

Table 2 Potency of CysLTRAs

Compounds	Potency (K_i μM)[a]	Rightward shift of LTD_4- dose-response curve	Subjects	Dose, route[b]
LY-171883	22.9	4.6–6.1	Asthmatic	400 mg O
L-649923	8.9	3.8	Nonasthmatic	1 g O
L-648051	6.2	4.0	Nonasthmatic	1.2 mg I
SKF-104353	0.04	12.3	Asthmatic	800 μg I
		10.0	Nonasthmatic	800 μg I
Pranlukast	0.0024	25.0	Nonasthmatic	900 mg O
RG-12525	0.003	7.5	Asthmatic	800 mg O
MK-571	0.009	44.0	Asthmatic	28 mg IV
		84.0	Asthmatic	277 mg IV
Zafirlukast	0.0003	117.0	Nonasthmatic	40 mg O
Montelukast	0.0009	[c]	Asthmatic	40 or 200 mg O

[a]Inhibition constant (K_i) determined by ^{3}[H]LTD_4 binding assay.
[b]Route of administration: O, oral; I, inhaled; IV, intravenous.
[c]Larger than the in vivo detectable range (>100) (237).

there is convincing evidence that cysLTRAs also possess anti-inflammatory effects, potentially reducing airway inflammation and AHR (18,212).

H. Effects of CysLTRAs in Human Models of Asthma

Pretreatment of atopic asthmatics with two oral doses of zafirlukast (20 mg) markedly protected against the EAR (0–2 hr) and the LAR (2–6 hr), reducing the maximal percentage fall in FEV_1 by an average of 88% and 54%, respectively, and significantly attenuated the AHR to histamine 6 hr postallergen (148). In subjects with exercise-induced asthma, inhaled zafirlukast (0.4 mg) decreased exercise-induced bronchoconstriction by an average 52%, while a single oral dose of 20 mg caused a mean reduction of 40% (242,243). Similarly, at this single oral dose, zafirlukast has been shown to attenuate sulfur dioxide–induced bronchoconstriction (244).

Intravenous administration of MK-571 (450 mg) starting 20 min before allergen and continuing until 8 hr postallergen provided similar protection, reducing the AUC (0–3 hr) during the EAR by 88% and the AUC (3–10 hr) during the LAR by 63% (245). Unfortunately, no data are published on the effect of MK-571 on allergen-induced AHR 24 hr after allergen challenge. In another study in asthmatic subjects, an intravenous dose of this cysLTRA (160 mg) effectively reduced exercise-induced bronchoconstriction by an average of 68%, independently of its bronchodilator effect (246).

Pretreatment with two oral daily doses (10 mg) of montelukast, a potent cysLTRA, resulted in a marked inhibition of the EAR, reducing the AUC (0–3 hr) by an average of 75% and the AUC (3–8 hr) during the LAR by a mean of 57% (247). However, this dose was not effective in reducing eosinophil counts or activation in induced sputum 24 hr after allergen challenge, which may also account for the incomplete inhibition of the LAR (247). In patients with mild persistent asthma, a similar dose of montelukast once daily for 12 weeks inhibited exercise-induced bronchoconstriction by an average of 47% (expressed as reduction in AUC), thereby substantially shortening the time until recovery as compared to placebo (248).

A comparable protection against exercise-induced bronchoconstriction (mean reduction of 45%) has been found after 2 weeks pretreatment with oral pranlukast (450 mg daily) (249). In patients with aspirin-sensitive asthma, a single oral dose of this cysLTRA (225 mg) provided a considerable inhibition of airway narrowing induced by dipyrone, a pyrazolone derivative (250). Given twice daily (450 mg) during 5.5 days, pranlukast has been shown to attenuate the EAR, reducing the mean maximal fall in FEV_1 by 48% and the mean maximal fall in FEV_1 during the LAR by 35% (251). Furthermore, there was a marked decrease (78%) in the allergen-induced AHR at 24 hr postchallenge (251). Two other cysLTRAs, MK-0679 and SKF-104353, have also attenuated the aspirin-induced bronchoconstriction in aspirin-sensitive asthmatic patients (252,253).

Finally, BAY-x7195, a novel cysLTRA, when inhaled by asthmatic males for 4.5 days in three daily doses of 4 mg, has been shown to reduce exercise-induced bronchoconstriction by 38% (254).

In summary, these studies provide convincing evidence that leukotriene modulators accomplish clinically relevant protection against exercise- and cold dry air–induced bronchoconstriction and against airway responses following challenges with allergen and with nonsteroidal anti-inflammatory drugs such as aspirin. The results indicate that, in most susceptible patients, these airway responses are predominantly mediated by cysteinyl leukotrienes. These findings led to long-term studies with antileukotriene drugs in patients with asthma of varying severity.

I. Effects of LTSIs on Clinical Asthma

As with the acute asthma models, the most commonly applied LTSI in long-term trials in asthma is the 5-LO inhibitor zileuton. After 4 weeks treatment with zileuton (600 mg qid), improvement in symptom scores and lung function parameters was noted, together with a decreased need for β_2-agonist use in 139 patients with mild to moderate persistent asthma (215). Comparable beneficial effects on clinical and lung function parameters have been established after 13 and 26 weeks of treatment with zileuton (400 or 600 mg qid) in 401 patients with moderate to severe persistent asthma and in 373 patients with mild to moderate persistent asthma, respectively (255,256). In both studies, dose-dependent improvements were noted in daytime (28–37%), and nighttime symptom scores (31–33%), and in FEV_1 (16%), together with a decrease in β_2-agonist use (26–31%) (255,256). Moreover, zileuton treatment established a substantially reduced need for corticosteroids in both studies (255,256). In another study in 10 patients with moderate persistent asthma, 13 weeks of pretreatment with zileuton at the same dosing regime provided adequate protection against the airway response to cold, dry air (145). Intriguingly, despite the relatively short half-life of zileuton (2.3 hr), the reduction in cold-air responsiveness persisted for up to 10 days after discontinuation of treatment (145). In addition, one single oral dose of zileuton 400 mg provided a marked protection against AHR to inhaled histamine (2.1 doubling doses) and to distilled water (1.3 doubling doses) in asthmatic patients treated with inhaled corticosteroids for at least 6 months (257). These findings suggest that leukotrienes are involved in the pathophysiology of AHR and that leukotriene modulators may have anti-inflammatory activity in asthma, which complements that provided by corticosteroids.

Until recently, very few long-term studies in asthma have been reported with FLAP inhibitors, probably due to the withdrawal from development of several leading drugs in this class. In a dose-finding study with the FLAP inhibitor MK-0591 (25 mg qid, or 25, 50, or 125 mg bid) for 6 weeks, modest though significant improvements were found in clinical symptoms and lung function parameters along with a decrease in β_2-agonist use in 239 patients with mild to moderate persistent asthma (258).

J. Effects of CysLTRAs on Clinical Asthma

Presently, an ever-increasing number of clinical studies in asthma are being performed with oral anti-leukotriene drugs, in particular with cysLTRAs. The most important placebo-controlled follow-up studies, many of which have not yet been published in full, are discussed below.

Six weeks of treatment with MK-571 (75 mg tid for 2 weeks, followed by 150 mg tid for 4 weeks) improved daytime symptom scores by 30% and FEV_1 by 8–14%, and decreased β_2-agonist use by 30% in 43 patients with mild to moderate persistent asthma (259). Six weeks of treatment of 276 patients with moderate to severe persistent asthma with various doses of zafirlukast (5, 10 or 20 mg bid) provided dose-dependent improvements in daytime (26%) and nighttime (46%) symptoms, increased FEV_1 by 11%, and decreased β_2-agonist use by 30% (260). The beneficial effects on clinical symptoms, β_2-agonist use, and lung function parameters have been confirmed in several long-term studies with zafirlukast in large numbers of patients with mild to severe persistent asthma, most of which have not been published in full (261,262). In two daily doses of 20 mg during

13 weeks, zafirlukast reduced the need for oral corticosteroids for exacerbations in patients with mild to moderate persistent asthma previously using inhaled β_2-agonists only (263). Accordingly, a single daily dose of zafirlukast (20 mg) during 12 weeks provided a steroid-sparing effect in 9 patients with moderate persistent asthma who were using inhaled beclomethasone (1500 μg daily) (264).

In 29 patients with moderate to severe persistent asthma, treatment with montelukast (200 mg tid), for 10.3 days produced marked improvements in daytime and nighttime symptoms and in FEV_1 (9–14%) together with a decrease in β_2-agonist use (265). Similarly, dose-related improvements of these clinical parameters have been reported after 3 weeks of treatment with different doses of montelukast (2,10, and 50 mg) (266) and after 6 weeks of treatment with 10 mg of this drug (267), respectively, in 273 and 361 patients with moderate to severe persistent asthma, most of whom were already using concomitant anti-asthma therapy. In two other studies in patients with moderate (n = 226) and moderate to severe (n = 681) persistent asthma, 12 weeks of treatment with oral montelukast (10 mg once daily) allowed safe tapering of inhaled corticosteroids and protected against asthma exacerbations (268,269).

Eight weeks of treatment with pranlukast (450 mg bid) decreased daytime (40%) and nighttime (60%) symptom scores and increased the morning and evening peak expiratory flow (PEF) by 16% in 42 patients with moderate to severe persistent asthma (270). Furthermore, dose-dependent improvements in symptom scores (34%), FEV_1 (8–12%), and decreases in rescue medication (36%) were observed after 12 weeks of treatment with pranlukast (150, 300, or 450 mg bid) in a group of 586 patients with moderate to severe persistent asthma (271). In addition, 12 weeks of treatment with this cysLTRA (300 mg bid), not only improved the lung function parameters but also the AHR to histamine in 47 patients with mild persistent asthma (272). In another study in 17 patients, the beneficial effect on the AHR was associated with a decrease in serum eosinophil cationic protein (ECP) after a 4-week treatment period (225 mg bid) with this compound (273). Finally, in a study in 79 patients with moderate to severe persistent asthma using inhaled beclomethasone (≥1500 μg daily), 6 weeks of treatment with pranlukast (450 mg bid) provided a substantial steroid-sparing effect (274).

K. Effects of Leukotriene Modulators on Inflammatory Parameters Within the Airways

Since LTs are capable of inducing inflammatory events within human airways in vivo (166,167), it is logical to postulate that leukotriene modulation will inhibit these inflammatory effects. Hence, several studies have been initiated in pursuit of this hypothesis, the majority of which are still ongoing.

In patients with mild to moderate persistent asthma, 7 days of pretreatment with zileuton (600 mg qid) produced marked reduction levels of LTB_4 and cysteinyl LTs in the BAL fluid, together with a decrease in urinary LTE_4 excretion, while a trend was observed for improvement in nocturnal lung function values. These beneficial effects were accompanied by a significant decrease in the percentage of eosinophils both in the BAL and in peripheral blood (169). Using a similar dosing regime for 8 days, this 5-LO inhibitor significantly reduced eosinophil numbers and LTE_4 production in the BAL of subjects with atopic asthma 24 hr after allergen challenge (275). In addition, a correlation was found between LTE_4 levels and eosinophil numbers, suggesting that the eosinophils are the source of the cysteinyl LTs released following allergen (275).

Comparable anti-inflammatory effects have been obtained with some cysLTRAs. After 7 days pretreatment with zafirlukast (160 mg bid), significant decreases in eosinophils (45%) and basophils (57%) were reported in the BAL fluid of atopic asthmatics 48 hr after segmental allergen challenge (168). Similarly, 4 weeks of treatment with montelukast 10 mg once daily reduced eosinophil counts in sputum by 48% in 40 patients with mild to moderate persistent asthma (276). Furthermore, a 4-week treatment with pranlukast (225 mg bid) resulted in a decreased AHR to methacholine in patients with mild to moderate persistent asthma, which was accompanied by a marked decrease in inflammatory cells ($CD3^+$ and $CD4^+$ lymphocytes, $EG2^+$ eosinophils, and mast cells) in bronchial biopsies (277). Also, a similar dose of this drug has been shown to reduce eosinophils in sputum and peripheral blood of 27 asthma patients after 8 weeks treatment (278).

A growing number of studies are now reporting anti-inflammatory effects of leukotriene modulators in asthma (273,279). According to recent evidence, the anti-inflammatory properties of cysLTRAs can be explained at least in part through their potential to induce apoptosis of peripheral blood T lymphocytes in asthma (280). Moreover, cysLTRAs may also exert beneficial effects on long-term airway remodeling in asthma, preventing airway wall thickening and the associated AHR, as has been shown in a study in guinea pigs (281). Whether this also applies for humans remains to be investigated.

VI. Positioning of Leukotriene Modulators in Asthma Management

In summary, antileukotriene drugs have been shown to have considerable efficacy in bronchoprovocation models of asthma, including challenges with allergen, nonsteroidal anti-inflammatory drugs (NSAIDs), and exercise/cold dry air, and, more recently, with sulfur dioxide. Both LTSIs and cysLTRAs block approximately 80% of the early bronchoconstrictor response to allergen and at least half of the late response, and increasing evidence suggests that they can significantly impair allergen-induced inflammatory cell influx (168,275). Leukotriene modulators markedly reduce the severity and duration of acute bronchoconstriction induced by exercise or challenge with cold, dry air. Studies comparing the effects of cysLTRAs with cromoglycate in exercise challenge have demonstrated that pobilukast and zafirlukast provide at least similar protection against exercise-induced bronchoconstriction in asthma, with a better recovery than cromoglycate (282,283). Moreover, in a study comparing the protective effects of montelukast with those of the long-acting β_2-agonist salmeterol against exercise-induced bronchoconstriction, the cysLTRA provided superior protection (284). Furthermore, leukotriene modulators have been shown to completely abolish bronchoconstriction in response to NSAID exposure in aspirin-sensitive individuals. In clinical asthma, long-term treatment with leukotriene modulators has been shown not only to improve symptoms and function but also to reduce airway hyperresponsiveness and the number of asthma exacerbations, thereby allowing reduction in asthma controller medications, including corticosteroids (285). The leukotriene modulators zafirlukast (Accolate), montelukast (Singulair), pranlukast (Ultair), and zileuton (Zyflo) have consequently entered clinical practice in several countries including the United States, Japan, and several European countries within 1996–1998.

Because they possess both reliever and controller properties, the place of leukotriene modifiers within existing asthma treatment guidelines is presently being reviewed (18,212,286). Based on international consensus, current guidelines for asthma management stress the importance of anti-inflammatory medication, principally inhaled corticosteroids (ICS), in all patients requiring regular use of inhaled β_2-agonists (8). Even early studies showed that the bronchodilation obtainable with leukotriene modifiers is additive to that obtainable with β_2-agonists (241) and with ICS (287), suggesting that blockade of the distinct action of leukotriene in the asthmatic lung would make leukotriene modulators a useful adjunct to existing treatments. The greater efficacy of cysLTRAs in blocking the late response to allergen when administered by mouth as compared with the inhaled route has led to the widespread development of oral formulations of leukotriene modulators. Clearly, despite their bronchodilator properties, these are too slow-acting for use as rescue reliever medications, and asthmatic patients need to be advised to have inhaled β_2-agonists available when receiving prophylactic leukotriene modulator therapy. In addition, leukotriene modulators appear to have anti-inflammatory effects on proinflammatory target cells within the airways including leukocytes (169) and possibly T lymphocytes as well (280) and to drastically reduce the need for emergency corticosteroid use during acute exacerbations (288). Moreover, preliminary evidence from animal studies suggests that these drugs may prevent at least some of the features of airway remodeling (281). Hence, antileukotriene drugs may possess steroid-sparing properties and may be particularly beneficial for patients with moderate to severe persistent asthma. However, they are unlikely to replace prophylactic corticosteroid use due to the much wider variety of therapeutic effects of corticosteroids on airway inflammation and airway remodeling.

Antileukotriene drugs are thus entering modified treatment guidelines as oral prophylactic treatment for patients with asthma of varying severity whose disease is not properly controlled by their existing therapy and are designed to be used in addition to existing treatment. The convenience of oral treatment is likely to ensure a high degree of compliance among patients who have difficulty operating metered dose inhalers correctly (e.g., the elderly, small children) or who are reluctant to use inhalers and/or their spacer devices at work or school. Once-daily formulations with a favorable pharmacokinetic profile (e.g., montelukast) are likely to have an advantage over shorter-acting drugs (e.g., zileuton) with regard to compliance, although slow-release formulations of zileuton are under development. The elementary fact that leukotriene modifiers are not steroid-based drugs may enhance compliance in patients anxious about the perceived dangers of corticosteroids, despite widespread evidence of the safety of corticosteroids even at high inhaled doses.

On the other hand, there is a greater theoretical possibility of systemic side effects occurring with routine daily use of oral prophylactic drugs compared to topical use. As a group, leukotriene modulators appear to be very well tolerated and to cause few adverse effects (212). Although mild headache and gastrointestinal upset have been reported in patients receiving cysLTRAs in clinical trials, the frequency of such symptoms is not significantly higher than in patients receiving placebo. Use of zileuton is associated in a small number of patients with mild elevations in serum hepatic transaminases (255,289), but these are usually reversible on cessation of treatment. In the United States, routine liver function testing is advised for the first months of treatment with zileuton. Treatment with cys LTRAs has been associated with a small number of cases of Churg-Strauss syndrome, a form of acute eosinophilic vasculitis, but this is thought to be due to an abrupt reduction in concurrent (usually oral) corticosteroid use, which may have allowed an underlying hypereosinophilia to be revealed (290). It is not thought to be directly related to cysLTRAs and has also been observed with other disease-modifying drugs (e.g., inhaled corticosteroids). The phenomenon stresses the need for gradual tapering down of corticosteroid dosing if a patient's asthma becomes better controlled during treatment with leukotriene modulators.

Two groups of asthma patients seem likely to derive special benefit from leukotriene modulators, either as monotherapy or in addition to existing treatment (212). The drugs may particularly benefit, first, patients with exercise-induced asthma, for whom current treatment is often ineffective, and, second, patients with aspirin-sensitive asthma, who appear to have a preponderantly leukotriene-dependent form of asthma. The latter may be explained by the finding of a significantly increased frequency of a polymorphic allele for LTC_4 synthase in the aspirin-sensitive asthma population (291), closely associated with enhanced expression of LTC_4 synthase and elevated cys-LT synthesis in their airways (292). At the other extreme are asthmatic patients who do not respond to leukotriene modulators such as zileuton (293), supporting the impression from anecdotal clinical experience that distinct ''responder'' and ''nonresponder'' subgroups exist. This may be explained by recently described polymorphisms in the 5-LO gene promoter in both normal and asthmatic subjects, which are thought to lead to reduced 5-LO enzyme expression (294). These patients may thus have a form of asthma in which airway smooth muscle tone is relatively independent on cysteinyl LTs. Further study of these subjects may provide important clues to the role of cysteinyl LTs in chronic airway inflammation and remodeling in asthma. The development of routine tests to genotype patients for polymorphic LTC_4 synthase and 5-LO alleles may help in the better targeting of leukotriene modulator drugs to the patient populations most likely to benefit.

References

1. Smith L, McFadden ER. Bronchial hyperreactivity revisited. Ann Allergy Asthma Immunol 1995; 74:454–469.
2. Crimi E, Spanevello A, Neri M, Ind PW, Rossi GA, Brusasco V. Dissociation between airway inflammation and airway hyperresponsiveness in allergic asthma. Am J Respir Crit Care Med 1998; 157:4–9.
3. Djukanovic R, Wilson JW, Lai CKW, Holgate ST, Howarth PH. The safety aspects of fibreoptic bronchoscopy, bronchoalveolar lavage, and endobronchial biopsy in asthma. Am Rev Respir Dis 1991; 143:772–777.
4. Corrigan CJ, Kay AB. Asthma. Role of T-lymphocytes and lymphokines. Br Med Bull 1992; 48:72–84.
5. Okayama Y, Petit Frere C, Kassel O, Semper A, Quint D, Tunon de Lara MJ, Bradding P, Holgate ST, Church MK. IgE-dependent expression of mRNA for IL-4 and IL-5 in human lung mast cells. J Immunol 1995; 155:1796–1808.
6. Laitinen LA, Laitinen A. Structural and cellular changes in asthma. Eur Respir Rev 1994; 4:348–351.
7. Ebina M, Takahashi T, Chiba T, Motomiya M. Cellular hypertrophy and hyperplasia of airway smooth muscle underlying bronchial asthma. Am Rev Respir Dis 1993; 148:720–726.
8. National Institutes of Health, National Heart, Lung and Blood Institute. Global Initiative for Asthma. Bethesda, MD: NIH, NHLBI, January 1995.
9. Kuitert L, Barnes NC. PAF and asthma—time for an appraisal? Clin Exp Allergy 1995; 25:1159–1162.
10. Curzen N, Rafferty P, Holgate ST. The effect of flurbiprofen, a cyclooxygenase inhibitor, and terfenadine, alone and in combination, on allergen-induced immediate bronchoconstriction. Thorax 1987; 42:946–952.
11. Skoner DP, Page R, Asman B, Gillen L, Fireman P. Plasma elevations of histamine and a prostaglandin metabolite in acute asthma. Am Rev Respir Dis 1988; 137: 1009–1014.

12. Szczeklik A. Aspirin-induced asthma: an update and novel findings. Adv Prostaglandin Thromboxane Leukot Res 1994; 22:185–198.
13. Twentyman OP, Ollier S, Holgate ST. The effect of H_1-receptor blockade on the development of early- and late-phase bronchoconstriction and increased bronchial responsiveness in allergen-induced asthma. J Allergy Clin Immunol 1993; 91: 1169–1178.
14. Wood-Baker R, Holgate ST. The comparative actions and adverse effect profile of single doses of H_1-receptor antihistamines in the airways and skin of subjects with asthma. J Allergy Clin Immunol 1993; 91:1005–1014.
15. Roquet A, Dahlen B, Kumlin M, Ihre E, Anstren G, Binks S, Dahlen SE. Combined antagonism of leukotrienes and histamine produces predominant inhibition of allergen-induced early and late phase airway obstruction in asthmatics. Am J Respir Crit Care Med 1997; 155:1856–1863.
16. Dale HH. Progress in autopharmacology: a survey of present knowledge of the chemical regulation of certain functions by natural constituents of tissue. Johns Hopkins Med J 1930; 53:297–347.
17. Hay DWP, Torphy TJ, Undem BJ. Cysteinyl leukotrienes in asthma: old mediators up to new tricks. Trends Pharmacol Sci 1995; 16:304–309.
18. Holgate ST, Bradding P, Sampson AP. Leukotriene antagonists and synthesis inhibitors: new directions in asthma therapy. J Allergy Clin Immunol 1996; 98:1–13.
19. Stossel TP, Mason RJ, Smith AL. Lipid peroxidation by human blood phagocytes. J Clin Invest 1974; 54:638–645.
20. Samuelsson B. Leukotrienes: mediators of immediate hypersensitivity reactions and inflammation. Science 1983; 220:568–575.
21. Galella G, Medini L, Stragliotto E, Stefanini P, Rise P, Tremoli E, Galli C. In human monocytes interleukin-1 stimulates a phospholipase C active on phosphatidylcholine and inactive on phosphatidylinositol. Biochem Pharmacol 1992; 44: 715–720.
22. Kennedy I, Coleman RA, Humphrey PPA, Levy GP, Lumley P. Studies on the characterisation of prostanoid receptors: a proposed classification. Prostaglandins 1982; 24:667–689.
23. Vane J. Towards a better aspirin. Nature 1994; 367:215–216.
24. Samuelsson B, Dahlen SE, Lindgren JA, Rouzer CA, Serhan CN. Leukotrienes and lipoxins: structures, biosynthesis, and biological effects. Science 1987; 237:1171–1176.
25. Dixon RA, Jones RE, Diehl RE, Bennett CD, Kargman S, Rouzer CA. Cloning of the cDNA for human 5-lipoxygenase. Proc Natl Acad Sci USA 1988; 85:416–420.
26. Rouzer CA, Bennett CD, Diehl RE, Jones RE, Kargman S, Rands E, Dixon RA. Cloning and expression of human leukocyte 5-lipoxygenase. Adv Prostaglandin Thromb Leukot Res 1989; 19:474–477.
27. Samuelsson B, Haeggstrom JZ, Wetterholm A. Leukotriene biosynthesis. Ann NY Acad Sci 1991; 629:89–99.
28. Rouzer CA, Matsumoto T, Samuelsson B. Single protein from human leukocytes possesses 5-lipoxygenase and leukotriene A_4 synthase activities. Proc Natl Acad Sci USA 1986; 83:857–861.

29. Malaviya R, Malaviya R, Jakschik BA. Reversible translocation of 5-lipoxygenase in mast cells upon IgE/antigen stimulation. J Biol Chem 1993; 268:4939–4944.
30. Bell RL, Young PR, Albert D, Lanni C, Summers JB, Brooks DW, Rubin P, Carter GW. The discovery and development of zileuton: an orally active 5-lipoxygenase inhibitor. Int J Immunopharmacol 1992; 14:505–510.
31. Dixon RA, Diehl RE, Opas E, Rands E, Vickers PJ, Evans JF, Gillard JW, Miller DK. Requirement of a 5-lipoxygenase-activating protein for leukotriene synthesis. Nature 1990; 343:282–284.
32. Miller DK, Gillard JW, Vickers PJ, Sadowski S, Leveille C, Mancini JA, Charleson P, Dixon RA, Ford-Hutchinson AW, Fortin R, Gauthier JY, Rodkey J, Rosen R, Rouzer C, Sigal IS, Strader CD, Evans JF. Identification and isolation of a membrane protein necessary for leukotriene production. Nature 1990; 343:278–281.
33. Reid GK, Kargman S, Vickers PJ, Mancini JA, Leveille C, Ethier D, Miller DK, Gillard JW, Dixon RA, Evans JF. Correlation between expression of 5-lipoxygenase-activating protein, 5-lipoxygenase, and cellular leukotriene synthesis. J Biol Chem 1990; 265:19818–19823.
34. Woods JW, Evans JF, Ethier D, Scott S, Vickers PJ, Hearn L, Heibein JA, Charleson S, Singer II. 5-lipoxygenase and 5-lipoxygenase-activating protein are localized in the nuclear envelope of activated human leukocytes. J Exp Med 1993; 178:1935–1946.
35. Pueringer RJ, Bahns CC, Monick MM, Hunninghake GW. A23187 stimulates translocation of 5-lipoxygenase from cytosol to membrane in human alveolar macrophages. Am J Physiol 1992; 262:L454–L458.
36. Peters-Golden M, McNish RW. Redistribution of 5-lipoxygenase and cytosolic phospholipase A_2 to the nuclear fraction upon macrophage activation. Biochem Biophys Res Commun 1993; 196:147–153.
37. Abramovitz M, Wong E, Cox ME, Richardson CD, Li C, Vickers PJ. 5-lipoxygenase-activating protein stimulates the utilization of arachidonic acid by 5-lipoxygenase. Eur J Biochem 1993; 215:105–111.
38. Ford-Hutchinson AW. FLAP: a novel drug target for inhibiting the synthesis of leukotrienes. Trends Pharmacol Sci 1991; 12:68–70.
39. Mancini JA, Prasit P, Coppolino MG, Charleson P, Leger S, Evans JF, Gillard JW, Vickers PJ. 5-Lipoxygenase-activating protein is the target of a novel hybrid of two classes of leukotriene biosynthesis inhibitors. Mol Pharmacol 1992; 41:267–272.
40. Samuelsson B, Funk CD. Enzymes involved in the biosynthesis of leukotriene B_4. J Biol Chem 1989; 264:19469–19472.
41. Orning L, Gierse JK, Fitzpatrick FA. The bifunctional enzyme leukotriene A_4 hydrolase is an arginine aminopeptidase of high efficiency and specificity. J Biol Chem 1994; 269:11269–11273.
42. Orning L, Gierse J, Duffin K, Bild G, Krivi G, Fitzpatrick FA. Mechanism-based inactivation of leukotriene A_4 hydrolase/aminopeptidase by leukotriene A_4: Mass spectrometric and kinetic characterization. J Biol Chem 1992; 267:22733–22739.
43. Lam BK, Gagnon L, Austen KF, Soberman RJ. The mechanism of leukotriene B_4 export from human polymorphonuclear leukocytes. J Biol Chem 1990; 265:13438–13441.

44. Yokomizo T, Izumi T, Chang K, Takuwa Y, Shimuzu T. A G-protein-coupled receptor for leukotriene B_4 that mediates chemotaxis. Nature 1997; 387:620–624.
45. Martin TR, Pistorese BP, Chi EY, Goodman RB, Matthay MA. Effects of leukotriene B_4 in the human lung: recruitment of neutrophils into the alveolar spaces without a change in protein permeability. J Clin Invest 1989; 84:1609–1619.
46. Sampson SE, Costello JF, Sampson AP. The effect of inhaled leukotriene B_4 in normal and in asthmatic subjects. Am J Respir Crit Care Med 1997; 155:1789–1792.
47. Evans DJ, Barnes PJ, Spaethe SM, van Alstyne EL, Mitchell MI, O'Connor BJ. Effect of a leukotriene B_4 receptor antagonist, LY293111, on allergen induced responses in asthma. Thorax 1996; 51:1178–1184.
48. Christie PE, Barnes NC. Leukotriene B_4 and asthma. Thorax 1996; 51:1171–1173.
49. Evans RB. Comparative results of leukotriene modifiers in COPD and asthma (abstr). Am J Respir Crit Care Med 1998; 157:A413.
50. Penrose JF, Gagnon L, Goppelt Struebe M, Myers P, Lam BK, Jack RM, Austen KF, Soberman RJ. Purification of human leukotriene C_4 synthase. Proc Natl Acad Sci USA 1992; 89:11603–11606.
51. Lam BK, Penrose JF, Freeman GJ, Austen KF. Expression cloning of a cDNA for human leukotriene C_4 synthase, an integral membrane protein conjugating reduced glutathione to leukotriene A_4. Proc Natl Acad Sci USA 1994; 91:7663–7667.
52. Lam BK, Penrose JF, Rokach J, Xu K, Baldasaro MH, Austen KF. Molecular cloning, expression and characterization of mouse LTC_4 synthase. Eur J Biochem 1996; 238:606–612.
53. Lam BK, Xu K, Atkins MB, Austen KF. Leukotriene C_4 uses a probenecid-sensitive export carrier that does not recognize leukotriene B_4. Proc Natl Acad Sci USA 1992; 89:11598–11602.
54. Snyder DW, Aharony D, Dobson P, Tsai BS, Krell RD. Pharmacological and biochemical evidence for metabolism of peptide leukotrienes by guinea-pig airway smooth muscle in vitro. J Pharmacol Exp Ther 1984; 231:224–229.
55. Koller M, Konig W, Brom J, Bremm KD, Schonfeld W, Knoller J. Functional characteristics of leukotriene C_4- and D_4-metabolizing enzymes (gamma-glutamyl transpeptidase, dipeptidase) within human plasma. Biochim Biophys Acta 1985; 836:56–62.
56. Conroy DM, Piper PJ, Samhoun MN, Yacoub M. Metabolism and generation of cysteinyl-containing leukotrienes by human airway preparations. Ann NY Acad Sci 1991; 629:455–457.
57. Kellaway CH, Trethewie WR. The liberation of a slow reacting smooth muscle-stimulating substance in anaphylaxis. Q J Exp Physiol 1940; 30:121–145.
58. Brocklehurst WE. The release of histamine and formation of slow-reacting substance (SRS-A) during anaphylactic shock. J Physiol 1960; 151:416–435.
59. Buckner CK, Krell RD, Lavaruso RB, Coursin DB, Bernstein PR, Will JA. Pharmacological evidence that human intralobar airways do not contain different receptors that mediate contractions to leukotriene C_4 and leukotriene D_4. J Pharmacol Exp Ther 1986; 237:558–562.
60. Gardiner PJ, Abram TS, Tudhope SR, Cuthbert NJ, Norman P, Brink C. Leuko-

triene receptors and their selective antagonists. Adv Prostaglandin Thromb Leukot Res 1994; 22:49–61.
61. Gorenne I, Norel X, Brink C. Cysteinyl leukotriene receptors in human lung: what's new? Trends Pharmacol Sci 1996; 17:342–345.
62. Keppler D, Huber M, Hagmann W, Ball HA, Guhlmann A, Kastner S. Metabolism and analysis of endogenous cysteinyl leukotrienes. Ann NY Acad Sci 1988; 524: 68–74.
63. Maltby NH, Taylor GW, Ritter JM, Moore K, Fuller RW, Dollery CT. LTC_4 elimination and metabolism in man. J Allergy Clin Immunol 1990; 85:3–9.
64. Weller PF, Lee CW, Foster DW, Corey EJ, Austen KF, Lewis RA. Generation and metabolism of 5-lipoxygenase pathway leukotrienes by human eosinophils: predominant production of leukotriene C_4. Proc Natl Acad Sci USA 1983; 80: 7626–7630.
65. Bruynzeel PL, Kok PT, Hamelink ML, Kijne AM, Verhagen J. Exclusive LTC_4 synthesis by purified human eosinophils induced by opsonized zymosan. FEBS Lett 1985; 189:350–354.
66. MacGlashan DW, Peters SP, Warner J, Lichtenstein LM. Characteristics of human basophil sulphidopeptide leukotriene release: releasability defined as the ability of the basophil to respond to dimeric cross-links. J Immunol 1986; 136:2231–2239.
67. Peters SP, MacGlashan DWJ, Schleimer RP, Hayes EC, Adkinson NFJ, Lichtenstein LM. The pharmacologic modulation of the release of arachidonic acid metabolites from purified human lung mast cells. Am Rev Respir Dis 1985; 132:367–373.
68. Freeland HS, Schleimer RP, Schulman ES, Lichtenstein LM, Peters SP. Generation of leukotriene B_4 by human lung fragments and purified human lung mast cells. Am Rev Respir Dis 1988; 138:389–394.
69. Bigby TD, Holtzman MJ. Enhanced 5-lipoxygenase activity in lung macrophages compared to monocytes from normal subjects. J Immunol 1987; 138:1546–1550.
70. Damon M, Chavis C, Godard P, Michel FB, Crastes-de-Paulet A. Purification and mass spectrometry identification of leukotriene D_4 synthesized by human alveolar macrophages. Biochem Biophys Res Commun 1983; 111:518–524.
71. Atluru D, Lianos EA, Goodwin JS. Arachidonic acid inhibits 5-lipoxygenase in human T cells. Biochem Biophys Res Commun 1986; 135:670–676.
72. Goldyne ME, Rea L. Stimulated T cell and natural killer (NK) cell lines fail to synthesize leukotriene B_4. Prostaglandins 1987; 34:783–795.
73. Jakobsson PJ, Odlander B, Steinhilber D, Rosen A, Claesson HE. Human B lymphocytes possess 5-lipoxygenase activity and convert arachidonic acid to leukotriene B_4. Biochem Biophys Res Commun 1991; 178:302–308.
74. Jakobsson PJ, Steinhilber D, Odlander B, Radmark O, Claesson HE, Samuelsson B. On the expression and regulation of 5-lipoxygenase in human lymphocytes. Proc Natl Acad Sci USA 1992; 89:3521–3525.
75. Odlander B, Jakobsson PJ, Rosen A, Claesson HE. Human B and T lymphocytes convert leukotriene A_4 into leukotriene B_4. Biochem Biophys Res Commun 1988; 153:203–208.
76. Samuelsson B, Claesson HE. Leukotriene B_4: biosynthesis and role in lymphocytes. Adv Prostaglandin Thromb Leukot Res 1990; 20:1–13.

77. Sun FF, McGuire JC. Metabolism of arachidonic acid by human neutrophils: characterization of the enzymatic reactions that lead to synthesis of LTB_4. Biochim Biophys Acta 1984; 794:56–64.
78. Sala A, Bolla M, Zarini S, Muller Peddinghaus R, Folco G. Release of leukotriene A_4 versus leukotriene B_4 from human polymorphonuclear leukocytes. J Biol Chem 1996; 271:17944–17948.
79. Pace-Asciak CR, Klein J, Spielberg SP. Metabolism of leukotriene A_4 into C_4 by human platelets. Biochim Biophys Acta 1986; 877:68–74.
80. Fitzpatrick F, Liggett W, McGee J, Bunting S, Morton D, Samuelsson B. Metabolism of LTA_4 by human erythrocytes: a novel cellular source of LTB_4. J Biol Chem 1984; 259:11403–11407.
81. Zhou S, Stark JM, Leikauf GD. Leukotriene B_4 formation: human neutrophil-airway epithelial cell interactions. J Appl Physiol 1995; 78:1396–1403.
82. Fitzpatrick F, Haeggstrom J, Granstrom E, Samuelsson B. Metabolism of LTA_4 by an enzyme in blood plasma: a possible leukotactic mechanism. Proc Natl Acad Sci USA 1983; 80:5425–5429.
83. Feinmark SJ, Cannon PJ. Endothelial cell LTC_4 synthesis results from intercellular transfer of leukotriene A_4 synthesized by polymorphonuclear leukocytes. J Biol Chem 1986; 261:16466–16472.
84. Claesson HE, Haeggstrom JZ, Odlander B, Medina JF, Wetterholm A, Jakobsson PJ, Radmark O. The role of leukotriene A_4 hydrolase in cells and tissues lacking 5-lipoxygenase. Adv Exp Med Biol 1991; 314:307–315.
85. Dahinden CA. Regulation of leukotriene production by cytokines. Adv Prostaglandin Thromb Leukot Res 1994; 22:327–339.
86. Daniels RH, Finnen MJ, Hill ME, Lackie JM. Recombinant human monocyte IL-8 primes NADPH-oxidase and phospholipase A_2 activation in human neutrophils. Immunology 1992; 75:157–163.
87. Samet JM, Fonteh AN, Galli SJ, Tsai M, Fasano MB, Chilton FH. Alterations in arachidonate metabolism in mouse mast cells induced to undergo maturation in vitro in response to stem cell factor. J Allergy Clin Immunol 1996; 97:1329–1341.
88. Hoeck WG, Ramesha CS, Chang DJ, Fan N, Heller RA. Cytoplasmic phospholipase A_2 activity and gene expression are stimulated by tumor necrosis factor: dexamethasone blocks the induced synthesis. Proc Natl Acad Sci USA 1993; 90:4475–4479.
89. Funk CD, Hoshiko S, Matsumoto T, Radmark O, Samuelsson, B. Characterization of the human 5-lipoxygenase gene. Proc Nat Acad Sci USA. 1989; 86:2587–2591.
90. Hoshiko S, Radmark O, Samuelsson B. Characterization of the human 5-lipoxygenase promoter. Proc Natl Acad Sci USA 1990; 87:9073–9077.
91. Kennedy BP, Diehl RE, Boie Y, Adam M, Dixon RA. Gene characterization and promoter analysis of the human 5-lipoxygenase-activating protein (FLAP). J Biol Chem 1991; 266:8511–8516.
92. Pouliot M, McDonald PP, Borgeat P, McColl SR. Granulocyte/macrophage colony-stimulating factor stimulates the expression of the 5-lipoxygenase-activating protein (FLAP) in human neutrophils. J Exp Med 1994; 179:1225–1232.
93. Mancini JA, Evans JF. Cloning and characterization of the human leukotriene A_4 hydrolase gene. Eur J Biochem 1995; 231:65–71.
94. Penrose JF, Spector J, Baldasaro M, Xu K, Boyce J, Arm JP, Austen KF, Lam BK.

Molecular cloning of the gene for human leukotriene C_4 synthase: organization, nucleotide sequence, and chromosomal localization to 5q35. J Biol Chem 1996; 271:11356–11361.
95. Pouliot M, McDonald PP, Khamzina L, Borgeat P, McColl SR. Granulocyte-macrophage colony-stimulating factor enhances 5-lipoxygenase levels in human polymorphonuclear leukocytes. J Immunol 1994; 152:851–858.
96. McDonald PP, Pouliot M, Borgeat P, McColl SR. Induction by chemokines of lipid mediator synthesis in granulocyte-macrophage colony-stimulating factor-treated human neutrophils. J Immunol 1993; 151:6399–6409.
97. Pueringer RJ, Bahns CC, Hunninghake GW. Alveolar macrophages have greater amounts of the enzyme 5-lipoxygenase than do monocytes. J Appl Physiol 1992; 73:781–786.
98. Boyce JA, Lam BK, Penrose JF, Friend DS, Parsons S, Owen WF, Austen KF. Expression of LTC_4 synthase during the development of eosinophils in vitro from cord blood progenitors. Blood 1996; 88:4338–4347.
99. Cowburn AS, Holgate ST, Sampson AP. IL-5 increases the expression of 5-lipoxygenase activating protein (FLAP) and translocates 5-lipoxygenase (5-LO) to the nucleus in human blood eosinophils. J Immunol 1999; 163:456–465.
100. Murakami M, Austen KF, Bingham CO, Friend DS, Penrose JF, Arm JP. Interleukin-3 regulates development of the 5-lipoxygenase/leukotriene C_4 synthase pathway in mouse mast cells. J Biol Chem 1995; 270:22653–22656.
101. Macchia L, Hamberg M, Kumlin M, Butterfield JH, Haeggstrom JZ. Arachidonic acid metabolism in the human mast cell line HMC-1: 5-Lipoxygenase gene expression and biosynthesis of thromboxane. Biochim Biophys Acta 1995; 1257:58–74.
102. Brach MA, de Vos S, Arnold C, Gruss HJ, Mertelsmann R, Herrmann F. Leukotriene B_4 transcriptionally activates interleukin-6 expression involving NK-kB and NF-IL6. Eur J Immunol 1992; 22:2705–2711.
103. Rola-Pleszczynski M, Chavaillaz PA, Lemaire I. Stimulation of interleukin 2 and interferon gamma production by leukotriene B_4 in human lymphocyte cultures. Prostaglandins Leukot Med 1992; 23:207–210.
104. Yamaoka KA, Kolb JP. Leukotriene B_4 induces interleukin-5 generation from human T lymphocytes. Eur J Immunol 1993; 23:2392–2398.
105. Yamaoka KA, Dugas B, Paul-Eugene N, Mencia-Huerta JM, Braquet P, Kolb JP. Leukotriene B_4 enhances IL-4-induced IgE production from normal human lymphocytes. Cell Immunol 1994; 156:124–134.
106. McCain RW, Holden EP, Blackwell TR, Christman JW. Leukotriene B_4 stimulates human polymorphonuclear leukocytes to synthesize and release interleukin-8 in vitro. Am J Respir Cell Mol Biol 1994; 10:651–657.
107. Devchand PR, Keller H, Peters JM, Vazquez M, Gonzalez FJ, Wahli W. The PPARalpha-leukotriene B_4 pathway to inflammation control. Nature 1996; 384:39–43.
108. Khan MA, Hoffbrand AV, Mehta A, Wright F, Tahami F, Wickremasinghe RG. MK 886, an antagonist of leukotriene generation, inhibits DNA synthesis in a subset of acute myeloid leukaemia cells. Leuk Res 1993; 17:759–762.
109. Atluru D, Gudapaty S, O'Donnell MP, Woloschak GE. Inhibition of human mono-

nuclear cell proliferation, interleukin synthesis, mRNA for IL-2, IL-6, and leukotriene B_4 synthesis by a lipoxygenase inhibitor. J Leukoc Biol 1993; 54:269–274.
110. Brock TG, McNish RW, Bailie MB, Peters-Golden M. Rapid import of cytosolic 5-lipoxygenase into the nucleus of neutrophils after in vivo recruitment and in vitro adherence. J Biol Chem 1997; 272:8276–8280.
111. Covin R, Baillie M, Peters-Golden M. Changes in the subcellular distribution of 5-lipoxygenase accompany macrophage differentiation in the lung (abstr). Am J Respir Crit Care Med 1997; 151:A677.
112. Hammarstrom S, Murphy RC, Samuelsson B. Structure of leukotriene C: identification of the aminoacid part. Biochem Biophys Res Commun 1979; 91:209–213.
113. Murphy RC, Hammarstrom S, Samuelsson B. Leukotriene C: a slow-reacting substance from murine mastocytoma cells. Proc Natl Acad Sci USA 1979; 76:4275–4279.
114. Lewis RA, Austen KF, Drazen JM, Clark DA, Marfat A, Corey EJ. Slow reacting substances of anaphylaxis: identification of leukotrienes C-1 and D from human and rat sources. Proc Natl Acad Sci USA 1980; 77:3710–3714.
115. Morris HR, Taylor GW, Piper PJ, Tippins JR. Structure of slow-reacting substance of anaphylaxis from guinea pig lung. Nature 1980; 285:104–107.
116. Weiss JW, Drazen JM, Coles N, McFadden ER, Lewis R, Weller P, Corey EJ, Austen KF. Bronchoconstrictor effects of leukotriene C in humans. Science 1982; 216:196–198.
117. Holroyde MC, Altounyan REC, Cole M, Dixon M, Elliott EV. Bronchoconstriction produced in man by leukotrienes C and D. Lancet 1981; 2:17–18.
118. Weiss JW, Drazen JM, McFadden ERJ, Weller P, Corey EJ, Lewis RA, Austen KF. Airway constriction in normal humans produced by inhalation of leukotriene D: potency, time course, and effect of aspirin therapy. JAMA 1983; 249:2814–2817.
119. Griffin M, Weiss JW, Leitch AG, McFadden ERJ, Corey EJ, Austen KF, Drazen JM. Effects of leukotriene D on the airways in asthma. N Engl J Med 1983; 308:436–439.
120. Davidson AB, Lee TH, Scanlon PD, Solway J, McFadden ERJ, Ingram RHJ, Corey EJ, Austen KF, Drazen JM. Bronchoconstrictor effects of leukotriene E_4 in normal and asthmatic subjects. Am Rev Respir Dis 1987; 135:333–337.
121. Barnes NC, Piper PJ, Costello JF. Comparative effects of inhaled leukotriene C_4, leukotriene D_4, and histamine in normal human subjects. Thorax 1984; 39:500–504.
122. Gardiner PJ, Cuthbert NJ. Characterisation of the leukotriene receptor(s) on human isolated lung strips. Agents Actions Suppl 1988; 23:121–128.
123. Bisgaard H, Groth S, Dirksen H. Leukotriene D_4 induces bronchoconstriction in man. Allergy 1983; 38:441–443.
124. O'Byrne PM. Leukotrienes, airway hyperresponsiveness, and asthma. Ann NY Acad Sci 1988; 524:282–288.
125. Arm JP, O'Hickey SP, Hawksworth RJ, Fong CY, Crea AE, Spur BW, Lee TH. Asthmatic airways have a disproportionate hyperresponsiveness to LTE_4, as compared with normal airways, but not to LTC_4, LTD_4, methacholine, and histamine. Am Rev Respir Dis 1990; 142: 1112–1118.

126. Soter NA, Lewis RA, Corey EJ, Austen KF. Local effects of synthetic leukotrienes (LTC_4, LTD_4, LTE_4, and LTB_4) in human skin. J Invest Dermatol 1983; 80:115–119.
127. Piper PJ. Pharmacology of leukotrienes. Br Med Bull 1983; 39:255–259.
128. Joris I, Majno G, Corey EJ, Lewis RA. The mechanism of vascular leakage induced by leukotriene E_4. Am J Pathol 1987; 126:19–24.
129. Woodward DF, Weichman BM, Gill CA, Wasserman MA. The effect of synthetic leukotrienes on tracheal microvascular permeability. Prostaglandins 1983; 25:131–142.
130. Obata T, Kobayashi T, Okada Y, Nakagawa N, Terawaki T, Aishita H. Effect of a peptide leukotriene antagonist, ONO-1078, on antigen-induced airway microvascular leakage in actively sensitised guinea pigs. Life Sci 1992; 51:1577–1583.
131. McIntyre TM, Zimmerman GA, Prescott SM. Leukotrienes C_4 and D_4 stimulate human endothelial cells to synthesize platelet-activating factor and bind neutrophils. Proc Natl Acad Sci USA 1986; 83:2204–2208.
132. Coles SJ, Neill KH, Reid LM, Austen KF, Nii Y, Corey EJ, Lewis RA. Effects of leukotrienes C_4 and D_4 on glycoprotein and lysozyme secretion by human bronchial mucosa. Prostaglandins 1983; 25:155–170.
133. Marom Z, Shelhamer JH, Bach MK, Morton DR, Kaliner M. Slow-reacting substances, leukotrienes C_4 and D_4 increase the release of mucus from human airways in vitro. Am Rev Respir Dis 1982; 126:449–451.
134. Ahmed T, Greenblatt DW, Birch S, Marchette B, Wanner A. Abnormal mucociliary transport in allergic patients with antigen-induced bronchospasm: role of slow-reacting substance of anaphylaxis. Am Rev Respir Dis 1981; 124:110–114.
135. Kaye MG, Smith LJ. Effects of inhaled leukotriene D_4 and platelet-activating factor on airway reactivity in normal subjects. Am Rev Respir Dis 1990; 141:993–997.
136. Arm JP, Spur BW, Lee TH. The effects of inhaled LTE_4 on the airway responsiveness to histamine in subjects with asthma and normal subjects. J Allergy Clin Immunol 1988; 82:654–660.
137. Christie PE, Hawksworth R, Spur BW, Lee TH. Effect of indomethacin on LTE_4-induced histamine hyperresponsiveness in asthmatic subjects. Am Rev Respir Dis 1992; 146:1506–1510.
138. Fujimura M, Sakamoto S, Saito M, Miyake Y, Matsuda T. Effect of a thromboxane A_2 receptor antagonist on bronchial hyperresponsiveness to methacholine in subjects with asthma. J Allergy Clin Immunol 1991; 87:23–27.
139. Sampson SE, Sampson AP, Costello JF. The effect of inhaled prostaglandin D_2 in normal and asthmatic subjects, and of pretreatment with leukotriene D_4. Thorax 1997; 52:513–518.
140. Kohno S, Tsuzuike N, Yamamura H, Nabe T, Horiba M, Ohata K. Important role of peptide leukotrienes (p-LTs) in the resting tonus of isolated human bronchi. Jpn J Pharmacol 1993; 62:351–355.
141. Wang CG, Du T, Xu LJ, Martin JG. Role of leukotriene D_4 in allergen-induced increases in airway smooth muscle in the rat. Am Rev Respir Dis 1993; 148:413–417.
142. Salmon M, Walsh DA, Huang TJ, Barnes PJ, Chung KF. Quantitative proliferative changes in the airways of sensitized and chronically challenged brown-norway rats:

effect of cysteinyl leukotriene receptor antagonist pranlukast (abstr). Am J Respir Crit Care Med 1998; 157:A839.

143. Barnes PJ. Asthma as an axon reflex. Lancet 1986; 1:242–245.
144. Leikauf GD, Claesson HE, Doupnik CA, Hybbinette S, Grafstrom RC. Cysteinyl leukotrienes enhance growth of human airway epithelial cells. Am J Physiol 1990; 259:L255–L261.
145. Fischer AR, McFadden CA, Frantz R, Awni WM, Cohn J, Drazen JM, Israel E. Effect of chronic 5-lipoxygenase inhibition on airway hyperresponsiveness in asthmatic subjects. Am J Respir Crit Care Med 1995; 152:1203–1207.
146. Taki F, Suzuki R, Torii K, Matsumoto S, Taniguchi H, Takagi K. Reduction of the severity of bronchial hyperresponsiveness by the novel leukotriene antagonist 4-oxo-8-[4-(4-phenyl-butoxy) benzoylamino]-2-(tetrazol-5-yl)-4H-1-benzopyran hemihydrate. Arzneimittelforschung 1994; 44:330–333.
147. Fujimura M, Sakamoto S, Kamio Y, Matsuda T. Effect of a leukotriene antagonist, ONO-1078, on bronchial hyperresponsiveness in patients with asthma. Respir Med 1993; 87:133–138.
148. Taylor IK, O'Shaughnessy KM, Fuller RW, Dollery CT. Effect of the cysteinyl-LT receptor antagonist ICI 204,219 on allergen-induced bronchoconstriction and airway hyperreactivity in atopic subjects. Lancet 1991; 337:690–694.
149. Rosenthal RR, Lavins BJ, Hanby LA. Effect of treatment with zafirlukast (''Accolate'') on bronchial hyperresponsiveness in patients with mild-to-moderate asthma. J Allergy Clin Immunol 1996; 97:250.
150. Hui KP, Taylor IK, Taylor GW, Rubin P, Kesterson J, Barnes NC, Barnes PJ. Effect of a 5-lipoxygenase inhibitor on leukotriene generation and airway responses after allergen challenge in asthmatic patients. Thorax 1991; 46:184–189.
151. Diamant Z, Timmers MC, Van der Veen H, Friedman BS, DeSmet M, Depre M, Hilliard D, Bel EH, Sterk PJ. The effect of MK-0591, a novel 5-lipoxygenase activating protein inhibitor, on leukotriene biosynthesis and allergen-induced airway responses in asthmatic subjects in vivo. J Allergy Clin Immunol 1995; 95:42–51.
152. Irvin CG, Tu YP, Sheller JR, Funk CD. 5-lipoxygenase products are necessary for ovalbumin-induced airway responsiveness in mice. Am J Physiol 1997; 272: L1053–L1058.
153. Djukanovic R, Wilson JW, Britten KM, Wilson SJ, Walls AF, Roche WR, Howarth PH, Holgate ST. Quantitation of mast cells and eosinophils in the bronchial mucosa of symptomatic atopic asthmatics and healthy control subjects using immunohistochemistry. Am Rev Respir Dis 1990; 142:863–871.
154. Corrigan CJ, Kay AB. T cells and eosinophils in the pathogenesis of asthma. Immunol Today 1992; 13:501–507.
155. Wang JM, Rambaldi A, Biondi A, Chen ZG, Sanderson CJ, Mantovani A. Recombinant interleukin-5 is a selective eosinophil chemoattractant. Eur J Immunol 1989; 19:701–705.
156. Wardlaw AJ. Eosinophils in the 1990s: new perspectives on their role in health and disease. Postgrad Med J 1994; 70:536–552.
157. Lopez AF, Sanderson CJ, Gamble JR, Campbell HR, Young IG, Vadas MA. Recombinant interleukin-5 is a selective activator of human eosinophil function. J Exp Med 1988; 167:219–224.

158. Ford-Hutchinson AW, Bray MA, Doig MV, Shipley ME, Smith MJH. Leukotriene B: a potent chemotactic and aggregating substance released from polymorphonuclear leukocytes. Nature 1980; 286:264–265.
159. Sehmi R, Wardlaw AJ, Cromwell O, Kurihara K, Waltmann P, Kay AB. Interleukin-5 selectively enhances the chemotactic response of eosinophils obtained from normal but not eosinophilic subjects. Blood 1992; 79:2952–2959.
160. Spada CS, Nieves AL, Krauss AH, Woodward DF. Comparison of leukotriene B_4 and D_4 effects on human eosinophil and neutrophil motility in vitro. J Leukoc Biol 1994; 55:183–191.
161. Chan CC, McKee K, Tagari P, Chee P, Ford-Hutchinson AW. Eosinophil-eicosanoid interactions: inhibition of eosinophil chemotaxis in vivo by a LTD_4-receptor antagonist. Eur J Pharmacol 1990; 191:273–280.
162. Underwood DC, Osborn RR, Newsholme SJ, Torphy TJ, Hay DW. Persistent airway eosinophilia after leukotriene (LT) D_4 administration in the guinea pig: modulation by the LTD_4 receptor antagonist, pranlukast, or an interleukin-5 monoclonal antibody. Am J Respir Crit Care Med 1996; 154:850–857.
163. Foster A, Chan CC. Peptide leukotriene involvement in pulmonary eosinophil migration upon antigen challenge in the actively-sensitised guinea pig. Int Arch Allergy Appl Immunol 1991; 96:279–284.
164. Turner CR, Smith WB, Andresen CJ, Swindell AC, Watson JW. Leukotriene D_4 receptor antagonism reduces airway hyperresponsiveness in monkeys. Pulm Pharmacol 1994; 7:49–58.
165. Abraham WM, Ahmed A, Cortes A, Sielczak MW, Hinz W, Bouska J, Lanni C, Bell RL. The 5-lipoxygenase inhibitor zileuton blocks antigen-induced late airway responses, inflammation and airway hyperresponsiveness in allergic sheep. Eur J Pharmacol 1992; 217:119–126.
166. Laitinen LA, Laitinen A, Haahtela T, Vilkka V, Spur BW, Lee TH. Leukotriene E_4 and granulocytic infiltration into asthmatic airways. Lancet 1993; 341:989–990.
167. Diamant Z, Hiltermann JT, Van Rensen EL, Callenbach PM, Veselic-Charvat M, Van der Veen H, Sont JK, Sterk PJ. The effect of inhaled leukotriene D_4 and methacholine on cell differentials in sputum from patients with asthma. Am J Respir Crit Care Med 1997; 155:1247–1253.
168. Calhoun WJ, Williams KL, Simonson SG, Lavins BJ. Effect of zafirlukast (Accolate) on airway inflammation after segmental allergen challenge in patients with mild asthma (abstr). Am J Respir Crit Care Med 1997; 155:A662.
169. Wenzel SE, Trudeau JB, Kaminsky DA, Cohn J, Martin RJ, Westcott JY. Effect of 5-lipoxygenase inhibition on bronchoconstriction and airway inflammation in nocturnal asthma. Am J Respir Crit Care Med 1995; 152:897–905.
170. Brocklehurst WE. Occurrence of an unidentified substance during anaphylactic shock in cavy lung. J Physiol 1953; 120:16–17.
171. Bjorck T, Dahlen SE. Leukotrienes and histamine mediate IgE-dependent contractions of human bronchi: pharmacological evidence obtained with tissues from asthmatic and non-asthmatic subjects. Pulmon Pharmacol 1993; 6:87–96.
172. Wenzel SE, Larsen GL, Johnston K, Voelkel NF, Westcott JY. Elevated levels of leukotriene C_4 in bronchoalveolar lavage fluid from atopic asthmatics after endobronchial allergen challenge. Am Rev Respir Dis 1990; 142:112–119.

173. Wenzel SE, Fowler AA, Schwartz LB. Activation of pulmonary mast cells by bronchoalveolar allergen challenge: in vivo release of histamine and tryptase in atopic subjects with and without asthma. Am Rev Respir Dis 1988; 137:1002–1008.
174. Wenzel SE, Westcott JY, Smith HR, Larsen GL. Spectrum of prostanoid release after bronchoalveolar allergen challenge in atopic asthmatics and in control groups: an alteration in the ratio of bronchoconstrictive to bronchoprotective mediators. Am Rev Respir Dis 1989; 139:450–457.
175. Wenzel SE, Westcott JY, Larsen GL. Bronchoalveolar lavage fluid mediator levels 5 minutes after allergen challenge in atopic subjects with asthma: relationship to the development of late asthmatic responses. J Allergy Clin Immunol 1991; 87: 540–548.
176. Maltby NH, Taylor GW, Ritter JM, Moore K, Fuller RW, Dollery CT. LTC_4 elimination and metabolism in man. J Allergy Clin Immunol 1990; 85:3–9.
177. Christie PE, Tagari P, Ford-Hutchinson AW, Black C, Markendorf A, Schmitz-Schumann M, Lee TH. Increased urinary LTE_4 excretion following inhalation of LTC_4 and LTE_4 in asthmatic subjects. Eur Respir J 1994; 7:907–913.
178. Taylor GW, Taylor IK, Black PN, Maltby N, Fuller RW, Dollery CT. Urinary leukotriene E_4 after allergen challenge and in acute asthma and allergic rhinitis. Lancet 1989; 1:584–588.
179. Sampson AP, Castling DP, Green CP, Price JF. Persistent elevation in plasma and urinary leukotrienes after acute asthma. Arch Dis Child 1995; 73:221–225.
180. Kumlin M, Dahlen B, Bjorck T, Zetterstrom O, Granstrom E, Dahlen SE. Urinary excretion of leukotriene E_4 and 11-dehydro-thromboxane B_2 in response to bronchial provocations with allergen, aspirin, leukotriene D_4, and histamine in asthmatics. Am Rev Respir Dis 1992; 146:96–103.
181. Kikawa Y, Miyanomae T, Inoue Y, Saito M, Nakai A, Shigematsu Y, Hosoi S, Sudo M. Urinary leukotriene E_4 after exercise challenge in children with asthma. J Allergy Clin Immunol 1992; 89:1111–1119.
182. Bellia V, Bonanno A, Cibella F, Cutitta G, Mirabella A, Profita M, Vignola AM, Bonsignore G. Urinary LTE_4 in the assessment of nocturnal asthma. J Allergy Clin Immunol 1996; 97:735–741.
183. Asano K, Lilly CM, O'Donnell WJ, Israel E, Fischer A, Ransil BJ, Drazen JM. Diurnal variation of urinary leukotriene E_4 and histamine excretion rates in normal subjects and patients with mild-to-moderate asthma. J Allergy Clin Immunol 1995; 96:643–651.
184. Christie PE, Tagari P, Ford Hutchinson AW, Charlesson S, Chee P, Arm JP, Lee TH. Urinary leukotriene E_4 concentrations increase after aspirin challenge in aspirin-sensitive asthmatic subjects. Am Rev Respir Dis 1991;143:1025–1029.
185. Smith CM, Hawksworth RJ, Thien FC, Christie PE, Lee TH. Urinary leukotriene E_4 in bronchial asthma. Eur Respir J 1992; 5:693–699.
186. Nasser SMS, Pfister R, Christie PE, Sousa AR, Barker J, Schmitz-Schumann M, Lee TH. Inflammatory cell populations in bronchial biopsies from aspirin-sensitive asthmatic subjects. Am J Respir Crit Care Med 1996;153:90–96.
187. Sladek K, Dworski R, Soja J, Sheller JR, Nizankowska E, Oates JA, Szczeklik A. Eicosanoids in bronchoalveolar lavage fluid of aspirin-intolerant patients with asthma after aspirin challenge. Am J Respir Crit Care Med 1994; 149:940–946.

188. Becher G, Beck E, Winsel K. Leukotriene C_4, D_4, E_4, F_4 in the breathing condensate of asthmatics in relation to bronchial challenge test (abstr). Am J Respir Crit Care Med 1995; 151:A679.
189. Sampson AP, Thomas RU, Costello JF, Piper PJ. Enhanced leukotriene synthesis in leucocytes of atopic and asthmatic subjects. Br J Clin Pharmacol 1992; 33:423–430.
190. Shindo K, Miyakawa K, Fukumura M. Plasma levels of leukotriene B_4 in asthmatic patients. Int J Tissue React 1993; 15:181–184.
191. Okubo T, Takahashi H, Sumitomo M, Shindo K, Suzuki S. Plasma levels of leukotrienes C_4 and D_4 during wheezing attack in asthmatic patients. Int Arch Allergy Appl Immunol 1987; 84:149–155.
192. Vachier I, Romagnoli M, Tarodo de la Fuente P, Bousquet J, Godard P, Chanez P. Sputum leukotrienes content in asthma (abstr). Am J Respir Crit Care Med 1998; 157:A615.
193. Pavord ID, Ward R, Woltmann G, Sheller JR, Dworski R. Induced sputum eicosanoid concentrations in asthma (abstr). Am J Respir Crit Care Med 1998; 157:A717.
194. Lam S, Chan H, LeRiche JC, Chan-Yeung M, Salari H. Release of leukotrienes in patients with bronchial asthma. J Allergy Clin Immunol 1988; 81:711–717.
195. Wardlaw AJ, Hay H, Cromwell O, Collins JV, Kay AB. Leukotrienes LTC_4 and LTB_4 in bronchoalveolar lavage in bronchial asthma and other respiratory diseases. J Allergy Clin Immunol 1989; 84:19–26.
196. Djukanovic R. Asthma ''of mice and men''—How do animal models help us understand human asthma? Clin Exp Allergy 1994; 24:6–9.
197. Sterk PJ, Fabbri LM, Quanjer PhH, Cockcroft DW, O'Byrne PM, Anderson SD, Juniper EF, Malo J-L. Airway responsiveness: Standardized challenge testing with pharmacological, physical and sensitizing stimuli in adults. Eur Respir J 1993; 6(suppl 16): 53–83.
198. Busse WW, Calhoun WJ, Dick EC. Effect of an experimental rhinovirus 16 infection on airway mediator response to antigen. Int Arch Allergy Immunol 1992; 99: 422–424.
199. Dahlén B, Zetterström O. Comparison of bronchial and per oral provocation with aspirin in aspirin-sensitive asthmatics. Eur Respir J 1990; 3:527–534.
200. Phillips GD, Foord R, Holgate ST. Inhaled lysine-aspirin as a bronchoprovocation procedure in aspirin-sensitive asthma: its repeatability, absence of a late-phase reaction, and the role of histamine. J Allergy Clin Immunol 1989; 84:232–241.
201. Gibson PG, Wong BJO, Hepperle MJE, Kline PA, Girgis-Gabardo A, Guyatt G, Dolovich J, Denburg JA, Ramsdale EH, Hargreave FE. A research method to induce and examine a mild exacerbation of asthma by withdrawal of inhaled corticosteroid. Clin Exp Allergy 1992; 22:525–532.
202. O'Byrne PM, Dolovich J, Hargreave FE. State of art: Late asthmatic responses. Am Rev Respir Dis 1987; 136:740–751.
203. Weersink EJM, Postma DS, Aalbers R, De Monchy JG. Early and late asthmatic reaction after allergen challenge. Respir Med 1994; 88:103–114.
204. Jarjour NN, Calhoun WJ, Schwartz LB, Busse WW. Elevated bronchoalveolar lavage fluid histamine levels in allergic asthmatics are associated with increased airway obstruction. Am Rev Respir Dis 1991; 144:3–7.

205. Liu MC, Bleecker ER, Lichtenstein LM, Kagey-Sobotka A, Niv Y, Mclemore TL, Permutt S, Proud D, Hubbard WC. Evidence for elevated levels of histamine, prostaglandin D_2, and other bronchoconstricting postaglandins in the airway of subjects with mild asthma. Am Rev Respir Dis 1990; 142:26–32.
206. Stenton SC, Court EN, Kingston WP, Goadby P, Kelly CA, Duddridge M, Ward C, Hendrick DJ, Walters EH. Platelet activating factor in bronchoalveolar lavage fluid from asthmatic subjects. Eur Respir J 1990; 3:408–413.
207. Lee TH, Mencia-Huerta JM, Shih C, Corey EJ, Lewis RA, Austen KF. Effects of exogenous arachidonic, eicosapentaenoic and docosahexaenoic acids on the generation of 5-lipoxygenase pathway products by ionophore-activated human neutrophils. J Clin Invest 1984; 74:1922–1933.
208. Arm JP, Horton CE, Spur BW, Mencia-Huerta J-M, Lee TH. The effects of dietary supplementation with fish oil lipids on the airways response to inhaled allergen in bronchial asthma. Am Rev Respir Dis 1989; 139:1395–1400.
209. Arm JP, Horton CE, Mencia-Huerta J-M, House F, Eiser NM, Clark TJH, Spur BW, Lee TH. Effect of dietary supplementation with fish oil lipids on mild asthma. Thorax 1988; 43:84–92.
210. Picado C, Castillo JA, Schinca N, Pujades M, Ordinas A, Coronas A, Agusti-Vidal A. Effects of a fish oil enriched diet on aspirin intolerant asthmatic patients: a pilot study. Thorax 1988; 43:93–97.
211. Thien FCK, Mencia-Huerta J-M, Lee TH. Dietary fish oil effects on seasonal hay fever and asthma in pollen-sensitive subjects. Am Rev Respir Dis 1993; 147:1138–1143.
212. O'Byrne PM, Israel I, Drazen JM. Antileukotrienes in the treatment of asthma. Ann Intern Med 1997; 127:472–480.
213. Carey F, Forder RA. Radioimmunoassay of LTB_4 and 6-trans LTB_4: Analytical and pharmacological characterization of immunoreactive LTB_4 in ionophore-stimulated human blood. Prostaglandins Leukot Med 1986; 22:57–70.
214. Tagari P, Ethler D, Carry M, Korley V, Charleson S, Girard Y, Zamboni R. Measurement of urinary leukotrienes by reversed-phase liquid chromatography and radio-immunoassay. Clin Chem 1989; 35:388–391.
215. Israel E, Rubin P, Kemp JP, Grossman J, Pierson W, Siegel SC, Tinkelman D, Murray JJ, Busse W, Segal AT. The effect of inhibition of 5-lipoxygenase by zileuton in mild-to-moderate asthma. Ann Intern Med 1993; 119:1059–1066.
216. Israel E, Dermarkarian R, Rosenberg M, Sperling R, Taylor G, Rubin P, Drazen J. The effects of 5-lipoxygenase inhibitor on asthma induced by cold, dry air. N Engl J Med 1990; 323:1740–1744.
217. Israel E, Fischer AR, Rosenberg MA, Lilly CM, Callery JC, Shapiro J, Cohn J, Rubin P, Drazen JM. The pivotal role of 5-lipoxygenase products in the reaction of aspirin-sensitive asthmatics to aspirin. Am Rev Respir Dis 1993; 148:1447–1451.
218. Meltzer SS, Hasday JD, Cohn J, Bleecker ER. Inhibition of exercise-induced bronchospasm by zileuton: a 5-lipoxygenase inhibitor. Am J Respir Crit Care Med 1996; 153:931–935.
219. Strek ME, Solway J, Saller L, Kowash K, Miller CJ. Effect of the 5-lipoxygenase inhibitor, ZD 2138, on cold-air-induced bronchoconstriction in patients with asthma (abstr). Am J Respir Crit Care Med 1995; 151:A377.

220. Nasser SMS, Bell GS, Foster S, Spruce KE, MacMillan R, Williams AJ, Lee TH, Arm JP. Effect of the 5-lipoxygenase inhibitor ZD2138 on aspirin-induced asthma. Thorax 1994; 49:749–756.
221. Nasser SM, Bell GS, Hawksworth RJ, Spruce KE, Macmillan R, Williams AJ, Lee TH, Arm JP. Effect of the 5-lipoxygenase inhibitor ZD2138 on allergen-induced early and late asthmatic responses. Thorax 1994; 49:743–748.
222. Van Schoor J, Joos GF, Kips JC, Pauwels RA, Drajesk JF, Carpentier PJ. The effect of ABT-761, a novel 5-lipoxygenase inhibitor, on exercise- and adenosine-induced bronchoconstriction in asthmatics (abstr). Am J Respir Crit Care Med 1995; 151: A376.
223. Lehnigk B, Rabe KF, Dent G, Herst RS, Carpentier PJ, Magnussen H. Effects of a 5-lipoxygenase inhibitor, ABT-761, on exercise-induced bronchoconstriction and urinary LTE_4 in asthmatic patients. Eur Respir J 1998; 11:617–623.
224. Friedman BS, Bel EH, Buntinx A, Tanaka W, Han Y-HR, Shingo S, Spector R, Sterk P. Oral leukotriene inhibitor (MK-886) blocks allergen-induced airway responses. Am Rev Respir Dis 1993; 147:839–844.
225. Dahlén S-E, Dahlén B, Ihre E, Kumlin M, Franzén L, Stensvad F, Larsson C, Blomqvist H, Björck T, Zetterström O. The leukotriene biosynthesis inhibitor BAY x1005 is a potent inhibitor of allergen-induced airway obstruction and leukotriene formation in man (abstr). Am Rev Respir Dis 1993; 147:A837.
226. Hamilton AL, Watson RM, Wylie G, O'Byrne PM. Attenuation of early and late phase allergen-induced bronchoconstriction in asthmatic subjects by a 5-lipoxygenase activating protein antagonist, BAYx-1005. Thorax 1997; 52:348–354.
227. Dahlén B, Kumlin M, Ihre E, Zetterström O, Dahlén S-E. Inhibition of allergen-induced airway obstruction and leukotriene generation in atopic asthmatic subjects by the leukotriene biosynthesis inhibitor BAYx-1005. Thorax 1997; 52:342–347.
228. Fischer AR, Rosenberg MA, Roth M, Loper M, Jungerwirth S, Israel E. Effect of a novel 5-lipoxygenase activating protein inhibitor, BAY x1005, on asthma induced by cold dry air. Thorax 1997; 52:1074–1077.
229. Williams J, Gierczak S, Meltzer S, Nadel A, Jungerwirth S, Bleecker E. Effect of the leukotriene synthesis inhibitor BAY y1015 on exercise-induced bronchospasm in patients with asthma (abstr). Am J Respir Crit Care Med 1996; 153:A803.
230. Holroyde MC, Altounyan RE, Cole M, Dixon M, Elliott EV. Selective inhibition of bronchoconstriction induced by leukotrienes C and D in man. Adv Prostaglandin Thromb Leukot Res 1982; 9:237–242.
231. Jones TR, Guindon Y, Young R, Champion E, Charette L, Denis D, Ethier D, Hamel R, Ford-Hutchinson AW, Fortin R, Letts G, Masson P, McFarlane C, Piechuta H, Rokach J, Yoakim C. L-648,051, sodium 4-[3-(4-acctyl-3-hydroxy 2 propyl-phenoxy)-propylsylfonyl]-τ-oxo-benzenebutanoate: a leukotriene D_4 receptor antagonist. Can J Physiol Pharmacol 1986; 64:1535–1542.
232. Barnes NC, Piper PJ, Costello J. The effect of an oral leukotriene antagonist L-649,923 on histamine and leukotriene D_4-induced bronchoconstriction in normal man. J Allergy Clin Immunol 1987; 79:816–821.
233. Phillips GD, Rafferty P, Robinson C, Holgate ST. Dose-related antagonism of leukotriene D_4-induced bronchoconstriction by p.o. administration of LY-171883 in nonasthmatic subjects. J Pharmacol Exp Ther 1988; 246:732–738.

234. Wood-Baker R, Phillips GD, Lucas RA, Turner GA, Holgate ST. The effect of inhaled LY-170680 on leukotriene D_4-induced bronchoconstriction in healthy volunteers. Drug Invest 1991; 3:239–247.
235. Wahedna I, Wisniewski AS, Tattersfield AE. Effect of RG 12525, an oral leukotriene D_4 antagonist, on the airway response to inhaled leukotriene D_4 in subjects with mild asthma. Br J Clin Pharmacol 1991; 32:512–515.
236. Joos GF, Kips JC, Pauwels RA, Van der Straeten ME. The effect of aerosolized SK&F 104353-Z_2 on the bronchoconstrictor effect of leukotriene D_4 in asthmatics. Pulmon Pharmacol 1991; 4:37–42.
237. Diamant Z. Experimental interventions in leukotriene- and allergen-induced airway responses in asthma in vivo, PhD thesis 1996, ISBN no. 90-9009332, chapter 2. University of Leiden, The Netherlands.
238. Gaddy JN, Margolskee DJ, Bush RK, Williams VC, Busse WW. Bronchodilation with a potent and selective leukotriene D_4 (LTD_4) receptor antagonist (MK-571) in patients with asthma. Am Rev Respir Dis 1992; 146:358–363.
239. Lammers J-WJ, Van Daele P, Van den Elshout FMJ, Decramer M, Buntinx A, De Lepeleire I, Friedman B. Bronchodilator properties of an inhaled leukotriene D_4 antagonist (verlukast—MK-0679) in asthmatic patients. Pulm Pharmacol 1992; 5: 121–125.
240. Impens N, Reiss TF, Teahan JA, De Smet M, Rossing TH, Shingo S, Zhang J, Schandevyl W, Verbesselt R, Dupont AG. Acute bronchodilation with an intravenously administered leukotriene D_4 antagonist, MK-679. Am Rev Respir Dis 1993; 147:1442–1446.
241. Hui KP, Barnes NC. Lung function improvement in asthma with a cysteinyl leukotriene receptor antagonist. Lancet 1991; 337:1062–1063.
242. Makker HK, Lau LC, Thomson HW, Binks SM, Holgate ST. The protective effect of inhaled leukotriene D_4 receptor antagonist ICI 204,219 against exercise-induced asthma. Am Rev Respir Dis 1993; 147:1413–1418.
243. Finnerty JP, Wood-Baker R, Thomson H, Holgate ST. Role of leukotrienes in exercise-induced asthma. Am Rev Respir Dis 1992; 145:746–749.
244. Lazarus SC, Wong HH, Watts MJ, Boushey HA, Lavins BJ, Minkwitz MC. The leukotriene receptor antagonist zafirlukast inhibits sulfur dioxide-induced bronchoconstriction in patients with asthma. Am J Respir Crit Care Med 1997; 156:1725–1730.
245. Rasmussen JB, Eriksson L-O, Margolskee DJ, Tagari P, Williams VC, Andersson K-E. Leukotriene D_4 receptor blockade inhibits the immediate and late bronchoconstrictor responses to inhaled antigen in patients with asthma. J Allergy Clin Immunol 1992; 90:193–201.
246. Manning PJ, Watson RM, Margolskee DJ, Williams VC, Schwartz JI, O'Byrne PM. Inhibition of exercise-induced bronchoconstriction by MK-571, a potent leukotriene D_4-receptor antagonist. N Engl J Med 1990; 323:1736–1739.
247. Diamant Z, Grootendorst DC, Veselic-Charvat M, Timmers MC, De Smet M, Leff JA, Seidenberg BC, Zwinderman AH, Peszek I, Sterk PJ. The effect of montelukast (MK-0476), a cysteinyl leukotriene receptor antagonist, on allergen-induced airway responses and sputum cell counts in asthma. Clin Exp Allergy 1999; 29: 42–51.

248. Leff JA, Busse WW, Pearlman D, Bronsky EA, Kemp J, Hendeles L, Dockhorn R, Kundu S, Zhang J, Seidenberg BC, Reiss TF. Montelukast, a leukotriene-receptor antagonist, for the treatment of mild asthma and exercise-induced bronchoconstriction. N Engl J Med 1998; 339:147–152.
249. Suguro H, Majima T, Ichimura K, Hashimoto N, Koyama S, Horie T. Effect of a leukotriene antagonist, pranlukast hydrate, on exercise-induced bronchoconstriction (abstr). Am J Respir Crit Care Med 1997; 155:A662.
250. Yamamoto H, Nagata M, Kuramitsu K, Tabe K, Kiuchi H, Sakamoto Y, Yamamoto K, Dohi Y. Inhibition of analgesic-induced asthma by leukotriene receptor antagonist ONO-1078. Am J Respir Crit Care Med 1994; 150:254–257.
251. Hamilton A, Faiferman I, Stober P, Watson RM, O'Byrne PM. Pranlukast, a cysteinyl leukotriene receptor antagonist, attenuates allergen-induced early- and late-phase bronchoconstriction and airway hyperresponsiveness in asthmatic subjects. J Allergy Clin Immunol 1998; 102:177–183.
252. Dahlén B, Kumlin M, Margolskee DJ, Larsson C, Blomqvist H, Williams VC, Zetterström O, Dahlén S-E. The leukotriene-receptor antagonist MK-0679 blocks airway obstruction induced by inhaled lysine-aspirin in aspirin-sensitive asthmatics. Eur Respir J 1993; 6:1018–1026.
253. Christie PE, Smith CM, Lee TH. The potent and selective sulfidopeptide leukotriene antagonist, SK&F 104353, inhibits aspirin-induced asthma. Am Rev Respir Dis 1991; 144:957–958.
254. Richter K, Jörres RA, Janicki S, Ulbrich E, Magnussen H. Protection against exercise-induced asthma by the inhaled leukotriene D_4-receptor antagonist BAY-x7195 (abstr). Am J Respir Crit Care Med 1998; 157:A409.
255. Israel E, Cohn J, Dube L, Drazen JM. Effect of treatment with zileuton, a 5-lipoxygenase inhibitor, in patients with asthma: a randomized controlled trial. JAMA 1996; 275:931–936.
256. Liu MC, Dubé LM, Lancaster J. Acute and chronic effects of a 5-lipoxygenase inhibitor in asthma: a 6-month randomized multicenter trial. J Allergy Clin Immunol 1996; 98:859–871.
257. Dekhuijzen PNR, Bootsma GP, Wielders PLML, Van den Berg LRM, Festen J, Van Herwaarden CLA. Effects of single-dose zileuton on bronchial hyperresponsiveness in asthmatic patients treated with inhaled corticosteroids. Eur Respir J 1997; 10:2749–2753.
258. Storms W, Friedman BS, Zhang J, Santanello N, Allegar N, Appel D, Beaucher W, Bronsky F, Busse W, Chervinsky P, Dockhorn R, Edwards T, Goldstein M, Grossman J, Hendeles L, Kemp J, Memon N, Noonan M, Owens G, Shapiro G, Spirn I, Strek M, Stricker W, Tinkelman D, Townley R, Wanderer A, Weisberg S, Winder J, Woehler T. Treating asthma by blocking the lipoxygenase pathway (abstr). Am J Respir Crit Care Med 1995; 151:A377.
259. Margolskee D, Bodman S, Dockhorn R, Israel E, Kemp J, Mansmann H, Minotti DA, Spector S, Stricker W, Tinkelman D, Townley R, Winder J, Williams V. The therapeutic effects of MK-571, a potent and selective leukotriene (LT) D_4 receptor antagonist, in patients with chronic asthma (abstr). J Allergy Clin Immunol 1991; 87:309.
260. Spector SL, Smith LJ, Glass M. Effects of 6 weeks of therapy with oral doses of

ICI 204,219, a leukotriene D_4 receptor antagonist, in subjects with bronchial asthma. Am J Respir Crit Care Med 1994; 150:618–623.

261. Howland W, Segal A, Glass M, Minkwitz MC. 6-week therapy with the oral leukotriene receptor antagonist ICI204219 in the treatment of asthma (abstr). J Allergy Clin Immunol 1994; 93:A259.

262. Spector S, Miller CJ, Glass M. 13-week dose-response study with Accolate™ (zafirlukast) in patients with mild-to-moderate asthma (abstr). Am J Respir Crit Care Med 1995; 151:A379.

263. Hassall SM, Miller C, Harris A. Zafirlukast (Accolate™) reduced the need for oral steroid bursts (abstr). Am J Respir Crit Care Med 1998; 157:A411.

264. Micheletto C, Turco P, Dal Negro R. Accolate 20 mg works as steroid sparing in moderate asthma (abstr). Am J Respir Crit Care Med 1997; 155:A664.

265. Reiss TF, Altman LC, Chervinsky P, Bewtra A, Stricker WE, Noonan G, Kundu S, Zhang J. Effects of montelukast (MK-0476), a new potent cysteinyl leukotriene (LTD_4) receptor antagonist, in patients with chronic asthma. J Allergy Clin Immunol 1996; 98:528–534.

266. Noonan MJ, Chervinsky P, Brandon M, Zhang J, Kundu S, McBurney J, Reiss TF. Montelukast, a potent leukotriene receptor antagonist, causes dose-related improvements in chronic asthma. Eur Respir J 1998; 11:1232–1239.

267. Reiss TF, Altman LC, Munk ZM, Seltzer J, Zhang J, Shingo S, Friedman B, Noonan N. MK-0476, an LTD_4 receptor antagonist, improves signs and symptoms of asthma with a dose as low as 10 mg, once daily (abstr). Am J Respir Crit Care Med 1995; 151:A378.

268. Leff JA, Israel E, Noonan MJ, Finn AF, Godard P, Lofdahl CG, Friedman BS, Connors L, Weinland DE, Reiss TF, Kundu S. Montelukast (MK-0476) allows tapering of inhaled corticosteroids (ICS) in asthmatic patients while maintaining clinical stability (abstr). Am J Respir Crit Care Med 1997; 155:A976.

269. Reiss TF, Chervinsky P, Dockhorn RJ, Shingo S, Seidenberg B, Edwards TB. Montelukast, a once-daily leukotriene receptor antagonist, in the treatment of chronic asthma: a multicenter, randomized, double-blind trial. Arch Intern Med 1998; 158: 1213–1220.

270. Suzuki N, Kudo K, Sano Y, Adachi M, Kanazawa M, Kudo S, Horie T, Kobayashi H, Konno K, Itoh K, Miyamoto T. Efficacy of oral pranlukast, a leukotriene receptor antagonist, in the treatment of asthma: an open study in Tokyo (abstr). Am J Respir Crit Care Med 1997; 155:A664.

271. Sahn S, Galant S, Murray J, Bronsky E, Spector S, Faiferman I, Stober P. Pranlukast (Ultair) improves FEV_1 in patients with asthma: results of a 12-week multicenter study vs nedocromil (abstr). Am J Respir Crit Care Med 1997; 155:A665.

272. Ramsay CF, Van Kan CI, Sterk PJ, Barnes NC. Pranlukast improves spirometry and bronchial hyperresponsiveness (BHR) in patients with mild asthma (abstr). Am J Respir Crit Care Med 1998; 157:A411.

273. Hozawa S, Haruta Y, Tamagawa K, Ishioka S, Yamakido M. Effect of a LT receptor antagonist, ONO-1078, on bronchial hyperresponsiveness and serum ECP in patients with asthma (abstr). Am J Respir Crit Care Med 1998; 157:A413.

274. Tamaoki J, Kondo M, Tagaya E, Takemura H, Nagai A, Takizawa T, Konno K. Leukotriene antagonist prevents exacerbation of asthma during reduction of

high-dose inhaled corticosteroid (abstr). Am J Respir Crit Care Med 1997; 155:A663.
275. Kane GC, Pollice M, Kim C, Cohn J, Dworski RT, Murray JJ, Sheller JR, Fish JE, Peters SP. A controlled trial of the effect of the 5-lipoxygenase inhibitor, zileuton, on lung inflammation produced by segmental antigen challenge in human beings. J Allergy Clin Immunol 1996; 97:646–654.
276. Leff JA, Pizzichini E, Efthimiadis A, Boulet LP, Wei LX, Weinland DE, Hendeles L, Hargreave FE. Effect of montelukast (MK-0476) on airway eosinophilic inflammation in mildly uncontrolled asthma: a randomized placebo-controlled trial (abstr). Am J Respir Crit Care Med 1997; 155:A977.
277. Nakamura Y, Hoshino M, Sim JJ, Ishii K, Hosaka K, Sakamoto T. Effect of the leukotriene receptor antagonist pranlukast on cellular infiltration in the bronchial mucosa of patients with asthma. Thorax 1998; 53:835–841.
278. Isogai S, Taniguchi M, Anzai K, Nakagawa C, Matsui K, Tanaka I, Kako K, Sato M, Okazawa M, Sakakibara H, Suetsugu S. Effects of peptido-leukotriene receptor antagonist pranlukast on eosinophil counts in peripheral blood and sputum in patients with chronic asthma (abstr). Am J Respir Crit Care Med 1998; 157:A412.
279. Kylstra JW, Sweitzer DE, Miller CJ, Bonuccelli CM. Zafirlukast (Accolate) in moderate asthma: patient-reported outcomes and peripheral eosinophil data from a 13-week trial (abstr). Am J Respir Crit Care Med 1998; 157:A410.
280. Melis M, Siena L, Pace E, Vignola AM, Garino G, Cibella F, Gjomarkaj M, Bonsignore G. Effect of zafirlukast on peripheral-blood T-lymphocytes (PBT) isolated from normal and asthmatic patients (abstr). Am J Respir Crit Care Med 1998; 157: A394.
281. Kurosawa M, Yodonawa S, Tsukagoshi H, Miyachi Y. Inhibition by a novel peptide leukotriene receptor antagonist ONO-1078 of airway wall thickening and airway hyperresponsiveness to histamine induced by leukotriene C_4 and leukotriene D_4 in guinea-pigs. Clin Exp Allergy 1994; 24:960–968.
282. Robuschi M, Riva E, Fuccella LM, Vida E, Barnabe R, Rossi M, Gambaro G, Spagnotto S, Bianco S. Prevention of exercise-induced bronchoconstriction by a new leukotriene antagonist (SK&F 104353): A double-blind study versus disodium cromoglycate and placebo. Am Rev Respir Dis 1992; 145:1285–1288.
283. Hofstra WB, Sterk PJ, Neijens HJ, Van der Weij AM, Van Zoest JGCM, Duiverman EJ. Two weeks treatment with zafirlukast (Accolate™), sodium cromoglycate or placebo on exercise-induced bronch constriction in asthmatic adolescents (abstr). Am J Respir Crit Care Med 1997; 155:A665.
284. Turpin JA, Edelman JM, DeLucca PT, Pearlman DS. Chronic administration of montelukast (MK-0476) is superior to inhaled salmeterol in the prevention of exercise-induced bronchoconstriction (EIB) (abstr). Am J Respir Crit Care Med 1998; 157:A456.
285. Suissa S, Dennis R, Ernst P, Sheehy O, Wood-Dauphinee S. Effectiveness of the leukotriene receptor antagonist zafirlukast for mild-to-moderate asthma: a randomized, double-blind, placebo-controlled trial. Ann Intern Med 1997; 126:177–183.
286. Sampson AP, Corne J, Holgate ST. Will the advent of anti-leukotriene therapy lead to changes in asthma treatment guidelines? BioDrugs 1997; 7:167–173.
287. Chapman KR, Friedman BS, Shingo S, Heyse J, Reiss T, Spector R. The efficacy

of an oral inhibitor of leukotriene synthesis (MK-0591) in asthmatics treated with inhaled steroids (abstr). Am J Respir Crit Care Med 1994; 149:A215.

288. Israel E, Cohn J, Dube L, Drazen J, and the Zileuton Study Group. Chronic 5-lipoxygenase (5-LO) inhibition by zileuton significantly decreases the requirement for acute steroid treatment of asthma (abstr). Am J Respir Crit Care Med 1995; 151:A678.
289. McGill KA, Busse WW. Zileuton. Lancet 1996; 348:519–524.
290. Wechsler ME, Garpestad E, Flier SR, Kocher O, Weiland DA, Polito AJ, Klinek MM, Bigby TD, Wong GA, Helmers RA, Drazen JM. Pulmonary infiltrates, eosinophilia, and cardiomyopathy following corticosteroid withdrawal in eight patients receiving zafirlukast treatment for asthma (abstr). Am J Respir Crit Care Med 1998; 157:A456.
291. Sanak M, Simon HU, Szczeklik A. Leukotriene C_4 synthase promoter polymorphism and risk of aspirin-induced asthma. Lancet 1997; 350:1599–1600.
292. Cowburn A, Sladek K, Soja J, Adamek L, Nizankowska E, Szczeklik A, Lam BK, Penrose JF, Austen KF, Holgate ST, Sampson AP. Over-expression of leukotriene C_4 synthase in bronchial biopsies of aspirin-intolerant asthmatics. J Clin Invest 1998; 101:834–846.
293. In K, Asano K, Busse W, Israel E, Fischer A, Kemp J, Ledford D, Murray JJ, Segal A, Tinkelman D, Drazen JM. Polymorphisms in the human 5-lipoxygenase gene sequence identified in normal and asthmatic subjects (abstr). Am J Respir Crit Care Med 1996; 153:A413.
294. In K, Asano K, Beler D, Grobholz J, Finn PW, Solverman EK, Silverman ES, Collins T, Fischer AR, Keith TP, Serino K, Kim SW, De Sanctis GW, Yandava C, Pillari A, Rubin P, Kemp J, Israel E, Busse W, Drazen JM. Naturally occurring mutations in the human 5-lipoxygenase gene promoter that modify transcription factor binding and reporter gene transcription. J Clin Invest 1997; 99:1130–1137.

11

The Anti-IgE Treatment Strategy for Asthma

JOHN V. FAHY

University of California
San Francisco, California

I. Introduction

A little over 30 years ago the Ishizakas and Hornbrook (1) reported that a unique immunoglobulin isotype, IgE, was the reaginic antibody responsible for immediate hypersensitivity reactions. Since that time IgE has been viewed as a logical target for novel drug development in asthma, because several lines of evidence suggest an important role for IgE in asthmatic airway inflammation. First, IgE levels are higher than normal in asthmatic subjects of all ages (2,3). Second, IgE-mediated type 1 hypersensitivity reactions are the likely mechanisms of acute bronchospasm in allergic asthmatic subjects exposed to aeroallergen (4). The specific mechanism is that allergen molecules cross-link adjacent Fab components of IgE on mast cells and basophils, causing secretion of mediators such as histamine, leukotrienes, tryptase, and chymase that results in airway narrowing. The resulting airflow obstruction is caused in part by smooth muscle contraction as well as by vascular leakage of plasma proteins and secretion of mucus from the airway epithelium. Third, IgE may have a role in maintaining chronic airway inflammation in asthma. For example, IgE-induced activation of mast cells causes secretion of preformed mediators, as described above, but also secretion of newly generated mediators such as cytokines and eicosanoids that can promote airway eosinophilia. Thus, chronic exposure to perennial aeroallergens such as that of the house dust mite might result in continuous mast-cell activation, continuous hypersecretion of eosinophil-active cytokines, and chronic airway eosinophilia. This is not the only mechanism by which IgE could mediate chronic airway inflammation in asthma, however, because there is increasing evidence that IgE can exert important proinflammatory effects on the airway through low-affinity IgE receptors (FcεR2) on resident cells such as dendritic cells, macrophages, and ciliated epithelial cells and on nonresident inflammatory cells such as mast cells, basophils, lymphocytes, and eosinophils (5,6).

Both Genentech and Novartis have developed monoclonal antibody research programs to target IgE, and both companies have succeeded in developing candidate antibodies for human testing. The Novartis antibodies (CGP 51901 and CGP 56901) and the Genentech antibody (rhuMAb-E25) have undergone Phase I trials in human subjects; based on these data, both companies have recently agreed to jointly develop rhuMAb-E25 as the most promising of these antibodies for further clinical trials. The challenge for the drug development process has been to engineer an anti-IgE antibody that reduces IgE levels without causing anaphylaxis. Below is a description of the successful strategy that has been developed to produce ''nonanaphylactogenic'' anti-IgE antibodies, together with a review of the early data on the safety and efficacy of this approach in patients with allergic airway disease, including asthma.

II. Development of Nonanaphylactogenic Anti-IgE Monoclonal Antibodies

Therapeutic anti-IgE antibodies need to block binding of IgE to the high-affinity IgE receptor (FCεR1) without cross-linking IgE and triggering degranulation of IgE-sensitized cells—i.e., the antibodies need to be nonanaphylactogenic. To achieve this, monoclonal antibodies against IgE have been developed that bind IgE at the same site as the high-affinity receptor (Fig. 1) (7). This particular binding affinity has two distinct advantages. First, the antibody will inhibit IgE effector functions by blocking IgE binding to high-affinity receptors on IgE effector cells such as mast cells and basophils. Second, the antibody will not cause mast-cell or basophil activation because it cannot bind to IgE on mast cells or basophils, since the FcεR1 receptor masks the anti-IgE epitope. Antibodies selected for blocking IgE-FcεR1 interaction also inhibit binding to FcεR2, because the binding site for FcεR2 is in the same Fc domain as the binding site for FcεR1.

The functional consequence of a therapeutic strategy based on systemic high-affinity anti-IgE antibody treatment is lower circulating IgE levels, unavailability of IgE for binding to IgE receptors on effector cells, and immediate bind-

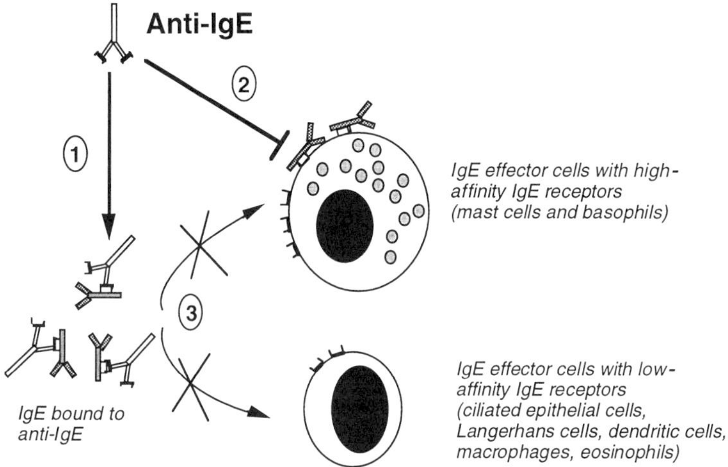

Figure 1 Schematic of the mechanism of action of nonanaphylactogenic anti-IgE antibodies. (1) Anti-IgE binds free IgE, and facilitates its removal via the reticuloendothelial system. (2) Anti-IgE *does not* bind IgE already bound to high- or low-affinity IgE receptors, and IgE effector cells are not activated; i.e., it is nonanaphylactogenic. (3) IgE complexed to anti-IgE is unavailable to bind to receptors on IgE effector cells, and these cells are thereby "disarmed" of IgE; IgE-mediated activation of these cells is prevented. Inhibition of IgE production by B cells as a consequence of anti-IgE binding to membrane-bound IgE on B cells has been demonstrated in mice (26,27), but it is not certain that anti-IgE decreases IgE production in humans.

ing of any IgE dissociating from FcεR1 and FcεR2 receptors on effector cells in tissue compartments; in this way, IgE effector cells are "disarmed," and IgE-dependent allergic reactions should be prevented. The antiallergic effect of anti-IgE cannot be expected to be immediate, because the disarming of effector cells of IgE will not be immediate. Current understanding of the kinetics of IgE binding to high-affinity receptors on mast cells and basophils is imperfect, but available data suggest that disarming high-affinity receptors on these cells is likely to take weeks rather than hours or days.

rhuMAb-E25 and CGP 56901 are nonanaphylactogenic murine antihuman IgE monoclonal antibodies that have been "humanized" by selective removal of murine residues not essential for binding of the antibody to IgE (7). The humanized versions of these murine monoclonal antibodies contain less than 5% murine residues and are thus rendered nonimmunogenic. In addition, these antibodies are selective for IgE and do not bind immunoglobulins of other isotype classes. Immune complex formation is therefore minimal, because the concentration of IgE in human blood is only 0.01% of total immunoglobulin levels.

III. The Role of IgE in Airway Inflammation: Lessons from Experiments Using Nonanaphylactogenic Anti-IgE

The availability of nonanaphylactogenic anti-IgE antibodies is allowing new investigations of the precise role of IgE in the airway eosinophilic inflammation characteristic of allergic airway diseases. In particular, these antibodies are facilitating study of the possible role of IgE in the secretion of Th2 cytokines and in recruitment of eosinophils to the airway after allergen challenge. For example, Coyle et al. (8) showed that giving anti-IgE Mab to sensitized mice 6 hr before airway challenge with house dust mite allergen significantly reduced the recovery of eosinophils from BAL 24 hr later, when these mice were compared with others that had been pretreated with a nonspecific IgG monoclonal antibody. Anti-IgE pretreatment also significantly inhibited the production of IL-4 and IL-5 but not interferon gamma by lung lymphocytes. Interestingly, allergen challenge of mice pretreated with anti-CD23 or of mice deficient in CD23 also caused little influx of eosinophils in BAL samples 24 hr later. In contrast, allergen challenge of mice deficient in mast cells led to the typical increase in eosinophils in BAL 24 hr later. These studies suggest that IgE-dependent mechanisms are important in the induction of the characteristic Th2 cytokine response to allergen and the subsequent infiltration of eosinophils into the airways. These studies further suggest that the low-affinity IgE receptor CD23, not FcεR1, may be the receptor most important for mediating allergen-induced airway eosinophilia initiated by antigen-IgE binding. Support for this idea comes from the finding that IgE-dependent antigen focusing by human B lymphocytes is mediated by CD23 (9). Thus, IgE interaction with CD23 may be an important step in antigen presentation to T lymphocytes by presenting cells, and anti-IgE treatment has the potential to disrupt this mechanism.

IV. Safety of the Anti-IgE Strategy

There are at least three safety concerns surrounding the anti-IgE treatment strategy: anti-IgE treatment may (1) cause anaphylaxis; (2) predispose to parasitic infections; and (3) provoke immune responses, including complement fixation or antibody formation.

The concern that anti-IgE antibodies may cause anaphylaxis has been eliminated by the development of nonanaphylactogenic antibodies, as described above. The concern that anti-IgE treatment may predispose to parasitic infections arises from data suggesting an important role for IgE in eliminating parasites (10). However, the role of IgE in host defense against parasitic infections such as *Schistosoma mansoni* is debated (11–13), and the debate has been intensified by conflicting reports of the role of IgE in eliminating parasites. For example, Amiri et al. (12) treated mice with a rabbit polyclonal antimouse anti-IgE or with an isotype control antibody and then infected them with *S. mansoni*. The result was surprising: reduction of the IgE response by anti-IgE antibody decreased the worm burden, the number of eggs per worm, and the number of hepatic granulomas. Amiri et al. (12) concluded that ". . . IgE plays a detrimental, rather than beneficial role for the host in schistosomiasis." Other authors do not agree. King et al. (13) infected normal mice and IgE-deficient mice (animals with a null mutation of the Cε gene, and thus incapable of making IgE) with *S. mansoni* and found that the IgE-deficient mice were significantly more susceptible to primary infection, developing worm burdens twofold greater than those of wild-type mice. In contrast to Amiri et al. (12), King et al. (13) concluded that ". . . IgE participates in parasite elimination in primary infection with *S. mansoni* and in the generation of humoral immunity and cytokine responses to the parasite." These conflicting data of the role of IgE in mouse models of *S. mansoni* are not easily resolved, but it is somewhat reassuring that the mouse model of IgE elimination that uses a monoclonal antibody appears safer than the mouse model that uses a gene knockout strategy. Overall, though, there is enough evidence for a potentially important role for IgE in host defense against parasites that clinical trials of anti-IgE treatments will need to monitor the incidence of parasitic infections closely.

The concern that anti-IgE may provoke an immune response is generic to all protein therapeutics but is considerably reduced by the "humanization step" in the engineering of anti-IgE molecules (7,14). Thus, for example, the development of antibodies against rhuMAb-E25 has not been detected in studies of over 1000 patients where the drug has been administered intravenously (15–18). Interestingly, the aerosol route of administration may be more immunogenic than the intravenous or subcutaneous route, because aerosolized rhuMAb-25 treatment in 20 patients was associated with development of an antibody to rhuMAb-E25 in 1 patient (19).

Although rhuMab-E25 has an IgG1 kappa structural framework, it does not fix complement. In addition, rhuMAb-E25:IgE complexes are of limited size (1 million MW or smaller) (20,21), and studies in cynomolgus monkeys indicate that these relatively small complexes do not accumulate in any body organs, including the kidney (21). To date, immune complex–mediated complications from rhuMAb-E25 treatment have not been reported in human studies and seem unlikely to occur based on the in vitro and animal data described above.

V. Effect of Anti-IgE Antibodies on Circulating Levels of IgE in Blood in Human Subjects

CGP 56901 and rhuMAb-E25 have been administered to human subjects, and pharmacokinetics data has been gathered. A single dose study of CGP 56901 in doses of 3, 10, 30, and 100 mg given intravenously to 33 pollen-sensitive subjects showed that this drug was well tolerated and resulted in a decrease in serum free

IgE (uncomplexed IgE) in a dose-dependent manner, with suppression after 100 mg reaching >96% (22). Total IgE (free IgE plus IgE complexed with CGP 51901) increased, reflecting slower clearance of the complexed IgE. Time to recovery of 50% of baseline IgE level ranged from a mean of 1.3 days for the 3-mg dose to 39 days for the 100-mg dose.

Treatment with intravenous rhuMAb-E25 results in a prompt reduction in free IgE levels after the first dose and a steady-state reduction is achieved after 42 days (Fig. 2) or longer (up to 84 days), depending on the dose of rhuMAb-E25 (15,18). The dose of rhuMAb-25 that causes a reduction in free IgE below the limits of detection of the IgE immunoassay has been examined in a study of 240 subjects with ragweed-induced allergic rhinitis who were treated with rhuMAb-25 intravenously or subcutaneously for 12 weeks (15). Pharmacodynamics data from this study revealed that consistent suppression of serum free IgE to the lowest levels of detection required an initial rhuMAb-E25 to total IgE ratio of approximately 1–15:1 (Fig. 3).

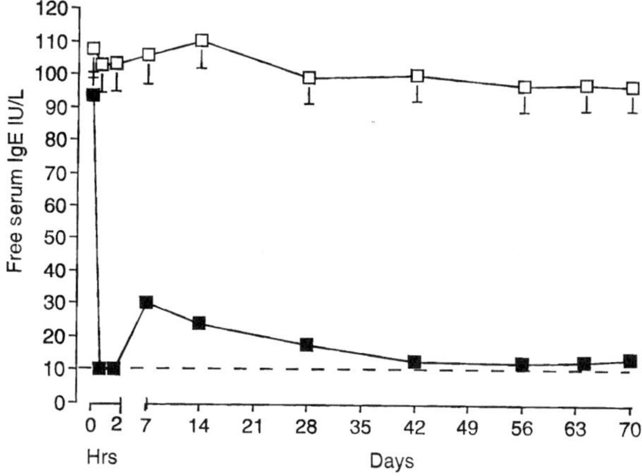

Figure 2 The effect of anti-IgE on serum levels of free IgE. The data are from a randomized placebo-controlled clinical trial of the effects of the nonanaphylactogenic anti-IgE antibody, rhuMAb-E25, in 19 allergic asthmatic subjects (18). Treatment consisted of weekly rhuMAb-E25 or placebo in a dose of 0.5 mg/kg for nine visits. The figure shows serum concentrations of free IgE (mean ± SEM) at baseline and during treatment with rhuMAb-E25 (closed squares; SEM values fall within the symbols) or placebo (open squares). Free IgE levels in the rhuMAb-E25 treated group were significantly lower in the rhuMAb-E25 group at the end of treatment ($p < 0.001$). The dashed line indicates the lower limit of detection for the free IgE assay (10 IU/L). Free IgE levels fell below this limit within 2 hr of rhuMAb-E25 administration in all nine subjects, and steady-state IgE levels were reached at day 42.

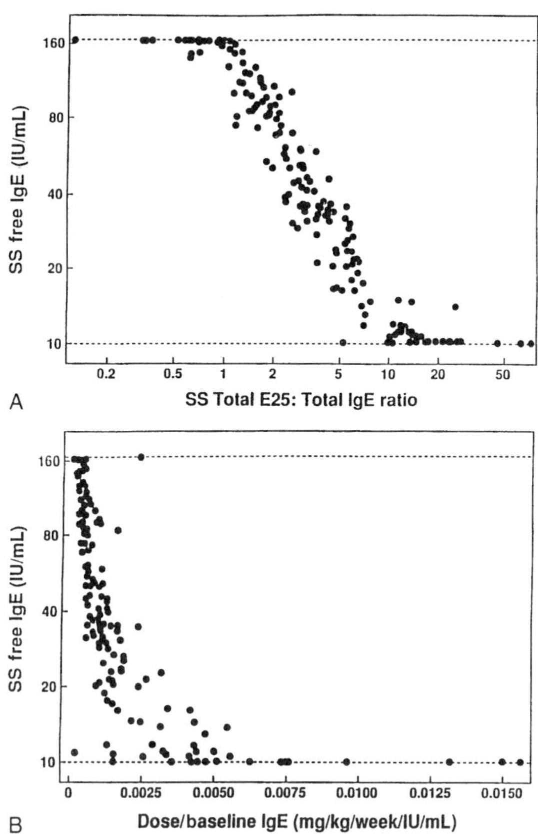

Figure 3 The relationship between the dose of anti-IgE and the level of free IgE in treated patients. The data are from a clinical trial of 240 subjects with ragweed-induced allergic rhinitis treated for 12 weeks with rhuMAb-E25 (15). Panel A: Steady-state (SS) free IgE plotted against steady state total rhuMAb-E25/total IgE (free IgE plus IgE complexed with rhuMAb-E25) ratio in treated patients. Steady-state concentrations are geometric means of predose values over days 42, 56, 70, and 84. Panel B: Steady-state free IgE against dose/baseline IgE in dosed patients. Steady-state free IgE is geometric mean of predose value over days 42, 56, 70, and 84. The data demonstrate that consistent suppression of serum free IgE requires an initial rhuMAb-E25/total IgE ratio of approximately 10–15:1. This analysis implied that dosing should be calculated on the basis of individual baseline IgE levels. Dosing of rhuMAb-E25 of approximately 0.005 mg/kg/week for each international unit per milliliter of baseline IgE suppressed serum free IgE to the lowest level of assay detection at steady state.

As with CGP 51901, total serum IgE (free and complexed IgE) increases in patients treated with rhuMAb-E25 because of slow clearance of the rhuMAb-E25:IgE complexes. Increases in total IgE depend on the dose of rhuMAb-E25 and can range up to sixfold higher than the baseline IgE (15,18). In one study with a 12-week treatment period, total IgE levels did not return to baseline following 8 weeks of follow-up (15), but other clinical studies of rhuMAb-E25, as yet unpublished, demonstrate that serum IgE levels return to baseline values by 16 weeks (after approximately five drug half-lives) (Robert B. Fick, Jr., Genentech Inc., personal communication).

VI. Effect of Anti-IgE Antibody on Allergic Rhinitis

The effect of rhuMAb-E25 on ragweed-induced allergic rhinitis has been tested in a multicenter study of 240 patients but was found not to significantly decrease mean daily eye and nose symptoms during the ragweed season (15). The lack of efficacy in this early Phase II trial may have been due to underdosing. Active treatment was administered for 12 weeks in doses of 0.15 mg/kg subcutaneously, 0.15 mg/kg intravenously, or 0.5 mg/kg intravenously. Thus, dose was adjusted for weight but not for baseline IgE levels, and baseline IgE levels emerged retrospectively as an important pharmacodynamic variable; the subjects with the greatest reduction in IgE levels were those with the low baseline IgE levels and low body weight. In fact, only 11 of the 181 actively treated patients had a reduction in free IgE to less than detectable levels. Another important finding to emerge from this study was that the subcutaneous route of administration was as effective as the intravenous route in suppressing free IgE levels. Because of the possibility that the original study used an insufficient dose of rhuMAb-25, the effects of rhuMAb-E25 in patients with allergic rhinitis is being studied again. This time the dose of rhuMAb-E25 is being adjusted for baseline IgE levels as well as baseline weight, and the drug will be administered subcutaneously; this repeat study should definitively determine the potential for anti-IgE treatment in allergic rhinitis.

VII. Effect of Anti-IgE Antibodies on Early and Late Asthmatic Responses to Aerosolized Allergen

The effects of rhuMAb-E25 treatment on the lower airway responses to aerosolized allergen challenge in asthmatic subjects has been studied in two clinical trials (17,18). In both studies a baseline allergen challenge was followed by intravenous rhuMAb-E25 or placebo for approximately 9 weeks, and the response to treatment was assessed by the effects of allergen on the early- or late-phase response or both. In both of these studies rhuMAb-E25 treatment was associated with a significant attenuation of the early-phase response. The change in the allergen PC15 was nearly three doubling doses, with evidence for a slightly greater effect 77 days than 27 days after treatment initiation (17). rhuMAb-E25 treatment was also associated with a 60% attenuation of the late-phase response (Fig. 4), which was statistically significant (18). A substantial reduction in the eosinophil percentage in induced sputum in the rhuMAb-E25 group was also seen (Fig. 5) (18). Although these eosinophil data were from a small number of subjects and the between-group differences did not reach statistical significance, they suggest that anti-IgE treatment in asthmatic subjects may result in a decrease in airway eosinophilia.

In both of these studies the effect of rhuMAb-E25 on methacholine reactivity was examined. One of the studies showed a statistically significant but modest

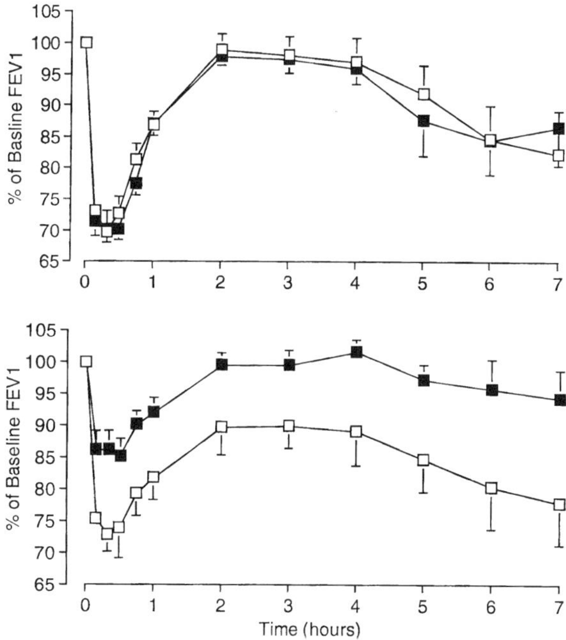

Figure 4 The effect of anti-IgE on the early- and late-phase responses to inhaled allergen. The data are from the study presented in Fig. 2. The figure shows the FEV_1 as a percent of baseline in the first hour after allergen challenge (early-phase response) and from 2–7 hr after allergen challenge (late-phase response) in the placebo (top panel) and rhuMAb-E25 (lower panel) groups at baseline (open squares) and at the end of treatment (closed squares). rhuMAb-E25 treatment significantly attenuated both the early- and late-phase responses.

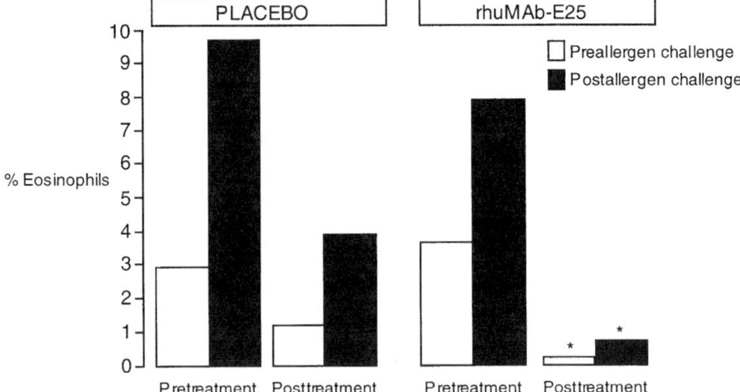

Figure 5 The effect of anti-IgE on the sputum eosinophils. The data are from the study presented in Figs. 2 and 4. Shown is median percentage of eosinophils in induced sputum collected before and after allergen challenge at baseline and at the end of treatment in the placebo group (left panel) and the rhuMAb-E25 group (right panel). The asterisk indicates that the median eosinophil value was significantly different from the corresponding value at baseline ($p < 0.05$) but not significantly different from the change in the corresponding values in the placebo group. Although these data are from a small number of subjects and the between-group differences do not reach statistical significance, they suggest that anti-IgE treatment in asthmatic subjects may result in a decrease in airway eosinophilia.

improvement in methacholine PC20 by day 76 after treatment initiation (17); in the other study, the baseline methacholine PC20 did not change significantly, but a significant attenuation in allergen-induced worsening in methacholine reactivity was observed (18). A recent report by Rabe et al. (23) suggests that large effects of anti-IgE on nonspecific airway hyperreactivity should not be expected. These investigators found that a nonanaphylactogenic anti-IgE monoclonal antibody inhibited allergen-induced contraction of passively sensitized human bronchial rings but had no effect on the histamine responsiveness of these sensitized rings. They concluded that "allergen responses in sensitized human airways are dependent on IgE levels in the sensitizing serum while non-specific (hyper)responsiveness depends on serum factors other than IgE."

These clinical studies of the effects of rhuMAb-E25 on lower airway response to allergen confirm a suspected role for IgE in mediating the early-phase response to allergen and demonstrate for the first time that IgE is also an important mediator of the late-phase response to allergen. Because inhibition of allergen-induced airway responses has proven to be a good indicator of efficacy in improving asthma control in clinical trials, these data provided the rationale for proceeding to a large multicenter trial to test the effects of rhuMAb-E25 on outcomes measuring asthma control. This trial has recently been completed, and preliminary results are encouraging (16).

VIII. Dose Selection of Anti-IgE

To achieve therapeutic efficacy with nonanaphylactogenic anti-IgE antibodies, it is necessary to use a dose that greatly decreases IgE levels. The experiments of MacGlashan and colleagues help explain this feature of the anti-IgE treatment strategy. First, FcεR1 densities on basophils from allergic and nonallergic persons range from 10^4 to 10^6 per cell, and several hundred thousand IgE receptors are usually occupied with IgE (24). Second, only about 2000 IgE molecules are required for a half maximal release of histamine from basophils exposed to specific allergen (25). This explains why anything less than near complete suppression of IgE levels will allow sufficient IgE binding to FcεR1 for full basophil activation. Thus, a little IgE goes a long way, and anti-IgE dosing for therapeutic efficacy will need to reduce IgE levels below a threshold value low enough to prevent IgE effector cell activation. From a practical therapeutic standpoint, this means that anti-IgE dosing needs to be individualized to a patient's total IgE level, and IgE levels on treatment need to undetectable or nearly so.

Also relevant to the discussion of anti-IgE dose and IgE level is the recent work of MacGlashan et al. (24), which suggests that FcεR1 receptor density on IgE effector cells is regulated by circulating levels of IgE. Specifically, these investigators examined the expression of IgE and FcεR1 on human basophils in 15 subjects receiving rhuMAb-E25 intravenously. They found that treatment with rhuMAb-E25 decreased free IgE levels to 1% of pretreatment levels and also resulted in a marked downregulation of FcεR1 on basophils; median receptor densities were approximately 220,000 receptors per basophil at baseline and fell to approximately 8300 receptors per basophil after 3 months of treatment. These data have important consequences for treatment with anti-IgE, because a reduction in IgE receptor density levels will magnify the functional consequences of a reduction in free IgE levels.

IX. Summary

Nonanaphylactogenic anti-IgE antibodies have been developed and have been shown to decrease serum IgE levels and to decrease allergen-induced bronchoconstriction during both the early- and late-phase responses to inhaled allergen. These results have prompted clinical trials of the effects of anti-IgE treatment on other outcomes, including FEV_1, peak flow, asthma symptoms, corticosteroid use, and quality of life. Although the early results from these trials are promising, it is still too early to predict the efficacy of anti-IgE in asthma relative to the efficacy of other asthma controller medications, and it is unclear if all asthmatic patients or just a subgroup will benefit from anti-IgE treatment. The anti-IgE approach to asthma treatment has several advantages, however, including concomitant treatment of other IgE-mediated disease (allergic rhinitis, allergic conjunctivitis, atopic dermatitis, and food allergies), a favorable side-effect profile (so far), and a twice-monthly dosing frequency. The disadvantages of anti-IgE treatment are those generic to recombinant protein therapeutics and include relatively high cost and requirement for injection therapy.

The successful development of nonanaphylactogenic anti-IgE antibodies is exciting, not only for asthma therapeutics but also because these molecules will allow the unraveling of the relative importance of IgE- and non-IgE–dependent mechanisms of airway inflammation in asthma. As the role of IgE in asthma is sorted out, the rational use of anti-IgE treatment in asthma should become clear. For the moment, we can be reasonably optimistic that a novel treatment for asthma will soon be available.

References

1. Ishizaka K, Ishizaka T, Hornbrook MM. Physio-chemical properties of human reaginic antibodies: IV. Presence of a unique immunoglobulin as a carrier of reaginic antibody. J Immunol 1966; 97:75–85.
2. Sears MR, Burrows B, Flannery EM, Herbison GP, Hewitt CJ, Holdaway MD. Relation between airway responsiveness and serum IgE in children with asthma and in apparently normal children. N Engl J Med 1991; 325:1067–1071.
3. Burrows B, Martinez F, Halonen RA, Barbee RA, Cline MG. Association of asthma with serum IgE levels and skin test reactivity to allergens. N Engl J Med 1989; 320: 271–277.
4. Church MK, Holgate ST, Shute JK, Walls AF, Sampson AP. Mast cell–derived mediators. In: Middleton E, Reed CE, Ellis EF, Adkinson NF, Yuninger JW, Busse WW, eds. Allergy Principles and Practices, 5th ed. St. Louis: Mosby-Year Book, 1998:146–167.
5. Sutton BJ, Gould HJ. The human IgE network. Nature 1993; 366:421–428.
6. Campbell AM, Vignola AM, Chanez P, Godard P, Bousquet P. Low affinity receptor for IgE on human bronchial epithelial cells in asthma. Immunology 1994; 82:506–508.
7. Heusser C, Jardieu P. Therapeutic potential of anti-IgE antibodies. Curr Opin Immunol 1997; 9:805–814.
8. Coyle AJ, Wagner K, Bertrand C, Tsuyuki S, Bews J, Heusser C. Central role of immunoglobulin (Ig) E in the induction of lung eosinophil infiltration and T helper 2 cell cytokine production: Inhibition by a non-anaphylactogenic anti-IgE antibody. J Exp Med 1996; 183:1303–1310.
9. Pirron U, Schlunck T, Prinz JC, Rieber EP. IgE-dependent antigen focusing by hu-

man B lymphocytes is mediated by the low affinity receptor for IgE. Eur J Immunol 1990; 20:1547–1551.
10. Finkelman FD, Pearce EJ, Urban JF, Sher A. Regulation and biological function of helminth-induced cytokine responses. Immunol Today 1991:462–467.
11. Capron M, Capron A. Immunoglobulin E and effector cells in schistosomiasis. Science 1994; 264:1876–1877.
12. Amiri P, Haak-Frendscho M, Robbins K, McKerrow JH, Stewart T, Jardieu P. Anti-immunoglobulin E treatment decreases worm burden and egg production in Schistosoma mansoni–infected normal and interferon γ knockout mice. J Exp Med 1994; 180:43–51.
13. King C, Xiangli J, Malhotra I, Liu S, Mahmoud AAF, Oettgen HC. Mice with targeted deletion of the IgE gene have increased worm burdens and reduced granulomatous inflammation following primary infection with Schistosoma mansoni. J Immunol 1997; 158:294–300.
14. Presta L, Lahr S, Shields R, Porter J, Gorman C, Fendley B, Jardieu P. Humanization of an Ab directed against IgE. J Immunol 1993; 151:2623–2632.
15. Casale TB, Bernstein L, Busse WW, Laforce CF, Tinkelman DG, Stolz RR, Dockhorn RJ, Reimann J, Su JQ, Fick RB, Adelman DC. Use of an anti-IgE humanized monoclonal antibody in ragweed-induced allergic rhinitis. J Allergy Clin Immunol 1997; 100:110–121.
16. Fick RB, Simon SJ, Su JQ, Zeiger R. Anti-IgE (rhuMAb) treatment of the symptoms of moderate-severe allergic asthma. Ann Asthma Allergy Immunol 1998; 80:80.
17. Boulet L-P, Chapman KR, Cote J, Kalra S, Bhagat R, Swystun VA, Laviolette M, Cleland LD, Deschesnes F, Su JQ, Devault A, Fick RB, Cockcroft DW. Inhibitory effects of an anti-IgE antibody E25 on allergen-induced early asthmatic response. Am J Respir Crit Care Med 1997; 155:1835–1840.
18. Fahy JV, Fleming HE, Wong HH, Liu JT, Su JQ, Reimann J, Fick RB, Boushey HA. The effect of an anti-IgE monoclonal antibody on the early and late phase responses to allergen inhalation in asthmatic subjects. Am J Respir Crit Care Med 1997; 155:1828–1834.
19. Fahy JV, Cockcroft DW, Boulet LP, Wong HH, Deschesnes F, Davis EE, Adelman DC. Effect of aerosolized anti-IgE (E25) on airway responses to inhaled allergen in asthmatic subjects. Am J Respir Crit Care Med 1998; 157:A410.
20. Liu J, Lester P, Builder S, Shire SJ. Characterization of complex formation by humanized anti-IgE antibody and monoclonal IgE. Biochemistry 1995; 34:10474–10482.
21. Fox JA, Hotaling TE, Struble C, Ruppel J, Bates DJ, Schoenhoff MB. Tissue distribution and complex formation with IgE of an anti-IgE antibody after intravenous administration in cynomolgus monkeys. J Pharmacol Exp Ther 1998; 279:1000–1008.
22. Corne J, Djukanovic R, Thomas L, Warner J, Botta L, Grandordy B, Gygax D, Heusser C, Patalano F, Richardson W, Kilchherr E, Staehelin T, Davis F, Gordon W, Sun L, Liuo R, Wang G, Chang T-W, Holgate S. The effect of intravenous administration of a chimeric anti-IgE antibody on serum IgE levels in atopic subjects: efficacy, safety and pharmacokinetics. J Clin Invest 1997; 99:879–887.
23. Rabe KF, Watson N, Dent G, Morton BE, Wagner KHM, Heusser CH. Inhibition

of human airway sensitization by a novel monoclonal anti-IgE antibody, 17-9. Am J Respir Crit Care Med 1998; 157:1429–1435.

24. MacGlashan DW, Bochner B, Adelman DC, Jardieu PM, Togias A, McKenzie-White J, Sterbinsky SA, Hamilton RG, Lichtenstein LM. Down-regulation of FcεR1 expression on human basophils during in vivo treatment of atopic patients with anti-IgE antibody. J Immunol 1997; 158:1438–1445.
25. MacGlashan DW. Releasability of human basophils: cellular sensitivity and maximal histamine release are independent variables. J Allergy Clin Immunol 1993; 91:605–615.
26. Bozelka BE, McCants ML, Salvaggio JE, Lehrer SB, Lehrer SB. IgE isotype suppression in anti-ε treated mice. Immunology 1982; 46:527–532.
27. Haak-Frenscho M, Robbins K, Lyon R, Shields R, Hooley J, Schoenhoff M, Jardieu P. Administration of an anti-IgE antibody inhibits CD23 expression and IgE production in vivo. Immunology 1994; 82:306–313.

12

Activity of T-Cell Subsets in Allergic Asthma

ANDRÉ BOONSTRA and HUUB F. J. SAVELKOUL

Erasmus University
Rotterdam, The Netherlands

I. Introduction

Atopic diseases like allergy and asthma are multifactorial conditions that are particularly strong in the development of the disease phenotype at a very young age (1). Allergy and asthma are generally considered complex disorders in which the disease expression (phenotype) results from an interaction between an individual's genetic makeup (genotype) and environmental factors. Atopic constitution is common, affecting up to 40% in Western populations (2). Indeed, atopy is considered to be a major risk factor for the development of asthma (3,4). In the last decades, asthma has been increasing both in prevalence and severity, especially among children. Although environmental factors, such as exposure to allergens, play an important role in the development of allergic diseases, there is also a strong genetic predisposition (5,6).

Atopy is characterized by the production of specific IgE antibodies directed against various allergens. Atopy has a strong genetic predisposition and underlies the development of allergic diseases in susceptible persons (7,8). Activation of T-helper type 2 (Th2) cells by allergens in genetically predisposed people is responsible for both the production of IgE antibodies and eosinophilia, which represent the hallmarks of allergic diseases (9–11). Early recognition of atopic diseases is particularly important, since a shorter duration of symptoms before diagnosis and subsequent avoidance of further exposures to the offending agents will result in a more favorable prognosis (12).

The vast majority of asthmatic patients suffer from allergic asthma. The allergic phenotype is associated with the presence of IgE antibodies to airborne allergens such as house dust mite, animal dander, and ragweed pollen (13). Other characteristics of asthma include an increased sensitivity of the airway smooth muscles to a variety of non-specific stimuli (airway hyperresponsiveness), and the presence of extensive inflammatory infiltrates within the airways, containing eosinophils, basophils, and T lymphocytes (14). In this chapter the selective activation of subsets of T-helper lymphocytes in relation to allergic asthma is discussed.

II. Th1-Th2 Subsets

Naive $CD4^+$ T-helper lymphocytes (Th0) undergo a priming step to develop into effector cells capable of modulating specific immune responses. Naive cells produce only small amounts of interleukin-2 (IL-2). Upon stimulation, these cells can develop into at least two subpopulations, each with a distinct cytokine profile (15–17). T-helper type 1 (Th1) cells secrete IL-2, interferon γ (IFN-γ), and tumor necrosis factor α (TNF-α) but not IL-4, IL-5, and IL-13, whereas T-helper type 2 (Th2) cells produce IL-4, IL-5, IL-6, IL-10, and IL-13 but not IL-2 and IFN-γ. Both subpopulations secrete IL-3 and granulocyte-macrophage colony-stimulating factor (GM-CSF). T-helper type 0 (Th0) cells have also been identified, secreting both Th1 and Th2 cytokines (Table 1) (15,16). It is still uncertain whether these

Table 1 Cytokine Production Profiles of Human T-Cell Clones

Cytokine	Th0	Th1	Th2
IL-2	++	++	+
IFN-γ	+	++	−
TNF-β	++	++	−
IL-3	++	++	++
IL-6	+	+	+
GM-CSF	++	++	++
TNF-α	++	++	++
IL-4	+	−	++
IL-5	+	−	++
IL-10	++	+	++
IL-13	++	+	++

Th0 cells are the common precursors of Th1 and Th2 cells or whether they comprise a third effector population. It should be stressed that Th1 and Th2 subsets are extremes and do not represent discrete subsets. Moreover, within a polarized Th1 or Th2 phenotype, individual T-helper cells possess differential rather than coordinated gene expression (18). For instance, expression of cytokines in T-helper cells purified directly from the lungs of influenza-infected mice revealed IFN-γ, IL-5, and IL-6 but not IL-4 mRNA (19).

Th1 cells efficiently induce cell-mediated responses, including phagocytosis and cytotoxicity, predominantly through the action of IFN-γ. Alternatively, Th2 cells provide help for antibody production (through IL-4) and enhance eosinophil proliferation and function (through IL-5) (20,21). The ratio of these T-helper cell subpopulations determines whether or not the immune system is able to respond appropriately to various stimuli. Disturbance of this balance may result in various clinical manifestations. Excessive Th1 stimulation results in enhanced rejection of grafts, inflammatory events, and some forms of autoimmunity (e.g., diabetes type I), whereas excessive Th2 activation induces enhanced antibody synthesis, including IgE (21,22). It has convincingly been shown that allergy is dependent on the presence of $CD4^+$ T-helper cells (22,23). Moreover, while one should be cautious about compartmentalization of (chronic) diseases and cytokine responses (e.g., intracellular infections generate Th1 responses and extracellular infections generate Th2 responses), atopy is commonly associated with a strong Th2 response, including the release of IL-4, IL-5, IL-9, and IL-13 (24,25).

Furthermore, polarization has also been demonstrated for the $CD8^+$ T lymphocytes. In general, activated $CD8^+$ T cells exhibit a cytokine pattern similar to that of Th1 cells, whereas a minor population has been shown to secrete Th2 cytokines (26). $CD8^+$ T cells activated in the presence of IL-4 can convert into Th2-like cells, which have lost their cytolytic activity. These cells produce IL-4, IL-5, and IL-10 and provide help for B cells identical to the Th2 cells (26).

Allergic asthma is generally considered a disease driven by Th2 type cells, where the presence of Th2 cells correlates with eosinophil infiltration and determines the severity of the disease (27,28). The Th2-derived cytokine IL-5 is a crucial cytokine: it accounts for the recruitment and activation of eosinophils, resulting in airway eosinophilia in allergic patients (29–31). In animal models, depletion of $CD4^+$ T cells results in abrogation of the airway eosinophilia and in subsequent reduction of airway hyperresponsiveness (32). Similarly, elevated serum IgE and allergen-specific IgE levels as observed in atopic patients can be explained in terms of excessive Th2 activation. Antigen-specific IgE responses against T cell–dependent antigens can be generated only by cognate interaction between B cells and Th2 cells, in which two signals are essential: CD40-CD40L interaction and the presence of IL-4 (33). The Th2-derived cytokine IL-4 is crucial as a growth factor for Th2 cells but also acts as an obligatory factor for the isotype switch to IgE through regulation of the transcription of germline-ε expression. Another clear indication that Th2 cells are involved in allergic asthma comes from an animal study in which an enhanced migration of Th2 cells was observed toward allergic as compared with nonallergic airways (34,35).

III. Cytokines

An important question is which events determine the induction of either a Th1 or Th2 response. There is general agreement that the outcome is influenced by tightly regulated, multifactorial events, such as the type of antigen, the antigen dose, the route of antigen entry, and the antigen-presenting cell (APC) (21). These factors influence the production of certain cytokines by APCs, thereby probably altering the microenvironment in which T-cell activation occurs. As described above, the balance between Th1 and Th2 cells is essential in mounting an appropriate immune response to a certain antigen. Cytokines play a key role in determining the subset polarization of T helper cells into either Th1 or Th2 responses (20).

Accumulating evidence suggests that the combined effects of a wide array of cytokines produced by different cell types, including activated T cells, could play a major part in regulating the successive steps leading to the characteristic eosinophil-rich airways inflammation (25,30,31,36–38). The numbers of IL-4 and IL-5 mRNA and protein product–positive cells were increased in asthmatics as compared to controls (39). There was also elevated expression of mRNA encoding IL-3, IL-13, GM-CSF, RANTES, and MCP-3 (36,40,41). This upregulation of eosinophil-active cytokines (IL-5, GM-CSF, and IL-3) and C-C chemokines (RANTES and MCP-3) within the bronchial mucosa was a characteristic feature of bronchial asthma (40).

IL-12 is a dominant factor promoting Th1 development. Dendritic cells (DC) and macrophages are able to produce this cytokine immediately after recognition of specific antigens, particularly microbial antigens (42). Apart from these professional APCs, which are the major producers of this cytokine, IL-12 can also be produced by monocytes, epithelial cells, B cells, and Langerhans cells. IL-12 is a potent inducer of IFN-γ production by natural killer (NK) cells and T cells (both $CD4^+$ and $CD8^+$) (42,43). Using IL-12 knockout mice, it was demonstrated that IL-12 is essential for the development of Th1 responses by its ability to induce the production of IFN-γ (Fig. 1) (44). However, IL-12 is unable to reverse an established Th2 phenotype to Th1 cells. This is probably due to differential expression of the IL-12 receptor subunits. Polarized Th1 cells express both the IL-12 β1 and β2 chains, whereas committed Th2 cells lack expression of the IL-12 receptor β2 chain, which is essential for IL-12 signaling (45,46). The nonresponsiveness of Th2 cells was also demonstrated using allergen-specific T-lymphocyte clones obtained from the peripheral blood of atopic patients (47).

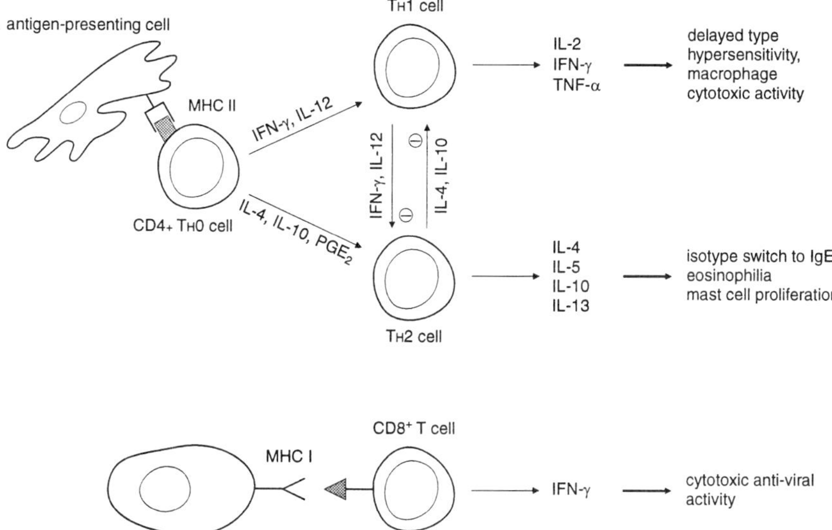

Figure 1 The regulation and function of T-cell subsets.

Other cytokines involved in Th1 polarization include IL-18 and IFN-γ. Apart from its growth-stimulatory properties, IL-18 has recently been shown to act synergistically with IL-12 to induce Th1 polarization (48,49). Furthermore, evidence has been provided that IL-12 is able to upregulate the expression of the IL-18 receptor, thereby rendering these cells permissive for the effects of IL-18. Alternatively, polarized Th2 cells lack expression of the IL-18 receptor (49).

IFN-γ can exert its effects by indirect and direct pathways. Indirectly, this cytokine has been shown to increase the production of IL-12 by dendritic cells and macrophages, and it has been suggested that IFN-γ may enhance the expression of functional IL-12 receptors on naive T cells (50). Furthermore, IFN-γ directly suppresses the proliferation of Th2 cells but not of Th1 cells, thereby favoring the outgrowth of Th1 cells. The role of IFN-γ in driving Th1 polarization is not entirely clear. In vitro studies have shown that addition of IFN-γ alone during priming of uncommitted, naive T cells is not sufficient for Th1 development. Besides, IFN-γ receptor knockout mice are still able to elicit Th1 responses (51). In addition, it has been reported that Th1 cells, in contrast to Th2 cells, are unable to respond to IFN-γ due to lack of the IFN-γ receptor α chain (52). This explains why IFN-γ inhibits the proliferation of Th2 cells but not of Th1 cells.

Polarization of Th2 cells is critically dependent on the presence of IL-4 (20). IL-4 knockout mice fail to mount Th2 responses (53). The source of initial endogenous IL-4 is still a matter of debate. Candidate cells include naive T cells,

NK1.1$^+$ T cells, and non-lymphoid cells like basophils and mast cells. Recently, APC-derived IL-6 has been shown to induce the synthesis of small amounts of IL-4 in CD4$^+$ T cells (54). IL-4 functions directly as a growth factor for Th2 cells, thereby clonally expanding Th2 cells and consequently augmenting the amount of IL-4 produced. On the other hand, IL-4 inhibits the production of IFN-γ and IL-12 (42). Besides IL-4, the Th2-derived cytokine IL-10 and the APC-derived prostaglandin E2 also inhibit Th1 proliferation and strongly reduce the production of IL-12 by APCs (55). Interestingly, IL-12 cannot inhibit priming for IL-4 production, demonstrating a dominant effect of IL-4 on the phenotype of the induced immune response. IL-13 is another Th2 cytokine capable of inhibiting Th1 cytokine synthesis, as was shown in animal models of infectious disease. Hence, this cytokine also inhibits progression to chronic infection. Besides, IL-13 is not merely a surrogate for IL-4 but potentially plays a critical role in both the induction and effector phases of the immune response.

The existence of positive and negative feedback mechanisms suggest that once a Th1- or Th2-type immune response is established, it is irreversibly committed to a particular cytokine profile. This holds true only for the Th2 phenotype, which is generally considered to be irreversible. However, in vitro polarized Th1 cells can be converted into IL-4–producing cells by exposure to exogenous IL-4 (56). It should be emphasized that these mechanisms were clarified in vitro. Under physiological conditions, it is likely that cytokines shift the balance along the Th1–Th2 axis only transiently, without permanently fixing the Th phenotype. The extreme situation of a fixed Th1 or Th2 phenotype is seen only in severe pathological conditions.

IV. Genetics of Atopy and Asthma

Most cases of asthma are associated with atopy, the IgE-mediated familial syndrome of allergic asthma, eczema, and rhinitis following exposure to common environmental allergens. Early studies have demonstrated associations between formation of specific IgE responses and certain HLA-DR antigens and alleles. The significance of this association with HLA class II molecules is based on their antigen presentation to CD4+ T cells, and, more generally, in regulating immune responses (57). Positive associations may reflect more efficient presentation of particular peptides to T-helper cells, thus promoting the T-cell switching to Th2 lymphocytes and a specific IgE response. Genomewide searches for genetic linkages associated with allergic asthma have now identified six potential linkages, including the cytokine gene cluster located on chromosome 5q31.1-q33 (12,58,59), the high-affinity Fc epsilon receptor on chromosome 11q13 (60), chromosome 12q14.3-q24.1 (61), and the HLA-DR alleles on chromosome 6p21.3 (62). Recently, however, other linkage profiles have been described involving potential linkages to autosomal markers on chromosomes 4, 6, 7, 11, 13, and 16. These data point to the significant heterogeneity of atopic status and possible heterogeneity of genetic predisposition, as the atopic phenotype may have a range of presentations from an asymptomatic individual to a patient with fully expressed skin, nasal, and/or bronchial symptoms.

It is generally appreciated that the prevalence of asthma is increasing; currently asthma affects one child in seven in western Europe. The reasons for this apparent increase are suggested to include a better and earlier diagnosis, more efficient treatment regimens, a shift from severe to milder disease, and increased exposure to environmental allergens (28). In recent years, the synthesis of IgE was shown to be dependent on a cytokine network. Activated Th2 cells, eosinophils, and basophils may produce IL-4. This cytokine has a unique role in directing immunoglobulin isotype switching toward synthesis of IgE. Moreover, IL-4 has a critical role in the regulation of differentiation of naive T cells into Th2 cells and the upregulation of IgE synthesis. IL-4 has been shown to be encoded on chromosome 5q in close proximity to other cytokine genes (IL-3, IL-5, IL-9, IL-13, and GM-CSF) contributing to the development of allergic inflammation and IgE production (58). It has been proposed that one or more polymorphisms in genes within human chromosome 5q31.1 are responsible for the differential regulation of overall IgE production. Indeed, genetic polymorphisms have been identified within the regulatory elements of the IL-3, IL-4, and IL-9 genes belonging to the IL-4 gene cluster. The transcription of the IL-4 gene is regulated by multiple promoter elements that either induce or suppress transcription. The positive enhancer element-1 (PRE-1) has been shown to play a key role in IL-4 expression. Its enhancer function is strongly suppressed by the activity of a silencer region containing two protein binding sites: negative regulatory elements (NRE) I and II. In addition, the murine IL-4 promoter region contains five purine-rich regions with binding specificity for NF-AT (nuclear factor of activated T cells). Binding of NF-AT in Th2 cells correlates with high IL-4 transcription (63). Selective expression in polarized Th2 cells and binding to the IL-4 promoter region of three additional transcription factors has been reported: STATa-6, c-maf, and GATA-3. C-maf and GATA-3 together with NF-AT have been implicated in facilitating the accessibility of the IL-4 locus, whereas STAT-6 binding induces enhanced expression of IL-4 production. Interestingly, the P region of the IL-4 promoter region shares homology with the corresponding IL-5 sequence, indicating one possible mechanism for the coordinated expression of the Th2 cytokines. Activity of the NRE regions as well as an IFN-stimulation response element (ISRE) inhibits the expression of the IL-4 gene. Thus, it has been demonstrated that the human IL-4 promotor region exists in multiple allelic forms, which differ in the level of IL-4 transcription and expression in T cells. Therefore, it is generally agreed that people with asthma produce abnormally high amounts of IL-4 (64).

Currently, two different IL-4 receptors (IL-4R) have been described. The type I IL-4R comprises a 140-kDa IL-4 binding protein (IL-4Rα/CDw124) that dimerizes with the common gamma chain shared with the IL-2, IL-7, IL-9, IL-13, and IL-15 receptors. Furthermore, the IL-4Rα is able to associate with one of the chains of the IL-13 receptor that comprises the type II IL-4R. The role of the type II receptors on different cell types is still subject of research. The presence of the common gamma chain in the type I receptor complex increases the binding affinity of IL-4 by two- to threefold and contributes to signal transduction. Receptor binding of IL-4 mobilizes the Janus tyrosine kinase (JAK) 1 and 3, which phosphorylate the IRS-2 substrate responsible for activating the growth-stimulatory activity of phosphoinositol 3 kinase (PI-3 kinase) as well as STAT-6 transcription factor.

Recently, a genetic polymorphism in the intracellular signaling part of the IL-4 receptor has been identified that is strongly associated with atopy; the underlying mutation may predispose persons to allergic diseases by altering the signaling function of the receptor (65). The presence of normal levels of IL-4 may therefore exert stronger biological effects resulting in higher levels of, for example, IgE, thereby predisposing suceptible persons to allergic disease.

V. Antigen Presentation

The effects of cytokines on the polarization of T-helper subsets are well studied. However, cells require instructions in order to mount the appropriate immune response to a particular pathogen. Stimulation of $CD4^+$ T cells is dependent on the interaction with the APCs, mostly dendritic cells, macrophages, and monocytes. The APCs present antigenic peptides on their MHC class II molecules to the T-cell receptor (TCR). The APCs also deliver costimulatory signals that are required for IL-2 production and optimal T-cell activation (66). The choice of whether a Th1 or Th2 response develops depends on the multifactorial process of antigen presentation. First of all, the dose of antigen is relevant. In an oversimplified statement, early experiments showed that low antigen dose favors Th1 responses, whereas high doses give rise to Th2 responses (67). One could explain this phenomenon by hypothesizing that at low antigen concentrations, the antigen has to be presented by dendritic cells or macrophages, both very efficient APCs that induce Th1 development through the production of IL-12. APCs that do not secrete IL-12 may present a high antigen dose. Currently, we know that the interaction is much more complex. Particularly in the atopic individual, there is a genetically based ability to react with antibody formation to a low dose of allergen that does not result in antibody formation in nonatopics.

Besides, the nature of the antigen (soluble or particulate antigen) as well as its route of entry (subcutaneous, inhaled, oral, or intravenous) also influences the outcome of the polarization process. In addition, the avidity of the TCR is also relevant, since it determines the strength of the signal delivered to the inside of the T cell. A high level of triggering is thought to favor Th1 activation, whereas low levels result in Th2 activation (68). Although initial studies demonstrated that different APCs selectively influenced T-cell polarization, it is now accepted that dendritic cells (DCs), macrophages, and B cells are capable of eliciting Th1 and Th2 responses in the presence of the appropriate cytokines.

Once activated, the APC is able to produce a plethora of cytokines that may influence T-cell polarization. The combination of APC-derived IL-1 and TNF-α as well as IL-12 and IL-18 are able to promote Th1 development, whereas prostaglandin E_2 (PGE_2) and IL-6 favor Th2 skewing (48,54,69). PGE_2 strongly inhibits the production of IL-2, IFN-γ, and IL-12, thereby directly inhibiting the development of Th1 cells. Indeed, monocytes from patients with atopic dermatitis show an increased production of PGE_2 and reduced levels of IL-12 (70). While monocytes can act as APCs for memory T cells, resident alveolar macrophages strongly suppress the APC function of DCs. Thereby, alveolar macrophages may induce a state of tolerance reflected in decreased (local) memory T-cell expression and suppression of IgE formation (71). The immunological outcome of initial T-cell activation events after inhaled allergens can be detected as T-cell anergy or tolerance (71). The balance between the potential immunoregulatory APC populations is a key factor in hypersensitivity and the pathogenesis of immunoinflammatory diseases (71).

Recent progress in the study of the phenotypic and functional heterogeneity of macrophages and DCs suggest the involvement of different subsets in skewing. However, temporal changes in the production of cytokines and the dominance of action of a particular cytokine could determine the outcome of immunomodulation.

Once the physical interaction between the T cell and the APC is established, costimulatory molecules stabilize the TCR-MHC complex and deliver additional signals, resulting in complete T-cell activation. The best-defined costimulatory molecules on the APC are B7-1 (CD80) and B7-2 (CD86), both of which interact with the T cell by interacting with their ligand CD28 on the T cell (66). Some studies have shown that B7-1 and B7-2 differentially influence the development of Th subsets (72). Antibodies to B7-1 and B7-2 inhibited Th1 and Th2 responses, respectively. However, the role of these molecules in skewing is probably more complex. First of all, their level of expression depends on the activation state of the APC; resting APCs have high B7-2 expression, whereas B7-1 is increased after triggering (66). The interaction between B7-1 and B7-2 on the APC and the T cell is still not entirely clear, since they both interact with the same ligand on the T cell. Most likely, they differ in the affinity for CD28, resulting in a variable strength of costimulation. This suggests that the timing of expression and the strength of the costimulatory signal are more important than the presence or absence of a particular molecule.

VI. Th2 Cells in the Airways of Patients with Asthma

In the bronchoalveolar lavage (BAL) and bronchial biopsies of patients with atopic asthma, cells expressing IL-4 and IL-5 were detected. The vast majority of these cells were activated T cells, whereas a minority consisted of mast cells and activated eosinophils (25). In contrast, T cells from airways of nonasthmatic individuals expressed only IL-2 and IFN-γ. IL-4 in combination with TNF-α has been shown to induce upregulation of VCAM-1 expression on vascular endothelium (73). VCAM-1 participates in the selective eosinophil adhesion via a VLA-4–dependent mechanism; therefore, the presence of IL-4 in the inflamed lung accounts for eosinophil recruitment at the allergic sites (73). Furthermore, the Th2-derived cytokine IL-5 is involved in the differentiation and maturation of eosinophils and exhibits chemotactic activity for these cells (29,74). Eosinophil accumulation and the development of airway hyperresponsiveness are abolished in IL-5–deficient mice (75). Other soluble factors that play an essential role in leukocyte trafficking toward and infiltration of the airways of allergic asthmatics include the chemokines. The superfamily of chemokines is traditionally divided into two subgroups based on the arrangement of the first two cysteins, which are either separated by one amino acid (C-X-C chemokines) or are adjacent (C-C chemokines) (37). In particular, the C-C chemokines have been implicated in the immunopathology of allergic asthma by their chemotactic and stimulatory activity and their ability to induce degranulation and histamine release from basophils (38,76). The C-C chemokines RANTES and MCP-3 act on eosinophils, whereas MCP-1, MCP-3, and RANTES affect basophil functions. Recently, some reports have described chemotactic proteins responsible for directing Th2 lymphocytes toward allergic airways. Interestingly, the major contributor to this process is not a traditional chemokine but IL-16, which is released in response to allergens, mitogen, histamine, or serotonin by $CD8^+$ T cells, eosinophils, airway epithelial cells, and possibly $CD4^+$ T cells (77). IL-16 chemotactically attracts $CD4^+$ T cells, eosinophils, and monocytes by interacting with the CD4 molecule. In asthmatic patients, IL-16 was detected in the BAL fluid 6 hr after allergen challenge (78). In fact, 80% of the chemotactic activity is ascribed to IL-16, whereas the remaining activity is due to the C-C chemokine MIP-1α. Similar RANTES levels were detected in the airways of asthmatic and healthy patients (79). In an ovalbumin-induced mouse model for allergic asthma, antibodies to IL-16 inhibited the development of airway hyperresponsiveness and suppressed the upregulation of ovalbumin-specific IgE (80). However, in this model, the numbers of eosinophils in BAL and airway tissue were not decreased due to in vivo treatment with antibodies to IL-16, although the presence and activity of IL-16 was determined in vitro.

Recently, the involvement of eotaxin in the process of Th2 trafficking has been proposed as well. It was shown that after in vitro polarization of $CD4^+$ T cells, the Th2 polarized cells showed a higher expression of the eotaxin ligand CCR3 (81). Hypothetically, this implies that once eotaxin is released within inflamed airways, Th2 cells (but not Th1 cells) are selectively attracted toward the site of inflammation, resulting in progressive polarization of the local Th2-cell response.

VII. The Induction of Tolerance

As outlined above, T-helper subset polarization is achieved by two basic principles. First, each subset produces its own autocrine growth factors, and, second, cytokines are produced that cross-regulate the outgrowth of the counteracting subset. However, the observed skewing in allergic asthmatics to the Th2 compartment may also result from other regulatory processes. The preferential activation of Th2 cells could be the result of active suppression of the Th1 subset due to the cytokine-related interaction between T-cell subsets and the APC. Indeed in many experimental systems of tolerance, the induction and activity of Th1 cells is preferentially blocked, as in insulin-dependent diabetes mellitus and following ultraviolet B treatment (82,83). Unresponsiveness can be achieved by different mechanisms, including clonal deletion, T-cell anergy, or active suppression mediated by regulatory cells (84–86). These mechanisms are not mutually exclusive but may act synergistically.

The process of T-cell anergy is best defined as a state of cellular unresponsiveness in which the cell is alive but unable to perform functional responses upon restimulation. Anergized cells are generated by antigen-specific T-cell activation in the absence of co-stimulatory molecules. This partial activation signal renders these cells unable to proliferate and secrete IL-2. The main contributors to the costimulatory signals are CD28 on the T cell and B7-1 and B7-2 on the APC (66). This interaction enhances the transcription rate and stabilization of IL-2 mRNA and increases the sensitivity of TCR triggering. The B7 molecules possess still another ligand, CTLA-4. This ligand has been shown to regulate T cell responses negatively and to evoke a complete block in cell-cycle progression and IL-2 production. CD28 expression on the T cell is constitutive, whereas CTLA-4 is induced early after T-cell activation (66). The differences in affinities and binding kinetics with B7-1 and B7-2 determine whether or not a cell becomes activated or remains unresponsive. The precise role of APC in tolerance induction is yet to be determined (87).

Clonal deletion of antigen-specific T cells and anergy are both passive mechanisms regulating immune responses. Active immunosuppression, on the other hand, is mediated by regulatory T cells (84). These T cells consist of classic Th2 cells (88), capable of inhibiting Th1 responses, but also alternative T-cell populations. One of the primary mechanisms of active immunosuppression is via secretion of immunosuppressive cytokines like IL-10, IL-4, and transforming growth factor-β (TGF-β). Recently, regulatory $CD4^+$ T-cell clones (human and murine) have been isolated from in vitro culture, which appeared to produce low levels of IL-2 and no IL-4 but high levels of IL-10 and TGF-β (89). When cocultured with naive $CD4^+$ T cells, these antigen-specific clones suppressed the proliferative response to the same antigen. The regulatory T-cell clones themselves exhibited a low proliferative capacity. Neutralization of IL-10 and TGF-β overcomes this proliferative block. The activity of TGF-β secreting regulatory T cells has been implicated as a component of oral tolerance, the recovery from experimental allergic encephalomyelitis, and in suppression of certain forms of inflammatory colitis (89). TGF-β–deficient mice suffer from inflammation that affects multiple organ systems—mainly the heart, liver, and lungs—whereas IL-10 knockout mice produce a chronic enterocolitis (90). This demonstrates the importance of these cytokines in regulating and dampening the immune response.

Regulatory T-cell subsets inhibiting Th2 type responses as well as Th1 mediated responses were recently found. At present, it is unknown whether these regulatory T cells are involved in the immunopathology of allergic asthma by provoking excessive suppression of the Th1 compartment.

VIII. Immunotherapy

It has been shown that allergen immunotherapy, through subcutaneous administration of increasing doses of allergen, greatly reduces IL-4 production by $CD4^+$ T cells from allergic patients (91). The underlying mechanisms are not fully elucidated, but it has been demonstrated that high levels of IL-4 are produced following stimulation with low doses of allergen in the presence of B cells. At high allergen concentrations, little IL-4 has been produced, especially when monocytes were used as APCs, suggesting that the antigen dose as well as the type of APC determine the cytokine profile of allergen-specific $CD4^+$ T cells and, consequently, the efficacy of immunotherapy. In this respect, administration of soluble antigen without adjuvant, administration of modified antigen peptides, or oral administration of soluble antigen leading to unresponsiveness has been suggested to induce a Th2-to-Th1 switch.

Several experimental approaches have been developed that may induce a state of inhibition or unresponsiveness of the allergen-specific immune response. This might be due to the induction of unresponsiveness to a particular allergen based on the modification of the T cell–APC interaction. The quantity and quality of the peptide can modulate the outcome of the interaction of the T-cell receptor with the peptide-MHC combination. When comparing the response of a Th2 clone after stimulation with a peptide that bears a single amino acid substitution with the normal peptide, specific T-cell responses are affected. The immunogenic peptide induces both IL-4 production as well as proliferation, whereas the altered peptide induces normal levels of IL-4 protein but no proliferation, probably related to the lack of IL-4R expression. Activation of Th1 clones by a particular altered peptide ligand induced normal cytotoxicity and upregulation of the IL-2R but no proliferation and cytokine production. This partial activation of Th1 and Th2 clones induced anergy in both cell types due to loss of IL-2 production and IL-4R expression, respectively. The hallmark of recent asthma research is to induce allergen-specific ''immune deviation'' to Th1 reactivity away from the default Th2 pathway (92). The reasons underlying the apparent failure of immune deviation in atopics remains to be clarified.

References

1. Holt PG, McMenamin C, Nelson D. Primary sensitisation to inhalant allergens during infancy. Pediatr Allergy Immunol 1990; 1:3–13.
2. Bjorksten B. Risk factors in early childhood for the development of atopic diseases. Allergy 1994; 49:400–407.
3. Croner S, Kjellman NIM. Development of atopic disease in relation to family history and cord blood IgE levels. Pediatr Allergy Immunol 1989; 1:14–20.
4. Kaufman HS, Frick OL. The development of allergy in infants of allergic parents: a prospective study concerning the role of heredity. Ann Allergy 1976; 37:410–415.
5. Woolcock AJ, Peat JK, Trevillion LM. Changing prevalence of allergies worldwide. In: Johansson SGO, ed. Progress in Allergy and Clinical Immunology. Gottingen, Germany: Hografe and Huber, 1995:167–171.
6. Sporik R, Holgate ST, Platts-Mills TAE, Cogswell JJ. Exposure to house-dust mite allergen (Der pI) and the development of asthma in childhood: a prospective study. N Engl J Med 1990; 323:502–507.
7. Rihoux J-P. The allergic reaction. Braine-l' Alleud, Belgium: UCB Pharmaceutical Sector, 1993:9–29.
8. Wüthrich B, Baumann E, Fries RA, Schnyder UW. Total and specific IgE (RAST) in atopic twins. Clin Allergy 1981; 11:147–154.
9. Hanson DG. Ontogeny of orally induced tolerance to soluble proteins in mice: I. Priming and tolerance in newborns. J Immunol 1981; 127:1518–1524.
10. Strobel S, Ferguson A. Immune responses to fed protein antigens in mice: 3. Systemic tolerance or printing is related to age at which antigen is first encountered. Pediatr Res 1984; 18:588–594.
11. Pfeiffer C, Murray J, Madri J, Bottomly K. Selective activation of Th1- and Th2-

like cells in in vivo response to human collagen IV. Immunol Rev 1991; 123:65–84.

12. Rosenwasser LJ. The genetics of allergy. Allergy 1998; 53(suppl 46):8–11.
13. Chapman MD. Environmental allergen monitoring and control. Allergy 1998; 53(45):48–53.
14. Menz G, Ying S, Durham SR, Corrigan CJ, Robinson DS, Hamid Q, Pfister R. Molecular concepts of IgE-initiated inflammation in atopic and nonatopic asthma. Allergy 1998; 53(45):15–21.
15. Mosmann TR, Coffman RL. Th1 and Th2 cells: Different patterns of lymphokine secretion lead to different functional properties. Annu Rev Immunol 1989; 7:145–173.
16. Romagnani S. The Th1/Th2 paradigm. Immunol Today 1997; 18:263–266.
17. Nakamura T, Kamogawa Y, Bottomly K, Flavell RA. Polarization of IL-4 and IFN-gamma-producing $CD4^+$ T cells following activation of naive $CD4^+$ T cells. J Immunol 1997; 158:1085–1094.
18. Kelso A. Th1 and Th2 subsets: paradigms lost? Immunol Today 1995; 16:374–379.
19. Baumgarth N, Kelso A. In vivo blockade of gamma interferon affects the influenza virus-induced humoral and the local cellular immune response in lung tissue. J Virol 1996; 70:4411–4418.
20. O'Garra A. Cytokines induce the development of functionally heterogeneous T helper cell subsets. Immunity 1998; 8:275–283.
21. Abbas AA, Murphy KM, Sher A. Functional diversity of helper T lymphocytes. Nature 1996; 363:787–793.
22. Romagnani S. Regulation of the development of type 2 T-helper cells in allergy. Curr Opin Immunol 1994; 6:838–846.
23. Robinson DS, Hamid Q, Ying S, Tsicopoulos A, Barkens J, Bentley AM, Corrigan C, Durham SR, Kay AB. Predominant Th2-like bronchoaleveolar T-lymphocyte population in atopic asthma. N Engl J Med 1992; 326:298–304.
24. Robinson D, Hamid Q, Bentley A, Ying S, Kay AB, Durham SR. Activation of CD4+ T cells, increased Th2-type cytokine mRNA, and eosinophil recruitment in bronchoalveolar lavage after allergen inhalation challenge in patients with atopic asthma. J Allergy Clin Immunol 1993; 92:313–324.
25. Ying S, Durham SR, Corrigan CJ, Hamid Q, Kay AB. Phenotype of cells expressing mRNA for Th2-type (interleukin-4 and interleukin-5) and Th1-type (interleukin-2 and interferon-gamma) cytokines in bronchoaleveolar lavage and bronchial biopsies from atopic asthmatic and normal control subjects. Am J Respir Cell Mol Biol 1995; 12:477.
26. Seder RA, Le Gros GG. The functional role of $CD8^+$ T helper type 2 cells. J Exp Med 1995; 181:5–7.
27. Romagnani S. Lymphokine production by human T cells in disease state. Annu Rev Immunol 1994; 12:227–257.
28. Romagnani S. The Th1/Th2 paradigm and allergic disorders. Allergy 1998; 53(suppl 46):12–15.
29. Lopez AF, Sanderson CJ, Gamble JR, Campbell HD, Young IG, Vadas MA. Recombinant human interleukin 5 is a selective activator of human eosinophil function. J Exp Med 1988; 167:219–224.

30. Corrigan CJ, Kay AB. T cells and eosinophils in the pathogenesis of asthma. Immunol Today 1992; 13:501–507.
31. Humbert M. Pro-eosinophilic cytokines in asthma. Clin Exp Allergy 1996; 26:123–127.
32. Gavett SH, Chen X, Finkleman F, Wills-Karp M. Depletion of murine CD4$^+$ T lymphocytes prevents antigen-induced airway hyperresponsiveness and pulmonary eosinophilia. Am J Respir Cell Mol Biol 1994; 10:587–593.
33. Spriggs MK, Armitage RJ, Strockbine L, Clifford KN, Macduff BM, Sato TA, Maliszewski CR, Fanslow WC. Recombinant human CD40 ligand stimulates B cell proliferation and immunoglobulin E secretion. J Exp Med 1992; 176:1543–1550.
34. Austrup F, Vetsweber D, Borges E, Lohning M, Brauer R, Herz U, Renz H, Hallman R, Scheffold A, Radbruch A, Hamann A. P- and E-selectin mediate recruitment of T-helper-1 but not T-helper-2 cells into inflammed tissues. Nature 1997; 385:81–83.
35. Kaplan AP, Kuna P. Chemokines and the late-phase reaction. Allergy 1998; 53(45): 27–32.
36. Powell N, Humbert M, Durham SR, Assoufi B, Kay AB, Corrigan C. Increased expression of mRNA encoding RANTES and MCP-3 in the bronchial mucosa in atopic asthma. Eur Respir J 1996; 9:2454–2460.
37. Baggiolini M, Dewald B, Moser B. Human chemokines: an update. Annu Rev Immunol 1997; 15:675–705.
38. Baggiolini M, Dahinden CA. CC chemokines in allergic inflammation. Immunol Today 1994; 15:127–133.
39. Ying S, Humbert M, Barkans J. Expression of IL-4 and IL-5 mRNA and protein product by CD4$^+$ and CD8$^+$ T cells, eosinophils and mast cells in bronchial biopsies obtained from atopic and nonatopic (intrinsic) asthmatics. J Immunol 1997; 158: 3549–3554.
40. Humbert M, Ying S, Corrigan C. Bronchial mucosal gene expression of the genes encoding C-C chemokines RANTES and MCP-3 in symptomatic atopic and nonatopic asthmatics: relationship to the eosinophil-active cytokines: IL-5, GM-CSF and IL-3. Am J Respir Cell Mol Biol 1997; 16:1–8.
41. Humbert M, Durham SR, Kimmitt P. Elevated expression of mRNA encoding interleukin-13 in the bronchial mucosa of atopic and non-atopic asthmatics. J Allergy Clin Immunol 1997; 99:657–665.
42. Trinchieri G. Interleukin-12: a pro-inflammatory cytokine with immuno-regulatory functions that bridge innate resistance and antigen-specific adaptive immunity. Annu Rev Immunol 1995; 13:251–276.
43. Hsieh CS, Macatonia SE, Tripp CS, Wolf SF, O'Garra A, Murphy KM. Development of Th1 CD4$^+$ T cells through IL-12 produced by Listeria-induced macrophages. Science 1993; 260:547–549.
44. Magram J, Connaughton SE, Warrier RR, Carvajal DM, Wu CY, Ferrante J, Stewart C, Sarmiento U, Faherty DA, Gately MK. IL-12 deficient mice are defective in IFN gamma production and type 1 responses. Immunity 1996; 4:471.
45. Rogge L, Barberis-Maino L, Biffi M, Passini N, Presky DH, Gubler U, Sinigaglia F. Selective expression of an interleukin-12 receptor component by human T helper 1 cells. J Exp Med 1997; 185:825–831.

46. Szabo S, Dighe AS, Gubler U, Murphy KM. Regulation of the interleukin (IL)-12β2 subunit expression in developing T helper (Th1) and Th2 cells. J Exp Med 1997; 185:817–824.
47. Hilkens CMU, Messer G, Tesselaar K, Van Rietschoten AGI, Kapsenberg ML, Wieringa EA. Lack of IL-12 signaling in human IL-12 allergen-specific Th2 cells. J Immunol 1996; 157:4316–4321.
48. Robinson D, Shibuya K, Mui A, Zonin F, Murphy E, Sana T, Hartley SB, Menon S, Kastelein R, Bazan F, O' Garra A. IGIF does not drive Th1 development but synergizes with IL-12 for interferon-gamma production and activates IRAK and NF kappa B. Immunity 1997; 7:571–581.
49. Ahn HJ, Maruo S, Tomura M, Mu J, Hamaoka T, Nakanishi K, Clark S, Kurimoto M, Okamura H, Fujiwara H. A mechanism underlying synergy between IL-12 and IFN-γ-inducing factor in enhanced production of IFN-γ. J Immunol 1997; 159:2125–2131.
50. Wenner CA, Guler ML. Macatonia SE, O'Garra A, Murphy KM. Roles of IFN-gamma and IFN-alpha in IL-12-induced T helper cell-1 development. J Immunol 1996; 156:1442–1447.
51. Schijns VE, Haagmans BL, Wierda CM, Kruithof B, Heijnen IA, Alber G, Horzinek MC. Mice lacking IL-12 develop polarized Th1 cells during viral infection. J Immunol 1998; 160:3958–3964.
52. Groux H, Sornasse T, Cottrez F, de Vries JE, Coffman RL, Roncarolo M-G, Yssel H. Induction of human T cell type I differentiation results in loss of IFN-γ receptor α-chain expression. J Immunol 1997; 158:5627–5631.
53. Kuhn R, Rajewski K, Muller W. Generation and analysis of interleukin-4 deficient mice. Science 1991; 254:707–710.
54. Rincon M, Anguita J, Nakamura T, Fikrig E, Flavell RA. Interleukin (IL)-6 directs the differentiation of IL-4-producing $CD4^+$ T cells. J Exp Med 1997; 185:461–469.
55. Gately MK, Renzetti LM, Magram J, Stern AS, Adorini L, Gubler U, Presky DH. The interleukin-12/interleukin-12-receptor system: role in normal and pathologic immune responses. Annu Rev Immunol 1998; 16:495–522.
56. Perez VL, Lederer JA, Lichtman AH, Abbas AK. Stability of Th1 and Th2 populations. Int Immunol 1995; 7:869–875.
57. Cookson WOCM. Genetic aspects of atopic allergy. Allergy 1998; 53:9–14.
58. Marsh DG, Neely JD, Breazeale DR, Ghosh B, Freidhoff LR, Ehrlich-Kautzky E, Schou C, Krishnaswamy G, Beaty TH. Linkage analysis of IL-4 and other chromosome 5q31.1 markers and total serum IgE concentrations. Science 1994; 264:1152–1155.
59. Meyers DA, Postma DS, Panhuysen CIM. Evidence for a locus regulating total serum IgE levels mapping to chromosome 5. Genomics 1994; 23:464–470.
60. Cookson WOCM, Sharp PA, Faux JA, Hopkin JM. Linkage between immunoglobulin E responses underlying asthma and rhinitis and chromosome 11q. Lancet 1989; 1:1292–1295.
61. Barnes KC, Neely JD, Duffy DL. Linkage of asthma and total serum IgE concentration to markers on chromosome 12q: evidence from Afro-Caribbean and Caucasian populations. Genomics 1996; 37:159–162.

62. Levine BB, Stremher RH, Fontino M. Rayweed hay fever: genetic control and linkage to HLA haplotypes. Science 1972; 178:1201–1203.
63. Paul WE, Seder RA. Lymphocyte responses and cytokines. Cell 1994; 76:241–251.
64. Rosenwasser LJ, Borish L. Genetics of atopy and asthma: the rationale behind promotor-based candidate gene studies (IL-4 and IL-10). Am J Respir Crit Care Med 1997; 156:S152–S155.
65. Hershey GKK, Friedrich MF, Esswein LA, Thomas ML, Chatila TA. The association of atopy with a gain of function mutation in the a subunit of the interleukin-4 receptor. N Engl J Med 1997; 337:1720–1725.
66. Lenschow DJ, Walumas TL, Bluestone JA. CD28/B7 system of T cell costimulation. Annu Rev Immunol 1996; 14:233–258.
67. Hosken NA, Shibuya K, Heath AW, Murphy KM, O'Garra A. The effect of antigen dose on CD4+ T helper cell phenotype development in a T cell receptor alpha/beta-transgenic model. J Exp Med 1995; 182:1579–1584.
68. Constant S, Pfeiffer C, Woodard A, Pasqualini T, Bottomly K. Extent of T cell receptor ligation can determine the functional differentiation of naive $CD4^+$ T cells. J Exp Med 1995; 5:1591–1596.
69. Snijdewint FGM, Kalinski P, Wierenga EA, Bos JD, Kapsenberg ML. Prostaglandin E2 differentially modulates cytokine secretion profiles of human T helper lymphocytes. J Immunol 1993; 150:5321–5329.
70. Chan SC, Kim JW, Henderson WR, Hanifin JM. Altered prostaglandin E2 regulation of cytokine production in atopic dermatitis. J Immunol 1993; 151:3345–3352.
71. Holt PG. Regulation of antigen-presenting cell function(s) in lung and airway tissues. Eur Respir J 1993; 6:120–129.
72. Kuchroo VK, Das MP, Brown JA, Ranger AM, Zamvil SS, Sobel RA, Weiner HL, Nabavi N, Glimcher LH. B7-1 and B7-2 costimulatory molecules activate differentially the Th1/Th2 developmental pathways: application to autoimmune disease therapy. Cell 1995; 80:707–718.
73. Carlos TM, Harlan JM. Leukocyte-endothelial adhesion molecules. Blood 1994; 84: 2068–2101.
74. Warringa RAJ, Schweizer RC, Maikoe T, Kuijper PHM, Bruijnzeel PLB, Koenderman L. Modulation of eosinophil chemotaxis by interleukin-5. Am J Respir Cell Mol Biol 1992; 7:631–636.
75. Foster PS, Hogan SP, Ramsay AJ, Matthaei KI, Young IG. Interleukin 5 deficiency abolishes eosinophilia, airways hyperactivity, and lung damage in a mouse asthma model. J Exp Med 1996; 183:195–201.
76. Lukacs NW, Strieter RM, Chensue SW, Kunkel SL. Activation and regulation of chemokines in allergic airway inflammation. J Leukoc Biol 1996; 59:13–17.
77. Center DM, Kornfeld H, Cruikshank WW. Interleukin 16 and its function as a CD4 ligand. Immunol Today 1996; 17:476–481.
78. Cruikshank WW, Long A, Tarpy RE, Kornfeld H, Caroll MP, Teran L, Holgate ST, Center DM. Early identification of interleukin-16 (lymphocyte chemoattractant factor) and macrophage inflammatory protein-1α (MIP-1α) in bronchoalveolar lavage fluid of antigen-challenged asthmatics. Am J Respir Cell Mol Biol 1995; 13: 738–747.
79. Fahy JV, Figueroa DJ, Wong HH, Liu JT, Abrams JS. Similar RANTES levels in

healthy and asthmatic airways by immunoassay and in situ hybridization. Am J Respir Crit Care Med 1997; 155:1095–1100.
80. Hessel EM, Cruikshank WW, Van Ark I, De Bie JJ, Van Esch B, Hofman G, Nijkamp FP, Center DM, Van Oosterhout AJ. Involvement of IL-16 in the induction of airway hyper-responsiveness and up-regulation of IgE in a murine model of allergic asthma. J Immunol 1998; 160:2998–3005.
81. Sallusto F, Mackay CR, Lanzavecchio A. Selective expression of the eotaxin receptor CCR3 by human T helper 2 cells. Science 1997; 277:2005–2007.
82. O'Garra A, Steinman L, Gijbels K. $CD4^+$ T-cell subsets in autoimmunity. Curr Opin Immunol 1997; 9:872–883.
83. Boonstra A, Savelkoul HFJ. The role of cytokines in ultraviolet-B induced immunosuppression. Eur Cytokine Net 1997; 8:117–123.
84. Whitacre CC, Gienapp IE, Orasz CG, Bitar DM. Oral tolerance in experimental autoimmune encephalomyelitis. J Immunol 1991; 147:2155–2163.
85. Friedman A, Weiner HL. Induction of anergy or active suppression following oral tolerance is mediated by antigen dose. Proc Natl Acad Sci USA 1994; 91:6688–6692.
86. Chen Y, Inobe J-I, Marks R, Gonnella P, Kuchroo VK, Weiner HL. Peripheral deletion of antigen-reactive T cells in oral tolerance. Nature 1995; 376:177–180.
87. Stobel S, Mowat AM. Immune responses to dietary antigens: oral tolerance. Immunol Today 1998; 19:173–181.
88. Yabuhara A, Macaubas C, Prescott SL. Th2-polarised immunological memory to inhalant allergens in atopics is established during infancy and early childhood. Clin Exp Allergy 1997; 27:1261–1269.
89. Letterio JJ, Roberts AB. Regulation of immune responses by TGF-beta. Annu Rev Immunol 1998; 16:137–162.
90. Asseman C, Powrie F. Interleukin 10 is a growth factor for a population of regulatory T cells. Gut 1998; 42:157–158.
91. Secrist H, DeKruyff RH, Umetsu DT. Interleukin 4 production by $CD4^+$ T cells from allergic individuals is modulated by antigen concentration and antigen-presenting cell type. J Exp Med 1995; 181:1081–1089.
92. Holt PG, Macaubas C. Development of long term tolerance versus sensitisation to environmental allergens during the perinatal period. Curr Opin Immunol 1997; 9: 782–787.

13

New Targets for Future Asthma Therapy

PETER J. BARNES

National Heart and Lung Institute
Imperial College
London, England

I. Introduction

Currently available therapy for asthma is highly effective and, if used appropriately, usually poses no problems in terms of adverse effects. However, some patients (~5–10% of asthmatic patients) remain poorly controlled despite what appears to be optimal therapy. There are some concerns about the safety of asthma therapy, particularly in the treatment of childhood asthma, as this treatment has to be given over a very long period (1). Compliance with inhaled therapy, particularly controller therapy, is very poor and might be improved with oral therapy (for example, a once-daily calendar pack). Yet oral therapy presents a problem of side effects, since the drug exerts effects throughout the body, whereas asthma is localized to the airways. This will necessitate the development of drugs that are *specific* for asthma and do not have effects on other systems or on normal physiological mechanisms (unlike β-agonists and corticosteroids). None of the currently available therapy is curative or has so far been shown to alter the natural history of the disease. Perhaps it is difficult to seek a cure for asthma until more about the molecular causes are known.

Despite considerable efforts by the pharmaceutical industry, it has been very difficult to develop new classes of therapeutic agents. This is partly because existing drugs are effective and safe and partly because animal models of asthma are very poor and do not predict clinical efficacy. Asthma is the most rapidly growing therapeutic market in the world, reflecting the world-wide increase in prevalence of asthma and the increasing recognition that chronic treatment is needed for many patients. The current worldwide asthma market exceeds $4 billion per year and is increasing rapidly. Because asthma is so prevalent and such a widespread problem, even a small percentage of this market is worth obtaining.

It is clearly important to understand more about the underlying mechanisms of asthma and also about how the currently used drugs work before rational improvements in therapy can be expected. A better understanding of the cellular and molecular mechanisms of asthma has identified new molecular targets for the developement of novel classes of drug, and there are several opportunities for new drug development in asthma; but whether these will revolutionize asthma treatment is unknown. This chapter focuses on some of these new targets, but in the context of existing drugs and drugs that are already in development. There are three major approaches to the development of new anti-asthma treatments:

- Improvement in existing classes of effective drug—e.g., long-acting inhaled β_2-agonists (salmeterol and formoterol) or long-acting anticholinergics (tiotropium bromide).
- Development of novel compounds, based on rational developments and improved understanding of asthma—e.g., antileukotrienes and IL-5 inhibitors.
- Development of novel compounds based on serendipity—e.g., furosemide (frusemide).

II. New Bronchodilators

Bronchodilators are presumed to act by reversing contraction of airway smooth muscle, although some may have additional effects on mucosal edema or inflammatory cells. The biochemical basis of airway smooth muscle relaxation has been studied extensively, yet no new types of bronchodilator have so far had any clinical impact. The molecular basis of bronchodilatation involves an increase in intracellular cyclic adenosine 3′, 5′ monophosphate (cAMP) and a reduction in cytosolic calcium ion concentration ([Ca^{2+}]) (Fig. 1). Recent studies suggest that the rise in cAMP is linked to the opening of Ca^{2+}-activated K^+ channels (maxi-K channels) in animal and human airway smooth muscle (2,3). However β-agonists may open maxi-K channels via a direct G-protein coupling to the channel, and this may occur at low concentrations of β-agonist that do not involve any increase in cAMP concentration (4). The molecular mechanisms underlying bron-

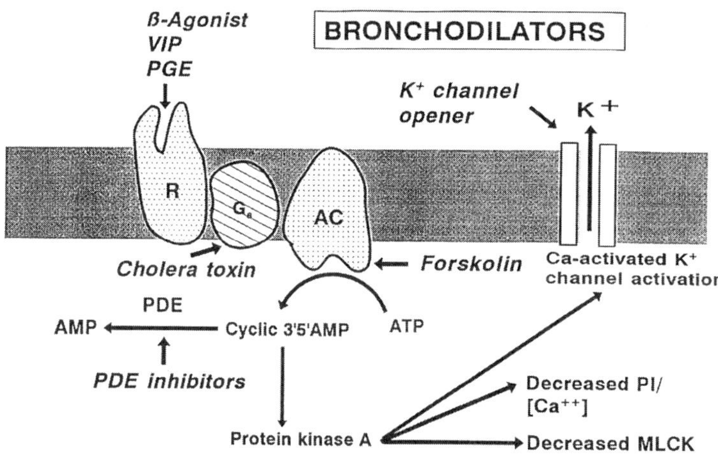

Figure 1 Bronchodilator mechanisms. By mimicking the molecular mechanisms of β_2-agonists, several other approaches to bronchodilatation are possible.

chodilatation may be exploited in the development of new bronchodilators, several of which are under development (Table 1).

Many selective β_2-agonists are now available and there has been a search for β-agonists that have even greater selectivity for β_2-receptors. However it is unlikely that any greater selectivity would be an advantage clinically, since, when the drugs are given by inhalation, a high degree of functional β_2-receptor selectivity is obtained. Furthermore, many of the side effects of β-agonists (tremor, tachycardia, hypokalemia) are mediated via β_2-receptors. There has been recent concern that inhaled β_2-agonists may be associated with increased asthma morbidity and mortality, but this is controversial, and there is little evidence that the nor-

Table 1 New Bronchodilators

Long-acting inhaled β_2-agonists (e.g., salmeterol, formoterol, TA2005)
Selective muscarinic antagonists (tiotropium)
Potassium channel openers (e.g., levcromakalim)
Selective phosphodiesterase inhibitors (PDE3, PDE4, PDE5 inhibitors)
Nitrovasodilators
VIP and analogues (Ro-25-1553)
Atrial natriuretic peptide, urodilatin, and analogues

mally used doses of inhaled β_2-agonists are a problem, particularly when these drugs are used as required for symptom relief rather than on a regular basis (5,6). The most important recent advance in bronchodilator therapy has been the introduction of the long-acting inhaled β_2-agonists, salmeterol and formoterol, which produce bronchodilatation and protection against bronchoconstriction for over 12 hr. These drugs have proved to be very useful clinically, provide additional control of asthma when added to inhaled glucocorticoids (7–9), and they are safe. This makes the development of new bronchodilators that would have any advantage extremely difficult.

A. Drugs That Increase Cyclic AMP

Understanding the molecular mechanism of β-agonists has prompted a search for other drugs than increase intracellular cAMP concentrations in airway smooth muscle cells. Several other receptors on airway smooth muscle, other than β-receptors, may activate adenylyl cyclase via a stimulatory G protcin (G_s).

Vasoactive Intestinal Peptide

VIP is a potent bronchodilator of human airways in vitro (10), but is ineffective in asthmatic patients in vivo (11). This may reflect degradation of the peptide by airway epithelial cells. A more stable cyclic analogue of VIP (Ro-25-1553) has a more prolonged effect in vitro and in vivo (12), but it is unlikely that VIP could be more effective that a β_2-agonist, as it would have a greater vasodilator effect and VIP receptors, unlike β_2-adrenoceptors, may not be expressed in peripheral airways (13).

Prostaglandins (PGs)

PGE_2 stimulates adenylyl cyclase and relaxes airways in vitro. However PGE_2 has not proved to be effective as a bronchodilator in vivo and may even lead to constriction and coughing in asthma patients, since PGE_2 also stimulates afferent nerve endings in airways (14). There is now evidence for at least four subtypes of PGE_2 (EP) receptor, and it is likely that the EP-receptor subtype on sensory nerves differs from the receptor subtype on airway smooth muscle, so that a selective agonist may be developed (15). In addition, there is evidence that PGE_2 has an inhibitory action on eosinophils and T lymphocytes and might therefore have anti-inflammatory potential. Inhaled PGE_2 inhibits the early and late responses to allergen and is involved in the refractory response to exercise in the airways, suggesting that PGE_2 may have some therapeutic potential (16). However, inhaled PGE_2 also induces coughing; therefore, in itself it would not be an appropriate therapy. Receptor subtype–selective PGE_2 agonists therefore have some potential and should be explored.

G-protein/Adenylyl Cyclase Stimulation

Receptor-mediated stimulation of adenylyl cyclase involves activation of G_s, which may be stimulated irreversibly by *cholera toxin*. Less toxic compounds that stimulate G_s are under investigation. Forskolin directly activates the catalytic subunit of adenylyl cyclase and large increases cAMP concentration in airway smooth muscle cells, but it has not proved to be effective as a bronchodilator in vitro (17). This may be because β_2-agonists are effective as bronchodilators via direct coupling to maxi-K channels via G_s in addition to a rise in cAMP that is seen with high concentrations of β-agonists (4).

B. Drugs That Increase Cyclic Guanosine Monophosphate (GMP)

Atrial Natriuretic Peptide

When given by intravenous infusion, atrial natriuretic peptide (ANP) produces a significant bronchodilator response and protects against bronchoconstrictor challenges (18,19). It is likely that the effects of ANP on airways are mediated by stimulation of *particulate* guanylyl cyclase and subsequent generation of cGMP (20). While ANP itself is not likely to be commercially valuable, it is possible that non-peptide agonists of ANP receptors may be developed in the future for inhaled use. ANP is being developed as an inhaled formulation for asthma. Urodilatin (ularitide), a related peptide, has a longer duration of action than ANP, as it is less susceptible to enzymatic breakdown and is as potent as salbutamol when given by intravenous infusion in asthmatic subjects (21).

Nitrovasodilators

Nitrovasodilators—such as isosorbide dinitrate, glyceryl trinitrate (GTN), and sodium nitroprusside—activate *soluble* guanylyl cyclase. A dose-dependent relaxant effect of various nitro compounds has been demonstrated on airway smooth muscle in a number of animal studies, and this effect appears to be mediated via stimulation of soluble guanylyl cyclase and subsequent generation of cGMP (20,22). Sublingual GTN and isosorbide dinitrate have been reported to have a bronchodilator effect in patients with asthma (23,24), although others have not confirmed these beneficial effects (25). It is now established that the endogenous neural bronchodilator in human airways is nitric oxide (NO) (26). Endogenous NO is derived from L-arginine by the action of NO synthase and under certain circumstances could be rate limiting in NO formation. This suggests that L-arginine may have bronchodilator potential under certain conditions. These studies suggest that bronchodilators with an alternative intracellular mechanism of action to β_2-agonists may be possible and that further investigation is warranted, particularly with inhaled formulations, in order to avoid vasodilator side effects.

It is not certain that drugs which elevate cGMP as opposed to cAMP would have any particular advantage as bronchodilators, although theroretically they could be additive with β_2-agonists, as they work via a different molecular mechanism. A major disadvantage is likely to be their vasodilator action (headache, palpitations), and this is likely to preclude their development. Furthermore, cGMP appears to have no effect in inflammatory cells, whereas cAMP in general has anti-inflammatory effects.

C. Selective Anticholinergics

There are several distinct subtypes of muscarinic receptor that have differing physiological roles in the airway, and there is some rationale for the development of selective antimuscarinics that block M_3 (and possibly M_1) receptors but avoiding blockade of prejunctional M_2 receptors, which would lead to an increase in the release of acetylcholine, as discussed elsewhere (27). A very promising new anticholinergic is *tiotropium bromide*, with a duration of action of >24 hr and kinetic selectivity for M_1 and M_3 receptors (28). Tiotropium bromide causes prolonged inhibition of cholinergic nerve-induced contraction of human airways in vitro (29) and provides prolonged bronchodilatation and protection against methacholine challenge (>36 hr) in asthmatic patients (30). While it is unlikely that a long-acting anticholinergic would have a major role in asthma therapy, this is likely to be a very valuable treatment in chronic obstructive pulmonary disease (COPD), where cholinergic tone is the major reversible element. Studies of inhaled tiotropium bromide have shown prolonged bronchodilatation in COPD after single doses, making once-daily administration possible (31).

D. K^+ Channel Openers

Potassium (K^+) channels play an important role in the recovery of excitable cells after activation and in maintaining cell stability. Opening of K^+ channels therefore results in relaxation of smooth muscle and inhibition of secretion. Many different types of K^+ channel have now been recognized electrophysiologically and with several selective toxins and drugs (32). K^+ channel openers (KCO) have been considered as possible new bronchodilators for asthma.

K_{ATP} Openers

Drugs that selectively activate an adenosine triphosphate (ATP) dependent K^+ channel (K_{ATP})—which opens in response to a fall in intracellular ATP concentration—in smooth muscle have been developed for the treatment of hypertension. The prototype of these drugs is cromakalim (BRL 3491). These drugs also inhibit spontaneous and induced tone in airway smooth muscle in vitro and might, therefore, have a role in normalizing ''hyperreactive'' airway smooth muscle (33).

K^+ channel openers are currently under investigation as potential antiasthma compounds (34,35). The active enantiomer of cromakalim, levcromakalim (BRL 38227), is a relatively effective relaxant of human bronchi in vitro and appears equally active against several spasmogens, suggesting that it works as a functional antagonist (36). This also suggests that it must have some inhibitory effect on intracellular Ca^{2+} release, possibly via changes in membrane potential. In vivo, it has no bronchodilator or protective effect against bronchoconstrictor challenge at maximally tolerated oral doses (37), but cromakalim has been shown to have a small protective effect against the fall in lung function at night in asthmatic patients (38). Several KCOs have been developed as possible bronchodilators, including aprikalim (RP-49356); HOE 234, which is more potent than levcromakalim in human airway smooth muscle (39); SDZ PCO400; and bimakalim (EMD 52692). Several of these KCOs have been in Phase I/II studies but the development of most of these compounds for asthma has now been halted (because of cardiovascular side effects).

Side effects include headache, flushing, and postural hypotension due to vasodilatation. It will therefore be necessary to develop these drugs for inhalational use in order to avoid these effects, although pilot studies with inhaled levcromakalim produced postural hypotension, presumably due to systemic absorption from the lung. It may be possible to develop K^+ channel openers that are more selective for airway than vascular smooth muscle in view of the diversity of K^+ channels. One such ''airway-selective'' KCO (BRL 55834) has already been described (40) and may be more selective because it also opens a large conductance Ca^{2+}-activated K^+ channel (K_{Ca}).

The future success of these compounds in asthma will probably depend on whether they have any additional effects not shared with β-agonists. K^+ channel openers inhibit the release of neuropeptides from sensory nerves and modulate neurotransmission in the airways (41,42), but whether they have effects on inflammatory cells is not certain. Cromakalim has an inhibitory effect on neurogenic inflammation in the airways and is able to block cigarette smoke–induced mucus secretion in guinea pigs (43). This suggests that these drugs may have a role in mucus hypersecretion.

Maxi-K Channel Openers

Many different types of K^+ channel have now been characterized. Relaxation of airway smooth muscle in response to β-agonists and theophylline appears to involve another type of channel (K_{Ca}), which is selectively blocked by charybdotoxin and iberiotoxin (3,44,45). Development of activators of this channel may therefore be an important target for future development, particularly since this channel may not be as important in relaxing vascular smooth muscle; therefore cardiovascular side effects may not be the major problem they appear to be with

K_{ATP} openers. One such drug, SCA40, is reported to be an opener of a charybdotoxin-sensitive K^+ channel in airway smooth muscle and to be a potent bronchodilator in guinea pig trachea in vitro (46). This has not been confirmed electrophysiologically, however (47), and other evidence suggests that it acts as a phosphodiesterase (PDE) inhibitor. Benzimidazole compounds, such as NS 1619, appear to be K_{Ca} openers (48); this has been documented in airway smooth muscle (47). K_{Ca} openers may also be effective as inhibitors of neuropeptide release, since K_{Ca} openers are involved in modulation of sensory nerves (42) and inhibition of sensory nerve activation (49).

III. Mediator Antagonists

Many different inflammatory mediators have now been implicated in asthma, and several specific receptor antagonists and synthesis inhibitors have been developed that will prove invaluable in working out the contribution of each mediator (Table 2). As many mediators probably contribute to the pathological features of asthma, it seems unlikely that a single antagonist will have a major clinical effect, as compared with nonspecific agents such as ß-agonists and glucocorticoids. However, until such drugs have been evaluated in careful clinical studies, it is not possible to predict their value. Conventional targets—such as histamine, leukotrienes, thromboxane, platelet-activating factor, adenosine, bradykinin, PDE IV

Table 2 Inflammatory Mediators and Inhibitors

Mediator	Inhibitor
Histamine	Terfenadine, loratadine, cetirizine
Leukotriene D_4	Zafirlukast, montelukast
Leukotriene B_4	Zileuton, Bay-x1005, ZD 2138, LY 293111
PAF	Apafant, modipafant, bepafant
Thromboxane	Ozagrel
Bradykinin	Icatibant, WIN 64338, FR167344
Adenosine	Theophylline
Reactive oxygen species	*N*-acetyl-cysteine, ascorbic acid, nitrones
Nitric oxide	Aminoguanidine, 1400W
Endothelin	Bosentan, SB 209670
IL-1β	Recombinant IL-1 receptor antagonist
TNF-α	TNF antibody, TNF soluble receptors
IL-4	IL-4 antibody, soluble IL-4 receptors
IL-5	IL-5 antibody
Mast-cell tryptase	APC366
Eosinophil basic proteins	Heparin

and tachykinins—are considered elsewhere in this book. New mediator targets include reactive oxygen species, NO, and endothelins and cytokines.

A. Antioxidants

The role of reactive oxygen species (ROS) in asthma is uncertain. ROS are generated from inflammatory cells, such as eosinophils and macrophages, and they may combine with oxide NO to form the more stable oxidant peroxynitrite ($ONOO^-$), which, in turn, generates hydroxyl radicals (OH^-). ROS activate the transcription factor nuclear factor-κB (NF-κB), which regulates the expression of many of the inflammatory proteins that are overexpressed in asthmatic airways (50). Antioxidants, such as *N*-acetylcysteine and ascorbic acid, have been tested in asthma but have not been shown to have any marked beneficial effects. However, these agents are relatively weak antioxidants. More potent antioxidants have now been developed, including the spin-trap antioxidants, such as nitrones (51), but these have not yet reached the stage of clinical development.

B. Nitric Oxide Synthase Inhibitors

NO, produced in large amounts from the inducible isoform of NO synthase (iNOS), which is overexpressed in asthmatic airways, may have proinflammatory effects in asthma by increasing plasma exudation in airways and amplifying eosinophilic inflammation (52,53). It follows that inhibition of iNOS may be beneficial in asthma. It is important to avoid inhibition of constitutive NOS, as this may cause hypertension and bronchoconstriction. Aminoguanidine has some selectivity for iNOS and reduces exhaled NO in asthmatic patients to a greater extent than in normal subjects (54). Whether regular treatment with aminoguanidine is beneficial in asthma has not yet been determined. More potent and selective iNOS inhibitors are now in clinical development (55).

C. Endothelin (ET) Antagonists

Endothelins are potent bronchoconstrictors and are abnormally expressed in asthmatic airways (56,57). Inhaled ET-1 is a potent constrictor of asthmatic airways (58). In addition, ET-1 causes proliferation of airway smooth muscle and stimulates fibrosis, suggesting that it may play a role on the remodeling of asthmatic airways. These effects are mediated via stimulation of ET_A and ET_B receptors. Several potent nonpeptidic endothelin antagonists, such as bosentan and SB209670, have now been developed (59,60). However, it may be difficult to test these compounds in asthma, as long-term studies would be needed to determine whether these drugs prevent the irreversible airway narrowing of chronic asthma.

D. Cytokines and Cytokine Inhibitors

A complex cytokine network is responsible for maintaining the chronic inflammation in asthma (61). Among the many cytokines involved in asthma, some may be more important in determining the nature of the inflammatory response or in amplifying the inflammatory state. There are several possible approaches to inhibiting specific cytokines. These range from drugs that inhibit cytokine synthesis (glucocorticoids, cyclosporin A, tacrolimus), blocking antibodies to cytokines or their receptors, soluble receptors to mop up secreted cytokines, receptor antagonists, or drugs that block the signal transduction pathways activated by cytokines (Fig. 2). Other cytokines appear to have an anti-inflammatory effect and may therefore be regarded as potentially therapeutic.

Anti-Interleukin-5

IL-5 plays a key role in orchestrating the eosinophilic inflammation of asthma (62). Blocking antibodies to IL-5 inhibit eosinophilic inflammation and airway hyperresponsiveness in animal models of asthma, including primates (63,64). This blocking effect may last for up to 3 months after a single injection. This

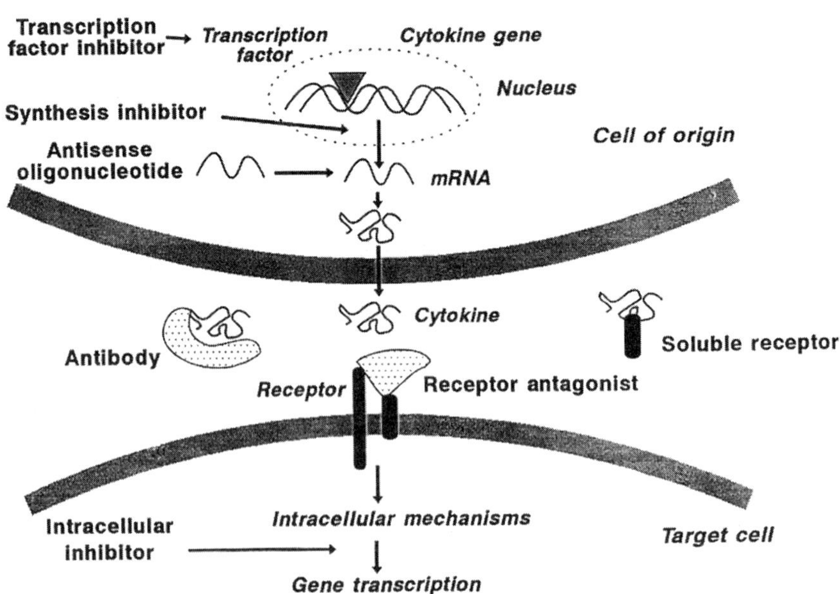

Figure 2 Cytokine inhibition. There are several points at which cytokines may be inhibited.

makes treatment of chronic asthma with such a therapy a feasible proposition. Humanized antibodies have now been developed and are in clinical trial in asthma. There is also a search for IL-5 receptor antagonists. One of the major beneficial effects of corticosteroids in asthma is inhibition of IL-5 gene transcription. Several transcription factors have now been identified in the regulation of mouse and human IL-5 gene (65,66). It has become clear that transcriptional control of mouse and human IL-5 are different, with marked differences in promoter sequences. NF-AT and GATA-4 are important in the human IL-5 promoter (66,67), and there is also an important suppressor element that probably normally keeps the gene repressed. Better understanding of the complex transcriptional control might lead to specific drugs that can selectively inhibit transcription. Another strategy is to block the signal transduction pathways activated by the IL-5 receptor in eosinophils. These have still not been well defined but predominantly involve the JAK-STAT signal transduction pathway, with involvement of STAT1, STAT3, and STAT5α (68–70). There is also a splice variant of STAT-3 (STAT-3β) that acts as a negative regulator that might be exploited therapeutically (71).

Anti-Interleukin-4

IL-4 is critical for the synthesis of IgE by β-lymphocytes and is also involved in eosinophil recruitment to the airways. Inhibition of IL-4 may therefore be effective in inhibiting allergic diseases, and anti-IL-4 receptors are now in clinical development as a strategy to inhibit IL-4. A peptide analogue of IL-4 with only a single amino acid substitution is reported to be an antagonist with only minimal agonist activity (72). Cell-specific IL-4 transcription appears to be activated by the protooncogene c-maf, which may provide another target for inhibition (73). IL-4 effects are predominantly mediated via STAT6, so that drugs that specifically block this transcription factor or its activating enzymes should also be effective (74).

Anti–Tumor Necrosis Factor (TNF)

TNF-α is expressed in asthmatic airways and may play a key role in amplifying asthmatic inflammation through the activation of nuclear factor-κB (NF-κB) and other transcription factors. In rheumatoid arthritis, blocking antibodies to TNF-α have produced remarkable clinical benefits, even in patients who were relatively unresponsive to steroids (75). Such antibodies or soluble TNF receptors are a logical approach to asthma therapy, particularly in patients with severe disease. One problem encountered in this therapy, however, is the development of antibodies that may limit the therapeutic effects after repeated administration.

Chemokine Inhibitors

C-C chemokines—such as RANTES, MCP-3, MCP-4, eotaxin, and eotaxin-2—may play a critical role in the recruitment of eosinophils into the airways of asthmatic patients. Fortunately all of these chemokines act on a common receptor, the CCR-3 receptor, which is expressed predominantly on eosinophils (76–78). Chemokine receptors are G protein–coupled receptors with the typical seven transmembrane-spanning segments and are therefore of a simpler structure than the receptors for most cytokines. Antibodies to CCR-3 receptors have now been developed (78), and it is likely that nonpeptide inhibitors will be discovered by random screening of chemical libraries.

Anti-Inflammatory Cytokines

Some cytokines appear to have anti-inflammatory effects in asthmatic inflammation and may therefore be considered to be potentially therapeutic. While it may not be feasible to administer these proteins as long term therapy, it may be possible to develop drugs that activate the same receptors or specific signal-transduction pathways activated by these receptors.

IL-1 receptor antagonist (IL-1ra) is a cytokine that binds to IL-1 receptors and blocks the action of IL1β. In experimental animals, it reduces airway hyperresponsiveness (79), but clinical studies of recombinant human IL-1ra in asthma have been disappointing.

Interferon gamma (IFN-γ) inhibits Th2 cells and should therefore theoretically reduce asthmatic inflammation. Administration of IFN-γ by nebulization to asthmatic patients has not been found to be effective, however, possibly due to the difficulty in obtaining a high enough concentration locally in the airways (80).

IL-12 is the endogenous regulator of Th1 cells and determines the balance between Th1 and Th2 cells (81). IL-12 administration to rats inhibits allergen-induced inflammation (82) and also inhibits sensitization to allergens. IL-12 produces some of its effects by releasing endogenous IFN-γ, but it also has additional effects. There appears to be a defect in IL-12 production in asthmatic patients (83). Recombinant human IL-12 has now been administered to humans and appears to be safe when administered in low doses. This is therefore a potential treatment for asthma that may reset a fundamental immunological switch.

IL-10 inhibits the synthesis of many inflammatory cytokines [tumor necrosis factor alpha (TNF-α), granulocyte-macrophage colony-stimulating factor (GM-CSF), chemokines] that are overexpressed in asthma. Its effects are partly mediated via inhibition of NF-κB (84). Indeed, there may be a defect in IL-10 secretion in asthma (85,86). Recombinant human IL-10 has proved to be remarkably effective in controlling inflammatory bowel disease, where similar cytokines are expressed, and may be given as a weekly injection (87).

IV. New Anti-Inflammatory Drugs

The recognition that asthma is a chronic inflammatory disease has prompted the earlier introduction of anti-inflammatory treatments. There has been an intensive search for anti-inflammatory treatments that are as effective as glucocorticoids but with fewer side effects. Several anti-inflammatory drugs for asthma are now in clinical development (Table 3). New steroids and PDE4 inhibitors are considered elsewhere in this book.

A. Transcription Factor Blockers

Transcription factors such as NF-κB and AP-1 play an important role in the orchestration of asthmatic inflammation (50,88), and this has prompted a search for specific blockers of these transcription factors or their activation pathways. It is now recognized that anti-inflammatory effects of corticosteroids are likely to be via direct inhibition of transcription factors, such as AP-1 and NF-κB, that are activated by asthma (89). Several new therapies based on interacting with specific transcription factors or their activation pathways are now in development for the treatment of chronic inflammatory diseases, and several drugs already in clinical use (corticosteroids, retinoic acid, cyclosporin A) work via transcription factors (90). One concern about this approach is the specificity of such drugs, but it is clear that transcription factors have selective effects on the expression of certain genes, and this may make it possible to be more selective. In addition, there are cell-specific transcription factors that may be targeted for inhibition, which could provide selectivity of drug action. One such example is nuclear factor of activated T cells (NF-AT), which is blocked by cyclosporin A and tacrolimus and has a restricted cellular distribution. In asthma it may be possible to target drugs to the airways by inhalation, as is currently done for inhaled corticosteroids to avoid any systemic effects.

Table 3 New Anti-Inflammatory Drugs for Asthma

New glucocorticoids (mometasone, cyclesonide, RP 106541)
Transcription factor blockers (NF-κB inhibitors, retinoic acid analogues)
Immunomodulators (inhaled oxeclosporin, tacrolimus, rapamycin, mycophenolate mofetil)
Phosphodiesterase-4 inhibitors (CDP 840, RP 73401, SB 207499)
Adhesion molecule blockers (VLA4 antibody, VLA4 blockers)
Cytokine inhibitors (humanized anti-IL-4, anti-IL5, anti-TNF antibodies)
Anti-inflammatory cytokines (IL-1ra, IFN-γ, IL-10, IL-12)
Anti-IgE antibody
Peptides for immunotherapy

Dissociated Steroids

The recognition that most of the anti-inflammatory effects of steroids are mediated by repression of transcription factors (transrepression)—whereas the endocrine and metabolic effects of steroids are likely to be mediated via DNA binding (transactivation)—has led to a search for novel corticosteroids that selectively transrepress, thus reducing the risk of systemic side effects. Since corticosteroids bind to the same glucocorticoid receptor (GR), this seems at first to be an unlikely possibility, but while DNA binding involves a GR homodimer, interaction with transcription factors AP-1 and NF-κB involves only a single GR. A separation of transactivation and transrepression has been demonstrated with reporter gene constructs in transfected cells using selective mutations of GR (91). Furthermore some steroids, such as the antagonist RU486, have a greater transrepression than transactivation effect. Indeed, the topical steroids used in asthma therapy today, such as fluticasone propionate and budesonide, appear to have more potent transrepression than transactivation effects, which may account for their selection as potent anti-inflammatory agents (92). Recently, a novel class of steroids has been described in which there is potent transrepression with relatively little transactivation. These ''dissociated'' steroids, including RU24858 and RU40066, have anti-inflammatory effects in vivo (93). The suggests that the development of steroids with a greater margin of safety is possible and may predict the development of oral steroids that may be safe to use in asthma.

NF-κB Inhibitors

Since NF-κB may play a pivotal role in asthma (50), this has suggested that specific NF-κB inhibitors might be beneficial in asthma therapy (94). Antioxidants have the ability to block activation of NF-κB in response to a wide variety of stimuli and drugs, such as pyrrolidine dithiocarbamate, have proved useful for in vitro studies, but are too toxic for in vivo development (95). Spin-trap antioxidants may be more effective, since they work at an intracellular level (96). However, antioxidants do not block all of the effects of NF-κB; this may require the development of novel drugs.

Some naturally occurring NF-κB inhibitors have already been identified. Thus gliotoxin, derived from *Aspergillus*, is a potent NF-κB inhibitor that appears to be relatively specific (97). The anti-inflammatory cytokine IL-10 also has an inhibitory effect on NF-κB via an effect on IκB-α (84), and is another therapeutic possibility, particularly as there appears to be a deficit in IL-10 secretion in airway macrophages from asthmatic patients which is correlated with increased secretion of proinflammatory cytokines and chemokines (86).

Novel approaches to inhibition of NF-κB would be to develop specific inhibitors of IκB kinases involved in the initial activation of NF-κB, so as to block the signal transduction pathways leading to activation of NF-κB. Now that IκB kinases have been identified, it may be possible to screen and design specific inhibitors. It may also be possible to inhibit the activity of the enzymes responsible for its degradation of the IκB complex, although the proteasome has many other important functions and its inhibition is likely to produce severe side effects. Recently it has been possible to block NF-κB function by targeting of a specific enzyme (ubiquitin ligase) involved in conjugation of ubiquitin (98). It may be more difficult to develop drugs to directly inhibit the components of NF-κB itself, but antisense oligonucleotides have been shown to be effective inhibitors in vitro and stable, cell-permeable phosphorothioate oligonucleotides are a therapeutic possibility in the future. Recently, adenovirus-mediated gene transfer of IκB-α has been reported to inhibit endothelial cell activation (99).

However, it may be unwise to block NF-κB for prolonged periods, as it plays such a critical role in immune and host defense responses. Targeted disruption (''knockout'') of p65 is lethal because of developmental abnormalities (100), whereas lack of p50 results in immune deficiencies and increased susceptibility to infection (101). Topical application of NF-κB inhibitors by inhalation may prove to be safe, however.

New Drug Interactions

One of the most important implications of research on transcription factors is that multiple and complex interactions between these proteins are possible and that this leads to cross-talk between different signal-transduction pathways. This might be exploited therapeutically by the combination of drugs that act on different transcription factors or pathways that may work together cooperatively. For example, NF-AT has a cytoplasmic component (NF-ATp) that is blocked by cyclosporine and tacrolimus, and a nuclear component AP-1, which is blocked by corticosteroids (Fig. 3). Combining steroids and cyclosporine may therefore have a synergistic inhibitory effect on the expression on genes such as IL-2, IL-4, and IL-5. This has indeed been demonstrated for IL-2 in human T cells, where a combination of both drugs has a much greater suppressive effect than either drug alone (102). This suggests that a dose of cyclosporin A too low to produce nephrotoxic side effects may be combined with an inhaled steroid, so that this synergistic interaction is confined to the airways.

Another interaction that may be exploited therapeutically is that between retinoic acid and steroids. Retinoic acid (vitamin A) binds to retinoic acid receptors, which, like GR, bind to cyclic AMP response element binding protein (CREB)–binding protein (CBP). There appears to be a synergistic interaction between steroids and retinoic acid in repression of transcription factors, such as NF-κB and AP-1, presumably because of competition for binding sites on CBP. A synergistic interaction between retinoic acid and steroids has been demonstrated in suppression of GM-CSF release from cultured epithelial cells, suggesting that retinoic acid may potentiate the anti-inflammatory effects of steroids (103). Novel retinoic acid derivatives activate a subtype of retinoic acid receptor

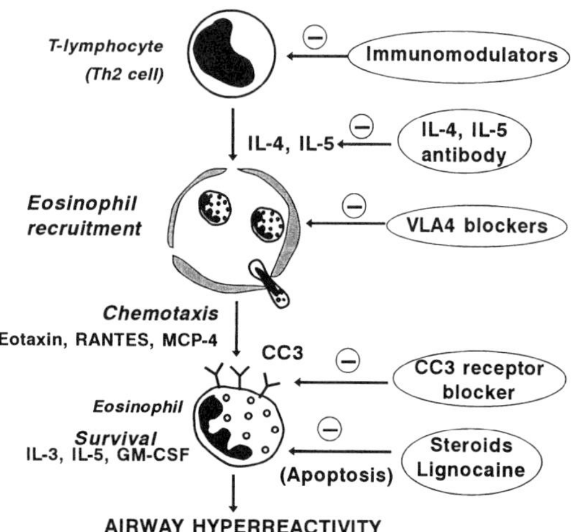

Figure 3 Nuclear factor of activated T cells regulates expression IL-2, IL-4, and IL-5. It is made up of a cytoplasmic component (NF-AT) and AP-1. Cyclosporine inhibits NF-AT by inhibiting the activity of calcineurin (CaN), which is needed for activation of NF-AT, whereas steroids inhibit by blocking the AP-1 component. This predicts a synergy between these two drugs.

(RXR) that interacts with these transcription factors, so that it may be possible to develop more selective retinoids for this purpose (104).

B. New Antiallergic Drugs

Cromones may be effective in controlling mild asthma in some patients. They appear to have a specific action on allergic inflammation, yet the molecular mechanism of action remains uncertain. Although it was believed that the primary mode of action involves inhibiting the release of mast-cell mediators, it has now been demonstrated that it has effects on several other inflammatory cells and on sensory nerves (105). There is now increasing evidence that cromones may act on certain types of chloride channels that are expressed in mast cells and sensory nerves (106). Both cromolyn sodium and nedocromil sodium must be given by inhalation; all attempts to develop orally active drugs of this type have been unsuccessful, possibly because topical administration is critical to their efficacy.

Diuretics

The loop diuretic furosemide (frusemide) shares many of the actions of cromones, inhibiting indirect bronchoconstrictor challenges (allergen, exercise, cold air, adenosine, metabisulfite) but not direct bronchoconstriction (histamine, methacholine) when given by inhalation (107,108). The mechanism of action of furosemide is not shared by the more potent loop diuretic bumetanide, suggesting that some other mechanism than the inhibition of the $Na^+/K^+/Cl^-$ cotransporter must be involved. This is most likely to involve inhibition of the same chloride channel that is inhibited by cromones. Furosemide itself does not appear to be very effective when given regularly by metered-dose inhaler in asthma (109), but it is possible that more potent and long-lasting chloride-channel blockers might be developed in the future.

Eosinophil Inhibitors

Asthma is characterized by eosinophilic inflammation; selective blockade of eosinophils is therefore a logical strategy. Indeed, there is unlikely to be any major side effect for such a therapeutic approach. Eosinophil infiltration into the airways and their activation may be blocked in several ways (Fig. 4). Eosinophil recruitment from the circulation may be blocked by antibodies to the adhesion molecules VCAM-1 (expressed on endothelial cells) and VLA-4 (expressed on eosinophils). Humanized VLA-4 antibodies are not in clinical trial in asthma and small molecules that may be suitable for oral absorption are also in development. IL-5 plays an important role in eosinophil recruitment; selective blockade of IL-5 may therefore be a valuable approach. Humanized IL-5 antibodies are now in clinical trial

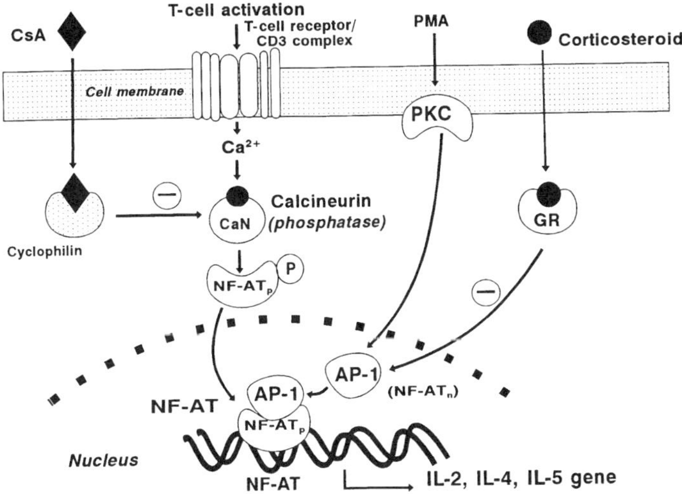

Figure 4 Eosinophil inhibition. There are several points at which eosinophilic inflammation may be blocked.

in asthma (as discussed above), but other approaches to blocking IL-5, such as transcription blockade and inhibitors of IL-5 receptors, are now under investigation. As discussed above, chemokines play a critical role in selectively attracting eosinophils into the airways and, although several chemokines (RANTES, MCP, MCP-4, eotaxin) are selective for eosinophils, they all work through a common receptor on the eosinophil, CCR-3. CCR3 inhibitors are therefore likely to be effective inhibitors of eosinophil inflammation.

Once recruited into the airways, eosinophils would normally undergo apoptotic death, but they survive owing to the effects of various growth factors, such as IL-3, IL-5, and granulocyte-GM-CSF. Blocking of these cytokines results in programmed cell death or apoptosis. This may be mediated in part by the Fas receptor (Apo-1, CD95), as anti-Fas antibody increased apoptosis and results in resolution of eosinophilic inflammation (110). This might be exploited therapeutically by selectively activating Fas on eosinophils. Unfortunately, Fas is expressed on many cells; therefore this will not provide any specificity. Corticosteroids increase eosinophil apoptosis, although the mechanisms involved in this are not yet understood (111). Other drugs may also have such an effect, and the complex biochemical pathways involved in apoptosis may provide opportunities for selective eosinophil deletion (112). It has recently been observed that the local anesthetic lidocaine increases eosinophil apoptosis (113); in an uncontrolled trial in steroid-dependent asthmatics, nebulized lidocaine appeared to have a steroid-sparing effect and improved asthma control (114).

T lymphocytes may play a critical role in initiating and maintaining the inflammatory process in asthma via the release of cytokines that result in eosinophilic inflammation, suggesting that T-cell inhibitors may be useful in controlling asthmatic inflammation. Corticosteroids suppress inflammation in asthma partly through an inhibitory action on T-cell cytokine production. PDE4 inhibitors also have an inhibitory action on T-cell function (115) and inhibit the secretion of IL-5 from allergen-driven T cells (116).

The nonspecific immunomodulator *cyclosporin A* has a steroid-sparing effect in steroid-dependent asthmatic patients (117,118), but its efficacy is limited and side effects, particularly nephrotoxicity, limit its widespread use (119). The possibility of using inhaled cyclosporin A is now being explored, since in experimental asthma in animals the inhaled drug is effective in inhibiting the inflammatory response (120). Immunomodulators such as *tacrolimus (FK506)* and rapamycin appear to be more potent but are also toxic and would offer no real advantage. Novel immunomodulators, such as mycophenolate mofetil, may be less toxic and therefore of greater potential value in asthma therapy (121,122). One problem with nonspecific immunomodulators, such as cyclosporin A, is that they inhibit both Th1 and Th2 cells and therefore do not reset the imbalance between these types of T cell. They also inhibit suppresser T cells that may modulate the inflammatory response. What is required is selective inhibition of Th2 cells, and there is now a search for such opportunities for intervention, as discussed elsewhere in this book.

Cell Adhesion Blockers

It is now recognized that the infiltration of inflammatory cells into tissues is dependent on the adhesion of blood-borne inflammatory cells to endothelial cells prior to migration to the inflammatory site (123). This depends upon specific glycoprotein adhesion molecules on both leukocytes and endothelial cells, which may be upregulated, showing increased binding affinity in response to various stimuli such as cytokines or mediators such as PAF or leukotrienes. Monoclonal antibodies, which inhibit these adhesion molecules, therefore may prevent inflammatory cell infiltration. Thus a monoclonal antibody to ICAM-1 on endothelial cells prevents the eosinophil infiltration into airways and the increase in bronchial reactivity after allergen exposure in sensitized primates (124). The interaction between the $\alpha 4$ integrin VLA-4 and VCAM-1 is important for eosinophil inflammation, however humanized antibodies to VLA-4 have not been developed (125). In contrast, several small molecule blockers of VLA-4 have now been developed that are effective in blocking eosinophilic inflammation in response to allergens in animal models of asthma (126). While the blocking of adhesion molecules is an attractive new approach to the treatment of inflammatory disease, there may be potential dangers in inhibiting immune responses, such as increased infections and increased risks of neoplasia.

IgE Inhibition

Inhibition of IgE using blocking antibodies that do not result in cell activation is considered elsewhere in this book. Clinical studies with a humanized anti-IgE antibody has shown impressive inhibitory effects in allergen-induced responses (127). While infusions of antibody may not be feasible for the long-term treatment of mild asthma, this could be a realistic therapy for patients with more severe forms of asthma. In the future, it may be possible to develop smaller molecules that inhibit IgE. IL-4 inhibitors should have a similar effect, since IgE is critically dependent on IL-4. This is an attractive possibility, as such therapies would be effective in other inflammatory diseases as well, such as rhinitis and atopic dermatitis.

Immunotherapy

Although immunotherapy as currently practiced has been disappointing in the therapy of asthma (128), it is likely that more effective vaccines will be developed in the future (129,130). As the complex mechanisms of antigen presentation and the interaction between antigen-presenting cells and T-lymphocyte receptors are elucidated, this may lead to the development of peptides that will block allergen-induced immune reactions (131). Such peptides are now in clinical trials in allergic diseases.

Vaccination

The vast majority of asthma is allergic, and allergy appears to be related to an imbalance between Th1 and Th2 cells. The development of allergic disease may be determined early in life by factors that affect this balance. There is a strong inverse association between a positive tuberculin test (indicating a Th1-mediated response) and atopy (132). This suggests that it might be possible to immunize children against the risk of developing allergic diseases by stimulating local Th1-mediated immunity in the respiratory tract before sensitization occurs (133).

V. Gene Therapy

Many genes are involved in asthma (134). Several genes determine atopic status, but—more importantly—genes may also determine the severity and pattern of asthma. Genetic polymorphisms of cytokine and other genes may determine the severity of asthmatic inflammation and the response to treatment, so it may be possible to predict the outcome of asthma by screening for such polymorphisms in the future. The diversity of genes involved in asthma makes gene therapy for asthma an unlikely prospect (135).

It is possible, however, that transfer of anti-inflammatory genes may provide anti-inflammatory or inhibitory proteins in a convenient manner. Such gene transfer has been shown to be feasible in animals, using viral vectors (136). Possible anti-inflammatory proteins relevant to asthma include IL-10, IFN-γ, IL-12, and IκB. Antisense oligonucleotides may switch off specific genes, but there are considerable problems in getting these molecules into cells. An inhaled antisense oligonucleotide directed against the adenosine A_1-receptor has been shown to reduce airway hyperresponsiveness in a rabbit model of asthma, demonstrating the feasibility of this approach in treating asthma (137). Considering all the practical problems encountered by gene therapy makes this approach unlikely in the foreseeable future other than for proof of concept studies.

VI. Conclusions

Many different new therapeutic approaches to the treatment of asthma are possible, yet few new drugs have reached the clinic. The β_2-agonists are by far the most effective bronchodilator drugs and lead to rapid symptomatic relief. Now that inhaled β_2-agonists with a long duration of action have been developed, it is difficult to imagine that more effective bronchodilators could be discovered. All new bronchodilators have suffered from the problem that they relax vascular smooth muscle to a greater extent than airway smooth muscle and therefore have vasodilator side effects that would preclude their use in asthma.

Similarly, inhaled corticosteroids are extremely effective as chronic treatment in asthma and suppress the underlying inflammatory process. There is increasing evidence that earlier use of inhaled glucocorticoids may not only control asthma effectively but also prevent irreversible changes in airway function. For most patients, a short acting β_2-agonist on demand and regular inhaled steroids are sufficient to provide excellent control of asthma (138). For some patients, a fixed combination of β_2-agonist and steroid inhaler may be a useful development, since they will improve compliance with inhaled-steroids regimens (which is poor because of the lack of immediate bronchodilator effect) (139).

The *ideal* drug for asthma would probably be a tablet that can be administered once daily to improve compliance. It should have no side effects, and this means that it should be specific for the abnormality of asthma (or allergy) (140).

Future developments in asthma therapy should be directed toward the inflammatory mechanisms, and perhaps more specific therapy may one day be developed. The possibility of developing a ''cure'' for asthma seems remote, but when more is known about the genetic abnormalities of asthma, it may be possible to search for such a therapy. Advances in molecular biology may aid the development of drugs that can specifically switch off relevant genes, but more must be discovered about the basic mechanisms of asthma before such advances become possible.

References

1. Barnes PJ. Current therapies for asthma: promise and limitations. Chest 1997; 111: 17S–22S.
2. Jones TR, Charette L, Garcia ML, Kaczorowski GJ. Interaction of iberiotoxin with β-adrenoceptor agonists and sodium nitroprusside on guinea pig trachea. J Appl Physiol 1993; 74:1879–1884.
3. Miura M, Belvisi MG, Stretton CD, Yacoub MH, Barnes PJ. Role of potassium channels in bronchodilator responses in human airways. Am Rev Respir Dis 1992; 146:132–136.
4. Kume H, Hall IP, Washabau RJ, Takagi K, Kotlikoff MI. Adrenergic agonists regulate K_{Ca} channels in airway smooth muscle by cAMP-dependent and -independent mechanisms. J Clin Invest 1994; 93:371–379.
5. Barnes PJ, Chung KF. Questions about inhaled β_2-agonists in asthma. Trends Pharmacol Sci 1992; 13:20–23.
6. Drazen JM, Israel E, Boushey HA, Chinchilli VM, Fahy JV, Fish JE, Lazarus SC,

Lemanske RF, Martin RJ, Peters SP, Sorkness C, Szefler SJ. Comparison of regularly scheduled with as needed use of albuterol in mild asthma. N Engl J Med 1996; 335:841–847.

7. Greening AP, Ind PW, Northfield M, Shaw G. Added salmeterol versus higher-dose corticosteroid in asthma patients with symptoms on existing inhaled corticosteroid. Lancet 1994; 344:219–224.
8. Woolcock A, Lundback B, Ringdal N, Jacques L. Comparison of addition of salmeterol to inhaled steroids with doubling the dose of inhaled steroids. Am J Respir Crit Care Med 1996; 153:1481–1488.
9. Pauwels RA, Lofdahl C-G, Postma DS, Tattersfield AE, O'Byrne PM, Barnes PJ, Ullman A. Effect of inhaled formoterol and budesonide on exacerbations of asthma. N Engl J Med 1997; 337:1412–1418.
10. Palmer JBD, Cuss FMC, Barnes PJ. VIP and PHM and their role in nonadrenergic inhibitory responses in isolated human airways. J Appl Physiol 1986; 61:1322–1328.
11. Barnes PJ, Dixon CMS. The effect of inhaled vasoactive intestinal peptide on bronchial hyperreactivity in man. Am Rev Respir Dis 1984; 130:162–166.
12. O'Donnel M, Garippa RJ, Rinaldi N, Selig WM, Smiko B, Renzetti L, Tanno SA, Wasserman MA, Welton A, Bolin DR. Ro25-1553: a novel long-acting vasoactive intestinal peptide agonist. Part 1: In vitro and in vivo bronchodilator studies. J Pharmacol Exp Ther 1994; 270:1282–1288.
13. Carstairs JR, Barnes PJ. Visualization of vasoactive intestinal peptide receptors in human and guinea pig lung. J Pharmacol Exp Ther 1986; 239:249–255.
14. Walters EH, Davies BH. Dual effect of prostaglandin E_2 on normal airways smooth muscle in vivo. Thorax 1982; 37:918–922.
15. Coleman RA, Smith WL, Narumiya S. International Union of Pharmacology classification of prostanoid receptors: Properties, distribution, and structure of the receptors and their subtypes. Pharmacol Rev 1994; 46:205–229.
16. Pavord ID, Tattersfield AE. Bronchoprotective role for endogenous prostaglandin E_2. Lancet 1995; 344:436–438.
17. Waldeck B, Widmark E. Comparison of the effects of forskolin and isoprenaline on tracheal, cardiac and skeletal muscles from guinea-pig. Eur J Pharmacol 1985; 112:349–353.
18. Angus RM, Mecallaum MJA, Hulks G, Thomson NC. Bronchodilator, cardiovascular and cyclic guanylyl monophosphate response to high dose infused atrial natriuretic peptide in asthma. Am Rev Respir Dis 1993; 147:1122–1125.
19. Angus RM, Millar EA, Chalmers GW, Thomson NC. Effect of inhaled atrial natriuretic peptide and a neutral endopeptidase inhibitor on histamine-induced bronchoconstriction. Am J Respir Crit Care Med 1995; 151:2003–2005.
20. Ishil K, Murad F. ANP relaxes bovine tracheal smooth muscle and increase cGMP. Am J Physiol 1989; 256:C495–500.
21. Fluge T, Fabel H, Wagner TO, Schneider B, Forssmann WG. Urodilatin (ularitide, INN): a potent bronchodilator in asthmatic subjects. Eur J Clin Invest 1995; 25: 728–736.
22. Gruetter CA, Childers CC, Bosserman MK, Lemke SM, Ball JG, Valentovic MA. Comparison of relaxation induced by glycerl trinitate, isosorbide dinitrate and

sodium nitroprusside in bovine airways. Am Rev Respir Dis 1989; 139:1192–1197.
23. Hirschleiter L, Arora Y. Nitrates in the treatment of bronchial asthma. Br J Dis Chest 1991; 39:275–283.
24. Okayama M, Sasaki H, Takishima T. Bronchodilator effect of subligual isosorbide dinitrate in asthma. Eur J Clin Pharmacol 1984; 26:151–155.
25. Miller WC, Shultz TF. Failure of nitroglycerin as a bronchodilator. Am Rev Respir Dis 1979; 120:471–472.
26. Belvisi MG, Stretton CD, Barnes PJ. Nitric oxide is the endogenous neurotransmitter of bronchodilator nerves in human airways. Eur J Pharmacol 1992; 210:221–222.
27. Barnes PJ. Muscarinic receptor subtypes in airways. Life Sci 1993; 52:521–528.
28. Barnes PJ, Belvisi MG, Mak JCW, Haddad E, O'Connor B. Tiotropium bromide (Ba 679 BR), a novel long-acting muscarinic antagonist for the treatment of obstructive airways disease. Life Sci 1995; 56:853–859.
29. Takahashi T, Belvisi MG, Patel H, Ward JK, Tadjkarimi S, Yacoub MH, Barnes PJ. Effect of Ba 679 BR, a novel long-acting anticholinergic agent, on cholinergic neurotransmission in guinea-pig and human airways. Am J Respir Crit Care Med 1994; 150:1640–1645.
30. O'Connor BJ, Towse LJ, Barnes PJ. Prolonged effect of tiotropium bromide on methacholine-induced bronchoconstriction in asthma. Am J Respir Crit Care Med 1996; 154:876–880.
31. Maesen FPV, Smeets JJ, Sledsens TJM, Wald FDM, Cornelissen JPG. Tiotropium bromide, a new long-acting antimuscarinic bronchodilator: a pharmacodynamic study in patients with chronic obstructive pulmonary disease (COPD). Eur Respir J 1995; 8:1506–1513.
32. Garcia M, Galvez A, Garcia-Calvo M, King VF, Vazquez J, Kaczorowski GJ. Use of toxins to study potassium channels. J Bioenerg Biomembr 1991; 23:615–646.
33. Morley J. K^+ channel openers and suppression of airway hyperreactivity. Trends Pharmacol Sci 1994; 15:463–468.
34. Black JL, Barnes PJ. Potassium channels and airway function: new therapeutic approaches. Thorax 1990; 45:213–218.
35. Buckle DR. Prospects for potassium channel activators in the treatment of airways obstruction. Pulm Pharmacol 1993; 6:161–169.
36. Black JL, Armour CL, Johnson PRA, Alouan LA, Barnes PJ. The action of a potassium channel activator BRL 38227 (lemakalim) on human airway smooth muscle. Am Rev Respir Dis 1990; 142:1384–1389.
37. Kidney JC, Fuller RW, Worsdell Y, Lavender EA, Chung KF, Barnes PJ. Effect of an oral potassium channel activator BRL 38227 on airway function and responsiveness in asthmatic patients: comparison with oral salbutamol. Thorax 1993; 48: 130–134.
38. Williams AJ, Lee TH, Cochrane GM, Hopkirk A, Vyse T, Chiew F, Lavender E, Richards DH, Owen S, Stone P, Church S, Woodcock AA. Attenuation of nocturnal asthma by cromakalim. Lancet 1990; 336:334–336.
39. Miura M, Belvisi MG, Ward JK, Tadjkarini M, Yacoub MH, Barnes PJ. Bronchodi-

latory effects of the novel potassium channel opener HOE 234 in human airways in vitro. Br J Clin Pharmacol 1993; 35:318–320.

40. Arch JR, Bowring NE, Buckle DR. Evaluation of the novel potassium channel activator BRL 55834 as an inhaled bronchodilator in guinea-pigs and rats: comparison with levcromakalim and salbutamol. Pulm Pharmacol 1994; 7:121–128.
41. Ichinose M, Barnes PJ. A potassium channel activator modulates both noncholinergic and cholinergic neurotransmission in guinea pig airways. J Pharmacol Exp Ther 1990; 252:1207–1212.
42. Stretton CD, Miura M, Belvisi MG, Barnes PJ. Calcium-activated potassium channels mediate prejunctional inhibition of peripheral sensory nerves. Proc Natl Acad Sci USA 1992; 89:1325–1329.
43. Kuo H, Rohde JAL, Barnes PJ, Rogers DF. K^+ channel activator inhibition of neurogenic goblet cell secretion in guinea pig trachea. Eur J Pharmacol 1992; 221: 385–388.
44. Jones TR, Charette L, Garcia ML, Kaczorowski GJ. Selective inhibition of relaxation of guinea-pig trachea by charybodotoxin, a potent Ca^{++}-activated K^+ channel inhibitor. J Pharmacol Exp Ther 1990; 225:697–706.
45. Jones TR, Charette L. Interaction of the Cab2+X-activated K^+ channel inhibitor iberiotoxin with beta adrenoceptor agonists on isolated guinea pig trachea. Am Rev Respir Dis 1992; 145:A203.
46. Laurent F, Michel A, Bonnet PA, Chapat JP, Boucard M. Evaluation of the relaxant effect of SCA40, a novel charybdotoxin-sensitive potassium channel opener, in guinea-pig isolated trachealis. Br J Pharmacol 1993; 108:622–626.
47. Macmillan S, Sheridan RD, Chilvers ER, Patmore L. A comparison of the effects of SCA40, NS 004 and NS 1619 on large conductance Ca(2+)-activated K+ channels in bovine tracheal smooth muscle cells in culture. Br J Pharmacol 1995; 116: 1656–1660.
48. Olesen SP, Munch E, Moldt P, Orejer J. Selective activation of Ca2+-dependent K+ channels by novel benzimidazolone. Eur J Pharmacol 1994; 251:53–59.
49. Fox AJ, Barnes PJ, Venkatesan P, Belvisi MG. Activation of large conductance potassium channels inhibits the afferent and efferent function of airway sensory nerves. J Clin Invest 1997; 99:513–519.
50. Barnes PJ, Karin M. Nuclear factor-κB: a pivotal transcription factor in chronic inflammatory diseases. N Engl J Med 1997; 336:1066–1071.
51. Thomas CE, Ohlweiler DF, Carr AA, Nieduzak TR, Hay DA, Adams G, Vaz R, Bernotas RC. Characterization of the radical trapping activity of a novel series of cyclic nitrone spin traps. J Biol Chem 1996; 271:3097–3104.
52. Barnes PJ. Nitric oxide and airway disease. Ann Med 1995; 27:389–393.
53. Barnes PJ, Liew FY. Nitric oxide and asthmatic inflammation. Immunol Today 1995; 16:128–130.
54. Yates DH, Kharitonov SA, Thomas PS, Barnes PJ. Endogenous nitric oxide is decreased in asthmatic patients by an inhibitor of inducible nitric oxide synthase. Am J Respir Crit Care Med 1996; 154:247–250.
55. Garvey EP, Oplinger JA, Furfine ES, Kiff RJ, Laszlo F, Whittle BJR, Knowles RG. 1400W is a slow tight binding and highly selective inhibitor of inducible nitric oxide synthase in vitro and in vivo. J Biol Chem 1997; 272:4959–4963.

56. Barnes PJ. Endothelins and pulmonary diseases. J Appl Physiol 1994; 77:1051–1059.
57. Hay DW, Henry PJ, Goldie RG. Is endothelin-1 a mediator in asthma? Am J Respir Crit Care Med 1996; 154:1594–1597.
58. Chalmers GW, Little SA, Patel KR, Thomson NC. Endothelin-1-induced bronchoconstriction in asthma. Am J Respir Crit Care Med 1997; 156:382–388.
59. Douglas SA, Meek TD, Ohlstein EH. Novel receptor antagonists welcome a new era in endothelin biology. Trends Pharmacol Sci 1994; 15:313–316.
60. Hay DW, Luttmann MA. Nonpeptide endothelin receptor antagonists: IX. Characterization of endothelin receptors in guinea pig bronchus with SB 209670 and other endothelin receptor antagonists. J Pharmacol Exp Ther 1997; 280:959–965.
61. Barnes PJ. Cytokines as mediators of chronic asthma. Am J Resp Crit Care Med 1994; 150:S42–S49.
62. Egan RW, Umland SP, Cuss FM, Chapman RW. Biology of interleukin-5 and its relevance to allergic disease. Allergy 1996; 51:71–81.
63. Mauser PJ, Pitman A, Witt A, Fernandez X, Zurcher J, Kung T, Jones H, Watnick AS, Egan RW, Kreutner W, Adams GK. Inhibitory effect of the TRFK-5 anti IL-5 antibody in a guinea pig model of asthma. Am Rev Respir Dis 1993; 148:1623–1627.
64. Mauser PJ, Pitman AM, Fernandez X, Foran SK, Adams GK, Kreutner W, Egan RW, Chapman RW. Effects of an antibody to interleukin-5 in a monkey model of asthma. Am J Respir Crit Care Med 1995; 152:467–472.
65. Zhang DH, Cohn L, Ray P, Bottomly K, Ray A. Transcription factor GATA-3 is differentially expressed in murine Th1 and Th2 cells and controls Th2-specific expression of the interleukin-5 gene. J Biol Chem 1997; 272:21597–21603.
66. Stranick KS, Zambas DN, Uss AS, Egan RW, Billah MM, Umland SP. Identification of transcription factor binding sites important in the regulation of the human interleukin-5 gene. J Biol Chem 1997; 272:16453–16465.
67. Yamagata T, Nishida J, Sakai R, Tanaka T, Yazaki Y, Hirai H. Of the GATA-binding proteins, only GATA-4 selectively regulates the human IL-5 gene promoter in IL-5 producing cells which express multiple GATA-binding proteins. Leukemia 1997; 11(suppl 3):501–502.
68. Pazdrak K, Stafford S, Alam R. The activation of the Jak-STAT 1 signalling pathway by IL-5 in eosinophils. J Immunol 1995; 155:397–402.
69. van der Bruggen T, Caldenhoven E, Kanters D, Coffer P, Raaijmakers JA, Lammers JW, Koenderman L. Interleukin-5 signaling in human eosinophils involves JAK2 tyrosine kinase and Stat1a. Blood 1995; 85:1442–1448.
70. Mui ALF, Wakao H, O'Farrell AM, Miyajima A. Interleukin-3, granulocyte-macrophage colony stimulating factor and interleukin-5 transduce signals through two STAT5 homologs. EMBO J 1995; 14:1166–1175.
71. Caldenhoven E, van Dijk TB, Solari R, Armstrong J, Raaijmakers JAM, Lammers J-WJ, Koenderman L, de Groot RP. STAT3b, a splice variant of transcription factor STAT3, is a dominant negative regulator of transcription. J Biol Chem 1996; 271: 13221–13227.
72. Kruse N, Tony HP, Sebald W. Conversion of human interleukin-4 into a high affinity antagonist by a single amino acid replacement. EMBO J 1992; 11:3237–3244.

73. Ho IC, Hodge MR, Rooney JW, Glimcher LH. The proto-oncogene c-maf is responsible for tissue-specific expression of interleukin-4. Cell 1996; 85:973–983.
74. Takeda K, Tanaka T, Shi W, Matsumoto M, Minami M, Kashiwamura S, Nakanishi K, Yoshida N, Kishimoto T. Essential role for Stat6 in IL-4 signalling. Nature 1996; 380:627–630.
75. Elliott MJ, Maini RN, Feldmann M, Kalden JR, Antoni C, Smolen JS, Leeb B, Breedveld FC, Macfarlane JD, Bijl H, Woody JN. Randomised double-blind comparison of diuretic monoclonal antibody to tumour necrosis factor a (cA2) versus placebo in rheumatoid arthritis. Lancet 1994; 344:1105–1110.
76. Adams DH, Lloyd AR. Chemokines: leucocyte recruitment and activation cytokines. Lancet 1997; 349:490–495.
77. Ponath PD, Qin S, Post TW, Wang J, Gerard NP, Newman W, Gerard C, Mackay CR. Molecular cloning and characterization of a human eotaxin receptor expressed selectively on eosinophils. J Exp Med 1996; 183:2437–2448.
78. Heath H, Qin S, Rao P, Wu L, LaRosa G, Kassam N, Ponath PD, Mackay CR. Chemokine receptor usage by human eosinophils: the importance of CCR3 demonstrated using an antagonistic monoclonal antibody. J Clin Invest 1997; 99:178–184.
79. Selig W, Tocker J. Effect of interleukin-1 receptor antagonist on antigen-induced pulmonary responses in guinea-pigs. Eur J Pharmacol 1992; 213:331–336.
80. Boguniewicz M, Martin RJ, Martin D, Gibson U, Celniker A. The effects of nebulized recombinant interferon-γ in asthmatic airways. J Allergy Clin Immunol 1995; 95:133–135.
81. Trinchieri G. Interleukin 12: a proinflammatory cytokine with immunoregulatory functions that bridge innate resistance and antigen-specific adaptative immunity. Annu Rev Imunol 1995; 13:252–276.
82. Gavett SH, O'Hearn DJ, Li X, Huang SK, Finkelman FD, Wills-Karp M. Interleukin 12 inhibits antigen-induced airway hyperresponsivness, inflammation and Th2 cytokine expression in mice. J Exp Med 1995; 182:1527–1536.
83. van der Pouw Kraan TC, Boeije LC, de Groot ER, Stapel SO, Snijders A, Kapsenberg ML, van der Zee JS, Aarden LA. Reduced production of IL-12 and IL-12-dependent IFN-gamma release in patients with allergic asthma. J Immunol 1997; 158:5560–5565.
84. Wang P, Wu P, Siegel MI, Egan RW, Billah MM. Interleukin(IL)-10 inhibits nuclear factor kappa B activation in human monocytes. IL-10 and IL-4 suppress cytokine synthesis by different mechanisms. J Biol Chem 1995; 270:9558–9563.
85. Borish L, Aarons A, Rumbyrt J, Cvietusa P, Negri J, Wenzel S. Interleukin-10 regulation in normal subjects and patients with asthma. J Allergy Clin Immunol 1996; 97:1288–1296.
86. John M, Lim S, Seybold J, Robichaud A, O'Connor B, Barnes PJ, Chung KF. Inhaled corticosteroids increase IL-10 but reduce MIP-1a, GM-CSF and IFN-γ release from alveolar macrophages in asthma. Am J Respir Crit Care Med 1998; 157: 256–262.
87. van Deventer SJ, Elson CO, Fedorak RN. Multiple doses of intravenous interleukin 10 in steroid-refractory Crohn's disease: Crohn's Disease Study Group. Gastroenterology 1997; 113:383–389.

88. Barnes PJ, Adcock IM. Transcription factors and asthma. Eur Respir J 1998; 12: 221–234.
89. Barnes PJ. Molecular mechanisms of steroid action in asthma. J Allergy Clin Immunol 1996; 97:159–168.
90. Manning AM. Transcription factors: a new frontier in drug discovery. Drug Dev Ther 1996; 1:151–160.
91. Heck S, Kullmann M, Grast A, Ponta H, Rahmsdorf HJ, Herrlich P, Cato ACB. A distinct modulating domain in glucocorticoid receptor monomers in the repression of activity of the transcription factor AP-1. EMBO J 1994; 13:4087–4095.
92. Adcock IM, Barnes PJ. Ligand-induced differentiation of glucocorticoid recepto(GR) transrepression and transactivation. Am J Respir Crit Care Med 1996; 153: A243.
93. Vayssiere BM, Dupont S, Choquart A, Petit F, Garcia T, Marchandeau C, Gronemeyer H, Resche-Rigon M. Synthetic glucocorticoids that dissociate transactivation and AP-1 transrepression exhibit antiinflammatory activity in vivo. Mol Endocrinol 1997; 11:1245–1255.
94. Barnes PJ, Adcock IM. NF-κB: a pivotal role in asthma and a new target for therapy. Trends Pharmacol Sci 1997; 18:46–50.
95. Schreck R, Rieber P, Baeuerle PA. Reactive oxygen intermediates as apparently widely used messengers in the activation of the NF-κB transcription factor and HIV-1. EMBO J 1991; 10:2247–2258.
96. Miyajima T, Kotake Y. Spin trapping agent, phenyl N-tert-butyl nitrone, inhibits induction of nitric oxide synthase in endotoxin-induced shock in mice. Biochem Biophys Res Commun 1995; 215:114–121.
97. Pahl HL, Krauss B, Schultze-Osthoff K, Decker T, Traenckner M, Myers C, Parks T, Warring P, Muhlbacher A, Czernilofsky A-P, Baeuerle PA. The immunosuppressive fungal metabolite gliotoxin specifically inhibits transcription factor NF-κB. J Exp Med 1996; 183:1829–1840.
98. Yaron A, Gonen H, Alkalay I, Hatzubai A, Jung S, Beyth S, Mercurio F, Manning AM, Ciechanover A, Ben-Neriah J. Inhibition of NF-κB cellular function via specific targeting of the IkB-ubiquitin ligase. EMBO J 1997; 16:6486–6494.
99. Wrighton CJ, Hofer-Warbinek R, Moll T, Eytner R, Bach FH, de Martin R. Inhibition of endothelial cell activation by adenovirus-mediated expression of IkBa, an inhibitor of transcription factor NF-κB. J Exp Med 1996; 183:1013–1022.
100. Beg AA, Sha WC, Bronson RT, Ghosh S, Baltimore D. Embroyonic lethality and liver degeneration in mice lacking the RelA component of NF-κB. Nature 1995; 376:167–170.
101. Sha WC, Liou HC, Tuomanen EI, Baltimore D. Targeted disruption of the p50 subunit of NF-κB leads to multifocal defects in immune responses. Cell 1995; 80: 321–330.
102. Wright LC, Cammisuli S, Baboulene L, Fozzard J, Adcock IM, Barnes PJ. Cyclosporin A and glucocorticoids interact synergistically in T lymphocytes: implications for asthma therapy. Am J Respir Crit Care Med 1995; 151:A675.
103. Wallace J, Adcock IM, Barnes PJ. Retinoic acid potentiates the inhibitory effects of dexamethasone on AP-1 DNA binding in epithelial cells. Am J Respir Crit Care Med 1996; 153:A209.

104. Rowe A. Retinoid X receptors. Int J Biochem Cell Biol 1997; 29:275–278.
105. Barnes PJ, Holgate ST, Laitinen LA, Pauwels R. Asthma mechanisms, determinants of severity and treatment: the role of nedocromil sodium. Clin Exp Allergy 1995; 25:771–787.
106. Heinke S, Szucs G, Norris A, Droogmans G, Nilius B. Inhibition of volume-activated chloride currents in endothelial cells by chromones. Br J Pharmacol 1995; 115:1393–1398.
107. Bianco S, Pieroni MG, Refini RM, Robuschi M, Vaghi A, Sestini P. Inhaled loop diuretics as potential new anti-asthmatic drugs. Eur Respir J 1993; 6:130–134.
108. Barnes PJ. Diuretics and asthma. Thorax 1993; 48:195–197.
109. Yates DH, O'Connor BJ, Yilmaz G, Aikman S, Chen-Worsdell M, Barnes PJ, Chung KF. Effect of acute and chronic inhaled furosemide on bronchial hyperresponsiveness in mild asthma. Am J Respir Crit Care Med 1995; 152:892–896.
110. Tsuyuki S, Bertrand C, Erard F, Trifilieff A, Tsuyuki J, Wesp M, Anderson GP, Coyle AJ. Activation of the Fas receptor on lung eosinophils leads to apoptosis and the resolution of eosinophilic inflammation of the airways. J Clin Invest 1995; 96:2924–2931.
111. Meagher LC, Cousin JM, Seckl JR, Haslett C. Opposing effects of glucocorticoids on the rate of apoptosis in neutrophilic and eosinophilic granulocytes. J Immunol 1996; 156:4422–4428.
112. Anderson GP. Resolution of chronic inflammation by therapeutic induction of apoptosis. Trends Pharmacol Sci 1996; 17:438–442.
113. Ohnishi T, Kita H, Mayeno AN, Okada S, Sur S, Broide DH, Gleich GJ. Lidocaine in bronchoalveolar lavage fluid (BALF) is an inhibitor of eosinophil-active cytokines. Clin Exp Immunol 1996; 104:325–331.
114. Hunt L, Swelund H, Frigas E, Gleich GH. Nebulized lidocaine can be used successfully as glucocorticoid sparing/replacing therapy in severe glucocorticoid-dependent asthma. Am J Respir Crit Care Med 1996; 153:A534.
115. Giembycz MA, Corrigan CJ, Seybold J, Newton R, Barnes PJ. Identification of cyclic AMP phosphodiesterases 3, 4 and 7 in human $CD4^+$ and $CD8^+$ T-lymphocytes. Br J Pharmacol 1996; 118:1945–1958.
116. Essayan DM, Huang S-K, Kagey-Sabotka A, Lichtenstein LM. Effects of nonselective and isoenzyme selective cyclic nucleotide phosphodiesterase inhibitors on antigen-induced cytokine gene expression in peripheral blood mononuclear cells. Am J Respir Cell Mol Biol 1995; 13:692–702.
117. Alexander AG, Barnes NC, Kay AB. Trial of cyclosporin in corticosteroid-dependent chronic severe asthma. Lancet 1992; 339:324–328.
118. Nizankowska E, Soja J, Pinis G, Bochenek G, Stadek K, Domgala B, Pajak A, Szczeklik A. Treatment of steroid-dependent bronchial asthma with cyclosporin. Eur Respir J 1995; 8:1091–1099.
119. Barnes PJ. Immunomodulators in asthma: Where do we stand? Eur Respir J 1996; 9:154S–159S.
120. Morley J. Cyclosporin A in asthma therapy: a pharmacological rationale. J Autoimmun 1992; 45(suppl A):265–269.
121. Thompson AG, Starzl TC. New immunosuppressive drugs: mechanistic insights and potential therapeutic advances. Immunol Rev 1993; 136:71–98.

122. Lipsky JJ. Mycophenolate mofetil. Lancet 1996; 348:1357–1359.
123. Pilewski JM, Albelda SM. Cell adhesion molecules in asthma: homing activation and airway remodeling. Am J Respir Cell Mol Biol 1995; 12:1–3.
124. Weg VB, Williams TJ, Lobb RR, Noorshargh S. A monoclonal antibody recognizing very late activation antigen-4 inhibits eosinophil accumulation in vivo. J Exp Med 1993; 177:561–566.
125. Yuan Q, Strauch KL, Lobb RR, Hemler ME. Intracellular single-chain antibody inhibits integrin VLA-4 maturation and function. Biochem J 1996; 818:591–596.
126. Lobb RR, Abraham WM, Burkly LC, Gill A, Ma W, Knight JA, Leone DR, Antognetti G, Pepinsky RB. Pathophysiologic role of alpha 4 integrins in the lung. Ann NY Acad Sci 1996; 796:113–123.
127. Fahy JV, Fleming HE, Wong HH, Liu JT, Su JQ, Reimann J, Fick RB, Boushey HA. The effect of an anti-IgE monoclonal antibody on the early and late phase responses to allergen inhalation in asthmatic subjects. Am J Respir Crit Care Med 1997; 155:1828–1834.
128. Barnes PJ. Immunotherapy for asthma: is it worth it? N Engl J Med 1996; 334: 531–532.
129. Hoyne G-F, Lamb J-R. Peptide-mediated regulation of the allergic immune response. Immunol Cell Biol 1996; 74:180–186.
130. Nelson HS. Does allergen immunotherapy have a role in the treatment of bronchial asthma? Allergy Asthma Proc 1997; 18:157–162.
131. Yssel H, Fasler S, Lamb J, de Vries JE. Induction of non-responsiveness in human allergen specific type 2 helper cells. Curr Opin Immunol 1994; 6:847–852.
132. Shirakawa T, Enomoto T, Shimazu S, Hopkin JM. The inverse association between tuberculin responses and atopic disorder. Science 1997; 275:77–79.
133. Holt PG. A potential vaccine strategy for asthma and allied atopic diseases during infancy. Lancet 1994; 344:456–458.
134. Sandford A, Weir T, Pare P. The genetics of asthma. Am J Respir Crit Care Med 1996; 153:1749–1765.
135. Demoly P, Mathieu M, Curiel DT, Godard P, Bousquet J, Michel FB. Gene therapy strategies for asthma. Gene Ther 1997; 4:507–516.
136. Xing Z, Ohkawara Y, Jordana M, Grahern FL, Gauldie J. Transfer of granulocyte-macrophage colony-stimulating factor gene to rat induces eosinophilia, monocytosis and fibrotic lesions. J Clin Invest 1996; 97:1102–1110.
137. Nyce JW, Metzger WJ. DNA antisense therapy for asthma in an animal model. Nature 1997; 385:721–725.
138. Barnes PJ. Inhaled glucocorticoids for asthma. N Engl J Med 1995; 332:868–875.
139. Barnes PJ, O'Connor BJ. Use of a fixed combination β_2-agonist and steroid dry powder inhaler in asthma. Am J Respir Crit Care Med 1995; 151:1053–1057.
140. Barnes PJ. New drugs for asthma. Clin Exp Allergy 1996; 26:738–745.

14

Current Practice and Future Trends in Clinical Trials in Asthma

JOHAN C. KIPS and ROMAIN A. PAUWELS

University Hospital Ghent
Ghent, Belgium

I. Introduction

Despite intensive research, asthma remains a poorly defined disease. This is reflected in current definitions, which remain largely descriptive (1). Although it is widely claimed and accepted that chronic airway inflammation is the crucial feature in the pathophysiology of the disorder (2), the exact functional contribution of the various cells and mediators possibly involved remains to be further established. It follows that no single parameter can be used as the ultimate outcome measure for clinical trials in asthma.

Several indices of disease activity can be evaluated. This includes recording of clinical symptoms, physiological measures, health-related quality-of-life measurement, treatment use, or evaluation of the underlying airway inflammation. The correlation between these various groups of outcome measures is generally rather low. This implies that combining different outcome measures will prove complementary rather than being redundant. In most clinical trials, this concept is being increasingly adopted. In this chapter an attempt is made to review the value of various outcome measures that can be used to assess the efficacy of novel treatment strategies being developed for asthma.

II. Outcome Measures in Asthma

Several indices of disease activity can be monitored in asthma (3). Attempts are currently made to standardize some of these outcome measures for asthma clinical research (4). This standardization process includes assessment of a given index of disease activity in terms of reliability and validity. The reliability is based on evaluation of inter- and intraobserver consistency in addition to the repeatability of the technique, which is examined by measuring the parameter on two or more occasions during a stable phase of the disease. Elements of validity assessment include evaluation of the conformity of a technique to other indices of disease activity, its ability to distinguish between asthma and other diseases, and its responsiveness to intervention. Only a relatively limited number of outcome measures have been fully validated according to these general principles (Table 1).

A. Symptom Scores

Recording of clinical symptoms is one of the most commonly used outcome measures in asthma. Symptoms are usually collected by means of questionnaires. Among these, two major groups can be recognized. The first group is specifically intended to record asthma symptoms in epidemiological research. These questionnaires have been designed to establish the prevalence of chronic lung diseases including asthma in certain populations. Well-validated examples include the In-

Table 1 Outcome Measures in Asthma

Validated
Symptom measures
Questionnaires for epidemiological surveys
Questionnaires for clinical studies
Pulmonary function tests
Pre- and postbronchodilator FEV_1*
Airway responsiveness testing
Peak flow recording
Assessment of airway inflammation
Induced sputum
Health-related quality-of-life assessment
Nonvalidated
Treatment regimens
Health care utilization outcomes
Health economic parameters

* Forced expiratory volume in 1 second.

ternational Union Against Tuberculosis and Lung Disease (IUATLD), Medical Research Council (MRC) and American Thoracic Society—Division of Lung Disease (ATS-DLD) questionnaires for adults and the University of Sidney questionnaire for population studies involving children (5–10). These questionnaires address the occurrence of symptoms such as wheezing, dyspnea, cough, chest tightness, nighttime awakenings, and sputum production. The reporting interval ranges from the last 12 months to ever in life. It has to be noted that these types of questionnaires are not sufficiently detailed to allow for accurate assessment of the current severity of asthma, and they have not been evaluated in terms of responsiveness to clinical interventions.

The second type of questionnaire is being used for the evaluation of asthma symptoms in subjects with established asthma in clinical trials during a certain time interval, providing more information on the intensity, duration, variability, and frequency of symptoms. The symptom-reporting interval in these questionnaires is shorter than in those intended for epidemiological studies. Various asthma symptom scores have been developed in this respect, generally expressing severity of symptoms on a four- to five-point response scale or visual analogue scale (VAS). The reliability and validity of these symptom questionnaires have, with a few exceptions (11,12), not been established nor has the appropriate time interval for data collection been determined (13). Moreover, an increase in symptom intensity is usually considered to be a less sensitive indicator of asthma deterioration than lung function changes (14,15). However, although some patients are indeed poor perceivers of airway obstruction, it has been suggested that carefully obtained symptom-based questionnaires can detect exacerbations more rapidly than peak-flow monitoring (16). In addition, it has to be noted that the occurrence of exacerbations, which is an important outcome measure, especially in longer-term clinical trials, does not clearly correlate to peak-flow variability or airway hyperresponsiveness (17–19).

B. Physiological Measures: Pulmonary Function Tests

The main physiological manifestation of asthma, as included in most definitions of the disease, is variable airway obstruction. It is therefore logical and compulsory to include pulmonary function tests as an objective measurement in evaluating the effectiveness of asthma intervention in a research setting. As the degree of airway obstruction in asthma is variable, lung function monitoring should include not only baseline function as a parameter of the current disease activity but also an evaluation of the airway "twitchiness" as a marker of the disease lability (20). Baseline lung function is usually assessed by performing spirometry and may also be estimated from the early-morning peak flow between clinic visits. Airway lability can be measured by ambulatory peak-flow monitoring or estimated from measurement of airway responsiveness.

Baseline Spirometry

The forced expiratory volume in 1 sec (FEV_1) derived from a properly performed spirometry is generally regarded as the best standardized pulmonary function parameter (21–23). FEV_1 is inversely and linearly related to the degree of airway obstruction. The short-term repeatability is very good. In a clinical trial setting, it is obviously important to minimize as much as possible the influence of factors that add to the variability of FEV_1 measurements. These include well-identifiable factors such as bronchodilator use or the time of day in addition to less controllable elements such as exposure to cold, dry air or other nonspecific irritants. Administration of a potent bronchodilator minimizes the effect of these interfering bronchoconstrictor factors. The postbronchodilator FEV_1 is therefore considered to be an even more stable measure in asthmatics than comparing visit-to-visit baseline FEV_1. Fluctuations in the degree of bronchodilator reversibility are usually not considered a useful asthma outcome measure.

The use of the FEV_1 as an outcome variable in multicenter studies necessitates careful standardization of the procedure in the different participating centers. The use of the same spirometric equipment and a central quality control further increases the reliability of the measurements (24).

Airway Responsiveness

The variability in airway obstruction is to a certain extent linked to the twitchiness of the airways or susceptibility to asthma attacks. The element of variability can be approached either by ambulatory lung-function monitoring or assessing airway responsiveness, which measures the sensitivity of the airways to inhaled nonallergic or nonsensitizing stimuli (25,26). A variety of clinical, physical, or physicochemical stimuli can be used to measure non-specific airway hyperresponsiveness, methacholine and histamine being among the most favored (27). A methacholine challenge is fairly reproducible if performed in the same center but is not very well standardized (28). There is no shortage of standards, but they are all different. This can be a problem in using the methacholine challenge as an outcome measure in multicenter studies.

A question that remains to a large extent unresolved is how to interpret methacholine challenges. The degree of methacholine responsiveness is usually expressed as the provocative concentration or dose causing a fall in FEV_1 of 20% (PC_{20} or PD_{20} FEV_1).* This represents the position of the methacholine dose-response curve but disregards the information that can be gained from other characteristics of this curve, such as the slope of the curve and the presence or absence of a plateau (29,30). The PC_{20} FEV_1 has been proposed as a marker of underlying

---

* Provocative concentration or dose to cause a fall of 20% in FEV_1.

airway inflammation in asthma. In some studies a correlation has indeed been found between PC_{20} FEV_1 and parameters of acute airway inflammation such as the number of activated eosinophils, T cells, or mast cells in bronchial biopsies (31,32). However, this has not been invariably confirmed (33,34); even if present, the correlation is usually weak. Others have postulated that the plateau of the dose-response curve represents a better functional correlate of airway remodeling, which is considered to result from more chronic inflammatory changes in the asthmatic airways (35–37). This issue remains, however, to be further explored.

An additional question relates to the choice of the bronchoconstrictor stimulus. Methacholine and histamine are thought to cause airway narrowing by direct stimulation of specific receptors on airway smooth muscle cells. In contrast, other stimuli, such as adenosine 5′ monophosphate (AMP) or exercise, cause airway constriction through the secondary release of mediators from inflammatory cells or neurons. This so-called indirect airway responsiveness has been suggested to be more specific for asthma and to be a better marker of asthma severity (38). Again, these claims have not been validated at present.

Ambulatory Monitoring

The major disadvantage of spirometry during scheduled clinic visits in clinical trials is that it offers only a ''snapshot'' of the degree of airway obstruction. Hence the need for ambulatory monitoring, providing multiple measurements of the degree of obstruction over a more prolonged period of time in the patient's natural setting. The most frequently used method to date is the peak-flow meter. Peak-flow monitoring is cheap, simple and safe. The disadvantages of peak-flow meters are that the readings are largely effort-dependent and less reproducible and that the instruments are poorly standardized. Peak-flow readings are therefore less accurate than FEV_1 measurements (39). The peak-flow meter generally gives reasonably accurate readings at low flows but overreads in the middle of the range and underreads in the high range. Hence, if a patient moves from the middle range to the higher range, the improvement might be underevaluated (40–42). It can be hoped that the hand-held spirometers currently being introduced will prove more accurate (43).

The diurnal variation in peak flow, calculated by measuring morning and evening peak flows over a number of days, also provides information on airway lability. This is less unpleasant, cheaper, and safer to perform than a provocation challenge and can be performed irrespective of the baseline lung function. Peak-flow variability has been shown to correlate with airway hyperresponsiveness. However, the correlation is usually weak, and it has been stressed that both markers provide slightly different information and therefore cannot be used interchangeably (44–46).

Assessment of Airway Inflammation

The presence of chronic mucosal airway inflammation is currently considered to be the central element in the pathophysiology of asthma. It would therefore seem logical to include a parameter of airway inflammation—in addition to symptoms and lung function criteria in clinical trials—especially in evaluating the potential effect of a number of the newer approaches described in the previous sections.

Several approaches can be adopted in this respect. The first, most direct approach is the histological examination of endobronchial (31–33,47–49) or even transbronchial biopsies (50) sampled with the fiberoptic bronchoscope. Although feasible in studies with a relatively limited sample size, this approach is obviously hampered by its invasiveness, especially when one is embarking into long-term studies on a large number of subjects. In addition, it must be realized that even this ''gold standard'' approach has not been well standardized. Many different techniques for sampling, processing, and analyzing tissue have been described and adopted, none of which has been validated (51,52).

A second approach, therefore, consists of monitoring airway inflammation by less invasive techniques on more readily available samples, such as serum, urine, or exhaled air. Various parameters have been proposed, ranging from cell-specific markers of activity such as eosinophil cationic protein (ECP) or the soluble IL-2 receptor in serum (53) to very broad markers of inflammation such as nitric oxide (NO) in exhaled air (54). In view of the importance attributed to eosinophils in the pathophysiology of asthma, it is not surprising that a lot of interest has focused on serum ECP. Again, as ECP measurements remain to be fully evaluated in terms of reliability and validity, it is unclear whether they provide additional information on asthma control beyond the monitoring of symptoms and pulmonary function tests (55).

A third approach, which has been thoroughly investigated over the past few years, consists of analyzing induced sputum (56,57). This technique is relatively noninvasive if properly performed and yet provides a direct sample from within the airways. As for bronchial biopsies, differences in techniques for inducing and processing sputum exist, none of them being invariably adopted as the ''gold standard.'' However, these different methods have in general been shown to be both reliable and valid (58). Induced sputum as a marker of airway inflammation, therefore, does appear promising, offering the possibility of repeated sampling in longer-term intervention studies in a larger group of patients.

Other Outcome Measures in Asthma

In addition to symptom scores, lung function measurements, and assessment of airway inflammation, a range of data can provide useful additional information as outcome measures in clinical asthma research.

Quality-of-Life Assessment

Health-related quality of life (HRQL) is increasingly being recognized as an important outcome measure (59). Moreover, it has clearly been shown that HRQL correlates poorly with functional outcome measures and therefore needs to be assessed by specifically designed and validated tools (59,60). A number of questionnaires have been validated in this respect. These include generic questionnaires such as the Medical Outcome Survey Short Form with 36 units (MOS-SF36), which include broadly applicable questions on the patient's social, mental, and physical status (61). Alternatively, disease-specific forms can be used, including the Asthma Quality of Life Questionnaire (AQLQ) or the St. George Respiratory Questionnaire (SGRQ) (62–64).

Treatment Regimen

In evaluating the effect of a therapeutic intervention in asthma, it is obviously important to record the medication needed by the patient, in addition to symptom intensity or lung function parameters. If, for the same intensity of symptoms, the patient requires more medication, be it a higher dose of controller medication or a higher amount of reliever medication, the severity of asthma has obviously increased. In clinical studies, treatment has to be included as an outcome measure. Medication use is frequently included in asthma diaries, together with symptom scores and peak-flow recordings. However, as for most other outcome measures, a well-validated medication score remains to be fully developed (65,66). The most widely adopted technique is to keep the controller medication constant and to allow and record changes in the use of a single rescue medication.

A particular consideration in recording medication use is estimating patient compliance (67). Methods to assess adherence to treatment include direct measures, such as biochemical analysis of medication in saliva or blood, in addition to a variety of indirect measures. These include clinician judgment, self-report by the patient, counting of pills, weighing of canisters, or, more recently, monitoring via electronic devices. Overall, compliance is generally considered to be low (68,69). In addition, the degree of concordance between standard adherence measurement and electronic records is rather poor, with self-report and medication measurement consistently overestimating adherence. One of the problems in nonelectronic measurement is that of medication "dumpers" (70). These patients appear to offer the best collaboration to the study, yet their adherence is generally lower than that of so-called noncompliant or moderately compliant subjects.

Asthma Mortality and Health Care Utilization Statistics

Mortality and health care utilization elements such as hospitalization or emergency department visits can be used for evaluating the long-term efficacy of pharmacological intervention in large groups of patients. However, one must bear in mind that—owing to differences in disease classification, referral pattern, organization, and delivery of care or access to care—the evaluation of these data is not always straightforward (3).

Health Economic Parameters

Asthma clearly has an important economic impact (71–73). In view of the need to limit health expenditures in many countries, it becomes increasingly important to add an economic evaluation to the efficacy assessment of therapeutic strategies in asthma (74). As for many other outcome measures, the economic evaluation of asthma treatment is hampered by the lack of standardized outcome measures. Estimations of indirect costs vary largely between groups, as does the direct cost related to hospital-based treatment (75). In addition, the absence of a single, well-identifiable clinical outcome measure complicates cost-effectiveness analyses in asthma. Hence the need to include composite scores, such as the "symptom-free days" or disease-specific quality-of-life questionnaires in health-economic analyses for asthma (76). Another approach consists of a cost-utility analysis, evaluating the effect of treatment mainly in terms of quality-adjusted life years (QALYs) (77). Although this technique allows for pharmacoeconomic comparisons with other diseases, the sensitivity of utility measures to clinically significant health changes in asthma seems limited (78).

III. Conclusion

One of the aspects that clearly illustrates the complexity of asthma is the difficulty of defining the severity of the disease (79). No single parameter unequivocally reflects the severity of asthma: baseline FEV_1, peak-flow variability, airway hyperresponsiveness, intensity of symptoms, markers of inflammation, and quality of life all reflect slightly different aspects of the disease. The correlation between these various outcome measures is insufficient that any one can freely substitute for another. Therefore, in evaluating the effect of a therapeutic regimen on the severity of asthma, different parameters should be evaluated. Most scoring systems record symptoms, treatment use, and lung function criteria, including baseline FEV_1 at clinic visits and ambulatory peak-flow measurements (80). We recommend the use of an aggregate score that reflects the objectives of asthma management—namely, the number of days with asthma under control. This implies the absence of asthma symptoms, lung function above 80% of predicted or personal best value, no need for rescue medication, and absence of medication-related side effects (19). An additional parameter that becomes increasingly important is HRQL, which can now be evaluated by validated questionnaires. Finally, especially in evaluating the effect of newer compounds that have the capacity to profoundly interfere with the inflammatory process underlying asthma, it becomes mandatory to include direct markers of airway inflammation in clinical trials. It can be argued that induced sputum would seem to be the most reliable and valid parameter in this respect.

References

1. Global initiative for asthma. Global Strategy for Asthma Management and Prevention. Publication no. 95-3659. Washington, DC: National Heart, Lung and Blood Institute, 1995.
2. Djukanovic R, Roche WR, Wilson JW, Beasley CRW, Twentyman OP, Howarth PH, Holgate ST. State of the art: mucosal inflammation in asthma. Am Rev Respir Dis 1990; 142:434–457.
3. Rose R, Weiss KB. An overview of outcomes measurement in asthma care. Immunol Allergy Clin North Am 1996; 16:841–858.
4. Bailey WC, Wilson SR, Weiss KB, Windsor RA, Wolle JM. Measures for use in asthma clinical research. Am J Respir Crit Care Med 1994; 149:s1–s8.
5. Medical Research Council, Committee on the Aetiology of Chronic Bronchitis. Standardised questionnaire on respiratory symptoms. Br Med J 1960; 2:1665.
6. Ferris BG. Epidemiology standardization project: II. Recommended respiratory disease questionnaires for use with adults and children in epidemiologic research. Am Rev Respir Dis 1978; 118:s7–s53.
7. Burney PGJ, Chinn S, Britton JR, Tattersfield AE, Papacosta AO. What symptoms predict the bronchial response to histamine? Evaluation of a community survey of the Bronchial Symptoms Questionnaire (1984) of the International Union Against Tuberculosis and Lung Disease. Int J Epidemiol 1989; 18:165–173.
8. Burney PGJ, Laitinen LA, Perdrizet S, Huckauf H, Tattersfield AE, Chinn S, Poisson N, Heeren A, Britton JR, Jones T. Validity and repeatability of the IUATLD (1984) Bronchial Symptoms Questionnaire: an international comparison. Eur Respir J 1989; 1:940–945.
9. Salome CM, Peat JK, Britton WJ, Woolcock AJ. Bronchial hyperresponsiveness in two populations of Australian schoolchildren. Clin Allergy 1987; 17:271–281.
10. Torren K, Brisman J, Järvholm B. Asthma and asthma-like symptoms in adults assessed by questionnaires. Chest 1993; 104:600–608.
11. Wasserfallen J-B, Gold K, Schulman KA, Baraniuk JN. Development and validation of a rhinoconjunctivitis and asthma symptom score for use as an outcome measure in clinical trials. J Allergy Clin Immunol 1997; 100:16–22.
12. Steen N, Hutchinson A, McColl E, Eccles MP, Hewison J, Meadows KA, Blades SM, Fowler P. Development of a symptom based outcome measure for asthma. Br Med J 1994; 309:1065–1068.

13. O'Connor GT, Weiss ST. Clinical and symptom measures. Am J Respir Crit Care Med 1994; 149:s21–s28.
14. Apter AJ, Affleck G, Reisine ST, Tennen HA, Barrows E, Wells M, Willard A, ZuWallack RL. Perception of airway obstruction in asthma: sequential daily analyses of symptoms, peak expiratory flow rate, and mood. J Allergy Clin Immunol 1997; 99:605–612.
15. Boulet LP, Deschesnes F, Turcotte H, Gignac F. Near fatal asthma: clinical and physiologic features, perception of bronchoconstriction, and psychologic profile. J Allergy Clin Immunol 1991; 88:838–846.
16. Gibson PG, Wong BJO, Hepperle MJE, Kline PA, Girgis-Gabardo A, Guyaat G, Dolovich J, Denburg JA, Ramsdale EH, Hargreave FE. A research method to induce and examine a mild exacerbation of asthma by withdrawal of inhaled corticosteroid. Clin Exp Allergy 1992; 22:525–532.
17. Josephs LK, Gregg I, Mullee MA, Holgate ST. Nonspecific bronchial reactivity and its relationship to the clinical expression of asthma. Am Rev Respir Dis 1989; 140: 350–357.
18. Johnston SL, Pattemore PK, Sanderson G, Smith S, Lampe F, Josephs L, Symington P, O'Toole S, Myint SH, Tyrrell DAJ, Holgate ST. Community study of role of viral infections in exacerbations of asthma in 9–11 year old children. Br Med J 1995; 310:1225–1229.
19. Pauwels RA, Löfdahl CG, Postma DS, Tattesrfield AE, O'Byrne P, Barnes PJ, Ullman A. Effect of inhaled formoterol and budesonide on exacerbations of asthma. N Engl J Med 1997; 337:1405–1411.
20. Enright PL, Lebowitz MD, Cockroft DW. Physiologic measures: pulmonary function tests. Am J Respir Crit Care Med 1994; 149:s9–s18.
21. Gardner RM, Hankinson JL, Clausen JL, Crapo RO, Johnson RL, Epler GR. Standardization of spirometry—1987 update. Official statement of the American Thoracic Society. Am Rev Respir Dis 1987; 136:1285–1298.
22. Quanjer PPH, ed. Standardization of lung function tests for the European Community for steel and coal. Bull Eur Physiopathol Respir 1983; 19(suppl 5): 1–95.
23. American Thoracic Society. Lung function testing: selection of reference values and interpretative strategies. Am Rev Respir Dis 1991; 144:1202–1218.
24. Anthonisen NR, Connett JE, Kiley JP, Altose MD, Bailey WC, Buist AS, Conway WA, Enright PL, Kanner RE, O'Hara P, Owens GR, Scanlon PD, Tashkin DP, Wise RA; for the Lung Health Study Research Group. Effects of smoking intervention and the use of an inhaled anticholinergic bronchodilator on the rate of decline of FEV_1: The Lung Health Study. JAMA 1994; 272:1497–1505.
25. Hargreave FE, Dolovich J, O'Byrne PM, Ramsdale EH, Daniel EE. The origin of airway hyperresponsiveness. J Allergy Clin Immunol 1986; 78:825–832.
26. Cockcroft DW. Nonallergic airway responsiveness. J Allergy Clin Immunol 1988; 81:111–119.
27. Cockcroft DW. Airway responsiveness. In Barnes PJ, Grunstein MM, Leff AR, Woolcock AJ, eds. Asthma. New York: Lippincott-Raven, 1997:1253–1266.
28. Sterk PJ, Fabbri LM, Quanjer PH, Cockcroft DW, O'Byrne PM, Anderson SD, Juniper EF, Malo J-L. Airway responsiveness: Standardized challenge testing with phar-

macological, physical and sensitizing stimuli in adults. Eur Respir J 1993; 6(suppl 16):53–83.
29. Woolcock AJ, Salome CM, Yan K. The shape of the dose-response curve to histamine in asthmatic and normal subjects. Am Rev Respir Dis 1984; 130:71–75.
30. Sterk PJ, Bel EH. The shape of the dose-response curve to inhaled bronchoconstrictor agents in asthma and in chronic obstructive pulmonary diseases. Am Rev Respir Dis 1991; 143:1433–1437.
31. Sont JK, van Krieken JHJM, Evertse CE, Hooijer R, Willems LNA, Sterk PJ. Relationship between the inflammatory infiltrate in bronchial biopsy specimens and clinical severity of asthma in patients treated with inhaled steroids. Thorax 1996; 51: 496–502.
32. Bentley AM, Menz G, Storz C, Robinson DS, Bradley B, Jeffery PK, Durham SR, Kay AB. Identification of T lymphocytes, macrophages, and activated eosinophils in the bronchial mucosa in intrinsic asthma. Am Rev Respir Dis 1992; 146:500–506.
33. Djukanovic R, Wilson JW, Britten KM, Wilson SJ, Walls AF, Roche WR, Howarth PH, Holgate ST. Quantitation of mast cells and eosinophils in the bronchial mucosa of symptomatic atopic asthmatics and healthy control subjects using immunohistochemistry. Am Rev Respir Dis 1990; 142:863–871.
34. Crimi E, Spanavello A, Neri M, Ind PW, Rossi GA, Brusasco V. Dissociation between airway inflammation and airway hyperresponsiveness in allergic asthma. Am J Respir Crit Care Med 1998; 157:4–9.
35. Lambert RK, Wiggs BR, Kuwano K, Hogg JC, Paré PD. Functional significance in increased airway smooth muscle in asthma and COPD. J Appl Physiol 1993; 74: 2771–2781.
36. Moreno RH, Hogg JC, Paré PD. Mechanics of airway narrowing. Am Rev Respir Dis 1986; 133:1171–1180.
37. Macklem PT. A theoretical analysis of the effect of airway smooth muscle load on airway narrowing. Am J Respir Crit Care Med 1996; 153:83–89.
38. Pauwels R, Joos G, Van Der Straeten M. Bronchial hyperresponsiveness is not bronchial hyperresponsiveness is not bronchial asthma. Clin Allergy 1988; 18:317–321.
39. Frischer T, Meinert R, Urbanek R, Kuehr J. Variability of peak expiratory flow rate in children: short and long term reproducibility. Thorax 1995; 50:35–39.
40. Miller MR, Dickinson SA, Hitchings DJ. The accuracy of portable peak flow meters. Thorax 1992; 47:904–909.
41. Sly PD, Cahill P, Willet K, Burton P. Accuracy of mini peak flow meters in indicating changes in lung function in children with asthma. Br Med J 1994; 308:572–574.
42. Miles JF, Tunnicliffe W, Cayton RM, Ayres JG, Miller MR. Potential effects of correction of inaccuracies of the mini-Wright peak expiratory flow meter on the use of an asthma self-management plan. Thorax 1996; 51:403–406.
43. Godschalk I, Brackel HJL, Peters JCK, Bogaards JM. Assessment of accuracy and applicability of a portable electronic diary card spirometer for asthma treatment. Respir Med 1996; 90:619–622.
44. Boezen HM, Postma DS, Schouten JP, Kerstjens HAM, Rijcken B. PEF variability, bronchial responsiveness and their relation to allergy markers in a random population (20–70 yr). Am J Respir Crit Care Med 1996; 154:30–35.

45. Brand PLP, Duiverman EJ, Postma DS, Waalkens HJ, Kerrebijn KF, van Essen-Zandvliet EEM, and the Dutch CNSLD Study Group. Peak flow variation in childhood asthma: relationship to symptoms, atopy, airways obstruction and hyperresponsiveness. Eur Respir J 1997; 10:1242–1247.
46. Kerstjens HAB, Brand PLP, de Jong PM, Koëter GH, Postma DS, and the Dutch CNSLD Study Group. Influence of treatment on peak expiratory flow and its relation to airway hyperresponsiveness and symptoms. Thorax 1994; 49:1109–1115.
47. Laitinen LA, Laitinen A, Haahtela T. Airway mucosal inflammation even in patients with newly diagnosed asthma. Am Rev Respir Dis 1993; 147:697–704.
48. Jeffery PK, Wardlaw AJ, Nelson FC, Collins JV, Kay AB. Bronchial biopsies in asthma: an ultrastructural, quantitative study and correlation with hyperreactivity. Am Rev Respir Dis 1989; 140:1745–1751.
49. Bousquet J, Chanez P, Lacoste JY, Barnéon G, Ghavanian N, Enander I, Venge P, Ahlstedt S, Simony-Lafontaine J, Godard P, Michel FB. Eosinophilic inflammation in asthma. N Engl J Med 1990; 323:1033–1039.
50. Kraft M, Djukanovic R, Wilson S, Holgate ST, Martin RJ. Alveolar tissue inflammation in asthma. Am J Respir Crit Care Med 1996; 154:1505–1510.
51. Workshop summary and guidelines: investigative use of bronchoscopy, lavage, and bronchial biopsies in asthma and other airway diseases. J Allergy Clin Immunol 1991; 88:808–814.
52. Laitinen A, Laitinen LA, Virtanen IT. Bronchial biopsies. In: Barnes PJ, Grunstein MM, Leff AR, Woolcock AJ, eds. Asthma. New York: Lippincott-Raven, 1997:209–224.
53. Venge P. Soluble markers of allergic inflammation. Allergy 1994; 49:1–8.
54. Barnes PJ, Kharitonov SA. Exhaled nitric oxide: a new lung function test. Thorax 1996; 51:233–237.
55. Kips JC, Pauwels RA. Serum eosinophil cationic protein in asthma: what does it mean? Clin Exp Allergy 1998; 28:1–3.
56. Pavord ID, Pizzichini MMM, Pizzichini E, Hargreave FE. The use of induced sputum to investigate airway inflammation. Thorax 1997; 52:498–501.
57. O'Byrne PM, Inman MD. Induced sputum to assess airway inflammation in asthma. Eur Respir J 1996; 9:2435–2436.
58. Kips JC, Peleman RA, Pauwels RA. Induced sputum: do differences matter? Eur Respir J 1998; 11:529–533.
59. Curtis JR, Martin DP, Martin TR. Patient-assessed health outcomes in chronic lung disease. Am J Respir Crit Care Med 1997;156:1032–1039.
60. Juniper EF. Quality of life in adults and children with asthma and rhinitis. Allergy 1997; 52:971–977.
61. Stewart AL, Hays R, Ware JE. The MOS short-form general health survey: reliability and validity in a patient population. Med Care 1988; 26:724–732.
62. Bousquet J, Khani J, Dhivert H, Richard A, Chicoye A, Ware JE, Michel FB. Quality of life in asthma: internal consistency and validity of the SF-36 questionnaire. Am J Respir Crit Care Med 1994; 149:371–375.
63. Juniper EF, Guyatt GH, Epstein RS, Ferrie PJ, Jaeschke R, Hiller TK. Evaluation of impairment of health-related quality of life in asthma: development of a questionnaire for use in clinical trials. Thorax 1992; 47:76–83.
64. Jones PW, Quirk FH, Baveystock CM, Littlejohns P. A self-completed measure of

health status for chronic airflow limitation: the St George's Respiratory Questionnaire. Am Rev Respir Dis 1992; 145: 1321–1327.

65. Busse WW, Maisiak R, Young KR. Treatment regimen and side effects of treatment measures. Am J Respir Crit Care Med 1994; 149:s44–s50.
66. Richards JM, Bailey WC, Windsor RA, Martin B, Soong S-J. Some simple scales for use in asthma research. J Asthma 1988; 25:363–371.
67. Rand CS, Wise RA. Measuring adherence to asthma medication regimens. Am J Respir Crit Care Med 1994; 149:s69–s76.
68. Horn CR. Compliance by asthma patients: how much of a problem? Res Clin Forum 1986; 8:47–53.
69. Rand CS, Wise RA, Nides M, Simmons, MS, Bleecker ER, Kusek TW, Li VC, Tashkin DP. Metered-dose inhaler adherence in a clinical trial. Am Rev Respir Dis 1992; 146:1559–1564.
70. Braunstein GL, Trinquet G, Harper AE, and a compliance working group. Compliance with nedocromil sodium and a nedocromil sodium/salbutamol combination. Eur Respir J 1996; 9:893–898.
71. Weiss KB, Gergen PJ, Hodgson TA. An economic evaluation of asthma in the United States. N Engl J Med 1992; 326:862–866.
72. Smith DH, Malone DC, Lawson KA, Okamoto LJ, Battista C, Saunders WB. A national estimate of the economic costs of asthma. Am J Respir Crit Care Med 1997; 156:787–793.
73. Barnes PJ, Jonsson B, Klim JB. The costs of asthma. Eur Respir J 1996; 9:636–642.
74. Sullivan SD, Weiss KB. Assessing cost-effectiveness in asthma care: building an economic model to study the impact of alternative intervention strategies. Allergy 1993; 48:146–152.
75. Buxton MJ. The economics of asthma—An introduction. Eur Respir Rev 1996; 6: 105–107.
76. Sullivan S, Elixhauser A, Buist AS, Luce BR, Eisenberg J, Weiss KB. National asthma education and prevention program working group report on the cost effectiveness of asthma care. Am J Respir Crit Care Med 1996; 154:s84–s95.
77. Jones PW. Quality of life, health economics and asthma. Eur Respir Rev 1995; 5: 279–283.
78. Rutten-van Mölken MPMH, Custers F, Van Doorslaer EKA, Jansen CCM, Heurman L, Maesen FPV, Smeets JJ, Bommer AM, Raaijmakers JAM. Comparison of performance of four instruments in evaluating the effects of salmeterol on asthma quality of life. Eur Respir J 1995; 8:888–898.
79. Woolcock AJ. Assessment of asthma severity. In: Barnes PJ, Grunstein MM, Leff AR, Woolcock AJ, eds. Asthma. New York: Lippincott-Raven, 1997:1499–1506.
80. Redier H, Daures J-P, Michel C, Proudhon H, Vervloet D, Charpin D, Marsac J, Dusser D, Brambilla C, Wallaert B, Kopferschmitt M-C, Pauli G, Taytard A, Cogis O, Michel F-B, Godard P. Assessment of the severity of asthma by an expert system. Am J Respir Crit Care Med 1995; 151:345–352.

AUTHOR INDEX

Italic numbers give the page on which the complete reference is listed.

A

Aaas P, 93, *111*
Aalbers R, 31, *45*, 65, 66, 67, *79*, 133, *149*, 298, *321*
Aarden LA, 372, *386*
Aarons A, 372, *386*
Aaronson AL, 156, *172*
Aas K, 65, 66, *79*
Abbas AA, 345, 346, *356*
Abbas AK, 348, *358*
Abraham WM, 29, *44*, 61, *76*, 295, *319*, 379, *389*
Abram TS, 289, *312*
Abramovitz M, 288, *311*
Abrams JS, 65, *78*, 352, *359*
Abzug MJ, 167, *179*
Adachi M, 305, *326*
Adam M, 291, *314*
Adamek L, 309, *328*
Adams DH, 372, *386*
Adams G, 369, 373, *384*
Adams GK, 43, *55*, 371, *385*
Adams T, 94, *112*
Adamus WS, 194, *201*
Adcock IM, 8, *21*, 158, *173*, 208, *224*, 373, 375, *387*
Adcock JJ, 219, *234*
Adelman DC, 333, 336, *341*
Adelman Dc, 339, *342*
Adelroth E, 36, *49*, 60, 71, *75*, *82*, 239, *271*
Adelstein AM, 143, *153*
Adkinson NFJ, 289, *313*
Adorini L, 348, *358*
Advenier C, 38, *51*, 120, *146*, 204, 209, 210, 213, 214, 215, 216, 218, 220, *223*, *225*, *227*, *228*, *229*, *230*, *231*, *232*, *234*, *235*, 244, 254, 261, *273*, *277*
Affleck G, 393, *399*
Affrime MB, 195, *202*
Agertoft L, 125, *147*, 161, 163, 164, 169, 171, *176*, *177*, *180*, *181*
Agrawal DK, 184, 186, 187, 188, 189, 191, *196*, *198*, *199*
Aguis RM, 59, *74*
Agusti-Vidal A, 298, *322*
Aharony D, 289, *312*
Ahlstedt S, 57, 65, *73*, 212, *227*, 396, *402*
Ahluwalia A, 217, *232*
Ahmad HR, 33, *46*
Ahmed A, 295, *319*
Ahmed MU, 243, 256, *272*
Ahmed T, 96, 100, *113*, 293, *317*

Ahn HJ, 347, 351, *358*
Ahrens R, 168, *179*
Aikawa T, 91, *109*, 220, *235*
Aikman S, 377, *388*
Aikman SL, 32, *45*, 125, 140, *147*, 266, *283*
Ain-Shoka AA, 94, *112*
Aishita H, 293, *317*
Aizawa H, 37, *50*, 218, *233*
Akimoto K, 211, *226*
Akkerman JW, 187, *198*
Al-Hage M, 186, *197*
Alabaster V, 102, *117*
Alam I, 185, *197*
Alam R, 371, *385*
Albelda SM, 379, *389*
Alber G, 347, *358*
Albert D, 288, *311*
Alessandrini F, 209, *224*
Alexander AG, 67, *80*, 378, *388*
Alexander R, 251, 257, 263, 267, 268, *276*, *283*
Alexander WJ, 126, 129, 135, 137, *148*
Alger LE, 214, 217, *229*, *232*
Ali H, 212, *226*
Ali M, 205, *223*
Aliakbar J, 209, *224*
Alkalay I, 375, *387*
Allal C, 141, *152*
Allegar N, 304, *325*
Allen DB, 164, 167, *178*, *179*
Allen KM, 208, *224*
Allen R, 250, 251, 253, 255, 257, 263, 267, 268, *275*, *276*, *278*
Allen S, 166, *178*
Allen SC, 96, *114*
Alley MR, 35, *48*
Allison A, 134, *150*
Alm P, 207, *223*
Alouan L, 212, *226*
Alouan LA, 367, *383*
Altiere RJ, 70, *82*
Altman LC, 305, *326*
Altose MD, 41, *55*, 394, *400*
Altounyan RE, 301, *323*
Altounyan REC, 292, *316*
Altraja A, 71, *82*
Alvarez R, 243, 256, *272*
Alves AC, 257, *279*
Alving K, 42, *55*, 212, *227*
Ambrosio G, 187, *198*
Amelung PJ, 11, *22*
Amiri P, 332, 333, *341*
Anastassious ED, 158, *174*
Andersen CJ, 217, *232*
Anderson G, 120, 122, 123, *146*, *147*
Anderson GA, 69, 78, *81*
Anderson GP, 378, *388*
Anderson HR, 1, 2, *20*
Anderson N, 254, *277*
Anderson SD, 30, 31, 36, 37, *44*, 125, 140, *147*, 297, 298, *321*, 394, *400*
Anderson W, 141, *152*
Andersson KE, 162, *176*, 302, *324*
Andersson N, 163, 170, *177*
Andersson P, 125, *147*
Ando M, 37, *51*
Ando R, 94, *112*
Ando RE, 38, *51*
Andresen CJ, 259, *280*, 295, *319*
Anguita J, 348, 351, *358*
Angus RM, 194, *201*, 365, *382*
Annunziato F, 65, *78*
Anstren G, 242, *271*, 286, *310*
Anthonisen NR, 394, *400*
Antognetti G, 379, *389*
Antognoni G, 12, *23*
Antoni C, 371, *386*
Antoniadou H, 101, *117*
Anzi K, 306, *327*
Apap CR, 37, *51*, 205, *223*
Appel D, 304, *325*
Appleman MM, 245, *273*
Apter AJ, 393, *399*
Aquilina AT, 100, 101, *116*
Araki S, 37, *51*
Arbesman CE, 156, *172*
Arbetter K, 94, *112*
Arch JR, 367, *384*
Archer RL, 251, *276*
Archibald E, 16, *24*

Arm JP, 291, 292, 294, 297, 298, 299, *314*, *315*, *316*, *317*, *320*, *322*, *323*
Armitage RJ, 345, *357*
Armour CL, 158, 169, *174*, 212, *226*, 367, *383*
Armstrong J, 371, *385*
Arnold C, 291, *315*
Arora Y, 365, *383*
Arrighi JF, 257, *279*
Arshad SH, 13, 18, *23*
Arvidsson P, 142, *152*
Aryana A, 88, 90, 91, *106*, *107*
Asano K, 297, 309, *320*, *328*
Ashe JH, 92, *110*
Ashton MJ, 248, 251, 256, 257, *275*, *276*
Asman B, 286, *309*
Asseman C, 359, *360*
Assoufi B, 57, 64, 67, *72*, *80*, 158, *174*, 346, *357*
Astolfi M, 213, 214, 215, *227*, *229*, *230*
Atkins MB, 289, *312*
Atkinson M, 143, 144, *153*
Atluru D, 289, 291, *313*, *315*
Aubert B, 133, *149*
Auphan N, 158, *173*
Aussel C, 243, 257, *273*
Austen KF, 58, 60, 61, *73*, *75*, 254, *277*, 288, 289, 291, 292, 293, 298, 309, *311*, *312*, *313*, *314*, *315*, *316*, *317*, *322*, *328*
Austin J, 2, *20*
Austrup F, 346, *357*
Autio P, 167, *179*
Avery AJ, 141, *152*
Avital A, 162, *177*
Awni WM, 294, 304, *318*
Ayala LE, 96, 100, *113*
Ayres JG, 395, *401*
Azzawi M, 57, 64, *72*

B

Baboulene L, 375, *387*
Bacci E, 140, *151*
Bach FH, 375, *387*
Bach MK, 293, *317*
Baeuerle PA, 374, *387*
Baggiolini M, 158, *174*, 346, 352, *357*
Baghat MS, 162, *176*
Baglioni C, 158, *173*
Bahna S, 12, *23*
Bahns CC, 288, 291, *311*, *315*
Bai TR, 29, 33, 34, 35, 36, 41, *44*, *46*, *47*, *49*, 208, *224*
Bailey D, 92, *110*
Bailey GS, 61, *75*
Bailey WC, 392, 394, 397, *399*, *400*, *402*
Baillie M, 292, *316*
Baillie MB, 292, *316*
Bakdach H, 209, 210, 215, *225*
Baker A, 90, *107*
Baker AJ, 242, 255, *271*
Baker DG, 87, 92, 94, *106*, *110*, *111*
Baker J, 216, *231*
Bakke O, 158, *174*
Bakker PF, 37, *51*, 215, *230*
Balcarek JM, 246, *274*
Baldasaro M, 291, *314*
Baldasaro MH, 289, *312*
Balder B, 125, 133, *148*
Baldwin AS, 158, *173*
Balfour-Lynn L, 164, *178*
Ball DI, 213, 215, *227*, *230*, 265, 267, *282*
Ball HA, 289, *313*
Ball JG, 365, *382*
Ball M, 143, 144, *153*
Ballard R, 101, *117*
Ballati J, 215, 220, *230*
Ballati L, 219, *234*
Balogh G, 96, *113*
Balow JE, 158, *174*
Baltimore D, 375, *387*
Baluk P, 217, *232*
Banks JB, 186, *197*
Banner KH, 255, *277*
Banner NR, 208, *224*
Bannon MJ, 203, *223*
Baran D, 162, *177*
Baraniuk J, 89, 90, *107*
Baraniuk JN, 38, *51*, 89, 90, 91, 92, *107*, 203, 204, 205, *223*, 393, *399*

Barbaro JF, 183, *196*
Barbee R, 11, *22*
Barbee RA, 329, *340*
Barber R, 141, *152*
Barbera JA, 191, 192, 193, *200*
Barberis-Maino L, 346, *357*
Barchasz E, 210, *225*
Barkans J, 57, 62, 67, *73*, *80*, 238, *270*, 346, *357*
Barker J, 297, *320*
Barlow RB, 86, *105*
Barnabe R, 307, *327*
Barnacle H, 169, *180*
Barnard J, 92, *110*
Barneon G, 57, 65, *73*, 396, *402*
Barnes CG, 268, *283*
Barnes KC, 348, *358*
Barnes N, 137, *151*
Barnes NC, 67, *80*, 192, 194, *201*, 286, 288, 292, 294, 295, 301, 305, 307, *309*, *312*, *316*, *318*, *323*, *324*, *326*, 378, *388*
Barnes P, 5, *21*, 90, 91, 92, 101, 102, *107*, *108*, *110*, *117*
Barnes PJ, 8, *21*, 27, 28, 29, 32, 35, 36, 37, 38, 40, 42, *44*, *45*, *48*, *50*, *51*, *53*, *55*, 58, 60, 70, *73*, *75*, *81*, 88, 89, 90, 91, 92, 94, 96, 97, *106*, *107*, *109*, *110*, *111*, *113*, *114*, 125, 131, 133, 137, 140, 141, 142, *147*, *149*, *151*, *152*, 158, 159, 160, *173*, *174*, *175*, 189, 190, 191, 192, 193, 194, 195, *199*, *200*, *201*, *202*, 203, 204, 205, 208, 210, 211, 214, 215, 216, 217, 220, *223*, *224*, *225*, *226*, *229*, *230*, *231*, *232*, *235*, 240, 241, 242, 243, 256, 257, 269, *271*, *272*, *279*, *280*, 288, 294, 295, *312*, *317*, *318*, 361, 362, 364, 365, 366, 367, 368, 369, 370, 372, 373, 374, 375, 376, 377, 378, 381, *381*, *382*, *383*, *384*, *385*, *386*, *387*, *388*, *389*, 393, 396, 398, *400*, *402*, *403*
Barnes VF, 210, *225*
Barnette MS, 250, 251, 253, 257, 265, 269, *276*, *279*, *282*
Baroody F, 105, *118*
Barr M, 2, *20*
Barrett JA, 243, 256, *272*
Barron R, 104, *117*
Barrows E, 393, *399*
Barthlow H, 90, *107*
Barthlow HG, 215, *230*
Basbaum CB, 87, 88, 89, 90, 92, *106*, *110*
Baskerville J, 162, 167, *176*, *179*
Baskerville JC, 166, 167, *178*
Bassett D, 94, *112*
Bast A, 93, *111*
Bastacky J, 35, *48*
Basterna J, 207, *223*
Bateman-Fite R, 251, 263, 268, *276*, *281*
Bates DJ, 333, *341*
Bates JHT, 32, *46*
Bates PJ, 15, *24*
Battista C, 398, *403*
Battisutta D, 9, *22*
Battram CH, 253, 260, 261, 263, 269, *276*
Batty D, 248, *275*
Batty EP, 137, 138, *151*
Bauer H, 264, *282*
Bauer PH, 254, *277*
Baumgarten CR, 208, *224*
Baumgarten HG, 264, *282*
Baumgarth N, 345, *356*
Baumgarttener C, 92, *110*
Baveystock CM, 397, *402*
Bazan F, 347, 351, *358*
Beach JR, 141, *152*
Beam WR, 158, *174*
Beasely R, 70, *82*, 142, 144, *152*
Beasley CR, 133, *149*
Beasley CRW, 35, 38, *48*, 58, 59, *73*, 239, *271*, 391, *399*
Beasley R, 59, 60, 67, 68, 69, 70, *74*, *75*, *80*, *81*, 135, 143, 144, *150*, *153*, *154*
Beaty TH, 348, 349, *358*
Beaucher W, 304, *325*
Beavo JA, 245, 246, 257, *273*, *274*, *279*
Becher G, 297, *321*
Beck E, 297, *321*
Beck GJ, 71, *83*
Beck JM, 217, *232*

Beck KC, 92, *110*
Beckendorf SK, 246, *274*
Becker AB, 141, *152*
Becker EL, 217, *231*
Becklake M, 394, *400*
Beg AA, 375, *387*
Behr N, 125, 133, *147*
Behrens BL, 259, *280*
Behtal R, 71, *83*
Beier N, 246, *274*
Bekele Z, 2, *20*
Bel EH, 30, 31, 33, 36, 37, 39, 40, 41, 42, *44*, *45*, *46*, *48*, *51*, *53*, *54*, *55*, 59, 66, *74*, 140, 141, *151*, 211, *226*, 295, 300, *318*, *323*, 394, *400*
Belanger M, 36, 42, *48*, 71, *83*
Beld AJ, 89, 91, 92, *107*, *108*, *110*
Beler D, 309, *328*
Beleta I, 258, *280*
Beleta J, 250, *275*
Bell GS, 299, *323*
Bell RL, 288, 295, *311*, *319*
Bellamy JF, 215, *230*
Bellia V, 43, *55*, 297, *320*
Bellini A, 8, *22*
Bellofiore S, 35, *47*
Belmonte K, 99, *115*
Belmonte KE, 94, *111*
Belvisi M, 102, *117*
Belvisi MG, 203, 204, 220, *223*, *235*, 362, 365, 366, 367, *381*, *383*, *384*
Ben-Jebria A, 210, *225*
Ben-Neriah J, 375, *387*
Bengtsson T, 256, *278*
Bennett CD, 288, *310*
Bennett J, 129, 131, 135, *149*
Bennett JA, 137, *150*
Bennett WA, 67, *80*
Bensch K, 89, *107*
Bentley A, 158, *174*, 345, 346, *356*
Bentley AM, 31, 38, *45*, *52*, 57, 62, 64, 67, *73*, *77*, *80*, 238, *270*, 395, 396, *401*
Benveniste J, 183, 185, *196*, *197*
Berdel D, 125, *147*
Berends C, 256, 257, *279*
Beresford IJM, 213, 215, *227*, *230*
Berga P, 250, *275*
Bergendal A, 120, 136, *146*
Bergren DR, 189, *199*
Bernareggi M, 220, *235*
Berne RM, 249, *275*
Berner P, 264, *282*
Berney C, 94, *112*
Bernotas RC, 369, 373, *384*
Bernstein A, 96, 104, *114*
Bernstein L, 333, 336, *341*
Bernstein PR, 289, *312*
Berrie CP, 86, *105*
Bertin L, 133, *149*
Berto JM, 36, *49*
Bertoerlli G, 169, *180*
Bertoncin P, 71, *83*
Bertorelli G, 36, 42, *49*, *55*
Bertrand C, 37, *51*, 65, *78*, 91, 92, *108*, 214, 215, 216, 217, *229*, *230*, *231*, *232*, 332, *340*, 378, *388*
Besson G, 214, *229*
Bettinger CM, 134, *150*
Beusenberg FD, 242, 255, *271*
Bews J, 332, *340*
Bewtra A, 305, *326*
Bewtra AK, 188, 189, 191, 195, *199*, *202*
Beyth S, 375, *387*
Bhagat R, 140, 141, *151*
Bhattarcharya S, 10, *22*
Biagi S, 58, 59, 60, 61, 64, 66, *73*
Biagiotti R, 65, *78*
Bianco S, 307, *327*, 377, *388*
Bichon D, 213, *227*
Bidani A, 242, *272*
Bidault J, 183, *196*
Bienenstock J, 212, *227*
Biffi M, 346, *357*
Bigby TD, 289, 308, *313*, *328*
Biggers MS, 265, 269, *282*
Biggs DF, 92, 93, *110*
Bijl H, 268, *283*, 371, *386*
Bild G, 288, *311*
Billah MM, 195, *202*, 371, 372, 374, *385*, *386*

Bingham CO, 291, *315*
Binks S, 242, *271*, 286, *310*
Binks SM, 302, *324*
Biochot E, 218, *233*
Birch S, 293, *317*
Birchmeier C, 246, *274*
Birdsall NJM, 86, *105*
Bisgaard H, 292, *316*
Bitar DM, 353, *360*
Bito H, 187, *198*
Bittinger F, 88, *106*
Biyah K, 216, *231*
Bjorck T, 210, *225*, 296, 301, *319*, *320*, *323*
Bjorksten B, 343, *355*
Bjorregaard-Anderson H, 162, *177*
Bkaer JE, 69, *81*
Blaber LC, 93, *111*
Black C, 296, *320*
Black DM, 166, *178*
Black J, 43, *56*
Black JL, 212, *226*, 367, *383*
Black PN, 296, *320*
Blackwell TR, 291, *315*
Blake DR, 268, *283*
Blake SM, 259, 261, 263, 267, 269, *280*
Blanchard DK, 257, *279*
Blanchard JC, 213, *227*
Blank ML, 183, *196*
Blanksteijn M, 89, 92, *107*, *110*
Blaser K, 38, *52*
Blazer K, 61, *76*
Blease K, 251, 257, 263, 267, *276*
Bleecker E, 301, *323*
Bleecker ER, 4, 6, 11, *21*, *22*, 42, *55*, 67, *79*, 298, *322*
Bleeker E, 101, *117*
Bleeker ER, 94, *112*
Bloemen PG, 256, *278*
Blogg T, 32, *46*
Blomjous FJ, 256, *278*
Blomqvist H, 301, 303, *323*, *325*
Bloom BR, 65, *78*
Bloom JW, 91, 92, *108*, *110*
Bloom SR, 210, *225*
Bloom TJ, 245, 257, *274*, *279*
Bloxham D, 251, 257, 263, 267, *276*
Bluestone JA, 63, *76*, 350, 351, 353, *359*
Blum AM, 209, *224*
Blumenthal M, 9, *22*
Blundell G, 162, *177*
Bochenek G, 378, *388*
Bochner B, 339, *342*
Bochner BS, 95, *113*
Bochnowicz S, 258, 261, 263, 269, *280*
Bodman S, 304, *325*
Bodner C, 15, *24*
Boeije LC, 372, *386*
Boezen HM, 395, *401*
Bogaard JM, 36, 37, *49*, *50*
Bogaards JM, 395, *401*
Boguniewicz M, 372, *386*
Boichot E, 38, *51*, 204, 213, 216, 218, *223*, *231*, *232*, *234*
Boie Y, 291, *314*
Bolado J, 158, *173*
Bolger G, 247, *275*
Bolin DR, 364, *382*
Bolivin JF, 167, *179*
Bolla M, 290, *314*
Bolliger CT, 125, 140, *147*
Bolser DC, 220, *235*
Bommer AM, 125, *147*, 398, *403*
Bonanno A, 297, *320*
Bond MW, 63, *77*
Bondy GP, 208, *224*
Bone MF, 194, *201*
Bonnet PA, 368, *384*
Bons J, 133, *149*
Bonsignore G, 297, 306, *320*, *327*
Bonsignore GB, 69, *81*
Bonstein HS, 156, *172*
Bonta IL, 242, 255, *271*
Bonuccelli CM, 306, *327*
Booms P, 39, 40, *53*, *54*
Boonsawat W, 35, 36, *47*, *49*
Boonstra A, 353, *360*
Boorsma M, 163, 170, *177*
Boorsma MM, 160, *175*
Booth H, 134, 141, *150*, *152*, 169, *180*
Boothman-Burrell D, 142, *152*
Bootsma GP, 171, *180*, 304, 308, *325*
Borgeat P, 291, *314*, *315*
Borges E, 346, *357*

Borish L, 27, 35, 38, *44*, 158, *174*, 349, *359*, 372, *386*
Borrello G, 135, *150*
Borson DB, 37, *50*, 89, 94, *107*, *112*
Bos JD, 351, *359*
Bosken C, 35, *48*
Bosserman MK, 365, *382*
Botta L, 333, *341*
Bottomly K, 343, 344, 351, *355*, *356*, *359*, 371, *385*
Bou J, 250, 258, *275*, *280*
Boucard M, 368, *384*
Bouchard TJ, 9, *22*
Boucher RC, 89, *106*
Boulet L, 97, *114*
Boulet L-Ph, 36, 37, 42, *48*, *49*, *50*
Boulet LP, 71, *83*, 134, *150*, 306, *327*, 333, 336, 338, *341*, 393, *399*
Boulet M, 134, *150*
Boullet C, 183, *196*
Boumpas DT, 158, *174*
Bourdon A, 205, 212, 213, 214, *223*
Boushey H, 58, *73*, 97, *114*
Boushey HA, 99, *115*, 221, *235*, 302, *324*, 333, 336, 337, *341*, 364, 379, *381*, *389*
Bouska J, 295, *319*
Bousquet J, 43, *55*, *56*, 57, 60, 64, 65, 66, 69, 71, *73*, *75*, *77*, *79*, *81*, *82*, *83*, 133, *149*, 217, 218, *231*, *233*, 266, *283*, 297, *321*, 380, *389*, 396, 397, *402*
Bousquet P, 330, *340*
Boutet M, 36, 37, 42, *49*, *50*
Bovers J, 193, *201*
Bowen-Page DF, 70, *82*
Bowring NE, 367, *384*
Boyce J, 291, *314*
Boyce JA, 291, *315*
Boyd E, 251, 257, 263, 267, *276*
Boyer V, 218, *233*
Bozelka BE, 339, *342*
Brach MA, 291, *315*
Brackeen MF, 251, 263, 268, *276*, *281*
Brackel HJL, 395, *401*
Bradding P, 60, 62, 63, 69, *75*, *76*, *77*, *81*, 134, *150*, 285, 286, 299, 300, 301, 302, 307, *309*, *310*
Bradley B, 57, 64, *72*, 395, 396, *401*
Bradley BL, 57, *72*, *73*
Bradley KL, 14, *24*
Brambilla C, 398, *403*
Bramley AM, 35, *47*, *48*
Brand PLP, 29, 42, *44*, *55*, 67, *79*, 165, *178*, 395, *401*
Brandon M, 305, *326*
Brann EG, 252, *276*
Brannan MD, 195, *202*
Braquet P, 217, *231*, 291, *315*
Braquet PG, 186, *198*
Brattsand R, 162, *176*
Brauer R, 346, *357*
Braun P, 38, *52*
Braunstein GL, 397, *403*
Braunstein J, 61, *76*
Brawley ES, 251, *276*
Bray MA, 295, *319*
Breazeale DR, 11, *22*, 348, 349, *358*
Brebner H, 156, *172*
Breedveld FC, 371, *386*
Breliere JC, 210, 213, 214, 215, *225*, *227*, *228*, *229*
Breliere JCG, 213, *227*
Bremm KD, 289, *312*
Bremner P, 135, *150*
Breton J, 263, *281*
Breukink H, 91, *109*
Brewster CE, 70, *82*
Brichant JF, 91, 93, *109*
Brick JJ, 134, *150*
Brideau C, 216, *231*
Briggs DB, 265, *282*
Brink C, 289, *312*, *313*
Brion JD, 220, *235*
Brisman J, 393, *399*
Bristol JA, 245, *273*
Brittain R, 122, *147*
Britten K, 38, *52*
Britten KM, 57, 59, 60, 62, 67, *72*, *76*, *80*, 160, *176*, 189, *199*, 295, *318*, 395, 396, *401*
Britton J, 2, 19, *20*, *26*
Britton JR, 141, *152*, 393, *399*
Britton MG, 127, *148*
Brobholz J, 309, *328*

Brock TG, 292, *316*
Brockbank W, 156, *172*
Brocklehurst WE, 289, 296, *312*, *319*
Brodde OE, 257, *279*
Broder I, 126, 129, 135, 137, *148*
Broide DH, 60, *75*, 378, *388*
Brokhoff CM, 126, 129, *148*
Brom J, 289, *312*
Bromberg PA, 89, *106*
Bromberger-Barnea B, 99, *115*
Bron A, 65, 66, 67, *79*
Bronsky E, 305, *326*
Bronsky EA, 105, *118*, 303, *324*
Bronsky F, 304, *325*
Bronson RT, 375, *387*
Brookman R, 89, *106*
Brooks B, 183, *196*
Brooks DW, 288, *311*
Brooks J, 104, *117*
Brostoff J, 59, 61, *74*
Brouard R, 221, *235*
Brouwer F, 91, *109*
Brouwers JW, 242, 255, *271*
Browman GW, 143, *153*
Brown CR, 158, *173*, 208, *224*
Brown HM, 157, *172*
Brown JA, 351, *359*
Brown JK, 90, 91, 94, *108*, *109*, *111*
Brown K, 2, 19, *21*, *26*
Brown KA, 32, *46*
Brown KE, 66, *79*
Brown PH, 66, 67, *79*, *80*, 162, *177*
Brown RH, 35, 39, *48*
Browner W, 166, *178*
Bruce MC, 35, *47*
Bruderman I, 96, *114*
Bruel JM, 43, *56*, 71, *83*
Brugess C, 143, *153*
Bruijnzeel P, 61, *76*
Bruijnzeel PLB, 352, *359*
Brunekreef B, 15, *24*
Brunelleschi S, 218, *233*
Brunelli G, 218, *233*
Bruning G, 264, *282*
Brunnee T, 212, *227*, 266, *283*
Brusasco V, 39, *53*, 285, *309*, 395, *401*
Bruynzeel I, 257, *279*
Bruynzeel PL, 187, 191, *198*, *200*, 289, *313*
Bryant T, 12, *23*
Bryce DK, 213, *227*
Brynes C, 5, *21*
Buckle DR, 367, *383*, *384*
Buckley SK, 264, *282*
Buckley TL, 218, *233*, *234*
Buckner CK, 94, 100, *112*, 214, 215, *229*, *230*, 289, *312*
Buettner P, 18, *25*
Builder S, 333, *341*
Buist AS, 143, 144, *153*, 394, 398, *400*, *403*
Bullock GR, 209, 212, *224*, *226*
Bunting S, 290, *314*
Buntinx A, 300, 301, *323*, *324*
Burcher E, 213, 214, *228*
Burgen ASV, 86, *105*
Burgers JA, 187, *198*
Burgess C, 135, 143, 144, *150*, *153*, *154*
Burgess CD, 135, *150*
Burke C, 160, *175*
Burke CM, 36, *49*, 65, *78*
Burke W, 194, *201*
Burkly LC, 379, *389*
Burman M, 247, 248, 250, 251, 253, 257, 265, *275*, *276*, *279*
Burney P, 1, 2, 4, *20*
Burney PGJ, 393, *399*
Burns FM, 255, *277*
Burns TL, 268, *283*
Burnstock G, 92, *110*
Burr M, 2, *20*
Burrows B, 5, 11, *21*, *22*, 329, *340*
Burrows SD, 245, *273*
Burton P, 395, *401*
Bury T, 188, 189, *199*, 266, *283*
Bush A, 5, *21*
Bush RK, 301, *324*
Busse W, 299, 303, 304, 309, *322*, *325*, *328*
Busse WW, 60, *75*, 94, 100, *112*, *116*, 169, *180*, 297, 298, 301, 303, 308, *321*, *324*, *328*, 333, 336, *341*, 397, *402*

Bustafsson P, 169, *180*
Butcher RW, 237, 238, 245, 269, *270*
Butland B, 2, 13, *20*, *23*
Butler JP, 34, 35, 39, *47*, *48*
Butterfield JH, 61, *76*, 291, *315*
Buxton MJ, 398, *403*
Buyatt G, 297, *321*
Byers D, 246, *274*
Byers LW, 183, *196*
Byorth PJ, 189, *199*
Byrd PK, 217, *232*
Byron KA, 158, *174*

C

Cahill P, 395, *401*
Cain MH, 245, *273*
Cairns J, 61, *76*
Caldenhoven E, 371, *385*
Calderon MA, 67, *80*, 159, 170, *174*
Calhoun WJ, 60, *75*, 134, *150*, 296, 297, 298, 306, *319*, *321*
Callahan S, 104, *117*
Callenbach PM, 296, 305, *319*
Callery JC, 192, *201*, 299, *322*
Calverley PM, 194, *201*
Calvo CF, 217, *232*
Calzetti F, 217, *232*
Calzoni P, 71, *83*
Cameron IR, 101, *117*
Cameron L, 43, *56*, 66, 71, *79*
Cammisuli S, 375, *387*
Campbell AM, 69, *81*, 330, *340*
Campbell EJ, 71, *83*
Campbell HD, 345, 352, *356*
Campbell HR, 295, *318*
Campbell J, 214, *229*
Campbell MJ, 41, *54*
Canal I, 266, *283*
Canet E, 220, *235*
Cannon PJ, 290, *314*
Canny G, 104, *117*
Capewell S, 167, *179*
Capron A, 332, *341*
Capron M, 332, *341*
Cardell LO, 208, *224*
Cardelus I, 250, *275*
Cardelus J, 258, *280*
Carey F, 299, *322*
Carey OJ, 19, *26*
Cargill RJ, 163, *177*
Carins J, 61, *76*
Carlberg C, 257, *279*
Carletti A, 140, *151*
Carlos TM, 352, *359*
Carlstedt-Duke J, 158, *173*
Caroll MP, 352, *359*
Carpenter DO, 265, *282*
Carpenter JR, 36, *50*, 266, *283*
Carpentier PJ, 299, 300, *323*
Carr AA, 369, 373, *384*
Carratu L, 187, *198*
Carrel AL, 167, *179*
Carrier G, 36, 42, *48*, 71, *83*
Carroll KN, 37, *50*
Carroll MP, 57, 61, 64, *74*, *77*
Carroll NG, 36, *49*
Carruette A, 213, *227*
Carry M, 299, *322*
Carryer HM, 155, *172*
Carson DA, 217, *232*
Carson SS, 217, *232*
Carstairs JR, 364, *382*
Carter CM, 243, 254, 256, *272*
Carter GW, 288, *311*
Carter L, 65, *78*
Cartier A, 36, 42, *49*, 125, 126, 129, 135, 137, 140, *147*, *148*
Carty TJ, 191, *200*
Carvajal DM, 346, *357*
Casale TB, 60, 61, *75*, 92, *110*, 333, 336, *341*
Casalini A, 42, *55*, 169, *180*
Cass D, 70, *81*
Cass GR, 16, 17, *25*
Cassatella MA, 217, *232*
Castillo JA, 298, *322*
Castle W, 127, 142, 143, *148*
Castleman W, 94, 99, *112*
Castleman WL, 38, *51*
Castling DP, 296, *320*
Catalioto RM, 213, *228*

Cato ACB, 374, *387*
Catterall C, 248, 251, 257, 263, 267, *275*, *276*
Catterall J, 101, *116*
Caughey GH, 60, 70, *75*, *82*
Cauley J, 166, *178*
Cavanaugh M, 104, *117*
Cavanaugh MJ, 99, 101, *115*
Cayton RM, 162, *176*, 395, *401*
Celniker A, 372, *386*
Center DM, 64, *78*, 352, 353, *359*, *360*
Cervantes C, 166, *178*
Ceska M, 217, *232*
Chakrin L, 90, *107*
Challis RAJ, 247, 252, *274*
Chalmers GW, 365, 369, *382*, *385*
Chambard JC, 158, *173*
Chambers DK, 96, 104, *114*
Chambers RJ, 265, 269, *282*
Champion E, 214, *229*, 301, *323*
Chan B, 219, *234*
Chan H, 60, *75*, 185, *196*, 297, *321*
Chan SC, 216, *231*, 268, *283*, 295, *319*, 351, *359*
Chan-Yeung M, 60, *75*, 297, *321*
Chandra RK, 13, *23*
Chanez P, 43, *55*, *56*, 57, 60, 64, 65, 66, 69, 71, *73*, *75*, *77*, *79*, *81*, *82*, *83*, 217, 218, *231*, *233*, 297, *321*, 330, *340*, 396, *402*
Chang DJ, 290, *314*
Chang K, 288, *312*
Chang TW, 43, *55*, 333, *341*
Chang-Yeung M, 185, *196*
Chap H, 186, *197*
Chapat JP, 368, *384*
Chapin DS, 251, *276*
Chapman K, 129, 131, 135, *149*
Chapman KR, 126, 129, 135, 137, *148*, 166, *178*, 307, *327*, 333, 336, 338, *341*
Chapman MD, 18, *26*, 344, 348, *356*
Chapman RW, 43, *55*, 370, 371, *385*
Charbonneau H, 246, *274*
Charette L, 301, *323*, 362, 367, *381*, *384*
Charitinov SA, 266, *283*
Charles P, 268, *283*
Charleson P, 288, *311*
Charleson S, 288, 292, 297, 299, *311*, *320*, *322*
Charpin D, 398, *403*
Charpin J, 99, 100, *115*, *116*
Chasson B, 221, *235*
Chatila TA, 350, *359*
Chattopadhyay U, 65, *78*
Chauhan AJ, 61, *76*
Chauret N, 268, *283*
Chavaillaz PA, 291, *315*
Chavanel G, 217, *232*
Chavis C, 289, *313*
Cheang M, 167, *179*
Chee P, 295, 297, *319*, *320*
Chen CN, 246, *274*
Chen J, 261, *281*
Chen X, 345, 346, *357*
Chen XR, 218, *233*
Chen Y, 353, *360*
Chen-Worsdell M, 377, *388*
Cheng JB, 88, *106*, 251, 255, 265, 268, 269, *276*, *278*, *282*, *283*
Chensue SW, 352, *359*
Chervinsky P, 126, 129, 135, 137, *148*, 169, *180*, 304, *325*
Cherwinski H, 63, *77*
Chestnut L, 17, *25*
Chetta A, 36, 42, *49*, *55*, 169, *180*
Cheung D, 35, 36, 37, 39, 40, *47*, *48*, *49*, *51*, *54*, 140, 141, *151*, 211, *226*
Chevinsky P, 305, *326*
Chi EY, 288, *312*
Chiappara G, 43, *55*
Chiba R, 35, *47*
Chiba T, 35, *47*, 286, 294, *309*
Chick T, 104, *117*
Chicoye A, 397, *402*
Chiew F, 367, *383*
Chignard M, 255, 268, *278*
Chikanza JC, 268, *283*
Child S, 43, *56*
Childers CC, 365, *382*
Chilton FH, 185, *197*, 242, 256, *271*, *272*, *278*, 290, *314*
Chilton JE, 137, *150*

Chilvers ER, 368, *384*
Chin TW, 167, *179*
Chinchilli VM, 364, *381*
Chinn CL, 2, 4, *20*
Chinn RA, 89, *107*
Chinn S, 2, 4, *20*, 393, *399*
Chiyotani A, 90, 104, *107*
Choquart A, 374, *387*
Chou SP, 91, *109*
Choudhury I, 265, *282*
Christensen SB, 250, 251, 253, 257, 265, *276*, *279*
Christian RM, 100, *116*
Christie G, 11, *22*
Christie PE, 5, *21*, 288, 294, 296, 297, 303, *312*, *317*, *320*, *325*
Christiensen SB, 265, 269, *282*
Christman JW, 291, *315*
Christopher JD, 195, *202*
Chu SS, 252, *276*
Chung FZ, 213, *227*, *228*
Chung KF, 36, 37, *48*, *50*, 140, 141, *151*, 160, *175*, 189, 190, 191, 192, 193, 194, *199*, *200*, *201*, 214, 216, 217, 220, *229*, *231*, *232*, *235*, 294, *317*, 364, 367, 372, 374, 377, *381*, *383*, *386*, *388*
Church MK, 61, 63, 66, *76*, *77*, *79*, 243, 257, *273*, 285, *309*, 329, *340*
Church S, 367, *383*
Cibella F, 297, 306, *320*, *327*
Cibulsky SM, 70, *82*
Cicutto L, 101, *117*
Ciechanover A, 375, *387*
Ciesla W, 92, *109*
Cieslinski LB, 246, 247, 250, 251, 253, 257, 265, *274*, *275*, *276*, *279*
Cink TM, 71, *83*
Claesson HE, 289, 290, 294, *313*, *314*, *318*
Clark ARF, 259, *280*
Clark DA, 292, *316*
Clark DJ, 163, 169, 170, *177*, *180*
Clark J, 61, *76*
Clark M, 129, 131, 135, *149*
Clark PO, 185, *197*
Clark RB, 141, *152*
Clark RL, 263, 268, *281*
Clark S, 347, *358*
Clark TJH, 157, *172*, 298, *322*
Clarke B, 210, *225*
Clausen JL, 394, *400*
Clayberger C, 65, *78*
Clayton DE, 94, *112*
Cleland LD, 333, 336, 338, *341*
Clifford KN, 345, *357*
Cline M, 11, *22*
Cline MG, 11, *22*, 329, *340*
Clough J, 94, 99, *112*
Clough JJ, 38, *51*
Cluzel M, 185, 195, *197*, *202*
Clyde WA, 100, *116*
Co E, 38, *52*
Cobos A, 192, 193, *200*
Coburn DA, 60, *75*
Cocchetto DM, 126, 129, 135, 137, *148*
Cochrane CG, 183, 187, *196*, *198*
Cochrane GM, 167, *179*, 367, *383*
Cockcroft D, 97, 100, *114*, *116*, 143, 144, *153*
Cockcroft DW, 30, 31, 36, 37, *44*, 97, *114*, 140, 141, *151*, 297, 298, *321*, 333, 336, 338, *341*, 393, 394, *400*
Codd SL, 35, *48*
Coffer P, 371, *385*
Coffman RL, 63, *77*, 238, *270*, 344, 347, *356*, *358*
Cogis O, 398, *403*
Cognon C, 213, *228*
Cogswell JJ, 343, *355*
Cogswell PC, 158, *173*
Cohan VL, 255, 268, *278*
Cohen-Aronovski R, 96, *114*
Cohn J, 192, *201*, 294, 296, 299, 304, 306, 307, 308, *318*, *319*, *322*, *325*, *326*, *327*
Cohn L, 371, *385*
Colby TV, 66, *79*
Cole M, 292, 301, *316*, *323*
Colella DF, 252, *276*
Coleman R, 122, *147*
Coleman RA, 213, 215, *227*, *230*, 265, *282*, 287, *310*, 364, *382*

Coles M, 292, *316*
Coles N, 292, *316*
Coles SJ, 293, *317*
Colicelli J, 246, *274*
Collier AM, 100, *116*
Collier C, 16, *24*
Collins JC, 69, *81*
Collins JV, 37, *50*, 57, 58, 59, 61, 64, 69, 70, *72*, *73*, 297, *321*, 396, *401*
Collins PD, 239, *271*
Collins T, 309, *328*
Colwell B, 12, *23*
Colwell BM, 12, *23*
Conley WG, 100, *116*
Conlon K, 65, *78*
Connaughton SE, 346, *357*
Connell MJ, 247, 252, 253, 258, 269, *274*
Connett JE, 41, *55*, 394, *400*
Connolly KM, 251, 263, 268, *276*, *281*
Connolly NL, 71, *83*
Conrad DJ, 60, *75*
Conradson RB, 210, *225*
Conroy DM, 289, *312*
Constant S, 351, *359*
Constantine JQ, 213, *227*
Conti M, 246, 247, *274*, *275*
Convit J, 65, *78*
Conway WA, 394, *400*
Cook DC, 251, *276*
Cook DG, 12, *23*
Cook RM, 266, *283*
Cooke C, 36, *49*
Cooke JP, 43, *56*
Cookson JB, 19, *26*
Cookson WO, 11, *22*, *23*
Cookson WOCM, 348, *358*
Coon JT, 129, 131, 135, *149*
Cooper D, 104, *117*
Cooper DM, 99, 101, *115*
Cooper K, 265, 269, *282*
Cooper S, 129, 131, 135, *149*
Coppolino MG, 288, *311*
Corderio RS, 257, *279*
Corey EJ, 60, *75*, 289, 292, 293, 298, *313*, *316*, *317*, *322*
Corhay JL, 188, 189, *199*, 266, *283*
Corne J, 43, *55*, 307, *327*, 333, *341*
Corne JM, 31, 36, *45*
Cornelissen JPG, 366, *383*
Cornelissen P, 104, *118*
Cornthwaite D, 18, *26*
Coronas A, 298, *322*
Corrigan C, 57, 62, *73*, 346, *357*
Corrigan CJ, 67, *80*, 238, 257, 269, *270*, *280*, 285, 295, *309*, *318*, 344, 345, 346, 352, *356*, *357*, 378, *388*
Corris P, 96, *113*
Corry D, 70, *81*
Cortes A, 295, *319*
Cortijo J, 258, *280*
Costello J, 265, 266, 267, *282*, 301, *323*
Costello JF, 192, *200*, *201*, 288, 292, 294, 297, *312*, *316*, *317*, *321*
Costello PS, 254, *277*
Costello R, 94, 95, 96, 99, *112*, *113*, *115*
Costello RW, 95, *113*
Costongs R, 127, *148*
Cotes JE, 30, *44*
Cotge J, 333, 336, 338, *341*
Cotton E, 104, *117*
Cotton MF, 167, *179*
Cottrez F, 347, *358*
Counihan H, 70, *82*
Coursin DB, 289, *312*
Court EN, 185, *196*, 298, *322*
Cousin JM, 378, *388*
Couture R, 203, *223*
Covin R, 292, *316*
Cowan DJ, 251, *276*
Coward GA, 141, *152*
Cowburn A, 309, *328*
Cowburn AS, 291, *315*
Cox G, 66, *79*
Cox ME, 288, *311*
Coyle AJ, 65, *78*, 332, *340*, 378, *388*
Cozzi Ph, 37, *50*
Crane J, 135, 142, 143, 144, *150*, *152*, *153*, *154*
Crapo RO, 394, *400*
Crastes-de-Paulet A, 218, *233*, 289, *313*
Crea AE, 185, *196*, 292, 294, *316*
Crea AEG, 238, *270*
Cree A, 140, *151*
Crepea SB, 156, *172*

Crimi E, 39, *53*, 285, *309*, 395, *401*
Crimi N, 210, 211, 212, *225*, *226*, *227*
Criscuoli M, 213, *228*
Croci T, 213, *228*
Croft M, 65, *78*
Crompton CK, 162, *177*
Crompton G, 104, *117*
Crompton GK, 158, *173*
Cromwell O, 295, 297, *319*, *321*
Croner S, 343, *355*
Cropp G, 104, *117*
Cross LJM, 212, *226*
Crossland L, 142, 144, *152*
Crotty TB, 66, *79*
Cruikshank WW, 64, *77*, *78*, 352, 353, *359*, *360*
Cruz A, 105, *118*
Cruz HN, 257, *279*
Cucchi P, 213, *228*
Cuello C, 205, *223*
Cullen K, 71, *83*
Culling C, 143, 144, *153*
Culp D, 89, *107*
Culpepper JA, 158, *174*
Cumming RG, 167, *179*
Cummings SR, 166, *178*
Cunningham CN, 254, *277*
Cuomo AJ, 60, *75*
Curiel DT, 380, *389*
Curtis JR, 396, 397, *402*
Cury JD, 71, *83*
Curzen N, 286, 294, *309*
Cuss FM, 91, *109*, 189, 193, *199*, 370, *385*
Cuss FMC, 364, *382*
Custers F, 398, *403*
Custovic A, 18, *26*
Cuthbert NJ, 289, 292, *312*, *316*
Cutitta G, 297, *320*
Cvietusa P, 372, *386*
Czernilofsky AP, 374, *387*

D

D'Agostino G, 93, *111*
D'Alonzo GE, 126, 129, 135, 137, *148*
D'Ortho MP, 218, *233*
D'Yachkova Y, 33, *46*
Da Ros B, 255, *277*
Daffonchio L, 218, *233*
Dahinden CA, 290, *314*, 346, 352, *357*
Dahl R, 137, *150*, 169, *180*
Dahl SG, 254, *277*
Dahlen B, 242, *271*, 286, 296, 297, 301, 303, *310*, *320*, *321*, *323*, *325*
Dahlen SE, 210, *225*, 242, *271*, 286, 287, 296, 301, 303, *310*, *319*, *320*, *323*, *325*
Dahlman K, 158, *173*
Dal Negro R, 305, *326*
Dale HH, 86, *105*, 286, *310*
Dale MM, 238, 240, 242, *270*
Dale TJ, 265, 267, *282*
Dales R, 104, *118*
Dallegri F, 243, *272*
Dalsgaard CJ, 217, *232*
Daly JW, 245, 248, 250, 264, *273*
Damon DB, 265, 269, *282*
Damon M, 217, *231*, 289, *313*
Dandurand RJ, 39, *53*
Daniel E, 97, *114*
Daniel EE, 31, 37, *45*, 91, *109*, 394, *400*
Daniels RH, 290, *314*
Daniels S, 10, *22*
Daniels SE, 11, *23*
Dannaeus A, 13, *23*
Dannenberg TB, 155, *172*
Daoui S, 213, *228*
Dapino P, 243, *272*
Dardenne AJ, 70, *81*
Dark J, 96, *113*
Das MP, 351, *359*
Daures JP, 43, *56*, 71, *83*, 398, *403*
Davidson AB, 292, *316*
Davidson R, 238, *270*
Davies AO, 137, *151*
Davies BH, 364, *382*
Davies R, 205, *223*
Davies RJ, 15, 17, *24*, *25*, 67, 70, *80*, *81*, 159, 170, *174*
Davis B, 61, *76*, 89, *106*, *107*
Davis EE, 333, *341*
Davis F, 43, *55*, 333, *341*
Davis JD, 89, *106*

Davis RL, 246, 263, 265, *274*, *281*
Dawes KF, 217, *232*
Daykin K, 91, *109*
De Bie JJ, 353, *360*
de Gouw HWFM, 32, 37, 42, *45*, *50*, *55*, 59, 66, *74*
de Graff CS, 129, 131, 135, *149*
de Groot ER, 372, *386*
de Groot RP, 371, *385*
de Jong JW, 41, *55*
de Jong PM, 42, *55*, 395, *401*
de Klerk EPA, 36, 38, *49*, *52*
de Klerk NH, 31, 37, *45*
de Lepeleire I, 301, *324*
de Martin R, 375, *387*
de Monchy GJR, 31, *45*
de Monchy JG, 57, 59, *74*, 256, 257, *279*, 298, *321*
de Monchy JGR, 133, *149*, 266, *283*
de Moraes VLG, 255, 268, *278*
De Pee S, 31, 37, *45*
De Sanctis GW, 309, *328*
De Smet M, 301, 303, *324*
de Stefano A, 67, *80*
de Vos C, 218, *233*
de Vos S, 291, *315*
de Vries JE, 347, *358*, 380, *389*
de Vries K, 160, *175*
de Zeeuw RA, 91, *108*
De-Marino V, 187, *198*
de-Santi MM, 71, *83*
Dea D, 214, *229*
Dean H, 101, *117*
DeBoisblanc BP, 169, *180*
Decker N, 121, *147*
Decker T, 374, *387*
Decramer M, 301, *324*
Degebrodt A, 63, *77*
DeGennaro FC, 220, *235*
Degroote D, 189, *199*
Dejong PM, 67, *79*
Dekhuijzen PNR, 67, *79*, 165, *178*, 304, 308, *325*
Dekhuijzen R, 29, *44*, 171, *180*
Dekhuyzen PNR, 42, *55*
Dekker FW, 30, *44*
DeKruyff RH, 359, *360*
Del Donno M, 36, 42, *49*, *55*, 169, *180*
Del Rio L, 166, *178*
Delacourt C, 218, *233*
Delespesse G, 158, *174*
Della Cioppa G, 128, *148*
DeLucca PT, 307, *327*
DeMarzo N, 57, *73*
Demoly P, 380, *389*
Demopoulus CA, 183, *196*
den Hartigh J, 36, 37, 39, *48*, *51*, 211, *226*
Denburg J, 58, *73*
Denburg JA, 297, *321*, 393, *400*
Denis D, 301, *323*
Denman AM, 18, *26*
Dennis M, 156, *172*
Dennis R, 307, *327*
Dennyh FW, 100, *116*
Denome S, 246, *274*
Dent G, 190, *199*, 242, 243, 256, 261, *272*, *279*, *281*, 300, *323*, 338, *341*
Dente FL, 140, *151*
Depre M, 295, 300, *318*
Derian CK, 243, 256, *272*
Derksen F, 93, *111*
Dermarkarian R, 192, *200*, 299, *322*
Derse CP, 66, *79*
Desai JC, 213, *227*
Desai MC, 213, 216, *227*, *231*
Deschesnes F, 333, 336, 338, *341*, 393, *399*
DeSmet M, 295, 300, *318*
DeToyer A, 97, *114*
Devalia J, 16, *24*
Devalia JL, 15, 17, *24*, *25*, 67, *80*, 159, 170, *174*
Devault A, 333, 336, 338, *341*
Devchand PR, 291, *315*
Devereaux G, 141, *152*
Devillier P, 209, 210, *225*
DeVos C, 188, *198*
Dewald B, 158, *174*, 346, 352, *357*
Dewar J, 139, *151*
Dey RD, 204, 209, *223*, *224*
Dhillon DP, 140, *151*

Dhillon P, 194, *201*
Dhivert H, 397, *402*
Di Benedetto G, 128, *148*
Di Franco A, 140, *151*
Diamant Z, 32, 37, *45*, *51*, 215, *230*, 295, 296, 300, 301, 303, 305, *318*, *319*, *324*
Diamond L, 70, *82*, 105, *118*
Diamond MI, 158, *173*
Diaz O, 192, 193, *200*
Diaz-Sanchez D, 65, *78*
Dichgans J, 263, *281*
Dick EC, 36, 37, 38, *49*, *50*, *52*, 94, 100, *112*, 297, *321*
Dickinson G, 104, *118*
Dickinson SA, 395, *401*
DiDonato JA, 158, *173*
Diehl RE, 288, 291, *310*, *311*, *314*
Dighe AS, 346, *358*
Dijkhuizen B, 256, 257, *279*
Dijkman JH, 30, 31, 35, 36, 37, 39, 40, 41, *44*, *45*, *47*, *48*, *49*, *51*, *53*, *54*, 140, 141, *151*, 211, *226*
Dillis JL, 218, *234*
Dimitrov-Szokodi D, 96, *113*
Dinarello CA, 255, *277*
Dinarevic S, 5, *21*
Ding DJ, 32, 33, 39, *46*
Diocee BK, 243, 244, 254, 256, *272*, *273*
Dirksen A, 41, *54*
Dirksen H, 292, *316*
Dishcuk J, 158, *174*
DiStefano A, 57, *73*
Dixon CM, 210, *225*
Dixon CMS, 96, *113*, 189, 193, *199*, 210, *225*, 364, *382*
Dixon M, 292, 301, *316*, *323*
Dixon RA, 288, 291, *310*, *311*, *314*
Diza BL, 257, *279*
Djeu JY, 257, *279*
Djokic TD, 37, *50*
Djukanovic R, 5, 15, *21*, *24*, 35, 38, 43, *48*, *52*, *55*, *56*, 57, 58, 59, 60, 61, 62, 64, 65, 66, 67, 68, 69, 70, *72*, *73*, *76*, *77*, 78, *78*, *79*, *80*, *81*, *82*, 133, *149*,
[Djukanovic R] 159, 160, *174*, *176*, 189, *199*, 208, *223*, 239, *271*, 285, 295, 297, *309*, *318*, *321*, 333, *341*, 391, 395, 396, *399*, *401*, *402*
Dlyle CA, 71, *83*
Dobson P, 289, *312*
Dockery DW, 17, *25*
Dockhorn R, 303, 304, 305, *324*, *325*, *326*
Dockhorn RJ, 126, 129, 135, 137, *148*, 333, 336, *341*
Doelman CJA, 93, *111*
Dohi Y, 190, *200*, 303, *325*
Doig MV, 295, *319*
Dolhain RJEM, 38, *52*
Doll R, 143, *153*
Dollery CT, 191, 193, *200*, *201*, 289, 295, 296, *313*, *318*, *320*
Dolovich J, 38, 42, *52*, 58, 66, *73*, *79*, 100, *116*, 160, *175*, 297, 298, *321*, 393, 394, *400*
Domanico PL, 251, *276*
Domenech T, 250, *275*
Domgala B, 378, *388*
Donaldson J, 247, *274*
Donnelly P, 35, *47*
Doods H, 92, *110*
Dougherty GJ, 63, *76*
Douglas B, 166, *178*
Douglas GJ, 259, *280*
Douglas J, 121, *146*
Douglas JJ, 66, *79*
Douglas N, 101, *116*
Douglas RG, 100, 101, *116*
Douglas SA, 369, *385*
Doull IJM, 164, *177*
Douma WR, 129, *149*
Doupnik CA, 294, *318*
Doutremepuich JD, 213, *227*
Dow E, 139, *151*
Downes H, 100, *115*
Downward J, 254, *277*
Drajesk JF, 299, *323*
Drapeau G, 209, 210, *225*
Drazen J, 299, 307, *322*, *327*

Drazen JM, 29, 35, 37, *44*, *48*, *51*, 60, *75*, 161, *176*, 192, *201*, 208, 214, *224*, *229*, 266, *283*, 292, 294, 297, 299, 300, 301, 302, 304, 307, 308, 309, *316*, *318*, *320*, *322*, *325*, *328*, 364, *381*
Drazen MB, 292, *316*
Droogmans G, 376, *388*
Drouin J, 158, *173*
Drozda SE, 213, *227*
Druce H, 105, *118*
Du T, 294, *317*
Dube J, 134, *150*
Dube L, 304, 307, 308, *325*, *327*
Dube LM, 304, 308, *325*
Dubois AE, 256, 257, *279*
Duce Gracia F, 128, *148*
Ducoux JP, 213, *227*, *228*
Duddle JM, 67, *80*, 159, 170, *174*
Duddridge M, 185, *196*, 298, *322*
Duell EA, 268, *283*
Duffin K, 288, *311*
Duffy D, 9, *22*
Duffy DL, 348, *358*
Dugas B, 291, *315*
Dugas M, 36, 42, *49*
Duhme H, 19, *26*
Duiverman EJ, 31, 37, 40, *45*, *54*, 160, 164, *175*, *178*, 307, *327*, 395, *401*
Dujkanovic R, 60, *75*
Dumont P, 91, 92, *108*
Dunlop K, 171, *181*
Dunnette S, 58, 59, 61, 69, 70, *73*
Dunnill MS, 69, 78, *81*
Duplantier AJ, 265, 269, *282*
Dupont AG, 301, *324*
Dupont S, 374, *387*
Durante S, 135, *150*
Durham S, 57, 64, *72*
Durham SR, 31, 38, *45*, *52*, 57, 62, 64, 67, *72*, *73*, *77*, *80*, 238, *270*, 344, 345, 346, 352, *356*, *357*, 395, 396, *401*
Dusser D, 398, *403*
Dusser DJ, 37, *50*
Dutoit J, 125, 140, *147*
Dutoit JI, 160, *175*
Dutton RW, 65, *78*
Dvorak AM, 60, *74*
Dworski R, 133, *149*, 297, *320*, *321*
Dworski RT, 306, *326*
Dwyer TM, 89, 90, *107*, *108*
Dyson C, 167, *179*
Dzau VJ, 43, *56*

E

Earnshaw JS, 127, *148*
Eastwood C, 194, *201*
Eaton M, 251, 257, 263, 267, *276*
Ebden P, 162, *176*
Ebina M, 35, *47*, 286, 294, *309*
Eccles MP, 393, *399*
Eckel SP, 195, *202*
Ecklund P, 92, *110*
Eda R, 195, *202*
Edelman JM, 307, *327*
Edmonds-Alt X, 209, 210, 214, 215, 216, 218, *225*, *228*, *230*, *231*, *234*
Edmunds L, 96, *114*
Edvinsson L, 208, *224*
Edwards C, 167, *179*
Edwards T, 305, *326*
Efthimiadis A, 38, 42, *52*, 306, *327*
Efthimiou J, 169, *180*
Egan RW, 43, *55*, 370, 371, 372, 374, *385*, *386*
Eggler JF, 265, 269, *282*
Eggleston P, 18, *26*
Eglen RM, 86, 87, *106*
Ehlert F, 92, *110*
Ehnert B, 18, *25*
Ehrlich-Kautzky E, 348, 349, *358*
Eidelman DH, 33, 35, 39, *46*, *47*, *52*, *53*
Eisenberg J, 398, *403*
Eiser N, 100, *116*
Eiser NM, 298, *322*
Eiyah K, 218, *234*
Ekstrom T, 128, *148*
Ekstrom-Jodal B, 99, 101, *115*
El-Fakahany EE, 91, 96, *108*, *113*
Elbon CL, 38, *52*, 93, 95, *111*, *113*

Elixhauser A, 398, *403*
Elliott EV, 292, 301, *316*, *323*
Elliott KRF, 255, *277*
Elliott MJ, 268, *283*, 371, *386*
Ellis EF, 163, *177*
Ellis JL, 204, 214, 215, *223*, *229*, *230*, 244, 261, *273*
Elsasser S, 125, 140, *147*
Elson CO, 372, 374, *386*
Elwood W, 37, *50*
Elzinga CR, 91, *108*, *109*
Elzinga CRS, 91, *108*, *109*
Emala C, 88, *106*
Emala CW, 90, 91, *107*
Emberlin J, 16, *24*
Emmett A, 141, *152*
Emonds-Alt X, 213, 214, 216, 220, *227*, *228*, *229*, *231*, *235*
Empey DW, 100, *116*
Enander I, 57, 65, *73*, 396, *402*
Endert E, 165, *178*
Endo Y, 37, *50*
Endres S, 255, *277*
Engel T, 41, *54*
Engels F, 256, *278*
Engels P, 248, *275*
Engelstatter R, 266, *283*
England PJ, 247, *274*
English AF, 168, *179*
Ennis M, 212, *226*
Enomoto T, 15, *24*, 380, *389*
Enright PL, 393, 394, *400*
Ensrud K, 166, *178*
Epler GR, 394, *400*
Epstein J, 97, 99, *114*, *115*
Epstein PM, 257, *279*
Epstein PN, 238, 244, *270*
Epstein RS, 397, *402*
Eran L, 61, *76*
Erard F, 65, *78*, 378, *388*
Erb KJ, 15, *24*
Eriksson LO, 302, *324*
Erle DJ, 70, *81*
Ernst P, 43, *56*, 64, 66, 71, *78*, *79*, 143, 144, *153*, 307, *327*
Eschenbacher WL, 208, *224*
Eskra JD, 191, *200*, 255, 268, *278*
Esqueda E, 92, *110*
Essayan DM, 255, 257, 265, 268, 269, *278*, *279*, *282*, 378, *388*
Esswein LA, 350, *359*
Ethier D, 288, 292, 299, 301, *311*, *322*, *323*
Ethier M, 91, *108*
Evangelista S, 215, 219, 220, *230*, *234*
Evans CM, 95, *113*
Evans DB, 245, *273*
Evans DJ, 195, *202*, 288, *312*
Evans DY, 264, *282*
Evans JF, 288, 291, 292, *311*, *314*
Evans JM, 192, *200*
Evans PM, 256, *279*
Evans R, 158, *173*
Evans RB, 288, *312*
Evans S, 38, 42, *52*
Evans TW, 210, *225*
Everaert E, 216, *231*
Evertse CE, 36, 38, 42, 43, *49*, *52*, 159, *174*, 395, 396, *400*
Evertse ChE, 38, *52*
Eytner R, 375, *387*
Ezeamuzie CI, 186, *197*

F

Fabbri L, 97, *114*
Fabbri LM, 30, 31, 36, 37, *44*, 57, 67, *73*, *80*, 94, 100, *112*, 297, 298, *321*, 394, *400*
Fabel H, 193, *201*, 365, *382*
Faherty DA, 346, *357*
Fahy J, 58, *73*
Fahy JV, 221, *235*, 333, 336, 337, *341*, 352, *359*, 364, 379, *381*, *389*
Faiferman I, 303, 305, *325*, *326*
Fairfax AJ, 194, *201*
Falnnery EM, 142, *152*
Fame TM, 93, 94, *111*
Fan N, 290, *314*
Fan TD, 238, 240, 242, *270*
Fanslow WC, 345, *357*
Fanta C, 104, *118*

Fantozzi R, 218, *233*
Faraone S, 187, *198*
Fardin V, 213, *227*
Farese RV, 70, *81*
Fargeas C, 158, *174*
Farley JM, 89, 90, *107*, *108*
Farmer J, 36, *49*, 65, *78*
Farrow GM, 59, 69, *74*
Fasano MB, 290, *314*
Fasler S, 380, *389*
Fauchere JL, 205, 212, 213, 214, *223*
Faul JL, 36, *49*, 65, *78*
Faulds D, 263, 265, *281*
Faulkner D, 93, *111*
Faurschou P, 126, 129, 135, 137, 146, *148*, *154*
Faux JA, 348, *358*
Fearon DT, 61, *75*
Feather I, 62, *76*
Feather IH, 69, *81*
Federman EC, 60, *75*
Fedorak RN, 372, 374, *386*
Fehlmann M, 243, 257, *273*
Feinberg SM, 155, *172*
Feinman R, 70, *82*
Feinmark SJ, 290, *314*
Feldman BMM, 89, 90, *107*
Feldman PL, 251, *276*
Feldmann M, 268, *283*, 371, *386*
Felez MA, 191, 192, 193, *200*
Fellerere K, 251, 264, *276*
Felten SY, 212, *227*
Fendley B, 333, *341*
Fenton G, 251, *276*
Ferguson A, 343, *355*
Ferguson EW, 247, 252, 253, 258, 269, *274*
Ferguson K, 245, *274*
Fernandez AG, 250, *275*
Fernandez LB, 91, *109*, 244, 261, *273*
Fernandez X, 43, *55*, 371, *385*
Ferrante J, 346, *357*
Ferraris L, 209, *224*
Ferrer SH, 266, *283*
Ferrie PJ, 397, *402*
Ferrigno L, 15, *24*
Ferris BG, 17, *25*, 393, *399*
Ferrua B, 243, 257, *273*
Festen J, 304, 308, *325*
Festin J, 171, *180*
Fewtrell CMS, 212, *226*
Fey MF, 158, *174*
Fichte K, 251, 264, *276*
Fick RB, 333, 336, 337, 338, 339, *341*, 379, *389*
Field J, 246, *274*
Fielding LE, 263, *281*
Figueroa DJ, 352, *359*
Fikrig E, 348, 351, *358*
Filley WV, 59, 68, *74*
Findlay BP, 67, *81*
Findlay GG, 67, *81*
Findlay SR, 105, *118*
Finkelman F, 345, 346, *357*
Finkelman FD, 63, *77*, 332, *341*, 372, *386*
Finkelstein FN, 144, *153*
Finlay AY, 167, *179*
Finn AF, 305, *326*
Finn PW, 309, *328*
Finnen MJ, 290, *314*
Finnerty J, 142, 144, *152*
Finnerty JP, 60, *75*, 249, *275*, 302, *324*
Finney MJB, 209, *225*
Finucane Th, 37, *50*
Fiocchi C, 209, *224*
Fireman P, 286, *309*
Fischer A, 219, *234*, 297, 309, *320*, *328*
Fischer AR, 192, *201*, 294, 299, 301, 304, 309, *318*, *322*, *323*, *328*
Fischer G, 251, 264, *276*
Fish JE, 39, *53*, 97, 100, *114*, 306, *326*, 364, *381*
Fishwick K, 141, *152*
Fitzpatrick F, 290, *314*
Fitzpatrick FA, 288, *311*
Fjelbirkeland L, 133, *149*
Flannery EM, 5, *21*, 329, *340*
Flatt A, 143, 144, *153*
Flavahan NA, 92, *110*
Flavell RA, 344, 348, 351, *356*, *358*
Fleischhacker WW, 264, *282*
Fleming HE, 333, 336, 337, *341*, 379, *389*

Flier SR, 308, *328*
Flint KC, 59, 61, *74*
Flores L, 92, *109*
Flower RJ, 217, *232*
Fluge T, 365, *382*
Fokkens PHB, 36, *49*
Fokkens WJ, 63, *77*
Folco G, 290, *314*
Folgering H, 96, *114*
Folkerts G, 37, *50*
Fong CY, 292, 294, *316*
Fong M, 255, 268, *278*
Fong T, 208, *224*
Fontana A, 263, *281*
Fonteh AN, 256, *278*, 290, *314*
Fontino M, 348, *359*
Foord R, 297, *321*
Foran SK, 43, *55*, 371, *385*
Ford S, 105, *118*
Ford-Hutchinson AW, 288, 295, 296, 297, 301, *310*, *311*, *319*, *320*, *323*
Forder RA, 299, *322*
Forderkunz S, 256, *278*
Foreman JC, 212, *226*, 238, 240, 242, *270*
Foresi A, 36, 37, 42, *49*, *51*, *55*, 169, *180*, 215, *230*
Forsberg K, 220, *235*
Forssmann WG, 365, *382*
Forster JK, 137, *150*
Forstner GG, 67, *81*
Forstner JF, 67, *81*
Fortin R, 288, 301, *311*, *323*
Foster A, 295, *319*
Foster DW, 289, *313*
Foster M, 248, 251, 256, 257, *275*
Foster PS, 352, *359*
Foster RW, 36, *50*, 266, *283*
Foster S, 299, *323*
Foucard T, 13, *23*
Foulon DM, 214, *229*
Fowler A, 60, *75*
Fowler AA, 296, *320*
Fox AJ, 220, *235*, 333, *341*, 368, 374, *384*
Fozzard J, 375, *387*
Fozzard JR, 248, *275*
Franchimont P, 189, *199*
Frank MI, 156, *172*
Franks FM, 86, *105*
Frantz R, 294, 304, *318*
Franzen L, 301, *323*
Fraser PM, 143, *153*
Fredberg JJ, 34, 39, *47*
Freedman IP, 158, *173*
Freeland HS, 66, *79*, 289, *313*
Freeman GJ, 289, *312*
Freezer NJ, 164, *177*
Freidhoff LR, 348, 349, *358*
Freidman B, 301, 305, *324*, *326*
Freidman BS, 295, 300, 304, 307, 308, *318*, *323*, *325*, *327*
Freidman J, 141, *152*
Freind DS, 291, *315*
Freitag A, 194, *201*
Freitas P, 104, *118*
Freudenthal Y, 125, *147*
Frew AJ, 57, 64, 67, 70, *72*, *80*, *81*, *82*
Frick OL, 100, *116*, 343, *355*
Frick WE, 100, *116*
Friedman A, 353, *360*
Friedrich MF, 350, *359*
Friend DS, 291, *315*
Fries RA, 343, *355*
Frigas E, 59, 69, *74*, 378, *388*
Frischer T, 395, *401*
Fritzsch C, 19, *26*
Frohlich JC, 193, *201*
Frolund L, 41, *54*, 160, *175*
Frossard N, 70, *81*, 218, *232*, *233*
Frost C, 129, 141, *148*, 164, *177*
Fryer A, 94, 95, 96, 99, *112*, *113*, *115*
Fryer AD, 38, *51*, *52*, 91, 92, 93, 94, 96, 98, 99, 100, 102, *108*, *109*, *110*, *111*, *112*, *113*, *114*, *116*
Fuccella LM, 307, *327*
Fugate MJ, 184, *196*
Fuglsang G, 162, *177*
Fujimoto K, 66, *79*
Fujimura M, 294, 295, *317*, *318*
Fujiwara H, 347, *358*
Fukuchi Y, 187, *198*
Fukuda T, 37, *50*, 187, *198*

Fukumura M, 297, *321*
Fulle HJ, 255, *277*
Fuller R, 127, 142, 143, *148*
Fuller RW, 42, *55*, 191, 193, *200*, *201*, 210, *225*, 242, 255, *271*, 289, 295, 296, *313*, *318*, *320*, 367, *383*
Funk CD, 288, 290, 295, *311*, *314*, *318*
Furdon PJ, 255, 268, *278*
Furfine ES, 369, *384*
Furkert J, 208, *224*

G

Gaarder PI, 17, *25*
Gaddy JN, 301, *324*
Gagnon L, 288, 289, *311*, *312*
Gagnon MA, 134, *150*
Galant S, 305, *326*
Galdes-Sebalt M, 104, *117*
Galella G, 287, *310*
Gallagher JP, 92, *110*
Galli C, 287, *310*
Galli SJ, 290, *314*
Galvez A, 366, *383*
Gambaro G, 307, *327*
Gamble JR, 295, *318*, 345, 352, *356*
Gambone LM, 95, *113*
Gandordy B, 120, *146*
Ganong A, 213, *227*
Ganstrom E, 290, *314*
Garbe E, 167, *179*
Garcia M, 366, *383*
Garcia ML, 362, 367, *381*, *384*
Garcia T, 374, *387*
Garcia-Calvo M, 366, *383*
Garcia-Sanz J, 65, *78*
Gardi C, 71, *83*
Gardiner PJ, 289, 292, *312*, *316*
Gardiner PV, 134, 141, *150*, *152*, 169, *180*
Gardner RM, 394, *400*
Garino G, 306, *327*
Garippa RJ, 364, *382*
Garland A, 38, *51*, 214, 217, 218, *229*, *232*, *233*
Garland LG, 219, *234*
Garpestad E, 308, *328*
Garret C, 213, *227*
Garvey EP, 369, *384*
Gately MK, 346, 348, *357*, *358*
Gatzy JT, 89, *106*
Gaudette R, 91, *109*
Gauldie J, 380, *389*
Gause WC, 63, *77*
Gauthier JY, 288, *311*
Gavett SH, 345, 346, *357*, 372, *386*
Gayard P, 100, *116*
Gayrard P, 99, *115*
Gearing AJH, 238, *270*
Gebremichael I, 189, *199*
Gelder C, 208, *224*
Gelder CM, 158, *173*
Gelfand EW, 14, *24*, 93, 94, *111*
Gelfand ML, 156, *172*
Gelich GH, 378, *388*
Genain GP, 263, 265, *281*
Genant HK, 166, *178*
George WHS, 157, *172*
Georges D, 133, *149*
Georgopoulos D, 101, *117*
Geppetti G, 214, *229*
Geppetti P, 37, *51*, 215, 216, 217, 219, 221, *230*, *231*, *232*, *234*, *235*
Geraint-James D, 59, 61, *74*
Gerard C, 372, *386*
Gerard NP, 372, *386*
Gergen PJ, 398, *403*
Gerlach W, 264, *282*
Germain N, 216, 218, *231*, *232*, *234*
German DF, 100, *116*
German V, 89, *107*
Germonpre PR, 203, 204, 209, 216, *223*, *224*, *231*
Gerogitis JN, 105, *118*
Gerristen J, 40, *54*, 160, *175*
Gerritsen J, 256, 257, *279*
Gerstin E, 92, *110*
Gertner A, 99, *115*
Gertner SB, 219, *234*
Gerzer R, 255, *277*
Gether U, 214, *228*
Geyer N, 251, 264, *276*
Ghaffar O, 64, *78*

Ghanekar SV, 215, *230*
Ghatei MA, 70, *82*
Ghavanian N, 57, 65, *73*, 396, *402*
Ghezzo H, 125, 140, *147*
Ghosh B, 348, 349, *358*
Ghosh S, 375, *387*
Ghosh SK, 188, *198*
Giachetti A, 204, 213, 214, 215, *223*, *227*, *228*, *229*, *230*
Giannarini L, 65, *78*
Giannini D, 140, *151*
Giannotti D, 213, *228*
Gibbons GH, 43, *56*
Gibbons WJ, 41, *54*
Gibson P, 58, *73*
Gibson PG, 297, *321*, 393, *399*
Gibson U, 372, *386*
Giedlin MA, 63, *77*
Gielen MH, 15, *24*
Giembycz MA, 217, *231*, 242, 243, 256, 257, 261, 269, *272*, *279*, *280*, *281*, 378, *388*
Gienapp IE, 353, *360*
Gierczak S, 301, *323*
Gierse J, 288, *311*
Gierse JK, 288, *311*
Gies JP, 91, 92, *108*
Gignac F, 393, *399*
Gijbels K, 353, *360*
Gilchrest HG, 195, *202*
Gill A, 379, *389*
Gill CA, 293, 294, *317*
Gillard JW, 288, *311*
Gillen L, 286, *309*
Gillen MS, 195, *202*
Gillespie CA, 167, *179*
Gillon RL, 188, *198*
Giotti A, 218, *233*
Girard V, 220, *235*, 244, 261, *273*
Girard Y, 299, *322*
Girgis-Gabardo A, 58, *73*, 297, *321*, 393, *399*
Gitter B, 214, *229*
Giudizin MG, 65, *78*
Giulekas D, 101, *117*
Giuliani DS, 213, *228*
Giuliani S, 213, 214, *227*, *228*
Gizycki MJ, 36, *49*
Gjomarkaj M, 306, *327*
Glass M, 60, *75*, 304, *325*, *326*
Gleich G, 95, *113*
Gleich GJ, 38, 42, *51*, *52*, 58, 59, 60, 61, 66, 68, 69, 70, *73*, *74*, *75*, *79*, 94, *112*, 239, 243, 257, *271*, 378, *388*
Glimcher LH, 351, *359*, 371, *386*
Glovsky MM, 16, 17, *25*
Gnosspelius Y, 137, *151*
Goadby P, 185, *196*, 298, *322*
Godard P, 57, 65, 66, 71, *73*, *79*, *82*, 217, 218, *231*, *233*, 289, 297, 305, *313*, *321*, *326*, 330, *340*, 380, *389*, 396, 398, *402*, *403*
Godard PH, 238, *270*
Godden D, 2, 15, *21*, *24*
Godfrey R, 71, *82*
Godfrey RC, 59, *74*
Godfrey S, 157, *173*
Godschalk I, 395, *401*
Goetzel EJ, 209, *224*
Goetzl E, 217, *232*
Goetzl EJ, 58, *73*, 217, *232*
Gold K, 393, *399*
Gold M, 169, *180*
Gold WM, 60, *75*, 100, *115*, *116*
Goldie RG, 369, *385*
Goldin JG, 96, *114*
Goldman AL, 248, *275*
Goldman D, 242, 256, *271*, *272*
Goldrich MS, 208, *224*
Goldstein H, 65, *78*
Goldyne ME, 289, *313*
Gomez FP, 192, 193, *200*
Gomm SA, 96, *114*
Gonen H, 375, *387*
Gonnella P, 353, *360*
Gontovnick L, 125, 140, *147*
Gonzalez FJ, 291, *315*
Gooding RC, 255, 268, *278*
Goodman RB, 288, *312*
Goodwin JS, 289, *313*
Goppelt Struebe M, 289, *312*
Gordon G, 89, *107*

Gordon RJ, 247, 252, 253, 258, 269, *274*
Gordon W, 43, *55*, 333, *341*
Gorenne I, 289, *313*
Gorman C, 333, *341*
Goso C, 213, 214, *227*, *229*
Gough KJ, 165, *178*
Goulaouic P, 213, *227*
Gould HJ, 330, *340*
Goulding D, 57, 61, 64, 67, *74*, *81*
Gourlay H, 105, *118*
Gozzard N, 217, 218, *232*, *234*, 251, 253, 257, 259, 261, 263, 267, 269, *276*, *277*, *280*
Graeff-Lonnevig V, 13, *23*
Graf P, 96, 97, *114*
Graf PD, 37, *51*, 94, 100, *112*, 214, 215, *229*, *230*
Grafstrom RC, 294, *318*
Grahern FL, 380, *389*
Grainger J, 143, 144, *153*
Grandgeorge S, 168, *179*
Grandordy B, 43, *55*, 121, *146*, 333, *341*
Grandordy BM, 91, *109*
Granstrom E, 296, *320*
Granzow CA, 195, *202*
Gras J, 250, *275*
Grast A, 374, *387*
Gratziou C, 57, 61, 62, 64, 67, *74*, *76*, *80*
Graves J, 93, 94, *111*
Green CP, 296, *320*
Green RM, 18, *26*
Green S, 11, *22*
Green SE, 192, *200*
Green WF, 1, *20*
Greenblatt DW, 293, *317*
Greening AP, 66, *79*, 128, 131, *148*, 158, 162, *173*, *177*, 364, *382*
Gregg I, 41, *54*, 393, *400*
Grembiale RD, 135, *150*
Grenier J, 218, *233*
Grettve L, 137, *150*
Grieco M, 101, *117*
Griffen M, 92, *110*
Griffin M, 60, *75*
Griffith WH, 92, *110*
Griffiths RJ, 255, 268, *278*
Griffiths-Johnson DA, 239, *271*
Griffiths-Johnson PA, 239, *271*
Grimaud C, 100, *116*
Grimes D, 263, 264, *281*, *282*
Gristwood R, 244, *273*
Gristwood RW, 250, 258, *275*, *280*
Griswold DE, 263, *281*
Gronemeyer H, 374, *387*
Grootendorst DC, 58, *73*, 303, *324*
Gross NJ, 38, *52*, 97, 104, *114*
Grossman J, 105, *118*, 126, 129, 135, 137, *148*, 299, 303, *322*
Grossman R, 129, 131, 135, *149*
Groth S, 292, *316*
Grous M, 250, 251, 253, 265, 269, *276*, *282*
Groux H, 347, *358*
Grove A, 137, 138, *151*, 163, *177*
Gruetter CA, 365, *382*
Grunberg K, 15, *24*, 37, 38, *50*, *52*
Grunstein MM, 211, *226*
Gruss HJ, 291, *315*
Gubler U, 346, 348, *357*, *358*
Gudapaty S, 291, *315*
Gueremy T, 255, *277*
Guevremont D, 216, *231*
Guhlmann A, 289, *313*
Guiliani S, 214, *230*
Guindon Y, 301, *323*
Guler ML, 347, *358*
Gulsvik A, 133, *149*
Gunst SJ, 32, 33, 34, *46*, *47*, 91, 93, *109*
Gunthert U, 69, *81*
Gustafsson JA, 158, *173*
Gustafsson LE, 210, *225*
Guyaat G, 393, *399*
Guyatt GH, 397, *402*
Guz A, 100, *116*
Gygax D, 43, *55*, 333, *341*

H

Haagmans BL, 347, *358*
Haahtela T, 69, 71, *81*, *83*, *84*, 159, 160, 161, *174*, *175*, *176*, 296, 305, *319*, 396, *401*

Haak-Frendscho M, 332, 333, *341*
Haak-Frenscho M, 339, *342*
Habbick B, 143, 144, *153*
Haby MM, 19, *26*
Hachsu R, 257, *279*
Haddad E, 89, 90, 91, *107*, *108*, 366, *383*
Haddad EB, 91, *108*
Haddox R, 105, *118*
Haeggstrom J, 290, *314*
Haeggstrom JZ, 288, 290, 291, *310*, *314*, *315*
Hagan RM, 213, 215, *227*, *230*
Hagermara DD, 133, *149*
Hagmann W, 289, *313*
Hahn H, 97, *114*
Hajer R, 91, *109*
Hakansson P, 71, *82*
Halayko AJ, 34, 39, *47*
Hale JJ, 216, *231*
Hall AE, 37, *51*, 208, *224*
Hall AK, 211, *226*
Hall I, 10, *22*, 91, *109*
Hall IP, 137, 139, *151*, 247, *274*, 362, 365, *381*
Hall J, 127, 142, 143, *148*
Hall WJ, 100, 101, *116*
Hallman R, 346, *357*
Halonen M, 11, 13, *22*, *23*, 91, 92, *108*, *110*
Halonen RA, 329, *340*
Ham EA, 242, 256, *272*
Hamann A, 346, *357*
Hamaoka T, 347, *358*
Hamberg M, 291, *315*
Hamel R, 301, *323*
Hameling ML, 191, *200*
Hamelink ML, 289, *313*
Hamelmann E, 14, *24*
Hamid Q, 36, 41, 43, *49*, *56*, 57, 62, 64, 66, 67, 71, *73*, *78*, *79*, *80*, 158, *174*, 238, *270*, 344, 345, 346, 352, *356*
Hamilton A, 303, *325*
Hamilton AL, 40, *53*, 301, *323*
Hamilton R, 208, *224*
Hamilton RG, 339, *342*
Hamilton SA, 67, *80*, 159, 170, *174*
Hammarstrom S, 292, *316*
Hammer R, 86, *105*
Hammond MD, 59, 61, *74*
Hampel FC, 105, *118*
Han YHR, 300, *323*
Hanahan DJ, 183, 185, *196*, *197*
Hanania NA, 166, *178*
Hanby LA, 295, *318*
Hancox B, 142, *152*
Hand JM, 254, 258, 261, 269, *277*
Hanifin JM, 268, *283*, 351, *359*
Hankinson JL, 394, *400*
Hanrahan J, 90, *107*
Hansel T, 61, *76*
Hanson B, 9, *22*
Hanson DG, 343, *355*
Hara M, 219, *234*
Hara N, 37, *50*, 218, *233*
Harbers H, 96, *114*
Harbinson PL, 265, 266, 267, *282*
Hardaker P, 16, *24*
Harding SM, 168, *180*
Hardman JG, 245, *273*
Harf A, 218, *233*
Hargreave F, 58, *73*, 97, 100, *114*, *116*
Hargreave FE, 31, 37, 38, 41, 42, *45*, *52*, *54*, 58, 60, 61, 66, *73*, *75*, *79*, 97, 100, *114*, *116*, 142, *153*, 160, *175*, 297, 298, 306, *321*, *327*, 393, 394, 396, *400*, *402*
Harkawat R, 141, *152*, 169, *180*
Harlan JM, 352, *359*
Harmid Q, 64, *77*
Harper AE, 397, *403*
Harre E, 142, *152*
Harris A, 305, *326*
Harris AL, 247, 252, 253, 258, 269, *274*
Harris JG, 125, 140, *147*
Harris K, 100, *115*
Harris SC, 221, *235*
Harrison DJ, 7, *21*
Harrison NK, 217, *232*
Harrison S, 259, *281*
Hartley JA, 63, *77*
Hartley SB, 347, 351, *358*

Hartmann R, 70, *82*
Hartung HP, 218, *233*
Haruta Y, 190, 195, *200*, *201*, 305, *326*
Harvath L, 243, 256, *272*
Hashimoto N, 303, *325*
Haskard DO, 57, 61, 64, *74*
Haslett C, 378, *388*
Hassall GK, 243, 254, 256, *272*
Hassall SM, 305, *326*
Hassan NAGM, 36, *50*
Hatzelmann A, 243, 256, 257, *272*, *273*, *278*
Hatzubai A, 375, *387*
Hauser C, 257, *279*
Hauser SL, 263, 265, *281*
Hausfeld J, 89, 90, *107*
Hawcock AB, 213, *227*
Hawksworth R, 61, *76*, 265, 266, 267, *282*, 294, *317*
Hawksworth RJ, 5, *21*, 292, 294, 297, 299, *316*, *320*, *323*
Haworth S, 91, *108*, 208, *224*
Hay DA, 369, 373, *384*
Hay DW, 295, *319*, 369, *385*
Hay DWP, 286, 295, *310*
Hay H, 297, *321*
Hayashi S, 208, *224*
Hayden F, 105, *118*
Hayes A, 212, *226*
Hayes EC, 289, *313*
Hays R, 397, *402*
Hazbun ME, 208, *224*
Hazeki K, 243, 256, *272*
Hazeki O, 243, 256, *272*
He S, 61, *76*
Head J, 251, 257, 263, 267, *276*
Heaf P, 143, *153*
Heaney LG, 212, *226*
Heard BE, 67, 71, *81*, *83*
Hearn L, 288, 292, *311*
Heaslip R, 242, 256, *272*
Heaslip RJ, 255, 264, 268, *278*, *282*
Heath AW, 350, *359*
Heath H, 372, *386*
Heath P, 265, 266, 267, *282*
Heaulme M, 213, *227*
Hebenstreit GF, 251, 264, *276*
Heck S, 374, *387*
Hedgpeth J, 263, 265, *281*
Hedlin G, 169, *180*
Hedner J, 137, *151*, 221, *235*
Heeren A, 393, *399*
Hegde SS, 86, 87, *106*
Hegele R, 208, *224*
Hegele RG, 15, *24*, 36, 41, *49*, 158, *173*
Heibein JA, 288, 292, *311*
Heijnen IA, 347, *358*
Heinig JH, 41, *54*
Heinke S, 376, *388*
Heino M, 69, *81*
Heinrich J, 17, *25*
Hekking PR, 242, 255, *271*
Helke CJ, 203, *223*
Heller RA, 290, *314*
Helmberg A, 158, *173*
Helmers RA, 308, *328*
Helms S, 158, *173*
Helweg D, 251, *276*
Helweg DA, 251, *276*
Heming TA, 242, *272*
Hemler ME, 379, *389*
Hendel-Kramer A, 17, *25*
Hendeles L, 303, 306, *324*, *327*
Henderson FW, 100, *116*
Henderson WR, 191, *200*, 268, *283*, 351, *359*
Hendrick DJ, 134, 141, *150*, *152*, 185, *196*, 298, *322*
Henochowicz S, 126, 129, 135, 137, *148*
Henricks P, 91, *109*
Henricks PA, 256, *278*
Henriksen JM, 125, *147*
Henrikson-DeStefano D, 70, *82*
Henry PJ, 369, *385*
Henson PM, 183, 185, 193, *196*, *197*, *201*
Hepperle MJE, 297, *321*, 393, *399*
Heravi J, 256, *278*
Herbert CA, 37, *50*
Herbert DA, 92, *110*
Herbison GP, 5, *21*, 329, *340*

Herd CM, 217, 218, *232*, *234*, 259, 261, 263, 267, 269, *280*
Herdman MJ, 17, *25*, 67, *80*, 159, 170, *174*
Hermans J, 31, 37, 40, 41, *45*, *54*
Hermanussen NW, 91, *108*
Hernandez A, 218, *233*
Herrlich P, 374, *387*
Herrmann F, 291, *315*
Hershenson MB, 38, *51*, 218, *233*
Hershey GKK, 350, *359*
Herst RS, 300, *323*
Heruman L, 398, *403*
Herz U, 346, *357*
Hess HJ, 213, *227*
Hess J, 305, *326*
Hessel EM, 353, *360*
Heuer HO, 194, *201*
Heusser C, 43, *55*, 330, 331, 332, 333, *340*, *341*
Heusser CH, 338, *341*
Hewison J, 393, *399*
Hewitt CJ, 5, *21*, 329, *340*
Hey JA, 220, *235*
Heyder J, 17, *25*
Heym J, 213, *227*
Heyse J, 307, *327*
Hida W, 221, *235*
Hide DW, 13, 18, *23*
Hidi R, 58, 59, 60, 61, 64, 66, *73*, *78*
Hiemstra PS, 36, 38, 42, *49*, *52*, *55*, 59, 66, *74*
Hieribson GP, 142, *152*
Higenbotham TW, 194, *201*
Higgins BG, 141, *152*
Higgins C, 194, *201*
Higgins KS, 220, *234*
Higgs G, 251, 253, 255, 257, 261, 263, 267, 268, 269, *276*, *277*, *278*
Higgs GA, 244, 259, 261, 263, 267, 269, *273*, *280*
Hilkens CMU, 346, *358*
Hill DJ, 12, *23*
Hill M, 93, 94, *111*
Hill ME, 290, *314*
Hill SJ, 244, 247, *273*, *274*
Hiller TK, 397, *402*
Hilliam C, 32, 33, *46*
Hilliam ChC, 31, *45*
Hilliard D, 295, 300, *318*
Hillman D, 33, *46*
Hillman L, 166, *178*
Hiltermann JT, 296, 305, *319*
Hiltermann TJN, 36, *49*
Hinterhuber H, 264, *282*
Hinton KL, 134, *150*
Hinz W, 295, *319*
Hirai H, 371, *385*
Hirai M, 70, *82*
Hirayama Y, 208, 215, 220, *224*, *230*, *235*
Hiroi J, 220, *235*
Hirose T, 218, *233*
Hirsch A, 215, *230*
Hirschleiter L, 365, *383*
Hirshman C, 88, 100, *106*, *115*
Hirshman CA, 90, 91, *108*, *109*
Hirst SJ, 34, 35, *47*
Hislop A, 91, *108*
Hislop AA, 208, *224*
Hitchings DJ, 395, *401*
Ho IC, 371, *386*
Hodge L, 19, *26*
Hodge MR, 371, *386*
Hodgson TA, 398, *403*
Hodlaway M, 4, *21*
Hoeck WG, 290, *314*
Hoekx JCM, 169, *180*
Hofer-Warbinek R, 375, *387*
Hoffbrand AV, 291, *315*
Hoffstein S, 242, *272*
Hofman G, 353, *360*
Hofstra WB, 307, *327*
Hogan SP, 352, *359*
Hogate ST, 60, *75*
Hogg JC, 31, 32, 33, 34, 35, 36, 41, *45*, *46*, *47*, *48*, *49*, *54*, 158, *173*, 395, *401*
Hogg N, 63, *76*
Hogger P, 168, *179*
Hohle K, 88, *106*
Hohman RJ, 208, *224*
Hoidel J, 95, 104, *113*

Hokfelt T, 205, 212, *223*, *227*
Holberg CJ, 13, *23*
Holbrook M, 251, 253, 257, 259, 261, 263, 267, 269, *276*, *277*, *280*
Holdaway MD, 5, *21*, 329, *340*
Holden EP, 291, *315*
Holgate S, 6, *21*, 333, *341*
Holgate ST, 15, 19, *24*, *26*, 27, 31, 35, 36, 37, 38, 41, 43, *44*, *45*, *48*, *50*, *52*, *54*, *55*, *56*, 57, 58, 59, 60, 61, 62, 63, 64, 65, 66, 67, 68, 69, 70, *72*, *73*, *74*, *75*, *76*, *77*, 78, *78*, *79*, *80*, *81*, *82*, 133, 134, 142, 144, *149*, *150*, *152*, 159, 160, 164, *174*, *176*, *177*, 189, 194, *199*, *201*, 208, *223*, 239, 244, 249, 265, 266, 267, *271*, *273*, *275*, *282*, 285, 286, 291, 295, 297, 299, 300, 301, 302, 307, 309, *309*, *310*, *315*, *318*, *321*, *323*, *324*, *327*, *328*, 329, *340*, 343, 352, *355*, *359*, 376, *388*, 391, 393, 395, 396, *399*, *400*, *401*, *402*
Holian A, 208, *224*
Holley LE, 59, 68, *74*
Hollingworth K, 169, *180*
Hollman GA, 167, *179*
Holloway JW, 15, *24*
Holloway L, 67, *81*
Holmes BJ, 65, *78*
Holness MA, 70, *82*
Holroyde MC, 292, 301, *316*, *323*
Holstin-Rathlou NH, 160, *175*
Holt PG, 28, 29, 40, *44*, 63, *77*, 343, 351, *355*, 359, *359*, *360*, 380, *389*
Holt PR, 165, *178*
Holtzman M, 97, *114*
Holtzman MJ, 60, *75*, 94, 99, *112*, *115*, 289, *313*
Homeyard S, 67, *80*
Honda Z, 187, *198*
Honeyman TW, 91, *108*
Hoogsteden HC, 36, 37, *49*, *50*, 63, *77*, 242, 255, *271*
Hooijer R, 38, *52*, 159, *174*, 395, 396, *400*
Hooley J, 339, *342*
Hopes E, 11, *22*
Hopkin JM, 15, *24*, 348, *358*, 380, *389*
Hopkirk A, 367, *383*
Hopp RJ, 188, 189, 191, 195, *199*, *202*
Hoppens CL, 185, *197*
Hopper J, 9, *22*
Hopper JD, 9, *22*
Hoppin GF, 32, 39, *46*
Horiba M, 294, *317*
Horie T, 185, *196*, 303, 305, *325*, *326*
Horn CR, 397, *402*
Hornbrook MM, 329, *340*
Horne SJ, 36, *49*, 65, *78*
Horowitz RI, 143, 144, *153*
Horsely MG, 96, 104, *114*
Horton CE, 298, *322*
Horzinek MC, 347, *358*
Hosaka K, 306, *327*
Hosford D, 186, *198*
Hoshiko S, 290, 291, *314*
Hoshino M, 306, *327*
Hosken NA, 350, *359*
Hosoi S, 297, *320*
Hossain S, 71, *83*
Hotaling TE, 333, *341*
Houghton C, 257, *280*
Hoult JRS, 256, *278*
House F, 298, *322*
Houslay MD, 237, 244, 245, *270*
Houston G, 162, *176*
Hovel C, 60, *75*
Howard L, 208, *224*
Howarth P, 18, *25*
Howarth PH, 35, 38, *48*, *52*, 57, 58, 59, 60, 61, 62, 64, 67, 69, *72*, *73*, *74*, *76*, *77*, *80*, *81*, 134, *150*, 160, *176*, 189, *199*, 208, *223*, 239, *271*, 285, 295, *309*, *318*, 391, 395, 396, *399*, *401*
Howarth PHG, 159, *174*
Howarth RH, 133, *149*
Howat D, 251, 257, 263, 267, *276*
Howbert J, 214, *229*
Howell CJ, 238, *270*
Howell DE, 263, *281*
Howell LL, 264, *282*
Howell RE, 91, *109*, 258, 263, 264, *280*, *281*, *282*

Howie SEM, 66, *79*
Howland W, 304, *325*
Hoyne GF, 379, *389*
Hozawa S, 190, 195, *200*, *201*, 305, *326*
Hsieh CS, 346, *357*
Hsieh KH, 190, 194, *199*, *201*
Hsieh SS, 63, *77*
Hsiue TR, 38, *51*, 218, *233*
Hsuan JJ, 239, *271*
Huang SK, 255, 257, 268, *278*, *279*, 372, 378, *386*, *388*
Huang TJ, 294, *317*
Huang XZ, 70, *81*
Huang Y, 95, 104, *113*
Hubbard WC, 298, *322*
Huber HL, 71, *83*
Huber M, 289, *313*
Huckauf H, 393, *399*
Hudak S, 238, *270*
Hudspith BN, 59, 61, *74*
Hughes B, 250, 251, 253, 257, 259, 261, 263, 267, 269, *275*, *276*, *277*, *280*
Hughes JM, 19, *26*, 158, 169, *174*
Hughes MD, 40, 42, *54*, *55*, 67, *79*, 160, *175*
Hughes P, 251, 257, 263, 267, *276*
Hugli TE, 61, *75*
Hui KP, 192, 194, *201*, 295, 301, 307, *318*, *324*
Hulks G, 365, *382*
Hulme EC, 86, *105*
Humbert M, 345, 346, *357*
Hummel S, 169, *180*
Humphrey PPA, 287, *310*
Hunninghake GW, 15, *24*, 58, 60, 61, *73*, *75*, 288, 291, *311*, *315*
Hunt L, 378, *388*
Hunt LW, 66, *79*
Hunter MK, 7, *21*
Hunter T, 7, *21*
Hurson B, 160, *175*
Hussack P, 66, *79*, 142, *153*
Husveti A, 96, *113*
Hutchinson A, 393, *399*
Hybbinette S, 294, *318*
Hyland RH, 126, 129, 135, 137, *148*
Hyma BA, 66, *79*

I

Ichikawa S, 217, *232*
Ichimura K, 303, *325*
Ichinose M, 36, 37, *49*, *50*, 208, 221, *224*, *235*, 367, *384*
Ida S, 59, *74*
Iglesia R, 192, 193, *200*
Ihre E, 242, *271*, 286, 301, *310*, *323*
Iikura Y, 211, *226*
Ikeda K, 94, *112*
Ikemura T, 186, *197*
Ikezawa K, 243, 257, *273*
Ikizler M, 37, *50*
Imai T, 220, *235*
Impens N, 301, *324*
In K, 309, *328*
in't Hout WG, 91, *108*
in't Veen JCCM, 42, *55*, 59, 66, *74*
Ind PW, 128, 131, *148*, 285, *309*, 364, *382*, 395, *401*
Ingenito EP, 39, *53*
Ingram CG, 140, *151*
Ingram DA, 217, *232*
Ingram R, 97, *114*
Ingram RH, 34, 39, *47*, *53*
Ingram RHJ, 292, *316*
Inman HMW, 143, *153*
Inman MD, 40, *53*, 396, *402*
Ino M, 186, *197*
Inobe JI, 353, *360*
Inoue H, 36, 37, *49*, *50*, 218, 221, *233*, *235*
Inoue Y, 297, *320*
Irani AMA, 57, *72*
Irvin C, 94, *112*
Irvin CG, 295, *318*
Irvin ChG, 38, *51*
Isaacs S, 96, *114*
Ishida K, 32, 33, 34, 35, *46*
Ishihara H, 89, 90, *107*
Ishihara T, 59, *74*
Ishii K, 306, *327*, 365, *382*
Ishii S, 187, *198*

Ishioka S, 190, 195, *200*, *201*, 305, *326*
Ishizaka K, 329, *340*
Ishizaka T, 329, *340*
Islam M, 100, *115*
Isogai S, 306, *327*
Israel E, 35, *48*, 161, *176*, 192, *200*, *201*, 214, *229*, 266, *283*, 294, 297, 299, 301, 303, 304, 305, 307, 308, 309, *318*, *320*, *322*, *323*, *325*, *326*, *327*, *328*, 364, *381*
Israel I, 299, 300, 301, 302, 307, 308, *322*
Itabashi S, 91, *109*
Itkin IH, 156, *172*
Ito K, 187, *198*
Ito Y, 93, 94, *111*
Itoh K, 194, *201*, 305, *326*
Ives JL, 251, *276*
Ivonnet P, 89, *106*
Iwamota P, 58, *73*
Izumi T, 187, *198*, 288, *312*

J

Jabbal I, 67, *81*
Jacboson M, 57, *72*
Jack RM, 289, *312*
Jackson J, 238, *270*
Jackson R, 143, 144, *153*
Jacob CO, 255, 268, *278*
Jacobitz S, 248, *275*
Jacobs F, 99, *115*
Jacobs L, 100, *116*
Jacoby D, 95, 99, 104, *113*, *115*
Jacoby DB, 37, 38, *50*, *51*, *52*, 93, 94, 95, 96, 100, *111*, *112*, *113*, *116*
Jacques L, 126, 129, 135, 137, *148*, 364, *382*
Jacques LA, 131, *149*
Jaeger EA, 167, *179*
Jaeschke R, 397, *402*
Jager R, 185, *196*
Jahnke V, 212, *227*
Jaklitsch H, 264, *282*
Jakobsson PJ, 289, 290, *313*, *314*
Jakschik BA, 288, *311*
James A, 10, *22*, 31, 33, 35, *45*, *46*, *48*
James AL, 32, 35, 36, *46*, *48*, *49*
James S, 92, *110*
James SD, 29, *44*
James T, 251, 253, 257, 261, 263, 267, 269, *276*, *277*
Jan Roorda RJ, 164, *177*
Janicki S, 303, *325*
Janiga KE, 35, *47*
Jankowski R, 105, *118*
Jansen CCM, 398, *403*
Jansen MAM, 41, *55*
Janssen LJ, 91, *109*
Jappy J, 248, *275*
Jardieu P, 330, 331, 332, 333, 339, *340*, *341*, *342*
Jardieu PM, 339, *342*
Jarjour NN, 60, *75*, 298, *321*
Jarnigan F, 89, *106*
Jarreau PH, 218, *233*
Jarvholm B, 393, *399*
Jarvinen M, 160, 161, *175*, *176*
Jarvis D, 2, 4, *20*, 208, *223*
Jawed SJ, 268, *283*
Jeffery P, 71, *82*
Jeffery PJ, 57, 64, *72*
Jeffery PK, 27, 36, 37, 38, *44*, *49*, *50*, *52*, 57, 69, *72*, *73*, *81*, 395, 396, *401*
Jenkins A, 162, *176*
Jenkins CR, 160, *176*
Jenkins LP, 263, *281*
Jenne J, 104, *117*
Jennings B, 162, *176*
Jenouri G, 36, *49*
Jensen MW, 32, *45*, 125, 140, *147*
Jenson T, 162, *177*
Jeppson A, 120, *146*
Jhall N, 67, *80*
Jhalli N, 159, 170, *174*
Jiang E, 34, 39, *47*
Jick H, 146, *154*
Johannson SA, 239, *271*
Johansen BV, 17, *25*
Johansen TE, 214, *228*
Johansson S, 71, *82*
Johansson SG, 13, *23*
John M, 372, 374, *386*

Johnsen HE, 243, 257, *273*
Johnson D, 104, *117*
Johnson JL, 251, *276*
Johnson L, 166, *178*
Johnson M, 121, 141, *147*, *152*
Johnson ME, 133, *149*
Johnson NM, 59, 61, *74*
Johnson PRA, 212, *226*, 367, *383*
Johnson RL, 394, *400*
Johnson WJ, 166, *178*
Johnston CC, 166, *178*
Johnston K, 296, *319*
Johnston M, 122, *147*
Johnston PR, 126, 129, *148*
Johnston S, 100, *116*
Johnston SL, 15, *24*, 194, *201*, 393, *400*
Jones A, 12, *23*
Jones AC, 12, *23*
Jones CA, 90, 91, *108*, *109*
Jones D, 4, *21*
Jones KA, 34, 39, *47*
Jones PW, 397, 398, *402*, *403*
Jones RE, 288, *310*
Jones T, 393, *399*
Jones TR, 214, *229*, 259, *280*, *281*, 301, *323*, 362, 367, *381*, *384*
Jong BM, 129, 131, 135, *149*
Jonkers GJ, 266, *283*
Jonsson B, 398, *403*
Joos G, 30, 31, 40, *45*, 210, 221, *225*, *235*, 395, *401*
Joos GF, 203, 204, 209, 210, 211, 212, 214, 215, 216, 221, *223*, *224*, *225*, *226*, *230*, *231*, 299, 301, *323*, *324*
Joos L, 125, 140, *147*
Jordan CC, 212, *226*
Jordan JE, 214, *229*
Jordan R, 253, 260, 261, 263, 269, *277*
Jordan SE, 67, *70*, *80*, *81*, 159, 170, *174*
Jordana M, 380, *389*
Joris I, 293, *317*
Jorres R, 125, 133, *147*
Jorres RA, 303, *325*
Jose PJ, 239, *271*
Joseph DR, 246, *274*
Josephs L, 393, *400*
Josephs LK, 41, *54*, 393, *400*
Jubber AS, 36, *50*
Judd M, 62, *76*
Julia-Serda G, 97, *114*
June CH, 63, *76*
Jung K, 61, *76*
Jung S, 251, *276*, 375, *387*
Jungerwirth S, 301, *323*
Junien JL, 263, *281*
Juniper E, 97, *114*
Juniper EF, 30, 31, 36, 37, *44*, 160, *175*, 297, 298, *321*, 394, 397, *400*, *402*

K

Kaczorowski GJ, 362, 366, 367, *381*, *383*, *384*
Kaegi MK, 38, *52*
Kagey-Sobotka A, 105, *118*, 255, 257, 265, 268, 269, *278*, *279*, *282*, 298, *322*, 378, *388*
Kageyama N, 221, *235*
Kagoshima M, 186, 195, *198*
Kahari VM, 71, *83*
Kahn RM, 38, *52*
Kaiser H, 105, *118*
Kako K, 306, *327*
Kalberg C, 141, *152*
Kalden JR, 371, *386*
Kaliner J, 101, *117*
Kaliner M, 89, 90, *107*, 205, *223*, 293, *317*
Kaliner MA, 61, *76*, 208, *224*
Kalinski P, 351, *359*
Kalra S, 333, 336, 338, *341*
Kaltreider HB, 217, *232*
Kamada AK, 169, *180*
Kambayashi T, 255, 268, *278*
Kaminsky DA, 296, 306, 307, *319*
Kaminuma O, 243, 257, *273*
Kamio Y, 295, *318*
Kammerman S, 242, *272*
Kamogawa Y, 344, *356*
Kampe M, 71, *82*
Kanazawa M, 305, *326*

Kane GC, 306, *326*
Kaneko T, 243, 256, *272*
Kanner RE, 41, *55*, 394, *400*
Kanno T, 93, *111*
Kanters D, 371, *385*
Kao BM, 214, *229*
Kaplan AP, 346, *357*
Kaplan HR, 247, 252, *274*
Kaplan MA, 156, *172*
Kaprio J, 9, *22*
Kapsenberg ML, 346, 351, *358*, *359*, 372, *386*
Kargacin ME, 91, *108*
Kargman S, 288, *310*, *311*
Karin M, 158, *173*, 369, 373, *384*
Karla S, 140, 141, *151*
Karlsson JA, 209, 220, *225*, *235*, 248, 251, 253, 254, 256, 257, 260, 261, 263, 269, *275*, *276*, *277*
Karlsson SED, 71, *82*
Karpel J, 104, *118*
Karrison T, 17, 18, *25*
Karrnaus W, 17, *25*
Kase H, 89, 90, *107*
Kashiwamura S, 371, *386*
Kassam N, 372, *386*
Kassel O, 62, *76*, 285, *309*
Kastelein R, 347, 351, *358*
Kastner S, 289, *313*
Kastumata U, 36, *49*
Katada T, 243, 256, *272*
Katai H, 70, *82*
Katayama H, 187, *198*
Kato M, 158, *174*
Katsumata U, 37, *50*
Kattan M, 18, *26*
Kauffman HF, 91, *109*
Kauffman HG, 57, 59, *74*, 256, 257, *279*
Kauffman HK, 133, *149*
Kaufman HS, 343, *355*
Kaulbach HC, 208, *224*
Kaulen P, 264, *282*
Kaur B, 2, *20*
Kava T, 69, *81*, 160, 161, *175*, *176*
Kawahara MS, 61, *75*
Kawano O, 37, *51*
Kay AB, 31, 37, 38, *45*, *50*, *52*, 57, 58, 59, 61, 62, 64, 67, 69, 70, *72*, *73*, *77*, *80*, *81*, 158, *174*, 238, *270*, 285, 295, 297, *309*, *318*, *319*, *321*, 345, 346, 352, *356*, *357*, 378, *388*, 395, 396, *401*
Kayahara H, 187, *198*
Kaye MG, 189, *199*, 294, *317*
Kayembe JM, 189, *199*
Kays JS, 215, *230*
Kazim F, 104, *117*
Keane A, 143, *153*
Keane-Myers AM, 63, *77*
Keene ON, 137, *150*
Keil U, 2, 19, *20*, *26*
Keith TP, 309, *328*
Kellaway CH, 289, *312*
Kelleher C, 18, *25*
Keller H, 291, *315*
Kelly CA, 185, *196*, 298, *322*
Kelly E, 38, *52*
Kelly JJ, 257, *279*
Kelly L, 99, *115*
Kelso A, 345, *356*
Kelvin D, 65, *78*
Kemeny DM, 65, *78*
Kemp AS, 12, *23*
Kemp J, 141, *152*, 303, 304, 309, *324*, *325*, *328*
Kemp JP, 126, 129, 135, 137, *148*, 162, *176*, 299, 303, *322*
Kennedy BP, 291, *314*
Kennedy I, 287, *310*
Kennedy T, 95, 104, *113*
Kent DC, 99, *115*
Kephart G, 95, *113*
Kephart GM, 59, 66, 68, *74*, *79*
Keppler D, 289, *313*
Kepron W, 94, *112*
Kerrebijn KF, 40, *54*, 141, *152*, 160, 164, *175*, *178*, 395, *401*
Kerrebijn KJ, 164, *177*
Kerrebjin KF, 129, 141, *148*
Kerstjens HAM, 29, 42, *44*, *55*, 67, *79*, 165, *178*, 395, *401*
Kessler GF, 100, *115*

Kesten S, 126, 129, 135, 137, *148*
Kester MH, 256, *278*
Kesterson J, 192, *201*, 295, *318*
Kestin S, 166, *178*
Khamzina L, 291, *315*
Khan MA, 291, *315*
Khani J, 397, *402*
Kharitonov S, 42, *55*
Kharitonov SA, 140, 141, *151*, 159, *174*, 369, *384*, 396, *402*
Khawaja A, 89, 90, *107*
Khimenko P, 92, *110*
Kidney JC, 192, *200*, 367, *383*
Kiff RJ, 369, *384*
Kiger JA, 246, *274*
Kijne AM, 289, *313*
Kikawa Y, 297, *320*
Kikkawa H, 243, 257, *273*
Kilbinger H, 93, *111*
Kilchherr E, 43, *55*, 333, *341*
Kiley JP, 394, *400*
Kilfeather S, 265, 266, 267, *282*
Killingsworth CR, 93, 94, *111*, *112*, 209, *224*
Kim AL, 93, *111*
Kim C, 306, *326*
Kim JW, 351, *359*
Kim SW, 309, *328*
Kimmitt P, 346, *357*
Kimura I, 190, *200*
Kimura K, 36, 37, *49*, *50*
King C, 332, 333, *341*
King CG, 39, *53*
King S, 2, *20*
King VG, 366, *383*
Kingaby R, 251, 257, 263, 267, *276*
Kings MA, 239, *271*
Kingston WP, 185, *196*, 298, *322*
Kinnier WJ, 264, *282*
Kino M, 185, *196*
Kips JC, 203, 204, 210, 214, 215, 216, 221, *223*, *225*, *230*, *231*, 299, 301, *323*, *324*, 396, *402*
Kirby DS, 268, *283*
Kirby JG, 58, 61, *73*
Kirkpatrick C, 88, *106*
Kishimoto S, 187, *198*
Kishimoto T, 371, *386*
Kishiyama JL, 217, *232*
Kita H, 378, *388*
Kiuchi H, 190, *200*, 303, *325*
Kiviranta K, 160, 161, *175*, *176*
Kjellman NIM, 343, *355*
Klaassen BM, 92, *110*
Klapproth H, 88, *106*
Klareskog L, 263, 268, *281*
Klassen BM, 89, 92, *107*
Klein J, 290, *314*
Klein JS, 209, *224*
Kliewer S, 158, *173*
Klim JB, 398, *403*
Kline PA, 160, *175*, 297, *321*, 393, *399*
Klinek MM, 308, *328*
Klink M, 11, *22*
Kluin Nelemans JC, 58, *73*
Kmetz P, 246, *274*
Knight A, 126, 129, 135, 137, *148*
Knight JA, 379, *389*
Knol EF, 257, *279*
Knol K, 40, *54*, 160, *175*
Knoller J, 289, *312*
Knowles G, 57, 64, *72*
Knowles RG, 369, *384*
Knox AJ, 34, 35, *47*, 141, *152*
Knox AP, 265, *282*
Knox RB, 17, *25*
Knudsen TE, 243, 257, *273*
Kobayashi DK, 71, *83*
Kobayashi H, 305, *326*
Kobayashi T, 293, *317*
Kobayashi Y, 185, *196*
Kobylarz DC, 245, *273*
Kobylarz-Singer DC, 247, 252, *274*
Kobzik L, 37, *51*
Koch B, 185, *196*
Kocher O, 308, *328*
Koe BK, 251, *276*
Koelsche GA, 155, *172*
Koenderman BL, 191, *200*
Koenderman L, 352, *359*, 371, *385*
Koenig JQ, 191, *200*
Koessler KK, 71, *83*

Koeter G, 129, *149*
Koeter GH, 29, 40, 41, *44*, *54*, *55*, 133, *149*, 160, 165, *175*, *178*, 395, *401*
Kohge S, 186, 195, *198*
Kohl A, 141, *152*
Kohno S, 186, *198*, 294, *317*
Kok PT, 289, *313*
Kok PTM, 191, *200*
Kok-Jensen A, 128, *148*
Kolb JP, 291, *315*
Kolendovic R, 58, *73*
Koller E, 100, *115*
Koller M, 289, *312*
Koltai M, 186, *198*
Konderman L, 371, *385*
Kondo M, 305, *326*
Konig P, 157, 166, *173*, *178*
Konig W, 289, *312*
Konno K, 90, 104, *107*, 305, *326*
Kopferschmitt MC, 398, *403*
Kopp C, 128, *148*
Korley V, 299, *322*
Kornfeld H, 352, *359*
Kornfield H, 64, *77*, *78*
Korts D, 105, *118*
Koskenvou M, 9, *22*
Koskinen S, 160, 161, *175*, *176*
Kotake Y, 374, *387*
Kotlikoff MI, 362, 365, *381*
Koto H, 37, *50*, 218, *233*
Kotsimbos TC, 36, 41, *49*
Kowash K, 299, *322*
Koyama S, 303, *325*
Kraan J, 40, *54*, 160, *175*
Kraft M, 43, *56*, 66, 78, *79*, 134, *150*, 396, *402*
Kramps JA, 36, 39, *48*
Kraneveld AD, 218, *234*
Kraus KG, 265, 269, *282*
Krause JE, 203, *223*
Krauss AH, 295, *319*
Krauss B, 374, *387*
Krausz T, 208, *224*
Krazonwski JJ, 257, *279*
Kreisman H, 126, 129, *148*
Krell RD, 214, *229*, 289, *312*
Kresten W, 100, *116*
Kreukniet J, 187, *198*
Kreutner W, 43, *55*, 371, *385*
Krishna MT, 61, *76*, 244, *273*
Krishnaswamy G, 348, 349, *358*
Krivi G, 288, *311*
Kroegel C, 217, *231*
Kroeger EA, 94, *112*
Kroes ACM, 37, *50*
Krouwels FH, 160, *175*
Krska K, 63, *77*
Kruithof B, 347, *358*
Kruse N, 371, *385*
Krzanowski JJ, 248, 252, 257, *275*, *276*, *279*
Kubo K, 66, *79*
Kubo T, 91, *108*
Kubota K, 137, 143, *150*
Kuchroo VK, 351, 353, *359*, *360*
Kudo S, 305, *326*
Kuehl F, 242, 256, *272*
Kuehr J, 395, *401*
Kuhn R, 347, *358*
Kuhr J, 17, *25*
Kuijper PHM, 352, *359*
Kuijpers EA, 32, *45*
Kuijpers EAP, 37, *51*, 215, *230*
Kuitert L, 286, 294, *309*
Kuitert LM, 194, *201*
Kukler J, 160, *175*
Kullmann M, 374, *387*
Kumar R, 166, *178*
Kume H, 362, 365, *381*
Kumlin M, 242, *271*, 286, 291, 296, 301, 303, *310*, *315*, *320*, *323*, *325*
Kummer W, 219, *234*
Kuna P, 346, *357*
Kundu S, 303, 305, *324*, *326*
Kunkel G, 208, 212, *224*, *227*, 266, *283*
Kunkel S, 65, *78*
Kunkel SL, 352, *359*
Kuo H, 367, *384*
Kuramitsu K, 303, *325*
Kurihara K, 295, *319*
Kurimoto F, 191, *200*
Kurimoto M, 347, *358*

Kurosawa M, 36, *48*, 191, *200*, 306, *327*
Kuwano K, 34, *47*, 395, *401*
Kwon OJ, 205, 217, *223*, *232*
Kwong T, 135, 143, 144, *150*, *153*
Kylstra JW, 306, *327*

L

la Rocca AM, 43, *55*
Labasi JM, 255, 268, *278*
Laberge S, 64, *78*
Lackie JM, 290, *314*
Lackie PM, 69, *81*
Lacoste JY, 57, 64, 65, 71, *73*, *77*, *82*, 396, *402*
Lacour M, 257, *279*
Ladenius AR, 218, *233*
Laduron PM, 213, *227*
Laemont K, 91, *109*
Laforce C, 126, 129, 135, 137, *148*
Laforce CF, 333, 336, *341*
Lafuma C, 218, *233*
Lag M, 15, *24*
Lagente V, 38, *51*, 204, 213, 216, 218, *223*, *231*, *232*, *233*, 254, 257, 263, *277*, *279*, *281*
Lahr S, 333, *341*
Lai CK, 189, *199*
Lai CKW, 57, *72*, 285, *309*
Lai E, 2, 4, *20*
Laitinen A, 69, 71, *81*, *82*, *83*, 159, *174*, 286, 296, 305, *309*, *319*, 396, *401*, *402*
Laitinen LA, 69, 71, *81*, *82*, *83*, 100, *116*, 159, 160, 161, *174*, *175*, *176*, 286, 296, 305, *309*, *319*, 376, *388*, 393, 396, *399*, *401*, *402*
Lake C, 155, *172*
Lakshminarayan S, 104, *118*
Laliberte G, 104, *118*
Lalloo UG, 220, *235*
Lam BK, 288, 289, 291, 309, *311*, *312*, *314*, *315*, *328*
Lam S, 60, *75*, 185, *196*, 297, *321*
Lamb J, 380, *389*
Lamb JR, 379, *389*
Lambert RK, 34, 35, *47*, *48*, 395, *401*
Lambert RY, 33, 35, *46*
Lammers J, 91, *108*
Lammers JW, 190, *199*, 371, *385*
Lammers JWJ, 38, *51*, 92, 96, *110*, *113*, 301, *324*, 371, *385*
Lampe F, 393, *400*
Lampe FC, 67, *81*
Lampert SI, 167, *179*
Lancaster J, 304, 308, *325*
Landau LI, 164, *178*
Landi M, 213, *228*
Landry Y, 91, 92, *108*
Lang PG, 268, *283*
Lange P, 71, *83*
Langley SJ, 137, 138, *151*
Lanni C, 288, 295, *311*, *319*
Lanser K, 100, *115*
Lanzavecchio A, 353, *360*
LaRosa G, 372, *386*
Larsen CS, 243, 257, *273*
Larsen G, 94, 104, *112*, *117*
Larsen GL, 38, *51*, 60, *74*, 93, 94, *111*, 259, *280*, 296, *319*, *320*
Larsson C, 301, 303, *323*, *325*
Larsson E, 263, 268, *281*
Larsson K, 39, *53*
Larsson P, 125, *147*, 163, 170, *177*
Larsson S, 142, *152*
Laszlo F, 369, *384*
Latimer K, 97, *114*, 160, *175*
Latimer KM, 160, *175*
Lau LC, 302, *324*
Lau-Schadendorf S, 18, *25*
Laubscher K, 142, *152*
Laude EA, 220, *234*
Laurent F, 368, *384*
Laurent GJ, 217, *232*
Laurenzi MA, 217, *232*
Lavaruso RB, 289, *312*
Lavender E, 367, *383*
Lavender EA, 367, *383*
Lavidette M, 134, *150*
Lavielle S, 213, 214, *228*
Lavins BJ, 295, 296, 302, 306, *318*, *319*, *324*

Laviolette M, 37, *50*, 333, 336, 338, *341*
Lawson KA, 398, *403*
Lawton PJ, 195, *202*
Lazarus SC, 60, *75*, 302, *324*, 364, *381*
Lazer L, 125, *147*
Le Fur G, 210, 213, 215, *225*, *227*, *228*
Le Gros G, 15, *24*, 65, *78*
Le Gros GG, 345, *356*
Leahy BC, 96, *114*
Lebel LA, 251, *276*
Lebel SW, 213, *227*
Leblanc P, 126, 129, *148*
Lebowitz MD, 393, *400*
Ledda F, 218, *233*
Ledered JA, 348, *358*
Ledford D, 309, *328*
Lee CW, 289, *313*
Lee F, 158, *174*
Lee LY, 94, *112*, 214, *229*
Lee NH, 100, *116*
Lee TH, 5, *21*, 61, 64, *76*, *77*, 185, *196*, 238, 265, 266, 267, *270*, *282*, 292, 294, 296, 297, 298, 299, 303, 305, *316*, *317*, *319*, *320*, *322*, *323*, *325*, 367, *383*
Lee WW, 41, *55*
Leeb B, 371, *386*
Leeder SR, 1, *20*, 167, *179*
Leen MG, 18, *25*
Leesnitzer MA, 251, *276*
Lefcoe NM, 157, 162, *172*, *176*
Lefebvre RA, 212, 215, *226*, *230*
Leff A, 94, *112*
Leff AR, 34, 37, 38, 39, *47*, *50*, *51*, *52*, 214, 217, 218, *229*, *232*, *233*
Leff JA, 303, 305, 306, *324*, *326*, *327*
Lefkowitz RJ, 137, *151*
Lefort J, 238, *271*
Legente V, 218, *234*
Leger S, 288, *311*
Lehnigk B, 300, *323*
Lehrer SB, 339, *342*
Lehtonen K, 160, 161, *175*, *176*
Lehtonen L, 169, *180*
Lei HY, 216, *230*
Lei M, 33, *46*
Lei YH, 215, *230*
Leikauf GD, 290, 294, *314*, *318*
Leitch GA, 60, *75*
Lelloch-Tubiana A, 238, *271*
LeLorier J, 167, *179*
Lemaire I, 291, *315*
Lemanske R, 94, 99, *112*
Lemanske RF, 38, *51*, 164, 167, *178*, *179*
Lemen RJ, 36, *48*
Lemke SM, 365, *382*
Lemoine H, 141, *152*
Lenfant C, 146, *154*
Lengel D, 214, *229*
Lenschow DJ, 350, 351, 353, *359*
Leonard C, 36, *49*, 65, *78*
Leonard EJ, 255, *277*
Leone DR, 379, *389*
LeRiche JC, 60, *75*, 297, *321*
Lester P, 333, *341*
Letarte M, 205, *223*
Letterio JJ, 354, *360*
Letts G, 301, *323*
Leuenberger P, 189, *199*
Leung DYM, 43, *56*, 65, 66, 67, 71, *79*, *80*, 155, *172*
Leung KBP, 59, 61, *74*, 212, *226*
Leveille C, 288, *311*
Levey AI, 93, *111*
Levine BB, 348, *359*
Levine C, 166, *178*
Levine E, 71, *83*
Levine JD, 217, *232*
Levine M, 88, *106*
Levine MA, 90, 91, *107*
Levinson H, 104, *117*
Levy GP, 287, *310*
Levy ML, 169, *180*
Lewis LD, 167, *179*
Lewis R, 292, *316*
Lewis RA, 289, 292, 293, 298, *313*, *316*, *317*, *322*
Lewis S, 2, 13, *20*, *23*, 129, 131, 135, *149*
Lewis SA, 253, 260, 261, 263, 269, *276*
Ley TJ, 71, *83*

Leyravaud S, 185, *197*
Li C, 268, *283*, 288, *311*
Li JCL, 164, *178*
Li M, 92, *109*, *110*
Li X, 36, *49*, 70, 71, *82*, *83*, 372, *386*
Li Y, 263, 265, *281*
Lianos EA, 289, *313*
Liberati N, 214, *229*
Lichtenfels R, 263, *281*
Lichtenstein L, 105, *118*
Lichtenstein LM, 60, *74*, 241, 242, 254, 255, 257, 268, *271*, *278*, *279*, 289, 298, *313*, *322*, 339, *342*, 378, *388*
Lichtman AH, 348, *358*
Liddle RF, 126, 129, 135, 137, *148*
Liekreski ES, 61, *75*
Liew FY, 369, *384*
Liggett S, 11, *22*
Liggett W, 290, *314*
Lilja G, 13, *23*
Lilly CM, 37, *51*, 192, *201*, 208, 214, *224*, *229*, 297, 299, *320*, *322*
Lim S, 372, 374, *386*
Linaker C, 144, *154*
Linden A, 120, 122, 123, 136, *146*, *147*, 219, *234*
Linden M, 239, *271*
Lindgren JA, 287, *310*
Lindley IJD, 66, *79*
Lindsay G, 70, *82*
Linscott V, 142, *152*
Liou HC, 375, *387*
Lipsky JJ, 378, *389*
Lipson E, 89, *106*
Lipworth BJ, 137, 138, 140, *151*, 163, 168, 169, 170, *177*, *180*
Lisel H, 251, 257, 263, 267, *276*
List SJ, 67, *81*
Litchfield T, 64, *77*
Little JW, 100, *116*
Little L, 61, *76*
Little SA, 369, *385*
Littlejohns P, 397, *402*
Liu J, 58, *73*, 333, *341*
Liu JT, 333, 336, 337, *341*, 352, *359*, 379, *389*
Liu MC, 298, 304, 308, *322*, *325*
Liu S, 332, 333, *341*
Liu X, 34, 39, *47*
Livi GP, 246, 248, *274*, *275*
Llenas J, 250, 258, *275*, *280*
Lloyd A, 65, *78*
Lloyd AR, 372, *386*
Llupia J, 250, *275*
Loader JE, 93, 94, *111*
Lobb RR, 95, *113*, 379, *389*
Lockhart A, 266, *283*
Loegering DA, 59, 69, *74*, 94, *112*
Lofdahl CG, 120, 131, 136, 142, *146*, *149*, *152*, 305, *326*, 364, *382*, 393, 398, *400*
Lofquist AK, 158, *173*
Loftus BG, 18, *25*
Lohning M, 346, *357*
Lois R, 266, *283*
Long A, 64, *77*, 352, *359*
Long-Fox A, 268, *283*
Longo KP, 213, *227*
Loper M, 301, *323*
Lopez AF, 295, *318*, 345, 352, *356*
Lopez M, 36, *49*
Lorentzen J, 263, 268, *281*
Lorimer S, 71, *82*
Loschmann PA, 263, *281*
Lotvall J, 125, *147*
Lotvall JO, 36, 37, *48*, *50*
Lotz M, 217, *232*
Lou UP, 214, *229*
Lou YP, 214, *229*
Lougheed D, 31, 41, *45*, *54*
Lougheed MD, 31, 37, *45*
Loughney K, 245, *274*
Louis R, 58, 59, 60, 61, 64, 66, *73*, *79*, 188, 189, *199*
Louis RE, 190, *200*
Louw SJ, 96, *114*
Lowe JA, 213, 214, *227*, *228*, 251, *276*
Lowell F, 100, *116*
Lowhagen O, 125, 133, *148*
Lubs ML, 9, *22*
Lucas RA, 301, *324*

Lucchesi A, 91, *108*
Luce BR, 398, *403*
Luchtel DL, 191, *200*
Luczynsak C, 2, *20*
Ludwig JC, 185, *197*
Luengo M, 166, *178*
Luio R, 333, *341*
Luisi BF, 158, *173*
Lukacs N, 65, *78*
Lukacs NW, 352, *359*
Lukert BP, 165, *178*
Lumb RH, 186, *197*
Lumb S, 251, 257, 263, 267, *276*
Lumley P, 287, *310*
Lundback B, 131, 137, *149*, *150*, 169, *180*, 364, *382*
Lundberg JM, 203, 204, 205, 207, 209, 212, 214, *222*, *223*, *225*, *227*, *229*
Lundberg JP, 220, *235*
Lunde H, 221, *235*
Lungarella G, 71, *83*
Lunn A, 18, *25*
Luria X, 266, *283*
Luts A, 207, *223*
Luttmann MA, 369, *385*
Lynch DA, 71, *83*
Lynch JR, 11, *22*
Lyon R, 339, *342*
Lyons H, 101, *117*

M

Ma W, 379, *389*
Maas KL, 96, *114*
Maayan CH, 162, *177*
Macatonia SE, 63, *77*, 346, 347, *357*, *358*
Macaubas C, 354, 359, *360*
Macchia L, 291, *315*
MacCoss M, 216, *231*
MacDermot J, 242, 255, *271*
MacDonald D, 259, 267 269, *280*
Macduff BM, 345, *357*
Macfarlane JD, 371, *386*
MacGlashan DW, 60, *74*, 241, 242, 254, *271*, 289, *313*, 339, *342*
Mackay CR, 353, *360*, 372, *386*
Mackay TW, 66, 71, *79*
Macklem PT, 29, 31, 32, 33, 34, 35, 37, 39, 41, *44*, *45*, *46*, *47*, *54*, 395, *401*
Maclagan J, 92, 93, 98, 99, 102, *110*, *111*, *114*, 211, *226*
Maclean DB, 221, *235*
MacLeod D, 265, 266, 267, *282*
Macmillan R, 299, *323*
Macmillan S, 368, *384*
Maconochie JG, 137, *150*
Macquin-Mavier I, 218, *233*
Macri F, 12, *23*
Madden J, 67, 70, *80*, *82*
Madison J, 91, *108*
Madison JM, 90, 91, *108*, *109*
Madri J, 343, *355*
Madsen F, 41, *54*, 160, *175*
Maeda A, 91, *108*
Maes RK, 94, *112*
Maesen BLP, 127, *148*
Maesen FPV, 125, *147*, 366, *383*, 398, *403*
Maeson F, 104, *118*
Maestrelli P, 57, *73*
Maffrand JP, 213, *228*
Maggi CA, 204, 209, 213, 214, 215, 218, 219, *223*, *224*, *227*, *228*, *229*, *230*, *233*, *234*
Maggi E, 65, *78*
Magnussen H, 34, 39, *47*, 122, 125, 133, *147*, 242, *272*, 300, 303, *323*, *325*
Magram J, 346, 348, *357*, *358*
Mahesh VK, 91, *108*
Mahmoud AAF, 332, 333, *341*
Maikoe T, 352, *359*
Maini RN, 268, *283*, 371, *386*
Mairon N, 120, *146*
Maisel AS, 257, *279*
Maisiak R, 397, *402*
Maj J, 205, *223*
Majima T, 303, *325*
Majno G, 293, *317*
Majumdar S, 71, *82*
Mak J, 89, 90, 91, *107*, *108*

Mak JCW, 88, 89, 90, 91, 92, *106*, *107*, *110*, 137, *151*, 366, *383*
Makajima N, 221, *235*
Makino S, 37, *50*, 187, 194, *198*, *201*
Makker HK, 38, *52*, 302, *324*
Malaviya R, 288, *311*
Malhotra I, 332, 333, *341*
Maliszewski CR, 345, *357*
Malkiel S, 155, *172*
Malmberg P, 39, *53*
Malo JL, 30, 31, 36, 37, 42, *44*, *49*, 125, 126, 129, 131, 135, 137, 140, *147*, *148*, *149*, 169, *180*, 297, 298, *321*, 394, *400*
Malone DC, 398, *403*
Malone T, 246, *274*
Maloney C, 166, *178*
Maltby N, 296, *320*
Maltby NH, 289, 296, *313*, *320*
Manara L, 213, *228*
Mancilla E, 95, 104, *113*
Mancini JA, 288, 291, *311*, *314*
Manetti R, 65, *78*
Mani R, 60, *75*
Manickam S, 208, *224*
Mann NM, 143, *153*
Mann RD, 137, 143, *150*
Manning AM, 373, 375, *387*
Manning CD, 257, *279*
Manning PJ, 302, *324*
Manolitsas ND, 67, 70, *80*, *81*, 159, 170, *174*
Mansmann H, 304, *325*
Mansmann HC, 167, *179*
Mant TGK, 61, *76*
Mantyh PW, 203, *223*
Manzini S, 213, 214, 215, 217, 218, 219, *227*, *229*, *230*, *232*, *233*, *234*
Mappe CE, 57, *73*
Marasco WA, 217, *231*
Marchandeau C, 374, *387*
Marchant J, 162, *177*
Marchette B, 293, *317*
Marfat A, 265, 269, *282*, 292, *316*
Margolskee D, 304, *325*
Margolskee DJ, 301, 302, 303, *324*, *325*
Marin M, 89, *106*, *107*
Marin MG, 61, *76*
Marini J, 104, *118*
Marini M, 8, *22*
Mark TW, 160, *175*
Markendorf A, 296, *320*
Markov AE, 166, 167, *178*, *179*
Marks R, 353, *360*
Marleau S, 239, *271*
Marom Z, 293, *317*
Marone G, 187, *198*
Marrades R, 192, 193, *200*
Marrelli F, 58, 59, 60, 61, 64, 66, *73*
Marron BE, 251, *276*
Marsac J, 398, *403*
Marsh DG, 11, *22*, 348, 349, *358*
Marshall PJ, 263, *281*
Martelli AN, 41, *54*
Marthan R, 210, *225*
Martin AJ, 164, *178*
Martin B, 397, *402*
Martin CAE, 214, 215, *229*, *230*, 244, 261, *273*
Martin D, 372, *386*
Martin DP, 396, 397, *402*
Martin JG, 32, 33, 39, *46*, *52*, *53*, 294, *317*
Martin MG, 32, *46*
Martin N, 9, *22*
Martin R, 11, *22*, 101, *117*, 263, *281*
Martin RJ, 43, *56*, 65, 66, 67, 71, 78, *79*, *80*, 158, *174*, 296, 306, 307, *319*, 372, *386*, 396, *402*
Martin RR, 35, *47*
Martin TR, 288, *312*, 396, 397, *402*
Martin W, 244, *273*
Martinez F, 11, *22*, 329, *340*
Martinez FD, 11, 12, 13, 19, *22*, *23*, *26*
Martins MA, 257, *279*
Martins T, 245, 247, *274*, *275*
Martling CR, 205, 207, 209, *223*, *225*
Maruo S, 347, 351, *358*
Mary D, 243, 257, *273*
Masamune H, 265, 269, *282*
Mascali JJ, 158, *174*
Maslen C, 248, 251, 256, 257, *275*

Maslen T, 169, *180*
Mason RJ, 286, *310*
Massarella GR, 69, 78, *81*
Masson P, 214, *229*, 301, *323*
Masterton CM, 137, 138, *151*
Mastronarde JG, 15, *24*
Masuda T, 89, 90, *107*
Mathieu M, 380, *389*
Mathur pN, 266, *283*
Maticardi PM, 15, *24*
Matsos G, 194, *201*
Matsuda T, 294, 295, *317*, *318*
Matsui K, 306, *327*
Matsumoto M, 186, *197*, 371, *386*
Matsumoto S, 93, *111*, 295, *318*
Matsumoto T, 288, 290, *310*, *314*
Matsuse T, 218, *233*
Matsuzaki M, 187, *198*
Matsuzawa Y, 66, *79*
Matthaei KI, 352, *359*
Matthay MA, 288, *312*
Matthews JK, 254, 258, 261, 263, 269, *277*, *280*
Matthews S, 13, 18, *23*
Mattoli S, 8, *22*
Matzinger P, 63, *77*
Mauser PJ, 43, *55*, 371, *385*
Maxwell DL, 210, *225*
Mayheno AN, 378, *388*
Maytum CK, 155, *172*
Mazurek N, 255, 268, *278*
Mazza JA, 126, 129, 135, 137, *148*, 169, *180*
McAllister K, 217, *232*
McAulay A, 67, *80*, 159, 170, *174*
McAulay AE, 70, *81*
McAuliffe M, 259, 267 269, *280*, *281*
McBride DE, 191, *200*
McBurney J, 305, *326*
McCaffrey T, 89, *106*
McCaig DJ, 94, *111*
McCain RW, 291, *315*
McCants ML, 339, *342*
McCarthy DS, 71, *83*
McColl E, 393, *399*
McColl SR, 291, *314*, *315*
McConnell RT, 255, 268, *278*
McConnochie KM, 13, *23*
McCrea KE, 244, *273*
McCubbin MM, 168, *179*
McCusker M, 38, *51*, 92, *110*, 190, *199*
McCusker MT, 96, *113*
McDevitt DG, 137, 138, *151*
McDonald D, 217, *232*
McDonald DM, 87, *106*
McDonald PP, 291, *314*, *315*
McDougall C, 11, *22*
McFadden CA, 294, 304, *318*
McFadden E, 97, 99, *114*, *115*
McFadden ER, 60, *75*, 285, 292, *309*, *316*
McFadden ERJ, 292, *316*
McFadden ETL, 101, *117*
McFarlane C, 259, 267 269, *280*, 301, *323*
McFarlane CS, 259, *281*
McGeady SJ, 167, *179*
McGee J, 290, *314*
McGill KA, 308, *328*
McGrath JL, 32, *45*, 266, *283*
McGregor GP, 210, 219, *225*, *234*
McGue M, 9, *22*
McGuire JC, 290, *314*
McHale MM, 246, *274*
McIntyre TM, 185, 186, *197*, 293, *317*
McIvor RA, 142, *153*
McKay K, 208, *224*
McKee K, 295, *319*
McKee KT, 214, *229*
McKenniff MG, 259, *280*
McKenzie-Whie J, 339, *342*
McKerrow JH, 332, 333, *341*
McLaughlin MM, 247, 248, *275*
McLean A, 137, *151*
McLean S, 213, *227*
Mclemore TL, 298, *322*
McLeod RL, 220, *235*
Mcmanus LM, 185, *197*
McMenamin C, 343, *355*
McMenamin PG, 63, *77*
McNaboe J, 171, *181*
McNamara AE, 43, *56*

McNamara P, 97, *114*
McNish RW, 288, 292, *311*, *316*
McNutt M, 143, 144, *153*
Meade CJ, 194, *201*
Meadows KA, 393, *399*
Meagher LC, 378, *388*
Mecallaum MJA, 365, *382*
Medina JF, 290, *314*
Medini L, 287, *310*
Meek TD, 369, *385*
Meeker SN, 261, *281*
Mehta A, 291, *315*
Meier CR, 146, *154*
Meier R, 158, *174*
Meinert R, 395, *401*
Meini S, 213, 214, *227*, *228*, *229*
Melander B, 137, 142, *150*, *152*
Melander E, 125, 133, *148*
Meldrum LA, 211, *226*
Melis M, 306, *327*
Mellis CM, 1, *20*
Melton LJ, 166, *178*
Meltz M, 251, *276*
Meltzer EO, 105, *118*, 162, *176*
Meltzer S, 301, *323*
Mencia-Huerta JM, 217, *231*, 291, 298, *315*, *322*
Menegazzi R, 71, *83*
Mengelers HJ, 187, *198*
Mengelers HJJ, 42, *55*, 67, *79*
Menius JA, 263, 268, *281*
Menkes CJ, 268, *283*
Menkes H, 97, 99, 100, *114*, *115*
Menon S, 347, 351, *358*
Mentzer RM, 249, *275*
Menz G, 38, *52*, 57, *73*, 344, 348, *356*, 395, 396, *401*
Mercurio F, 375, *387*
Merendino A, 43, *55*
Merini S, 215, *230*
Merkus PJFM, 164, *178*
Merrimam M, 251, 257, 263, 267, *276*
Mertelsmann R, 291, *315*
Merus H, 217, *232*
Messer G, 346, *358*
Messer JW, 67, *80*
Metters KM, 214, *229*
Metwali A, 209, *224*
Metzen J, 88, *106*
Metzger SJ, 58, *73*
Metzger WJ, 249, *275*, 380, *389*
Meurs H, 91, *108*, *109*
Meya U, 251, 264, *276*
Meyermann R, 263, *281*
Meyers DA, 4, 6, *21*, 348, *358*
Meyrick B, 89, *107*
Michaeli T, 245, 246, 247, *274*, *275*
Michel A, 368, *384*
Michel C, 398, *403*
Michel F, 218, *233*
Michel FB, 43, *56*, 57, 65, 69, 71, *73*, *81*, *82*, *83*, 217, 218, *231*, *233*, 289, *313*, 380, *389*, 396, 397, 398, *402*, *403*
Michel MC, 257, *279*
Micheletto C, 305, *326*
Michl U, 185, *196*
Miguel AG, 16, 17, *25*
Miller CJ, 304, *326*
Miki H, 221, *235*
Miki I, 187, *198*
Milani GF, 57, *73*
Milavetz G, 168, *179*
Miles E, 12, *23*
Miles EA, 12, *23*
Miles JF, 395, *401*
Milic-Emil J, 32, *46*
Millar EA, 365, *382*
Millar L, 214, *229*
Miller C, 305, *326*
Miller CJ, 299, 306, *322*, *327*
Miller DK, 242, 256, *272*, 288, *311*
Miller I, 89, *106*
Miller L, 89, *107*
Miller M, 100, *115*
Miller MR, 395, *401*
Miller S, 214, *229*
Miller WC, 365, *383*
Milligan G, 237, 244, 245, *270*
Mills J, 100, *116*
Mills JE, 100, *115*
Milner JN, 158, *173*

Miloux B, 213, *227*
Minami M, 187, *198*, 371, *386*
Minette P, 38, *51*, 92, 94, *110*, *111*
Minette PJ, 96, *113*
Mingfu Y, 93, *111*
Minkwitz MC, 302, 304, *324*, *325*
Minotti DA, 304, *325*
Minshall E, 36, 41, *49*
Minshall EM, 43, *56*, 66, 71, *79*, 259, *280*
Minton NA, 137, *150*
Mionami M, 187, *198*
Mirabella A, 297, *320*
Miralpeix M, 250, *275*
Mishina M, 91, *108*
Misso NL, 188, *198*
Mistretta A, 210, 211, 212, *225*, *226*, *227*
Mitchell EB, 18, *25*
Mitchell H, 18, *26*
Mitchell HW, 36, *48*
Mitchell MI, 288, *312*
Mitchell P, 167, *179*
Mitchell R, 94, *112*
Mitchell RA, 87, 92, *106*, *110*
Mitchell RW, 34, 38, 39, *47*, *52*, 94, *112*
Mitchelson F, 91, *109*
Mitzner W, 35, 39, *48*
Miura M, 36, 37, *49*, *50*, 208, 221, *224*, *235*, 362, 367, *381*, *383*, *384*
Miwa M, 186, *197*
Miyachi Y, 36, *48*, 306, *327*
Miyajima A, 371, *385*
Miyajima T, 374, *387*
Miyakawa K, 297, *321*
Miyake M, 245, 248, 250, 264, *273*
Miyake Y, 294, *317*
Miyamoto T, 187, 194, *198*, *201*, 305, *326*
Miyanomae T, 297, *320*
Miyayasu K, 220, *235*
Modlin RL, 65, *78*
Moffatt MF, 11, *22*, *23*
Moldt P, 368, *384*
Molfino N, 97, *114*
Molfino NA, 41, *54*
Molimard M, 209, 210, 215, 216, *225*, *230*, *231*, 244, 261, *273*
Molinari JF, 61, *76*
Moll H, 15, *24*
Moll T, 375, *387*
Moller GM, 36, *49*, 63, *77*
Molnar-Kimber KL, 255, 268, *278*
Monaco L, 247, *275*
Monick M, 58, *73*
Monick MM, 15, *24*, 288, *311*
Montefort S, 37, *50*, 57, 61, 62, 64, 67, 68, 69, *74*, *76*, *80*, *81*
Montmimy L, 37, *50*
Moodie SA, 244, *273*
Moodley I, 263, *281*
Moore B, 33, *46*
Moore BJ, 31, 39, *45*, *53*
Moore K, 289, 296, *313*, *320*
Moore KA, 219, *234*
Moore T, 92, *110*
Moore WR, 61, *76*
Moote DW, 126, 129, 135, 137, *148*
Moqbel R, 67, *80*, 239, *271*
Morcillo E, 258, *280*
More PF, 251, *276*
Moreau J, 210, *225*
Moreno R, 32, 33, *46*
Moreno RH, 31, 32, 35, *45*, *46*, 395, *401*
Morgan RK, 167, *179*
Morgan WJ, 13, *23*
Mori A, 243, 257, *273*
Morice AH, 220, *234*
Moriggi E, 255, *277*
Morimoto C, 65, *78*
Morley J, 239, *271*, 366, 378, *383*, *388*
Morone MP, 243, *272*
Morris HG, 163, *177*
Morris HR, 292, *316*
Morris MM, 38, 42, *52*, 60, *75*
Morris RJ, 126, 129, 135, 137, *148*
Morrison BJ, 12, *23*
Morrison J, 101, *117*
Morton BE, 338, *341*
Morton D, 290, *314*
Morton DR, 293, *317*

Mosbech H, 41, *54*
Moseler M, 17, *25*
Moseley P, 58, *73*
Moser B, 346, 352, *357*
Mosimann BL, 208, *224*
Mosko MM, 156, *172*
Mosmann TR, 344, *356*
Mossmann TR, 63, *77*
Motojmima S, 37, *50*
Motomiya M, 35, *47*, 286, 294, *309*
Mott GE, 185, *197*
Motulsky HJ, 257, *279*
Moussaoui S, 213, *227*
Mowat AM, 353, *360*
Mu J, 347, *358*
Mudholkar GS, 100, *116*
Mue S, 194, *201*
Muehsam WT, 264, *282*
Muhlbacher A, 374, *387*
Mui A, 347, 351, *358*
Mui ALF, 371, *385*
Muir JF, 133, *149*
Muirhead EE, 183, *196*
Muis T, 218, *234*
Mul FP, 257, *279*
Mulder PG, 63, *77*
Mulder PGH, 37, *50*, 63, *77*, 171, *180*
Mullee MA, 41, *54*, 393, *400*
Muller KM, 257, *279*
Muller N, 43, *56*
Muller Peddinghaus R, 290, *314*
Muller T, 248, 255, *275*, *277*
Muller W, 347, *358*
Mullikin-Kilpatrick D, 91, *108*
Mullol J, 89, 90, *107*
Munch E, 368, *384*
Munch M, 88, *106*
Mungai M, 2, *20*
Murad F, 365, *382*
Murakami M, 291, *315*
Murdoch S, 63, *76*
Murphy E, 347, 351, *358*
Murphy KM, 63, *77*, 345, 346, 347, 350, *356*, *357*, *358*, *359*
Murphy RC, 193, *201*, 292, *316*
Murray AB, 12, *23*
Murray J, 305, *326*, 343, *355*
Murray JJ, 133, *149*, 299, 303, 306, 309, *322*, *326*, *328*
Musk AW, 31, 37, *45*
Musk B, 31, *45*
Mussener A, 263, 268, *281*
Mutoh H, 187, *198*
Myers A, 93, *111*
Myers AC, 90, *107*
Myers C, 374, *387*
Myers P, 289, *312*
Myint SH, 393, *400*
Myles DD, 265, 267, *282*

N

Nabavi N, 351, *359*
Nabe M, 189, *199*
Nabe T, 186, *198*, 294, *317*
Naclerio R, 105, *118*
Nadel A, 301, *323*
Nadel J, 89, 90, 96, 97, 99, *106*, *107*, *114*, *115*
Nadel JA, 37, 39, *50*, *51*, *53*, 60, 61, *75*, *76*, 88, 89, 90, 92, 94, 99, 100, *106*, *107*, *112*, *115*, *116*, 205, 214, 215, 216, 217, 219, 221, *223*, *229*, *230*, *231*, *232*, *234*, *235*, 243, 256, *272*
Nadler LM, 63, *76*
Nagain A, 305, *326*
Nagase T, 187, *198*
Nagata M, 190, *200*, 303, *325*
Nagayama T, 93, *111*
Nagtegaal JE, 93, *111*
Nakagawa C, 306, *327*
Nakagawa N, 293, *317*
Nakagawa T, 187, *198*
Nakai A, 297, *320*
Nakai J, 211, *226*
Nakajima N, 208, *224*
Nakajima S, 194, *201*
Nakajima T, 158, *174*
Nakamata M, 187, *198*
Nakamura M, 187, *198*
Nakamura T, 344, 348, 351, *356*, *358*
Nakamura Y, 306, *327*

Nakanishi K, 347, *358*, 371, *386*
Nakanishi S, 214, *228*
Nakhosteen JA, 185, *196*
Naline E, 120, *146*, 209, 210, 213, 214, 215, 220, *225*, *227*, *228*, *229*, *230*, *235*, 254, 261, *277*
Nannini LJ, 41, *54*
Narumiya S, 364, *382*
Nasser SMS, 297, 299, *320*, *323*
Nathan M, 34, 39, *47*
Nathan RA, 126, 129, 135, 137, *148*
Naty S, 135, *150*
Nayak A, 305, *326*
Naylor B, 69, *81*
Ndukuw I, 94, *112*
Neas LM, 17, *25*
Neate MS, 168, *179*
Necheles J, 214, 217, *229*, *232*
Neeley SP, 217, *232*
Neely JD, 11, *22*, 348, 349, *358*
Neeskens P, 36, 42, *49*
Negri J, 372, *386*
Neijens HJ, 141, *152*, 160, *175*, 307, *327*
Neild JE, 101, *117*
Neill KG, 293, *317*
Neliat G, 213, 214, *227*, *228*
Nelson D, 158, *174*, 343, *355*
Nelson FC, 37, *50*, 69, *81*, 396, *401*
Nelson HS, 164, *177*, 379, *389*
Neri M, 285, *309*, 395, *401*
Nevitt M, 166, *178*
Newball HH, 60, *74*
Newell JD, 71, *83*
Newhouse M, 162, *176*
Newland AC, 194, *201*
Newman DJ, 252, *276*
Newman GB, 104, *117*
Newman LS, 71, *83*
Newman W, 372, *386*
Newman-Taylor A, 2, *21*
Newnham CM, 137, 138, *151*
Newnham DM, 137, *151*
Newsholme SJ, 254, 258, 261, 269, *277*, 295, *319*
Newson R, 16, *24*
Newton R, 257, 269, *280*, 378, *388*
Ng CK, 190, *199*
Ng'ang'a L, 2, *20*
Ng'ang'a LW, 2, *20*
Nguyen MH, 263, 265, *281*
Nguyen QT, 214, *228*
Nials A, 122, *147*
Nials AT, 265, 267, *282*
Nichol GM, 190, *199*
Nicholson CD, 247, 250, 252, *274*, *275*
Nicolai T, 19, *26*
Nicoll-Griffith D, 268, *283*
Nides M, 397, *403*
Nieber K, 208, *224*
Nieduzak TR, 369, 373, *384*
Nielsen JA, 251, *276*
Nielson CP, 242, 256, *272*
Nielson NH, 160, *175*
Niemann M, 9, *22*
Nieminen MM, 169, *180*
Nieves AL, 295, *319*
Nii Y, 293, *317*
Nijkamp F, 91, *109*
Nijkamp FP, 37, *50*, 218, *233*, *234*, 256, *278*, 353, *360*
Nikander K, 161, *176*
Nikawa J, 246, *274*
Nikolaizik W, 162, *177*
Nilander K, 160, *175*
Nilius B, 376, *388*
Nilsson G, 212, *227*
Ninan TK, 1, *20*, 163, *177*
Nishida J, 371, *385*
Nishikawa M, 137, *151*
Nishima S, 218, *233*
Niv Y, 298, *322*
Nizankowska E, 297, 309, *320*, *328*, 378, *388*
Noble A, 65, *78*
Noel LS, 251, 263, 268, *276*, *281*
Nonaka H, 89, 90, *107*
Noonan G, 305, *326*
Noonan M, 169, *180*
Noonan N, 305, *326*
Noorshargh S, 379, *389*
Norel X, 289, *313*

Norman P, 100, *116*, 289, *312*
Norman PS, 39, *53*, 97, 100, *114*
Noronha-Blob L, 91, *109*
Norris A, 376, *388*
Northfield M, 128, 131, *148*, 364, *382*
Northoff GH, 263, *281*
Nourshargh S, 256, *278*
Novak LB, 254, 258, 261, 269, *277*
Nowak D, 125, 133, *147*
Numa S, 91, *108*
Nunan LM, 91, *108*
Nunn AJ, 67, *81*
Nussbaum E, 167, *179*
Nyberg L, 125, *147*
Nyce JW, 249, *275*, 380, *389*
Nyman U, 263, 268, *281*

O

O'Brian T, 105, *118*
O'Byrne P, 131, 142, *149*, 393, 398, *400*
O'Byrne PM, 30, 31, 36, 37, 40, *44*, *49*, *53*, 58, 60, 61, *73*, *75*, 94, 100, *112*, 160, *175*, 194, *201*, 292, 297, 298, 299, 300, 301, 302, 303, 307, 308, *316*, *321*, *322*, *323*, *324*, *325*, 364, *382*, 394, 396, *400*, *402*
O'Connell J, 248, *275*
O'Connor B, 102, *117*, 366, 372, 374, *383*, *386*
O'Connor BJ, 32, 42, *46*, *55*, 125, 140, *147*, 191, 194, 195, *200*, *201*, *202*, 266, *283*, 288, *312*, 366, 377, 381, *383*, *388*, *389*
O'Connor G, 259, *281*
O'Connor GT, 41, 42, *54*, *55*, 393, *399*
O'Connor T, 18, *25*
O'Donnel M, 364, *382*
O'Donnell MP, 291, *315*
O'Donnell S, 123, *147*
O'Donnell WJ, 297, *320*
O'Driscoll BR, 96, 104, *114*
O'Fallon WM, 164, *178*
O'Farrell AM, 371, *385*
O'Flaherty JT, 186, *197*
O'Garra A, 63, *77*, 345, 346, 347, 350, 351, 353, *356*, *357*, *358*, *359*, *360*
O'Hara P, 394, *400*
O'Hearn DJ, 372, *386*
O'Hickey SP, 292, 294, *316*
O'Leary C, 63, *77*
O'Malley G, 242, 255, *271*
O'Neill K, 246, *274*
O'Reilly S, 220, *235*
O'Shaughnessy KM, 295, *318*
O'Toole S, 265, 266, 267, *282*, 393, *400*
Oates JA, 297, *320*
Obata T, 293, 294, *317*
Obrone J, 129, 131, 135, *149*
Oda M, 185, *197*
Odhiambo J, 2, *20*
Odlander B, 289, 290, *313*, *314*
Oehme P, 208, 212, *224*, *226*
Oettgen HC, 332, 333, *341*
Offord KP, 164, 166, *177*, *178*
Ogra PL, 14, *24*
Ohaja Y, 245, 248, 250, 264, *273*
Ohashi Y, 37, *50*
Ohata K, 294, *317*
Ohkawara Y, 380, *389*
Ohkubo K, 205, *223*
Ohlstein EH, 369, *385*
Ohlweiler DF, 369, 373, *384*
Ohnishi T, 378, *388*
Ohrui T, 91, *109*
Ohuchi Y, 221, *235*
Oikarinen A, 167, *179*
Okada S, 378, *388*
Okada Y, 293, *317*
Okamoto LJ, 398, *403*
Okamoto Y, 186, *197*
Okamura H, 347, *358*
Okaniami OA, 38, *52*
Okayama M, 89, 90, *107*, 365, *383*
Okayama Y, 62, *76*, 285, *309*
Okazaki H, 185, *196*
Okazawa M, 32, 33, 35, 43, *46*, *48*, *56*, 306, *327*
Okdao H, 187, *198*
Okhrogi H, 37, *51*

Okubo T, 297, *321*
Okudaira H, 243, 257, *273*
Older SA, 158, *174*
Olesen SP, 368, *384*
Oliveri R, 210, 211, 212, *225*, *226*, *227*
Olivieri D, 36, 42, *49*, *55*, 169, *180*
Ollerenshaw SL, 208, *223*
Ollier S, 286, *310*
Oman H, 13, *23*
Omini C, 218, *233*
Omoigui N, 43, *56*
Omwega MJ, 2, *20*
Ono S, 187, *198*
Oosterhoff Y, 41, *55*
Oosting H, 165, *178*
Opas E, 288, *311*
Oplinger JA, 369, *384*
Oppenheim J, 65, *78*
Orasz CG, 353, *360*
Ordinas A, 298, *322*
Orehek J, 99, 100, *115*, *116*
Orejer J, 368, *384*
Orgel HA, 105, *118*, 162, *176*
Ormstad H, 17, *25*
Orning L, 288, *311*
Orr LM, 32, *45*
Ortaldo J, 65, *78*
Ortaldo JR, 65, *78*
Osborn RR, 254, 258, 261, 263, 269, *277*, *280*, 295, *319*
Osborne J, 65, *78*
Osterman K, 137, *150*
Ostro B, 17, *25*
Ottonello L, 243, *272*
Otwinowski Z, 158, *173*
Ouchi Y, 187, *198*
Overbeek SE, 36, 37, 42, *49*, *50*, *55*, 63, 67, *77*, *79*
Overholt R, 96, *113*
Overlack C, 141, *152*
Owen S, 367, *383*
Owen WF, 291, *315*
Owens R, 250, 251, 253, 257, 263, 267, *275*, *276*
Owens RJ, 248, *275*
Oxender DL, 213, *227*, *228*
Oyake T, 221, *235*

P

Pace E, 43, *55*, 306, *327*
Pace-Asciak CR, 290, *314*
Pack RJ, 35, *48*
Padfield PL, 165, *178*
Padrid Ph, 37, *50*
Pagani ED, 247, 252, 253, 258, 269, *274*
Paganin F, 43, *56*, 71, *83*
Page C, 43, *56*
Page CP, 217, 218, *232*, *234*, 255, 259, 261, 263, 265, 266, 267, 269, *277*, *280*, *281*, *282*
Page R, 286, *309*
Paggiaro PL, 140, *151*
Pahdi H, 18, *26*
Pahl HL, 374, *387*
Pain MC, 71, *83*
Pajak A, 378, *388*
Pak J, 11, *22*, 134, *150*
Palacios JM, 250, *275*
Palermo B, 210, 211, *225*
Palermo F, 210, 211, 212, *225*, *226*, *227*
Palermo L, 166, *178*
Palfreyman MN, 248, 251, 256, 257, *275*, *276*
Palmer J, 127, 142, 143, *148*
Palmer JB, 91, *109*
Palmer JBD, 127, 133, 144, 146, *148*, *149*, *154*, 364, *382*
Palmer JD, 91, *108*
Palmer KNV, 96, 105, *114*
Palmqvist M, 125, 133, *147*, *148*
Palombella VJ, 70, *82*
Panhuysen CI, 6, *21*
Panhuysen CIM, 348, *358*
Papacosta AO, 393, *399*
Papakosta D, 101, *117*
Papi A, 15, *24*
Paradis L, 66, *79*
Pare P, 32, *46*, 380, *389*

Pare PD, 29, 31, 32, 33, 34, 35, 39, 41, 43, *44*, *45*, *46*, *47*, *48*, *53*, *54*, *56*, 395, *401*
Parham WM, 39, *53*
Park H, 61, *76*
Parks T, 374, *387*
Parronchi P, 65, *78*
Parry E, 2, *20*
Parsons S, 291, *315*
Parton T, 268, *283*
Pasqualini T, 351, *359*
Passini N, 346, *357*
Patacchini R, 213, 214, *227*, *228*, *229*, *230*
Patalano F, 43, *55*, 333, *341*
Patel H, 102, *117*, 366, *383*
Patel K, 100, *116*
Patel KR, 188, *198*, 369, *385*
Patmore L, 368, *384*
Patriarca P, 71, *83*
Patrick D, 104, *118*
Pattemore P, 100, *116*
Pattemore PK, 393, *400*
Patterson DK, 217, *232*
Patterson R, 100, *115*, 189, 193, *199*, *201*
Paubert-Braquet M, 218, *232*, *233*
Paul WE, 63, *77*, 349, *359*
Paul-Eugene N, 291, *315*
Paulauskis JD, 209, *224*
Pauli G, 91, 92, *108*, 398, *403*
Pauwels R, 30, 31, 40, *45*, 210, 221, *225*, *235*, 376, *388*, 395, *401*
Pauwels RA, 131, 142, *149*, 203, 204, 209, 210, 211, 212, 214, 215, 216, 221, *223*, *224*, *225*, *226*, *230*, *231*, 299, 301, *323*, *324*, 364, *382*, 393, 396, 398, *400*, *402*
Pavone V, 213, 214, *227*, *229*
Pavord ID, 137, 141, *150*, *152*, 297, *321*, 364, *382*, 396, *402*
Pavord JD, 127, *148*
Payan DG, 217, *232*
Payne AN, 254, *277*
Pazdrak K, 371, *385*
Pazoles CJ, 255, 268, *278*
Peachell PT, 241, 242, 254, *271*, *277*
Pearce EJ, 332, *341*
Pearce FL, 59, 61, *74*, 212, *226*
Pearce G, 137, 143, *150*
Pearce N, 2, *20*, 135, 142, 143, 144, *150*, *152*, *153*, *154*
Pearce-Pinto G, 31, 33, 37, *45*, *46*
Pearlman D, 303, *324*
Pearlman DS, 126, 129, 135, 137, *148*, 307, *327*
Pearson JDM, 86, *105*
Pearson S, 101, *117*
Peat JK, 1, 18, 19, *20*, *26*, 29, *44*, 71, *83*, 343, *355*, 393, *399*
Pedersen OF, 30, *44*
Pedersen S, 125, *147*, 161, 162, 163, 164, 165, 169, 171, *176*, *177*, *178*, *180*, *181*
Pedersen SE, 162, *176*
Pedersen W, 169, *180*
Pedone C, 213, 214, *227*, *229*
Peglion JL, 220, *235*
Pela R, 128, *148*
Pelaia G, 135, *150*
Peleman RA, 203, 204, *223*
Pellegrino R, 36, 39, *49*, *53*
Pendry YD, 215, *230*
Pengelly CDR, 156, *172*
Penrose JF, 289, 291, 309, *312*, *314*, *315*, *328*
Pepinsky RB, 379, *389*
Peppel K, 158, *173*
Perdizet S, 393, *399*
Peretti M, 217, *232*
Perez VL, 348, *358*
Perini AF, 264, *282*
Peris A, 36, *49*
Perkkanen J, 17, *25*
Perleman RA, 396, *402*
Permutt S, 39, *53*, 97, 100, *114*, *116*, 298, *322*
Peroni D, 62, 67, *76*, *80*
Peroni DG, 69, *81*
Perot S, 268, *283*
Perretti F, 215, 218, 219, 220, *230*, *233*, *234*
Perruchoud AP, 125, 140, *147*

Perry JD, 268, *283*
Perry M, 248, 250, 251, 253, 257, 263, 267, *275*, *276*
Persaud MP, 167, *179*
Persson CGA, 209, *225*
Persson G, 125, *147*
Persson GGA, 220, *235*
Persson MA, 217, *232*
Persson T, 160, 161, *175*, *176*
Pert CB, 217, *231*
Pesci A, 36, 42, *49*, *55*, 169, *180*
Peslin R, 30, *44*
Peszek I, 303, *324*
Peters A, 17, *25*
Peters GA, 67, *80*
Peters JCK, 395, *401*
Peters JM, 291, *315*
Peters M, 208, *224*
Peters MJ, 158, *173*
Peters SP, 60, 66, *74*, *79*, 289, 306, *313*, *326*
Peters-Golden M, 288, 292, *311*, *316*
Petit C, 220, *235*
Petit F, 374, *387*
Petit-Frere C, 62, *76*, 285, *309*
Petrie GR, 96, 105, *114*
Petterson T, 164, *178*
Pettipher ER, 255, 268, *278*
Peyronel JF, 213, *227*
Pezet S, 218, *233*
Pfeiffer C, 343, 351, *355*, *359*
Pfister A, 238, *271*
Pfister R, 297, *320*, 344, *356*
Pflug B, 264, *282*
Phelan PD, 164, *178*
Pheng Lui K, 36, *48*
Philip G, 105, *118*
Philippin B, 219, *234*
Phillips D, 251, *276*
Phillips E, 96, *113*
Phillips GD, 297, 301, *321*, *323*, *324*
Phillips GH, 168, *180*
Phillips MJ, 63, *77*
Phipps R, 89, 90, *107*
Piantadosi C, 95, 104, *113*
Picado C, 298, *322*
Picard D, 158, *173*
Piccinni MP, 65, *78*
Piechuta H, 259, 267 269, *280*, *281*, 301, *323*
Piedimonte G, 216, *231*
Pieroni MG, 377, *388*
Pierson R, 101, *117*
Pierson W, 299, 303, *322*
Pilewski JM, 379, *389*
Pillar JS, 265, 269, *282*
Pillari A, 309, *328*
Pin I, 58, *73*
Pinckard RN, 183, 185, *196*, *197*
Pinis G, 378, *388*
Pinnas J, 169, *180*
Piotrowska B, 194, *201*
Piper PJ, 192, *200*, 289, 292, 293, 297, 301, *312*, *316*, *317*, *321*, *323*
Pircher H, 65, *78*
Pires AL, 257, *279*
Pirron U, 332, *340*
Pistorese BP, 288, *312*
Pitman A, 371, *385*
Pitman AM, 43, *55*
Pittulainen E, 137, *150*
Pivirotto F, 57, *73*
Pizzichini E, 38, 42, *52*, 142, *153*, 306, *327*, 396, *402*
Pizzichini MMM, 38, 42, *52*, 396, *402*
Planquois JM, 254, *277*
Platts-Mills TAE, 343, *355*
Pliss LB, 39, *53*
Plozza T, 63, *77*
Pocock SJ, 160, *175*
Poisson N, 393, *399*
Polak JM, 70, *82*, 208, *223*, *224*
Polito AJ, 308, *328*
Pollice M, 306, *326*
Polonsky J, 183, *196*
Polosa R, 57, 61, 64, 67, 69, *74*, *80*, *81*, 210, 211, 212, *225*, *226*, *227*
Polson JB, 248, 252, 257, *275*, *276*, *279*
Ponath PD, 372, *386*
Poncelet M, 213, *227*, *228*
Pons F, 166, *178*
Ponta H, 374, *387*

Pool GL, 186, *197*
Popa V, 61, *76*
Pope CAD, 17, *25*
Porsius A, 92, *110*
Porter J, 333, *341*
Post M, 92, *110*
Post TW, 372, *386*
Postema JB, 91, *109*
Postlethwaite AE, 70, *82*
Postma DS, 4, 6, 11, *21*, *22*, 29, 31, 41, 42, *44*, *45*, *55*, 63, 67, *77*, *79*, 129, 131, 133, 135, 142, *149*, 165, *178*, 298, *321*, 348, *358*, 364, *382*, 393, 395, 398, *400*, *401*
Poston RN, 64, *77*
Pouliot M, 291, *314*, *315*
Poulter LW, 36, *49*, 65, *79*, 160, *175*
Pouw EM, 165, *178*
Powell JA, 268, *283*
Powell N, 346, *357*
Power C, 160, *175*
Power RF, 208, *224*
Powrie F, 359, *360*
Prabhakar U, 265, 269, *282*
Prahl P, 162, *177*
Prakash YS, 34, 39, *47*
Prasit P, 288, *311*
Prefontaine KE, 158, *173*
Prens EP, 63, *77*
Prescott SL, 354, *360*
Prescott SM, 185, 186, *197*, 293, *317*
Presky DH, 346, 348, *357*, *358*
Presta L, 333, *341*
Price CP, 296, *320*
Price JF, 296, *320*
Prickman LE, 155, *172*
Prieto L, 36, *49*
Primhak R, 169, *180*
Prinz JC, 332, *340*
Profita M, 297, *320*
Proietto V, 213, *227*, *228*
Promwong C, 65, *78*
Prossnitz ER, 187, *198*
Proud D, 61, *75*, 105, *118*, 298, *322*
Proudhon H, 398, *403*
Prummel MF, 165, *178*
Pruniaux MP, 263, *281*
Pueringer RJ, 288, 291, *311*, *315*
Puig J, 250, *275*
Pujades M, 298, *322*
Pujol JL, 218, *233*, 238, *270*
Purdie G, 135, *150*

Q

Qian Y, 120, *146*, 215, 216, *230*, *231*, 244, 254, 261, *273*, *277*
Qin S, 372, *386*
Qiu YH, 246, *274*
Quade DC, 245, *273*
Quanjer PH, 164, *178*, 394, *400*
Quanjer pH, 29, *44*
Quanjer PhH, 30, 31, 36, 37, *44*, 297, 298, *321*
Quanjer PPH, 394, *400*
Quartara L, 213, 214, *227*, *229*
Quebe-Fehling E, 128, *148*
Quennedey M, 121, *147*
Quinonez G, 212, *227*
Quint D, 62, *76*, 285, *309*
Quint DJ, 12, *23*, 168, *179*
Quirk FH, 397, *402*

R

Raaijmakers JA, 371, *385*
Raaijmakers JAM, 125, *147*, 371, *385*, 398, *403*
Rabe K, 122, 123, *147*
Rabe KF, 34, 39, *47*, 125, 133, *147*, 242, 256, *272*, *279*, 300, *323*, 338, *341*
Rabier M, 217, *231*
Raboudi S, 34, 39, *47*
Racke K, 88, *106*
Radbruch A, 346, *357*
Radermecker M, 188, *199*
Radermecker MF, 189, 190, *199*, *200*
Radford M, 169, *180*
Radmark O, 289, 290, 291, *313*, *314*
Radner DB, 156, *172*
Radwanski E, 195, *202*

Raeburn D, 37, *50*, 248, 251, 253, 254, 256, 257, 260, 261, 263, 269, *275*, *276*, *277*
Rafferty P, 61, *76*, 188, *198*, 286, 294, 301, *309*, *323*
Raghow R, 70, *82*
Rahnsdorf HJ, 374, *387*
Raines EW, 70, *82*
Raisz LG, 165, *178*
Raizenne ME, 17, *25*
Rajewski K, 347, *358*
Rakshi K, 266, *283*
Ram JS, 29, *44*
Ramage L, 140, *151*
Ramesha CS, 290, *314*
Ramhamadany E, 194, *201*
Ramnarine S, 89, 90, *107*
Ramnarine SI, 216, *231*
Ramsay AJ, 352, *359*
Ramsay CF, 305, *326*
Ramsay CM, 142, *152*
Ramsdale EH, 41, *54*, 160, *175*, 297, *321*, 393, 394, *400*
Rand CS, 397, *402*, *403*
Randolph TG, 155, *172*
Rands E, 288, *310*, *311*
Rangarajan P, 158, *173*
Ranger AM, 351, *359*
Ransil BJ, 297, *320*
Ransone LJ, 158, *173*
Rao G, 95, 104, *113*
Rao K, 34, 39, *47*
Rao P, 372, *386*
Rao PE, 243, 256, *272*
Rapecki S, 255, 268, *278*
Rasmussen JB, 302, *324*
Ratcliffe AJ, 251, *276*
Rathsack R, 208, *224*
Ratner P, 105, *118*, 126, 129, 135, 137, *148*
Ray A, 158, *173*, 371, *385*
Ray DW, 38, *51*, 218, *233*
Ray P, 371, *385*
Raynor M, 91, *109*
Rea L, 289, *313*
Rebuck AS, 143, 144, *153*
Record M, 186, *197*
Reddel HK, 29, *44*
Redermecker M, 266, *283*
Redier H, 398, *403*
Redington AE, 60, 63, 69, 70, *75*, *77*, *81*, *82*, 208, *223*
Redline S, 14, *24*
Reed CE, 66, *79*, 156, 164, *172*, *177*, *178*
Reed G, 105, *118*
Refini RM, 377, *388*
Regoli D, 205, 209, 210, 212, 213, 214, *223*, *225*, *229*
Regruson K, 247, *275*
Rehder K, 91, 92, 93, *109*, *110*
Reid GK, 288, *311*
Reid L, 89, 90, *107*
Reid LM, 67, *80*, 293, *317*
Reifsnyder DH, 245, *273*
Reimann J, 333, 336, 337, *341*, 379, *389*
Reimer LG, 163, *177*
Reinhardt D, 141, *152*
Reinheimer T, 88, *106*
Reinikainen K, 125, *147*, 160, *175*
Reis JM, 221, *235*
Reisine ST, 393, *399*
Reisman J, 104, *117*
Reisman RE, 156, *172*
Reiss T, 307, *327*
Reiss TF, 301, 303, 305, *324*, *326*
Rennard SI, 126, 129, 135, 137, *148*
Renner H, 212, *226*
Rennick DM, 238, *270*
Renz H, 93, 94, *111*, 346, *357*
Renzetti AR, 213, 214, *227*, *229*
Renzetti L, 364, *382*
Renzetti LM, 348, *358*
Resche-Rigon M, 374, *387*
Reves JT, 193, *201*
Rex MD, 65, 66, *79*
Reynolds LS, 213, *227*
Reynolds S, 167, *179*
Rhind G, 101, *116*
Rhoden KJ, 70, *81*
Ribbes G, 186, *197*
Riboux JP, 343, *355*
Riccio MM, 259, *280*

Richard A, 397, *402*
Richards DH, 367, *383*
Richards G, 142, *152*
Richards JM, 397, *402*
Richards W, 195, *202*
Richardson CD, 288, *311*
Richardson P, 89, *107*
Richardson PS, 99, *115*
Richardson W, 43, *55*, 333, *341*
Richerson HB, 29, *44*, 58, 60, 61, *73*, *75*
Riches V, 64, *78*
Richmond I, 169, *180*
Richter K, 303, *325*
Richter L, 246, *274*
Rickard K, 141, *152*
Rickard KA, 144, *154*
Ridge SM, 42, *55*, 192, *200*
Rieber EP, 332, *340*
Rieber P, 374, *387*
Rieger CH, 185, *196*
Riemersma RA, 129, 131, 135, *149*
Riethmuller A, 263, *281*
Riggs BL, 166, *178*
Riggs M, 245, 246, 247, *274*, *275*
Riis BJ, 165, *178*
Rijcken B, 42, *55*, 395, *401*
Rijnbeek PR, 37, *50*
Rijntjes E, 63, *77*
Riker WF, 86, *105*
Rinaldi N, 364, *382*
Rincon M, 348, 351, *358*
Ringdal N, 131, *149*, 364, *382*
Ringden O, 217, *232*
Rise P, 287, *310*
Risee A, 41, *54*
Riska H, 125, 126, 129, 135, 137, *147*, *148*
Risteli J, 167, *179*
Risteli L, 167, *179*
Ritter JM, 289, 296, *313*, *320*
Riva E, 307, *327*
Rizzo A, 43, *55*
Road J, 32, *46*
Robbins JD, 243, 256, *272*
Robbins K, 332, 333, 339, *341*, *342*
Roberts AB, 354, *360*
Roberts CR, 35, *48*
Roberts JA, 59, 60, 62, 68, 69, 70, *74*, *76*, *80*, 134, *150*
Roberts JM, 88, 89, 90, 92, *106*
Roberts NM, 190, *199*
Roberts R, 97, *114*
Roberts RS, 160, *175*
Roberts T, 263, 265, *281*
Robichaud A, 265, *282*, 372, 374, *386*
Robineau P, 220, *235*
Robinson C, 37, *50*, 60, *75*, 301, *323*
Robinson D, 158, *174*, 347, 351, *358*
Robinson DS, 38, *52*, 57, 62, 64, 67, *73*, *77*, *80*, 238, *270*, 344, 345, 346, *356*, 395, 396, *401*
Robinson G, 213, *227*
Robinson GA, 237, *270*
Robinson N, 93, *111*
Robinson NE, 93, 94, *111*, *112*
Robinson NJ, 42, *55*, 67, *79*
Robinson PJ, 15, *24*
Robiscek SA, 257, *279*
Robuschi M, 307, *327*, 377, *388*
Roca J, 191, 192, 193, *200*
Roche WR, 5, *21*, 35, 38, *48*, *52*, 57, 58, 59, 60, 67, 68, 69, 70, *72*, *73*, *74*, *80*, *81*, *82*, 133, *149*, 160, *176*, 239, *271*, 295, *318*, 391, 395, 396, *399*, *401*
Rodarte JR, 36, *49*
Rodenstein D, 97, *114*
Rodger IA, 214, *229*
Rodger IW, 214, 216, *229*, *231*, 259, 265, 267 269, *280*, *281*, *282*
Rodgers L, 245, 247, *274*, *275*
Rodkey J, 288, *311*
Rodregues de Miranda JF, 93, *111*
Rodreguez R, 71, *83*
Rodrigues de Miranda JF, 89, 91, 92, *107*, *108*, *110*
Rodriguez-Roisin R, 191, 192, 193, *200*
Roell G, 19, *26*
Roffel AF, 91, *108*, *108*, *109*
Rogers AV, 36, *49*
Rogers D, 89, 90, *107*

Rogers DF, 215, 216, *230*, *231*, 367, *384*
Rogge L, 346, *357*
Roghmann KJ, 13, *23*
Rohde JAL, 367, *384*
Rohdewald P, 168, *179*
Roitman-Johnson B, 9, *22*
Rokach J, 289, 301, *312*, *323*
Rola-Pleszczynski M, 291, *315*
Roldaan AC, 37, *51*, 205, *223*
Rolfe FG, 158, 169, *174*
Rollins JP, 155, *172*
Romagnani S, 65, *78*, 344, 345, 346, 349, *356*
Romagnoli M, 297, *321*
Romano FD, 91, *108*
Rombout PJA, 36, *49*
Roncarolo MG, 347, *358*
Rooklin AR, 167, *179*
Rooney JW, 371, *386*
Roorda RJ, 129, 141, *148*
Roos CM, 165, *178*
Roos D, 257, *279*
Roquet A, 242, *271*, 286, *310*
Rose D, 251, *276*
Rose M, 208, *224*
Rose R, 392, 397, *399*
Rosen A, 289, 290, *313*
Rosen R, 288, *311*
Rosen T, 213, *227*
Rosenberg M, 192, *200*, 299, *322*
Rosenberg MA, 192, *201*, 301, *323*
Rosenborg J, 125, *147*
Rosenhall L, 239, *271*
Rosenthal R, 100, *116*
Rosenthal RR, 97, 100, *114*, 295, *318*
Rosenwasser LJ, 27, 35, 38, *44*, 158, *174*, 349, *359*
Rosette C, 158, *173*
Rosimini F, 15, *24*
Rosina C, 67, *80*
Rosner B, 42, *55*
Ross R, 70, *82*
Rossenwasser LJ, 344, 348, *356*
Rossetti M, 210, *225*
Rossi GA, 285, *309*, 395, *401*
Rossi M, 307, *327*
Rossing TH, 301, *324*
Rostrup J, 126, 129, 135, 137, *148*
Rotger M, 191, 192, 193, *200*
Roth M, 301, *323*
Rottman FM, 158, *173*
Rouissi N, 214, *228*
Rouot B, 121, *147*
Roux F, 121, *146*
Rouzer C, 288, *311*
Rouzer CA, 287, 288, *310*
Rovero P, 213, 214, *227*, *228*, *229*
Rowe A, 376, *388*
Rozanski E, 94, *112*
Rubin AE, 189, *199*
Rubin AHE, 193, *201*
Rubin P, 192, *200*, *201*, 288, 295, 299, 303, 309, *311*, *318*, *322*, *328*
Rubinstein I, 37, *50*
Rubio R, 249, *275*
Ruff MR, 217, *231*
Ruffin R, 100, *116*
Ruffin-Morin Y, 254, *277*
Rufin RE, 97, *114*
Ruhlmann E, 34, 39, *47*
Rumbyrt J, 372, *386*
Ruoss SJ, 70, *82*
Ruppel J, 333, *341*
Rush JA, 265, 269, *282*
Rushton L, 129, 131, 135, *149*
Rusin LG, 268, *283*
Russell A, 248, 251, 257, 263, 267, *275*, *276*
Russell AA, 243, 256, *272*
Russell G, 163, *177*
Russo LL, 251, *276*
Rusznak C, 15, 17, *24*, *25*
Rutten-van Mooken MPMH, 398, *403*
Ryan G, 31, 37, *45*, 160, *175*
Ryan M, 7, *21*
Ryan MF, 171, *181*

S

Saarelainen P, 169, *180*
Saccomano NA, 251, *276*

Sackett DL, 143, *153*
Sadowski S, 288, *311*
Saetta M, 57, 67, *73*, *80*
Sagara H, 187, *198*
Sahn S, 305, *326*
Said SI, 204, *223*
Saito K, 185, 186, *196*, *197*
Saito M, 294, 297, *317*, *320*
Sakai DD, 158, *173*
Sakai K, 218, *233*
Sakai N, 90, 104, *107*
Sakai R, 371, *385*
Sakakibara H, 306, *327*
Sakamato T, 214, *229*
Sakamoto S, 294, 295, *317*, *318*
Sakamoto T, 216, *231*, 306, *327*
Sakamoto Y, 190, *200*, 303, *325*
Sakanaka C, 187, *198*
Sala A, 290, *314*
Salari H, 60, *75*, 185, *196*, 218, *233*, 297, *321*
Salathe M, 89, *106*
Salcedo C, 250, *275*
Salem H, 99, *115*
Salgame P, 65, *78*
Saller L, 299, *322*
Sallusto F, 353, *360*
Salmon M, 294, *317*
Salome C, 35, *47*
Salome CM, 19, *26*, 29, 31, 36, 37, *44*, *45*, *49*, 160, *175*, 393, 394, *399*, *400*
Salter H, 238, *270*
Salvaggio JE, 339, *342*
Samet JM, 6, *21*, 290, *314*
Samhoun MN, 289, *312*
Sampognaro S, 65, *78*
Sampson AP, 192, *201*, 286, 288, 291, 294, 296, 297, 299, 300, 301, 302, 307, 309, *310*, *312*, *315*, *317*, *320*, *321*, *327*, *328*, 329, *340*
Sampson AS, 91, *109*
Sampson K, 61, *76*
Sampson SE, 192, *201*, 288, 294, *312*, *317*
Samuelsson B, 287, 288, 289, 290, 291, 292, *310*, *311*, *313*, *314*, *316*
Sanak M, 308, *328*
SanaT, 347, 351, *358*
Sanderson CJ, 238, *270*, 295, *318*, 345, 352, *356*
Sanderson G, 100, *116*, 393, *400*
Sandford AJ, 11, *23*
Sandfored AJ, 11, *23*
Sanford A, 380, *389*
Sanjar S, 239, *271*
Sankary RM, 91, *109*
Sano Y, 305, *326*
Santanello N, 304, *325*
Santicioli P, 214, *229*
Santos C, 191, 192, 193, *200*
Santucci V, 213, *227*
Santulli RJ, 243, 256, *272*
Sardar N, 257, *280*
Sareen M, 168, *179*
Sargent C, 168, *179*
Saria A, 203, 204, 205, 209, 219, *222*, *223*, *225*, *234*
Sarmieneto U, 346, *357*
Sarpong SB, 17, 18, *25*
Sarter M, 264, *282*
Sasaki H, 89, 90, 91, *107*, *109*, 220, *235*, 365, *383*
Sasaki T, 89, 90, *107*
Saski M, 259, *280*
Sass P, 246, *274*
Sastre-y-Hernandez M, 251, 264, *276*, *282*
Sathe GM, 246, *274*
Satkus S, 88, 92, *106*, *109*
Satkus SA, 90, 91, *107*
Sato M, 306, *327*
Sato TA, 345, *357*
Satoh H, 214, *229*
Satoh K, 185, *197*
Satoh M, 89, 90, *107*
Satouchi K, 185, *196*, *197*
Saunders KB, 104, *117*
Saurat JH, 257, *279*
Savelkoul JFH, 353, *360*
Savineau JP, 210, *225*
Savoie C, 216, *231*
Scanlon PD, 292, *316*

Scentivanyi A, 248, *275*
Schachter E, 104, *118*
Schachter EN, 71, *83*
Schade FU, 255, 256, 268, *278*
Schaefer O, 91, *108*
Schall T, 65, *78*
Schandevyl W, 301, *324*
Schauer U, 185, *196*
Schbert H, 264, *282*
Scheerens H, 218, *234*
Scheffold A, 346, *357*
Scheid CR, 91, *108*
Scheinman RI, 158, *173*
Schellenberg R, 35, *47*
Schellenberg RR, 15, *24*, 32, 33, 34, 35, *46*, *48*, 218, *233*
Schermers HP, 242, 255, *271*
Schierhorn K, 212, *227*
Schijns VE, 347, *358*
Schiller I, 100, *116*
Schilling JG, 194, *201*
Schinca N, 298, *322*
Schinnar R, 143, *153*
Schioppacassi G, 255, *277*
Schleimer RP, 60, 66, 67, *74*, *79*, *80*, 158, *174*, 241, 242, 254, *271*, 289, *313*
Schlosser R, 89, *106*
Schlunck T, 332, *340*
Schmeding-Wiegel H, 264, *282*
Schmidt AW, 213, *227*
Schmidt D, 242, 256, *272*
Schmidt TJ, 158, *173*
Schmiott-Grohe S, 125, *147*
Schmitz-Schumann M, 296, 297, *320*
Schneider B, 365, *382*
Schneider HH, 264, *282*
Schneider R, 93, *111*
Schnemann M, 88, *106*
Schnyder UW, 343, *355*
Schoenen FJ, 251, *276*
Schoenhoff M, 339, *342*
Schoenhoff MB, 333, *341*
Schofield B, 95, *113*
Schon-Hegrad MA, 63, *77*
Schonfeld W, 289, *312*
Schony W, 251, 264, *276*
Schoonbrood DFME, 42, *55*, 67, *79*
Schork A, 268, *283*
Schot R, 35, 37, *47*, *50*
Schou C, 18, *25*, 348, 349, *358*
Schouten JP, 42, *55*, 395, *401*
Schratzer M, 251, 264, *276*
Schreck R, 374, *387*
Schrier AC, 30, *44*
Schudt C, 243, 254, 255, 256, 257, 268, *272*, *273*, *277*, *278*
Schuh S, 104, *117*
Schuiling M, 217, *232*
Schule R, 158, *173*
Schulman ES, 60, *74*, 289, *313*
Schulman KA, 393, *399*
Schultheis A, 94, *112*
Schultz KD, 212, *227*
Schultz-Weringhaus G, 100, *116*
Schultze-Osthoff K, 374, *387*
Schwabe U, 245, 248, 250, 264, *273*
Schwartz J, 121, *147*
Schwartz JI, 302, *324*
Schwartz LB, 57, 60, 61, *72*, *75*, 296, 298, *320*, *321*
Schwartz T, 214, *228*
Schwartz TW, 214, *228*
Schwarze J, 14, *24*
Schwarze PE, 15, *24*
Schweizer RC, 352, *359*
Scott AIF, 264, *282*
Scott J, 166, *178*
Scott S, 288, 292, *311*
Scott W, 96, *113*
Scypinski L, 218, *233*
Seager K, 59, 61, *74*
Seamon KB, 243, 256, *272*
Sears M, 4, *21*, 66, *79*
Sears MR, 5, *21*, 129, 131, 135, 142, *149*, *153*, 329, *340*
Seaton A, 2, 15, 19, *21*, *24*, *26*
Sebald W, 371, *385*
Seckl JR, 378, *388*
Secrist H, 359, *360*
Seder RA, 63, *77*, 345, 349, *356*, *359*
Seeds EAM, 259, *280*

Seeman E, 166, *178*
Segal A, 304, 309, *325*, *328*
Segal M, 259, *281*
Segal MR, 14, *24*, 41, *54*
Segal NL, 9, *22*
Sehmi R, 295, *319*
Seidenberg BC, 303, *324*
Seitz M, 158, *174*
Sekiguchi M, 66, *79*
Sekisawa K, 91, *109*
Sekizawa K, 60, *75*, 220, *235*
Sekut L, 251, 263, 268, *276*, *281*
Selig W, 372, *386*
Selig WM, 219, *234*, 364, *382*
Selroos O, 160, 161, *175*, *176*
Seltzer J, 305, *326*
Seltzer JM, 126, 129, 135, 137, *148*
Semeraro C, 255, *277*
Semper A, 62, *76*, 285, *309*
Semper AE, 63, *77*
Seneterre E, 43, *56*, 71, *83*
Senik A, 217, *232*
Senior R, 71, *83*
Senior RJ, 100, *116*
Senior RM, 71, *83*
Sepizer FE, 14, *24*
Serhan CN, 287, *310*
Serino K, 309, *328*
Serra MC, 217, *232*
Serra MF, 257, *279*
Service J, 32, 34, *46*
Sestini P, 377, *388*
Severinghaus JW, 87, *106*
Sewell WA, 158, 169, *174*
Seyama Y, 187, *198*
Seybold J, 257, 269, *280*, 372, 374, 378, *386*, *388*
Seymour ML, 291, *315*
Seymour PA, 213, *227*
Seymour WP, 238, *270*
Sha WC, 375, *387*
Shahid M, 247, 252, *274*
Shaikh WA, 167, *179*
Sham JSK, 215, *230*
Shannon HS, 143, *153*
Shannon VR, 60, *75*
Shapiro C, 101, *116*
Shapiro J, 192, *201*, 299, *322*
Shapiro S, 71, *83*
Shardonofsky FR, 39, *52*
Sharma A, 41, *54*
Sharma S, 253, 260, 261, 263, 269, *277*
Sharp PA, 11, *22*, 348, *358*
Shaw G, 128, 131, *148*, 364, *382*
Shaw MJ, 140, 141, *151*
Sheaffer CI, 100, *116*
Sheehy O, 307, *327*
Sheldrick RLG, 213, 215, *227*, *230*
Shelhamer JH, 293, *317*
Shelhammer J, 89, 90, 101, *107*, *117*
Sheller JR, 295, 297, 306, *318*, *320*, *321*, *326*
Shen X, 34, *47*
Shenoi PM, 162, *176*
Shenvi A, 214, *229*
Shepard RH, 39, *53*
Shepherd GL, 146, *154*
Sheppard D, 17, *25*, 70, *81*, 97, 99, *114*, *115*, 218, *233*
Sher A, 332, *341*, 345, 346, *356*
Sher ER, 67, *80*
Sheridan RD, 368, *384*
Shering PA, 264, *282*
Shi W, 371, *386*
Shibuya K, 347, 350, 351, *358*, *359*
Shida T, 194, *201*
Shields MD, 171, *181*
Shields R, 333, 339, *341*, *342*
Shigematsu Y, 297, *320*
Shih C, 298, *322*
Shimadzu W, 187, *198*
Shimazu S, 15, *24*, 380, *389*
Shimizu T, 93, *111*, 187, *198*
Shimura S, 89, 90, *107*
Shimuzu T, 288, *312*
Shindo K, 297, *321*
Shindoh Y, 59, *74*
Shinebourne E, 5, *21*
Shingo S, 300, 301, 305, 307, *323*, *324*, *326*, *327*
Shinnick-Gallagher P, 92, *110*
Shipley ME, 295, *319*

Shirakawa T, 15, *24*, 380, *389*
Shiraki K, 211, *226*
Shirasaki H, 158, *173*, 208, *224*
Shirato K, 208, 221, *224*, *235*
Shire SJ, 333, *341*
Shirley JT, 251, 265, 269, *276*, *282*
Shiue P, 37, *50*
Shore SA, 34, 39, *47*, 208, 209, *224*
Showell JH, 217, *231*, 255, 268, *278*
Shrestha M, 105, *118*
Shuckett EP, 167, *179*
Shukla SD, 185, 186, *197*
Shult P, 94, *112*
Shultz TF, 365, *383*
Shute J, 58, 59, 60, 61, 64, 65, 66, *73*, *76*, *78*
Shute JK, 66, *79*, 243, 257, *273*, 329, *340*
Shuttleworth D, 167, *179*
Sickels BD, 258, 264, *280*, *282*
Sieck GC, 34, 39, *47*
Siefken H, 93, *111*
Siegel MI, 372, 374, *386*
Siegel SC, 299, 303, *322*
Siegler PB, 158, *173*
Sielczak MW, 295, *319*
Siena L, 306, *327*
Sigal IS, 288, *311*
Sigurdson M, 71, *83*
Sillastu H, 71, *82*
Silva J, 268, *283*
Silver MJ, 185, *197*
Silver PJ, 247, 252, 253, 258, 269, *274*
Silverman ES, 309, *328*
Silverstein MD, 164, *178*
Silvert BD, 128, *148*
Sim JJ, 306, *327*
Simhandl C, 264, *282*
Simon HU, 308, *328*
Simon MT, 238, *271*
Simon SJ, 333, 339, *341*
Simons FER, 129, 141, *149*, *152*, 167, *179*
Simonson SG, 296, 306, *319*
Simonsson B, 99, 101, *115*
Simonsson BG, 71, *82*
Simony-Lafontaine J, 396, *402*
Simpson A, 18, *26*
Singer II, 288, 292, *311*
Singer M, 255, 268, *278*
Sinha B, 255, *277*
Sinigaglia F, 346, *357*
Sinon GT, 212, *227*
Sinony-Lafontaine J, 57, 65, *73*
Siok C, 213, *227*
Sisson JH, 185, *197*
Sjoerdsman K, 58, *73*
Skinner C, 162, *176*
Skloot G, 39, *53*
Skoner DP, 286, *309*
Skoogh BE, 99, 101, *115*, 120, 136, *146*
Skorodin MS, 38, *52*, 97, 104, *114*
Skuta GL, 167, *179*
Sladek K, 297, 309, *320*, *328*
Slater JE, 61, *76*
Sledsens T, 104, *118*
Sledsens TJM, 366, *383*
Slemenda CW, 166, *178*
Sloan SI, 65, 66, *79*
Sluiter HJ, 29, 42, *44*, *55*, 67, *79*, 160, *175*
Slutsky A, 97, *114*
Slutsky AS, 41, *54*
Sly PD, 28, 29, 32, 40, *44*, *46*, 395, *401*
Small P, 126, 129, 135, 137, *148*
Small RC, 36, *50*, 266, *283*
Smeal T, 158, *173*
Smeets J, 104, *118*
Smeets JJ, 125, *147*, 366, *383*, 398, *403*
Smeets SJ, 127, *148*
Smiko B, 364, *382*
Smith AL, 286, *310*
Smith B, 248, 251, 257, 263, 267, *275*, *276*
Smith CA, 7, *21*
Smith CM, 5, *21*, 297, 303, *320*, *325*
Smith D, 239, *271*
Smith DH, 398, *403*
Smith G, 35, *48*
Smith H, 101, *117*, 259, 260, *281*
Smith HR, 60, *74*, 296, *320*
Smith JB, 185, *197*

Smith L, 99, 101, *115*, *117*, 285, *309*
Smith LJ, 189, 193, *199*, *201*, 294, 304, *317*, *325*
Smith MJH, 60, *75*, 295, *319*
Smith PG, 35, *47*
Smith S, 393, *400*
Smith WB, 259, *280*, 295, *319*
Smith WL, 364, *382*
Smits HH, 15, *24*, 38, 42, *52*, *55*, 59, 66, *74*
Smolen JS, 371, *386*
Smorzik J, 96, *114*
Smyth ET, 127, 137, *148*, *150*
Snider GL, 156, *172*
Snider RM, 213, 214, 216, *227*, *228*, *231*
Snijders A, 372, *386*
Snijdewint GFM, 351, *359*
Snook S, 37, *50*
Snyder DW, 289, *312*
Snyder F, 183, *196*
Sobeck A, 15, *24*
Sobel RA, 351, *359*
Soberman RJ, 288, 289, *311*, *312*
Soderman DD, 242, 256, *272*
Sofia M, 187, *198*
Soja J, 297, 309, *320*, *328*, 378, *388*
Solari R, 371, *385*
Soler M, 125, 140, *147*
Solley GO, 59, 69, *74*
Solomon HF, 243, 256, *272*
Solverman EK, 309, *328*
Solway J, 37, 38, *50*, *51*, 217, *232*, 292, 299, *316*, *322*
Somers S, 167, *179*
Sommer N, 263, *281*
Song Y, 36, 41, *49*
Song YL, 43, *56*, 66, 71, *79*
Songsiridej V, 94, 100, *112*
Sont JK, 32, 36, 37, 38, 39, 40, 42, 43, *45*, *49*, *51*, *52*, *53*, *54*, *55*, 58, 59, 66, *73*, *74*, 159, *174*, 205, *223*, 296, 305, *319*, 394, *400*
Soong SJ, 397, *402*
Sorkness R, 38, *51*, 94, 99, *112*
Sornasse T, 347, *358*
Sorva R, 169, *180*
Soter NA, 293, *317*
Sotiropoulou E, 101, *117*
Soubrie P, 213, *227*, *228*
Soukop W, 251, 264, *276*
Souness JE, 243, 244, 248, 251, 253, 254, 255, 256, 257, 260, 261, 263, 269, *272*, *273*, *275*, *276*, *277*, *280*
Sousa AR, 297, *320*
Soutar A, 19, *26*
Southern DL, 126, 129, 135, 137, *148*
Sovijarvi A, 160, 161, *175*, *176*
Sovijarvi AR, 125, *147*
Spaan WJM, 36, *49*
Spada CS, 295, *319*
Spaethe SM, 288, *312*
Spagnola B, 92, *109*
Spagnotto S, 307, *327*
Spahn JD, 155, *172*
Spainhour DC, 252, *276*
Spanavello A, 395, *401*
Spanevello A, 285, *309*
Sparrow D, 41, 42, *54*, *55*, 259, *281*
Sparrow MP, 36, *48*
Spector J, 291, *314*
Spector R, 300, 307, *323*, *327*
Spector S, 304, 305, *325*, *326*
Spector SL, 60, *75*, 304, *325*
Speers DM, 100, *116*
Speilberg SP, 290, *314*
Speizer FE, 17, *25*, 143, *153*
Spence DP, 194, *201*
Spencer DA, 192, *200*
Spencer RW, 213, *227*
Spengler JD, 17, *25*
Sperling R, 192, *200*, 299, *322*
Sperner-Uterweger B, 264, *282*
Spessotto P, 71, *83*
Spina D, 259, *280*, *281*
Spitzer WO, 143, 144, *153*
Sporik R, 343, *355*
Spriggs MK, 345, *357*
Springall DR, 70, *82*, 208, *223*, *224*
Springer C, 162, *177*
Sprong RC, 93, *111*
Spruce KE, 299, *323*

Spur BW, 292, 294, 296, 298, 305, *316*, *317*, *319*, *322*
Squillace D, 38, 42, *52*
Sreedharan SP, 209, 217, *224*, *232*
Sreena S, 160, *175*
St. John T, 247, *275*
Stableforth DE, 162, *176*
Stacey MA, 8, *22*
Staczek J, 220, *235*
Stadek K, 378, *388*
Stadel JM, 247, *275*
Staehelin T, 43, *55*, 333, *341*
Stafford JA, 251, *276*
Stafford S, 371, *385*
Stahl EG, 39, *53*
Stalenheim G, 137, *150*
Stanciu L, 58, 59, 60, 61, 64, 66, *73*
Stanciu LA, 65, *78*
Stanford CF, 212, *226*
Stapel SO, 372, *386*
Stark JM, 290, *314*
Stark R, 104, *118*
Starzl TC, 378, *388*
Stawiski MA, 268, *283*
Stead RH, 212, *227*
Steeber AS, 95, *113*
Steel D, 90, *107*
Steen N, 393, *399*
Stefanini P, 287, *310*
Steffen RP, 247, 252, *274*
Steffensen I, 126, 129, 135, 137, *148*
Steinbach JP, 263, *281*
Steinberg R, 213, *227*
Steinbrecher A, 263, *281*
Steiner B, 247, *275*
Steinhilber D, 289, *313*
Steinijans VW, 266, *283*
Steinman L, 353, *360*
Steller JR, 133, *149*
Stendahl O, 256, *278*
Stenius-Aarniala B, 160, 161, *175*, *176*
Stensvad F, 301, *323*
Stenton SC, 185, *196*, 298, *322*
Stephens NL, 34, 39, *47*, 94, *112*
Sterbinsky SA, 339, *342*
Sterk P, 300, *323*
Sterk PH, 205, *223*
Sterk PJ, 28, 30, 31, 32, 33, 35, 36, 37, 38, 39, 40, 41, 42, 43, *44*, *45*, *46*, *47*, *48*, *49*, *50*, *51*, *52*, *53*, *54*, *55*, 58, 59, 66, *73*, *74*, 140, 141, *151*, 159, *174*, 211, 215, *226*, *230*, 295, 296, 297, 298, 300, 303, 305, 307, *318*, *319*, *321*, *324*, *326*, *327*, 394, 395, 396, *400*
Stern AS, 348, *358*
Stevens RL, 254, *277*
Stevenson C, 169, *180*
Stewart AL, 397, *402*
Stewart C, 346, *357*
Stewart GA, 188, *198*
Stewart JM, 212, *226*
Stewart T, 332, 333, *341*
Sticker WE, 305, *326*
Stimpson SA, 251, 255, 263, 268, *276*, *278*, *281*
Stinson-Fisher C, 214, *229*
Stobel S, 353, *360*
Stober P, 303, 305, *325*, *326*
Stolk J, 36, *49*
Stoll C, 255, *277*
Stolley PD, 143, *153*
Stolz RR, 333, 336, *341*
Stone P, 367, *383*
Stoof TJ, 257, *279*
Storey G, 157, *172*
Storms W, 304, 308, *325*
Storz C, 57, *73*, 395, 396, *401*
Storz Chr, 38, *52*
Stossel TP, 286, *310*
Strachan D, 2, *20*
Strachan DP, 1, 12, *20*, *23*
Strada SJ, 238, 244, *270*
Strader CD, 288, *311*
Stragliotto E, 287, *310*
Strahcan D, 16, *24*
Stranick KS, 371, *385*
Strassmann G, 255, 268, *278*
Strath M, 238, *270*
Strauch KL, 379, *389*
Street NE, 63, *77*
Strek ME, 299, *322*

Strember RH, 348, *359*
Stretton CD, 362, 365, 367, *381*, *383*, *384*
Stretton D, 244, 261, *273*
Stricker W, 304, *325*
Strickland AB, 251, 255, 268, *276*, *278*
Strieter RM, 352, *359*
Strobel S, 343, *355*
Strockbine L, 345, *357*
Strominger N, 265, *282*
Stropp JQ, 32, 34, *46*
Struble C, 333, *341*
Stuart AM, 146, *154*
Stupfel M, 87, *106*
Sturgess J, 90, *107*
Sturm RJ, 242, 256, *272*
Sturtridge WC, 166, *178*
Su JQ, 333, 336, 337, 338, 339, *341*, 379, *389*
Sudo M, 297, *320*
Suetsugu S, 306, *327*
Sugatani J, 186, *197*
Suguro H, 303, *325*
Suh EM, 251, *276*
Suissa S, 143, 144, *153*, 167, *179*, 307, *327*
Suko M, 243, 257, *273*
Sullivan CE, 208, *223*
Sullivan PJ, 265, 266, 267, *282*
Sullivan S, 398, *403*
Sullivan SD, 398, *403*
Sumitomo M, 297, *321*
Summer W, 100, *116*
Summer WR, 97, 100, *114*
Summers JB, 288, *311*
Summers QA, 96, *114*
Sun FF, 290, *314*
Sun G, 8, *22*
Sun L, 43, *55*, 333, *341*
Sun YL, 158, *173*
Sundblad BM, 39, *53*
Sundler F, 207, *223*
Sung TC, 91, *109*
Suphioglu C, 16, 17, *24*, *25*
Suppli Ch, 41, *54*
Sur S, 66, *79*, 378, *388*
Sussman HS, 140, 141, *151*
Sutherland EW, 237, 238, 245, 269, *270*
Sutton BJ, 330, *340*
Suzuki N, 305, *326*
Suzuki R, 295, *318*
Suzuki S, 297, *321*
Suzuki Y, 186, *197*
Svahn T, 160, 161, *175*, *176*
Svedmyr N, 125, 133, 137, 142, *148*, *151*, *152*, 221, *235*
Svendsen UG, 160, *175*
Swain SL, 65, *78*
Sweitzer DE, 306, *327*
Swelund H, 378, *388*
Swenson C, 70, *82*
Swindell AC, 295, *319*
Swinkles LMJW, 171, *180*
Swinnen JV, 246, *274*
Swystun A, 140, 141, *151*
Swystun VA, 333, 336, 338, *341*
Sy MLT, 167, *179*
Symington P, 393, *400*
Synek M, 67, *81*
Szabo S, 346, *358*
Szalai JP, 166, *178*
Szczeklik A, 286, 297, 308, *310*, *320*, *328*, 378, *388*
Szefler S, 101, *117*
Szefler SJ, 65, 66, 67, *79*, *80*, 155, 169, *172*, *180*
Szentivanyi A, 252, 257, *276*, *279*
Szucs G, 376, *388*

T

Tabe K, 190, *200*, 303, *325*
Tadjikarimi S, 102, *117*, 366, *383*
Tadjkarimi M, 367, *383*
Tagari P, 295, 296, 297, 299, 302, *319*, *320*, *322*, *324*
Tagaya E, 90, 104, *107*, 305, *326*
Tager IB, 14, *24*
Tahami F, 291, *315*
Tai HH, 242, *272*
Takagi K, 295, *318*, 362, 365, *381*

Takahashi H, 297, *321*
Takahashi T, 35, 36, 37, *47*, *49*, *50*, 102, *117*, 221, *235*, 286, 294, *309*, 366, *383*
Takami M, 187, *198*
Takashima T, 36, *49*
Takata S, 37, *50*, 218, *233*
Takeda K, 14, *24*, 371, *386*
Takemuira H, 305, *326*
Taki F, 295, *318*
Takishama T, 221, *235*
Takishima T, 37, *51*, 59, *74*, 89, 90, 91, *107*, *109*, 194, *201*, 365, *383*
Takizawa T, 71, *83*, 305, *326*
Takuwa Y, 288, *312*
Tamagawa K, 305, *326*
Tamaoki J, 94, *112*, 305, *326*
Tammeling GJ, 30, *44*
Tammivaara R, 160, 161, *175*, *176*
Tamoki J, 90, 104, *107*
Tamplin B, 99, *115*
Tamura G, 194, *201*, 218, 221, *233*, *235*
Tamura K, 89, 90, *107*
Tamura N, 184, *196*
Tan KS, 137, *151*
Tan S, 139, *151*
Tanaka D, 94, *112*
Tanaka DT, 38, *51*, 211, *226*
Tanaka I, 306, *327*
Tanaka R, 61, *76*
Tanaka T, 371, *385*, *386*
Tanaka W, 300, *323*
Tanemura M, 35, *47*
Tang ML, 12, *23*
Taniguchi H, 295, *318*
Taniguchi M, 306, *327*
Taniguchi Y, 218, *233*
Tanno SA, 364, *382*
Tarala RA, 96, *114*
Tariq S, 13, 18, *23*
Tarodo de la Fuente P, 297, *321*
Tarpy RE, 64, *77*, 352, *359*
Tarraf H, 17, *25*
Tashkin D, 266, *283*
Tashkin DP, 41, *55*
Tattersall FD, 265, *282*
Tattersfield AE, 19, *26*, 127, 129, 131, 135, 137, 141, 142, *148*, *149*, *150*, *152*, 301, *324*, 364, *382*, 393, 398, *399*, *400*
Taub D, 65, *78*
Taussig LM, 13, *23*
Taylor A, 92, *110*
Taylor B, 12, *23*
Taylor D, 259, *281*
Taylor DA, 32, *45*, 125, 140, *147*
Taylor DP, 246, *274*
Taylor DR, 142, *152*
Taylor G, 192, *200*, 299, *322*
Taylor GE, 219, *234*
Taylor GW, 191, 192, 193, *200*, *201*, 289, 292, 295, 296, *313*, *316*, *318*, *320*
Taylor IK, 191, 192, 193, *200*, *201*, 295, 296, *318*, *320*
Taylor JD, 255, 268, *278*
Taylor P, 17, *25*
Taylor RJ, 96, 104, *114*
Taytard A, 398, *403*
Teahan JA, 301, *324*
TeBiesebeek J, 92, *110*
Tech M, 160, *175*
Tedder TF, 95, *113*
Teelucksingh S, 165, *178*
Tence M, 183, *196*
Tennen HA, 393, *399*
Tenor H, 58, 59, 60, 61, 64, 66, *73*, 243, 254, 255, 257, *272*, *273*, *277*
Tepper RS, 34, *47*
Teran L, 64, *77*, 352, *359*
Terasaki WL, 238, 244, *270*
Terasawa M, 186, 195, *198*
Terce F, 186, *197*
Terwaki T, 293, *317*
Tesselaar K, 346, *358*
Testi R, 42, *55*, 169, *180*
Thagat R, 333, 336, 338, *341*
Thaideio PF, 251, *276*
Thein FCK, 298, *322*
Theodorsson E, 220, *235*
Theodorsson-Norheim E, 205, 207, 209, *223*, *225*
Thiemann HH, 19, *26*

Thien FC, 5, *21*, 297, *320*
Thiene G, 67, *80*
Thiruchelvam R, 144, *154*
Thomas CE, 369, 373, *384*
Thomas L, 43, *55*, 333, *341*
Thomas ML, 350, *359*
Thomas PS, 369, *384*
Thomas RU, 297, *321*
Thompson AG, 378, *388*
Thompson CB, 63, *76*
Thompson DC, 70, *82*
Thompson JR, 144, *154*
Thompson N, 97, *114*
Thompson PJ, 188, *198*
Thompson WJ, 238, 244, 245, *270*, *273*
Thomson H, 60, *75*, 302, *324*
Thomson HW, 302, *324*
Thomson NC, 160, *175*, 365, 369, *382*, *385*
Thomson RJ, 33, 34, 35, *46*, *47*, *48*, 218, *233*
Thorburn J, 12, *23*
Thurairatnam S, 251, *276*
Thurlbeck WM, 71, *83*
Tibi L, 165, *178*
Tierney DF, 39, *53*
Tijhuis GJ, 266, *283*
Timmermans A, 91, *109*
Timmers MC, 15, *24*, 31, 36, 37, 38, 39, 40, 41, *45*, *49*, *51*, *52*, *53*, *54*, 140, 141, *151*, 211, *226*, 295, 300, 303, *318*, *324*
Timonen KL, 17, *25*
Tinkelman D, 299, 303, 304, 309, *322*, *325*, *328*
Tinkelman DG, 99, 101, *115*, 164, *177*, 333, 336, *341*
Tippins JR, 292, *316*
Tobler A, 158, *174*
Tocker J, 372, *386*
Tocker JE, 219, *234*
Toda T, 246, *274*
Todd G, 171, *181*
Todwell LJ, 125, 140, *147*
Toelle BG, 18, *26*
Tofte SJ, 268, *283*
Togias A, 39, *53*, 105, *118*, 339, *342*
Toh H, 187, *198*
Tokiwa Y, 99, *115*
Tom-Moy M, 91, *109*
Tom-moy M, 90, *108*
Tomaki M, 208, 221, *224*, *235*
Tomioka M, 59, *74*, 212, *227*
Tomkin S, 18, *25*
Tomkinson A, 253, 254, 260, 261, 263, 269, *277*
Tomura M, 347, *358*
Tony HP, 371, *385*
Toogood JH, 157, 162, 165, 166, 167, *172*, *176*, *178*, *179*
Tool AT, 257, *279*
Tori K, 295, *318*
Tormey VJ, 36, *49*, 65, *78*
Torphy TJ, 241, 242, 246, 247, 254, 256, 258, 261, 263, 265, 269, *271*, *274*, *275*, *277*, *278*, *280*, *282*, 286, 295, *310*, *319*
Torren K, 393, *399*
Toteson TD, 14, *24*
Totty NF, 239, *271*
Toty L, 209, 210, 215, *225*
Tousignant C, 216, *231*
Tovey E, 18, *26*
Town GI, 142, *152*
Townley R, 304, *325*
Townley RG, 88, *106*, 184, 188, 189, 191, 195, *196*, *199*, *202*
Towse L, 102, *117*
Towse lJ, 366, *383*
Toyka KV, 218, *233*
Traenckner M, 374, *387*
Trampitsch E, 251, 264, *276*
Tranfa CME, 135, *150*
Traystman R, 99, *115*
Tremoli E, 287, *310*
Treppiari S, 215, *230*
Trethewie WR, 289, *312*
Trevillion LM, 343, *355*
Tricopo Ulos A, 238, *270*
Triflieff A, 378, *388*
Trigg CJ, 17, *25*, 67, 70, *80*, *81*, 159, 170, *174*

Triggiani M, 187, *198*
Trimble L, 268, *283*
Trinchieri G, 346, *357*, 372, *386*
Trinquet G, 397, *403*
Tripp CS, 63, *77*, 346, *357*
Trophy T, 242, 256, *272*
Trophy TJ, 248, 250, 251, 253, 257, 263, 265, *275*, *276*, *279*, *281*
Trudeau C, 125, 140, *147*
Trudeau JB, 296, 306, 307, *319*
Truong O, 239, *271*
Truong VH, 255, *277*
Tsai BS, 289, *312*
Tsai JJ, 67, *80*
Tsai M, 290, *314*
Tsai MJ, 158, *173*
Tsai SY, 158, *173*
Tsanakas J, 169, *180*
Tschomper BA, 71, *83*
Tse KS, 185, *196*
Tsicopoulos A, 57, 62, *73*
Tsokos GC, 158, *174*
Tsukagoshi H, 214, *229*, 306, *327*
Tsukakoshi H, 36, *48*
Tsukioka K, 187, *198*
Tsuyuki J, 378, *388*
Tsuyuki S, 332, *340*, 378, *388*
Tsuzuike N, 294, *317*
Tu YP, 295, *318*
Tuch T, 17, *25*
Tudhope SR, 289, *312*
Tunnicliffe W, 395, *401*
Tunon-de-Lara JM, 62, 63, *76*, *77*, 285, *309*
Tuomanen EI, 375, *387*
Turck CW, 209, *224*
Turco P, 305, *326*
Turcotte H, 36, 37, 42, *49*, *50*, 134, *150*, 393, *399*
Turki J, 11, *22*
Turner CR, 217, *232*, 255, 259, 268, *278*, *280*, 295, *319*
Turner GA, 301, *324*
Turner M, 66, *79*, 254, *277*
Turner MO, 129, 131, 135, 142, *149*, *153*
Turner NC, 243, 254, 255, 256, *272*, *277*
Turner S, 194, *201*
Turpin JA, 307, *327*
Turpin MP, 213, 215, *227*, *230*
Twentyman OP, 35, 38, *48*, 58, 59, *73*, 133, *149*, 239, *271*, 286, *310*, 391, *399*
Twort C, 205, *223*
Twort CHC, 34, 35, *47*
Tybulewicz VLG, 254, *277*
Tyers MB, 213, *227*
Tyrrell DAJ, 393, *400*

U

Uccelli A, 263, 265, *281*
Uddman R, 207, 208, *223*, *224*
Uden S, 191, 194, *200*, *201*
Ueki I, 89, *107*
Ueki IF, 94, *112*, 243, 256, *272*
Uffmann J, 193, *201*
Ui M, 243, 256, *272*
Ujiie Y, 220, *235*
Ulbrich E, 303, *325*
Ullah MI, 104, *117*
Ullman A, 120, 131, 136, 137, 142, *146*, *149*, *151*, 163, 170, *177*, 364, *382*, 393, 398, *400*
Ulmer W, 100, *115*
Ulrich V, 256, *278*
Ulrik CS, 71, *83*, 128, *148*
Umeno E, 218, *233*
Umetsu DT, 359, *360*
Umland JP, 265, 269, *282*
Umland SP, 370, 371, *385*
Unanue ER, 63, *76*
Undem B, 93, *111*, 242, 256, *272*
Undem BJ, 90, *107*, 185, *197*, 204, 214, 215, 218, *223*, *229*, *230*, *234*, 241, 242, 244, 247, 254, 258, 261, 269, *271*, *273*, *275*, *277*, *281*, 286, 295, *310*
Underwood DC, 254, 258, 261, 263, 269, *277*, *280*, 295, *319*
Underwood SL, 253, 260, 261, 263, 269, *276*
Urban JF, 332, *341*
Urbanek R, 395, *401*

Uss AS, 371, *385*
Utell MJ, 100, 101, *116*
Uthayarkumar S, 194, *201*

V

v/d Mark ThW, 40, *54*
Vachier I, 297, *321*
Vachier L, 66, *79*
Vadas MA, 295, *318*, 345, 352, *356*
Vagaggini B, 140, *151*
Vaghi A, 377, *388*
Valentine MD, 105, *118*
Valentovic MA, 365, *382*
Vamvalis C, 101, *117*
Van Aalderen WMC, 160, *175*
van Alystyne EL, 288, *312*
Van Amsterdam GM, 91, *109*
Van Amsterdam JG, 242, 255, *271*
Van Amsterdam RG, 91, *108*
Van Ark I, 353, *360*
van As A, 126, 129, 135, 137, *148*
Van Broeck D, 213, *227*, *228*
Van Daele P, 301, *324*
Van den Berg LRM, 304, 308, *325*
Van den Elshout FMJ, 301, *324*
van der Bruggen T, 371, *385*
Van der Laag H, 164, *177*
van der Laag H, 129, 141, *148*
van der Linde HJ, 37, *50*
van der Loo PG, 256, *278*
Van Der Mark TW, 160, *175*
van der Meer van Roomen W, 91, *109*
van der Molen T, 129, 131, 135, *149*
van der Pouw Kraan TC, 372, *386*
van der Raaij LM, 257, *279*
van der Straeten M, 30, 31, 40, *45*, 210, *225*, 395, *401*
van der Straeten ME, 211, *226*, 301, *324*
van der Tweel MC, 256, *278*
van der Veen H, 36, 37, 39, *48*, *51*, 211, 215, *226*, *230*, 295, 300, *318*
van der Weig AM, 307, *327*
van der Zee JS, 372, *386*
van der Zee SC, 15, *24*
van Deventer SJ, 372, 374, *386*
van Dijk TB, 371, *385*
van Doormaal JJ, 165, *178*
van Doorslaer EKA, 398, *403*
van Esch B, 353, *360*
van Essen-Zandvliet EE, 40, *54*, 160, *175*
van Essen-Zandvliet EEM, 141, *152*, 160, 164, *175*, *178*, 395, *401*
van Ginneken CAM, 89, 92, *107*, *110*
van Haarst JMW, 63, *77*
van Helden-Meeuwsen CG, 36, *49*, 63, *77*
van Herwaarden CLA, 171, *180*, 304, 308, *325*
van Houwelingen HC, 164, *178*
van Kan CI, 305, *326*
van Klink HCJ, 205, *223*
van Koppen CJ, 89, 91, 92, *107*, *108*, *110*
van Krieken JHJM, 36, 37, 38, 42, *49*, *51*, *52*, 58, *73*, 159, *174*, 205, *223*, 395, 396, *400*
van Loveren H, 218, *234*
van Noord JA, 125, 133, *147*
van Oosterhout AJ, 353, *360*
van Oosterhout AJM, 218, *234*
van Rensen EL, 296, 305, *319*
van Rietschoten AGI, 346, *358*
van Rooij H, 92, *110*
van Schadewijk WAAM, 36, *49*
van Schayck CP, 96, *114*
van Schoor J, 210, 221, *225*, *235*, 299, *323*
van Steen CJ, 15, *24*
van Tits LJH, 257, *279*
van Weel C, 96, *114*
van Wijnen JH, 15, *24*
van Zanten AK, 165, *178*
van Zoest JGCM, 307, *327*
Vandenbergh RH, 1, *20*
Vandenbroucke JP, 38, 39, 42, 43, *52*, *53*
Vanderheyden P, 91, 92, *108*
Vane J, 287, *310*
VanGinneken CAM, 91, *108*

Vanhoutte PM, 67, *81*
vanKlink HCJ, 37, *51*
Vanni L, 218, *233*
vanNieuwstadt R, 91, *109*
Vanzieleghem MA, 160, *175*
Vardey C, 122, *147*
Varenne P, 183, *196*
Vargaftig BB, 238, 255, 268, *271*, *278*
Varigos G, 158, *174*
Varley J, 60, *75*
Varosanec S, 251, 264, *276*
Vartanian MA, 213, *227*, *228*
Vassalli G, 8, *22*
Vathenen AS, 141, *152*
Vaughan LM, 168, *179*
Vaughan-Williams E, 2, *20*
Vauthan JH, 217, *232*
Vayssiere BM, 374, *387*
Vaz R, 369, 373, *384*
Vazquez J, 366, *383*
Vazquez M, 291, *315*
Vedal S, 31, 35, *45*, *48*
Velly J, 121, *147*
Velvisi MG, 367, 368, 374, *383*, *384*
Venable ME, 185, 186, *197*
Venburgt L, 35, *48*
Venge P, 57, 59, 65, 71, *73*, *74*, *82*, 239, *271*, 396, *402*
Venkatesan P, 368, 374, *384*
Venn A, 2, *20*
Verberne AAPH, 129, 141, *148*, 164, *177*
Verbesselt R, 301, *324*
Verbrugt L, 41, 43, *54*, *56*
Verburgt LM, 31, 39, *45*, *53*
Verghese MW, 251, 255, 268, *276*, *278*
Verhagen J, 191, *200*, 289, *313*
Verhoeven AJ, 257, *279*
Verman IM, 158, *173*
Vervloet D, 128, *148*, 398, *403*
Veselic-Charvat M, 58, *73*, 296, 303, 305, *319*, *324*
Vestal RE, 242, 256, *272*
Vetsweber D, 346, *357*
Vetterman J, 92, *110*
Vic P, 66, 71, *79*, *82*
Vicini E, 247, *275*
Vicker N, 251, *276*
Vickers PJ, 288, 292, *311*
Vida E, 307, *327*
Vignola AM, 43, *55*, 66, 69, *79*, *81*, 297, 306, *320*, *327*, 330, *340*
Vik DT, 61, *75*
Vikka V, 296, 305, *319*
Vilain P, 210, 213, 214, 215, 220, *225*, *227*, *228*, *229*, *235*
Vilcek J, 70, *82*
Vinci JM, 158, *173*
Vinick FJ, 213, *227*, 251, *276*
Violante B, 39, *53*
Virtanen I, 71, *82*
Virtanen IT, 396, *402*
Viskum K, 146, *154*
Voelkel NF, 193, *201*, 296, *319*
Voet B, 264, *282*
Voivin JF, 143, 144, *153*
von Berg A, 125, *147*
von Mutius E, 19, *26*
Vons C, 37, *50*
Vonsignore G, 43, *55*
Voorhees JJ, 268, *283*
Vroom TM, 63, *77*
Vrugt B, 65, 66, 67, *79*
Vuchinich T, 134, *150*
vVncheri C, 210, 211, 212, *225*, *226*
Vyse T, 367, *383*

W

Waage A, 158, *174*
Waalkens HJ, 40, *54*, 160, *175*, 395, *401*
Wachtel H, 264, *282*
Wadsworth J, 12, *23*
Waeldele F, 91, 92, *108*
Wagenmann M, 105, *118*
Wagner E, 99, *115*
Wagner EM, 35, 39, *48*
Wagner HW, 166, *178*
Wagner K, 332, *340*
Wagner KHM, 338, *341*
Wagner PD, 192, 193, *200*

Wagner TO, 365, *382*
Wahedna I, 141, *152*, 301, *324*
Wahl SM, 217, *231*
Wahlander L, 125, 133, 142, *148*, *152*
Wahli W, 291, *315*
Wahn U, 18, *25*
Wakao H, 371, *385*
Waku K, 187, *198*
Wald F, 104, *118*
Wald FDM, 366, *383*
Waldeck B, 120, *146*, 365, *382*
Wales M, 251, 257, 263, 267, *276*
Walker B, 208, *224*
Walker C, 38, *52*, 61, *76*
Wall S, 92, *109*, *110*
Wallace AM, 247, 252, 253, 258, 269, *274*
Wallace J, 375, *387*
Wallace WAH, 66, *79*
Wallaert B, 398, *403*
Waller RE, 16, *25*
Walls A, 61, 62, *76*
Walls AE, 134, *150*
Walls AF, 38, *52*, 57, 59, 60, 61, 67, 69, *72*, *76*, *80*, *81*, 160, *176*, 295, *318*, 329, *340*, 395, 396, *401*
Walsh DA, 294, *317*
Walsh DM, 213, 215, *227*, *230*
Walsh DT, 239, *271*
Walsh KA, 246, *274*
Walters AE, 254, *277*
Walters EH, 94, 100, *112*, 134, 141, *150*, *152*, 169, *180*, 185, *196*, 298, *322*, 364, *382*
Walti S, 65, *78*
Waltmann P, 295, *319*
Walumas TL, 350, 351, 353, *359*
Wang CG, 294, *317*
Wang CZ, 242, *272*
Wang G, 43, *55*, 333, *341*
Wang J, 67, *80*, 159, 170, *174*
Wang JH, 70, *81*
Wang P, 372, 374, *386*
Wang Z, 93, *111*
Wanner A, 29, *44*, 89, *106*, 293, *317*
Want J, 372, *386*
Ward C, 134, *150*, 169, *180*, 185, *196*, 298, *322*
Ward J, 102, *117*
Ward JK, 366, *383*
Ward PS, 191, 193, *200*, *201*
Ward R, 297, *321*
Ward TK, 367, *383*
Wardell J, 90, *107*
Wardell JR, 252, *276*
Wardlaw AJ, 37, *50*, 57, 58, 59, 61, 64, 69, 70, *72*, *73*, *81*, 295, 297, *318*, *319*, *321*, 396, *401*
Ware JE, 397, *402*
Ware JH, 17, *25*
Warner A, 91, *109*
Warner DO, 33, *46*, 91, 93, *109*
Warner J, 12, *23*, 43, *55*, 162, *177*, 289, *313*, 333, *341*
Warner JA, 12, *23*
Warner JO, 2, 12, *20*, *23*
Warnock ML, 217, *232*
Warrellow G, 250, 251, 253, 257, 263, 267, 268, *275*, *276*, *283*
Warrier RR, 346, *357*
Warring P, 374, *387*
Warringa RAJ, 352, *359*
Washabau RJ, 362, 365, *381*
Wasrren DJ, 238, *270*
Wasserfallen JB, 393, *399*
Wasserman MA, 293, 294, *317*, 364, *382*
Wasserman SI, 58, 60, *73*, *75*
Watanabe T, 187, *198*
Waters SD, 143, *153*
Watson JW, 255, 259, 265, 268, 269, *278*, *280*, *282*, 295, *319*
Watson N, 86, 87, *106*, 338, *341*
Watson R, 40, *53*
Watson RM, 194, *201*, 301, 302, 303, *323*, *324*, *325*
Watts MJ, 302, *324*
Webb EF, 263, *281*
Webber S, 248, 251, 256, 257, *275*
Webber SE, 37, *50*, 253, 260, 261, 263, 269, *277*
Weber PC, 255, *277*

Wechsler ME, 308, *328*
Wecker M, 105, *118*
Weeke B, 160, *175*
Weersink EJM, 31, *45*, 129, 133, *149*, 298, *321*
Weg VB, 379, *389*
Wegener T, 126, 129, 135, 137, *148*, *150*
Wei LX, 306, *327*
Weichman BM, 255, 268, *278*, 293, 294, *317*
Weichmann H, 19, *26*
Weigel NL, 158, *173*
Weiland DA, 308, *328*
Weiland S, 2, *20*
Weiland SK, 19, *26*
Weinberger M, 137, *151*, 168, *179*
Weiner ES, 268, *283*
Weiner HL, 351, 353, *359*, *360*
Weinland DE, 306, *327*
Weinreich D, 90, *107*, 219, *234*
Weinstein GD, 268, *283*
Weinstock JV, 209, *224*
Weir T, 208, *224*, 380, *389*
Weisberg SC, 169, *180*
Weishaar RE, 245, 247, 252, *273*, *274*
Weiss J, 17, *25*
Weiss JW, 292, *316*
Weiss KB, 392, 397, 398, *399*, *403*
Weiss S, 259, *281*
Weiss ST, 4, 13, 14, *21*, *23*, *24*, 41, 42, *54*, *55*, 97, *114*, 393, *399*
Weiss WJ, 60, *75*
Weissmann G, 242, *272*
Weisstein J, 92, *109*
Welch MJ, 162, *176*
Welgus HG, 71, *83*
Weller M, 263, *281*
Weller P, 292, *316*
Weller PF, 59, *74*, 289, *313*
Welliver RC, 14, *24*, 100, *116*
Wells JN, 245, *273*
Wells M, 393, *399*
Welton A, 364, *382*
Welton AF, 219, *234*
Wemer J, 92, *110*
Wenner CA, 347, *358*
Wenzel S, 372, *386*
Wenzel SE, 60, 65, 66, *74*, *75*, *79*, 296, 306, 307, *319*, *320*
Wescoe WC, 86, *105*
Wesp M, 378, *388*
Wessler I, 88, *106*
Westcott JY, 60, *74*, 296, 306, 307, *319*, *320*
Weston MC, 254, *277*
Wetterholm A, 288, 290, *310*, *314*
Whalen WM, 251, *276*
Whalley LJ, 264, *282*
Wharton J, 208, *224*
Whitacre CC, 353, *360*
White JR, 247, 263, *275*, *281*
White MV, 61, *76*, 208, *224*
White R, 71, *83*
White SR, 217, *232*
Whittle BJR, 369, *384*
Whorton R, 95, 104, *113*
Wichmann H, 17, *25*
Wickremasinghe RG, 291, *315*
Widdicombe J, 87, *106*
Widdicombe JG, 99, 100, *115*, 220, *234*
Widdicombe JH, 94, *112*
Widdop S, 91, *109*
Widmark E, 120, *146*, 365, *382*
Wielders PLML, 304, 308, *325*
Wierda CM, 347, *358*
Wierenga EA, 351, *359*
Wieringa EA, 346, *358*
Wiggs B, 41, *54*
Wiggs BR, 31, 32, 33, 34, *45*, *46*, *47*, 395, *401*
Wiggs SR, 35, *48*
Wigler M, 245, 246, 247, *274*, *275*
Wild M, 65, *78*
Wilding P, 129, 131, 135, *149*
Wilding PJ, 137, *150*
Wilkens H, 193, *201*
Wilkens JH, 193, *201*
Wilkinson R, 144, *154*
Will JA, 289, *312*
Willard A, 393, *399*

Willem J, 91, *108*
Willems LNA, 36, 37, 38, 42, 43, *49*, *51*, *52*, 58, *73*, 159, *174*, 205, *223*, 395, 396, *400*
Willemze R, 257, *279*
Willet K, 395, *401*
Williams AJ, 162, *176*, 299, *323*, 367, *383*
Williams C, 142, 144, *152*
Williams HL, 155, *172*
Williams IH, 251, *276*
Williams J, 127, *148*, 301, *323*
Williams JH, 70, *82*
Williams KL, 296, 306, *319*
Williams PV, 191, *200*
Williams TJ, 239, *271*, 379, *389*
Williams V, 304, *325*
Williams VC, 301, 302, 303, *324*, *325*
Wills-Karp M, 38, *52*, 63, *77*, 94, 98, *112*, 345, 346, *357*, 372, *386*
Wilson J, 57, *72*
Wilson JW, 5, *21*, 35, 36, 38, *48*, *49*, *52*, 57, 58, 59, 60, 64, 67, 70, 71, *72*, *73*, *77*, *80*, *82*, *83*, 133, *149*, 159, 160, *174*, *176*, 189, *199*, 239, *271*, 285, 295, *309*, *318*, 391, 395, 396, *399*, *401*
Wilson MC, 259, *280*
Wilson O, 36, *49*
Wilson P, 92, *110*
Wilson S, 43, *56*, 66, 78, *79*, 396, *402*
Wilson SJ, 38, *52*, 57, 59, 60, 67, *72*, *80*, 160, *176*, 189, *199*, 295, *318*
Wilson SR, 392, *399*
Wilton L, 137, 143, *150*
Winder J, 304, *325*
Winder S, 256, *278*
Windom H, 143, 144, *153*
Windom HH, 135, *150*
Windsor RA, 392, 397, *399*, *402*
Winkler JD, 256, *278*
Winning A, 194, *201*
Winsel K, 297, *321*
Winter J, 194, *201*
Wise RA, 41, *55*, 397, *402*, *403*
Wisniewski AF, 141, *152*
Wisniewski AFZ, 127, *148*
Wisniewski AS, 301, *324*
Wispe JR, 7, *21*
Withnall MT, 257, *280*
Witt A, 371, *385*
Woeppel SL, 258, *280*
Wolf B, 242, *272*
Wolf D, 93, *111*
Wolf SF, 63, *77*, 346, *357*
Wolfe B, 88, 92, *106*, *109*, *110*
Wolfe BB, 90, 91, *107*
Wolk R, 264, *282*
Wolle JM, 392, *399*
Woloschak GE, 291, *315*
Wolthers OD, 163, 165, *177*, *178*
Woltmann G, 297, *321*
Wolway J, 34, 39, *47*, 214, 218, *229*, *233*
Wong BJO, 297, *321*, 393, *399*
Wong CS, 127, 141, *148*, *152*
Wong E, 288, *311*
Wong GA, 308, *328*
Wong H, 58, *73*
Wong HH, 221, *235*, 302, *324*, 333, 336, 337, *341*, 352, *359*, 379, *389*
Wong HR, 7, *21*
Wong L, 89, *106*
Wood CC, 105, *118*
Wood D, 60, 61, *75*
Wood LJ, 243, 254, 255, 256, *272*, *277*
Wood P, 105, *118*
Wood-Baker R, 60, *75*, 286, 301, 302, *310*, *324*
Wood-Dauphinee S, 307, *327*
Woodard A, 351, *359*
Woodcock A, 18, *26*, 137, 138, *151*
Woodcock AA, 367, *383*
Woodman K, 135, 143, 144, *150*, *153*, *154*
Woodman VR, 253, 260, 261, 263, 269, *276*
Woods JW, 288, 292, *311*
Woodward DF, 293, 294, 295, *317*, *319*
Woody HA, 213, *227*
Woody JN, 268, *283*, 371, *386*

Woolcock A, 131, *149*, 364, *382*
Woolcock AJ, 1, 19, *20*, *26*, 29, 31, 35, 36, 37, *44*, *45*, *47*, *49*, 71, *83*, 160, *175*, *176*, 208, *223*, 343, *355*, 393, 394, 398, *399*, *400*, *403*
Wooton A, 158, *174*
Worden K, 58, *73*
Wordsell M, 141, *152*
Wordsell Y, 367, *383*
Wren GPA, 215, *230*
Wright AL, 13, *23*
Wright F, 291, *315*
Wright JL, 41, *54*
Wright LC, 375, *387*
Wright MG, 268, *283*
Wright PF, 37, *50*
Wrighton CJ, 375, *387*
Wroth H, 141, *152*
Wrothen S, 193, *201*
Wu CY, 158, *174*, 346, *357*
Wu JF, 70, *81*
Wu L, 372, *386*
Wu LH, 213, *227*, *228*
Wu MF, 34, *47*
Wu P, 372, 374, *386*
Wutrich B, 343, *355*
Wykle RL, 186, *197*
Wylie G, 301, *323*

X

Xhou XD, 63, *77*
Xiangli J, 332, 333, *341*
Xiao HQ, 93, 100, *111*, *116*
Xing Z, 380, *389*
Xu K, 289, 291, *312*, *314*
Xu LH, 39, *53*
Xu LJ, 294, *317*
Xu WX, 158, *173*
Xu X, 42, *55*
Xuan TD, 266, *283*
Xuan W, 19, *26*

Y

Yabuhara A, 354, *360*
Yacoub M, 102, *117*, 289, *312*
Yacoub MH, 208, *224*, 362, 366, 367, *381*, *383*
Yaegashi H, 35, *47*
Yager D, 35, *48*
Yamagata T, 371, *385*
Yamaguchi H, 91, *108*
Yamaguchi S, 186, 195, *198*
Yamaguchi T, 37, *51*
Yamakido M, 190, 195, *200*, *201*, 305, *326*
Yamamoto H, 190, *200*, 303, *325*
Yamamoto K, 190, *200*, 303, *325*
Yamamoto KR, 158, *173*
Yamamura H, 186, *198*, 294, *317*
Yamamura HI, 91, 92, *108*, *110*
Yamaoka KA, 291, *315*
Yamasaki M, 93, *111*
Yamashita T, 191, *200*
Yamauchi H, 208, 221, *224*, *235*
Yamawaki I, 216, *231*
Yamomoto KR, 158, *173*
Yan K, 31, 37, *45*, 394, *400*
Yancey SW, 126, 129, 135, 137, *148*
Yandava C, 309, *328*
Yang B, 89, *106*
Yang CM, 89, 90, 91, *107*, *108*, *109*
Yang KJ, 92, 93, *110*
Yang N, 158, *173*
Yang-Yen HF, 158, *173*
Yarkony KA, 96, 100, *113*
Yarnall D, 263, 268, *281*
Yarnall DP, 255, 268, *278*
Yaron A, 375, *387*
Yaroshe CA, 92, *110*
Yasuda R, 88, 92, *106*, *109*, *110*
Yasuda RP, 90, 91, *107*
Yasumitsu R, 220, *235*
Yasunaga K, 185, *197*
Yates DH, 140, 141, *151*, *152*, 159, *174*, 369, 377, *384*, *388*
Yazaki Y, 371, *385*
Ye RD, 187, *198*
Yeates D, 89, *106*
Yergey J, 268, *283*
Yermaneberham H, 2, *20*
Yernault J, 97, *114*

Yernault JC, 30, *44*
Ying S, 57, 62, 64, 67, *73*, *77*, *80*, 158, *174*, 238, *270*, 344, 345, 346, 352, *356*, *357*
Yiulmaz G, 377, *388*
Yoakim C, 301, *323*
Yodonawa S, 36, *48*, 306, *327*
Yokomizo T, 288, *312*
Yokota Y, 214, *228*
Yonno L, 255, 268, *278*
Yoshida N, 371, *386*
Yoshihara S, 219, *234*
Yoshinaga SK, 158, *173*
Yoshitomi T, 93, *111*
Yost BY, 95, *113*
Young CL, 141, *152*
Young G, 104, *118*
Young H, 65, *78*
Young HA, 65, *78*
Young IG, 295, *318*, 345, 352, *356*, *359*
Young KR, 397, *402*
Young PR, 288, *311*
Young R, 301, *323*
Young RP, 11, *22*, *23*
Young SG, 70, *81*
Yssel H, 347, *358*, 380, *389*
Yu DYC, 100, *115*
Yu M, 93, *111*
Yuan Q, 379, *389*
Yunginger JW, 164, *178*

Z

Zaagsma J, 91, *108*, *109*, 217, *232*
Zaagsman J, 257, *279*
Zabko-Potapovich B, 252, *276*
Zabucchi G, 71, *83*
Zagers H, 35, *47*
Zalavary S, 256, *278*
Zambas DN, 371, *385*
Zamboni R, 299, *322*
Zamel N, 31, 37, *45*
Zamvil SS, 351, *359*
Zanetti ME, 242, 256, *272*
Zarini S, 290, *314*
Zavala D, 58, 60, 61, *73*, *75*
Zawada E, 251, 264, *276*
Zehr B, 60, 61, *75*
Zeiger R, 333, 339, *341*
Zeng XP, 213, 214, *228*
Zetterstrom O, 137, *150*, 296, 297, 301, 303, *320*, *321*, *323*, *325*
Zhang DH, 371, *385*
Zhang J, 301, 303, 304, 305, *324*, *325*, *326*
Zhang Y, 120, *146*
Zhiping W, 39, *53*
Zhou D, 208, *224*, 255, 268, *278*
Zhou S, 290, *314*
Zimmerman D, 164, *178*
Zimmerman GA, 185, 186, *197*, 293, *317*
Zimmermann I, 100, *115*
Zochling R, 251, 264, *276*
Zonin F, 347, 351, *358*
Zou A, 187, *198*
Zuccati G, 65, *78*
Zuidhof AB, 217, *232*
Zurier RB, 242, *272*
ZuWallack FL, 393, *399*
Zvaifler NJ, 183, *196*
Zwinderman AH, 35, 40, *47*, *53*, *54*, 140, 141, *151*, 211, *226*, 303, *324*

SUBJECT INDEX

A

Adenosine
- antisense oligonucleotide to A1 receptor, 249
- effects in asthma, 249, 368
- release after antigen challenge, 249

Adhesion molecules
- blockers as novel anti-inflammatories, 373
  - VLA4 antagonists, 379
  - VLA4 antibodies, 373

Adrenaline, 120, 122

Afterload, 33

Airway hyperresponsiveness, relationship to mast cell mediators, 61

Airway inflammation, assessment methods, 58, 395, 396
- cellular infiltrate, 57
- cytokines/chemokines in (*see also* Cytokines/chemokines), 370
- effect of corticosteroids, 65
- eosinophilia, 57, 65, 238, 243, 377, 378
- in fatal asthma, 67
- immunoregulation of, 62
  - antigen presentation in, 62
  - antigen-presenting cells, 62
  - dendritic cells and, 63
  - lymphocytes in, 63, 64, 345
  - macrophages in, 63
  - release of NO from, 63

[Airway inflammation]
- induction by allergen challenge, 28, 58, 238
- mast cells, 59
- neurogenic, 203, 216
- neutrophilia, 58, 66
  - in exacerbations, 66
- regulation by immune system, 238

Airway smooth muscle, 32, 71
- hyperplasia in excessive airway narrowing, 34, 35
- hypertrophy in excessive airway narrowing, 34, 35
- hysteresis, 34
- limits to contraction of, 32
- muscarinic receptors, 91

Allergen challenge in asthma, 58, 95, 133, 184, 194, 297, 298
- allergic mice, 332
- allergic rats, IL12, effect of, 372
- cytokine levels in, 64
- effect of PAF antagonist, 194
- hyperresponsiveness in rabbits, adenosine A1 receptor antisense oligonucleotide, 380
- inflammatory consequences, 58
- muscarinic receptor dysfunction, 94–95
- rhuMAb-E25, effect in humans, 336–338

Allergic rhinitis, anti-IgE Mab effects, 334–336

Allergy
allergens, 17
genetics, 5, 6, 10
prenatal influences, 11, 12, 13
prevalence, 1,2
Th1/Th2, 12, 14, 15, 350
Alveolar macrophages
as antigen-presenting cells, 350
GMCSF release, 238
leukotriene release, 238
mediator release, effect of theophylline, 242
as source of PAF acetylhydrolase, 187
thromboxane release, 242
Aminoguanidine, 368
Angiotensin-converting enzyme, 205
Anticholinergic agents, 86, 86–98, 100, 101
atropine, 96–101, 104
darifenacin, 102–103
ipratropium, 96–98, 102, 104, 105
revatropate, 102–103
scopolamine, 12
tiotropium, 102, 104, 105, 362, 363, 366
Antigen-presenting cells, 62, 63, 346, 350–354
alveolar macrophages, 350
dendritic cells, 346
monocytes, 350, 354
role of CD23 in, 332
Anti-inflammatory approaches to asthma (*see also* Inhaled glucocorticosteroids)
adenosine receptor ligands, 368
adhesion molecule blockers, 95, 373
antagonists of individual mediators (list), 368
anti-oxidants, 368, 369
bradykinin antagonists, 368
chemokine blockers, 372
cytokine strategies, 370–373
endothelin antagonists, 368, 369
gene therapy, targets for viral vectors in asthma, 380
IL-1β blockers, 368, 372
[Anti-inflammatory approaches to asthma]
IL4 blockers, 368, 371, 373
IL5 blockers, 43, 95, 368, 370, 371, 373
immunomodulators, 373
cyclosporin A, 374, 378
mofetil, 373
mycophenolate, 373
oxeclosporin, 373
rapamycin, 373, 378
tacromlimus, 373
LTB_4 antagonists (*see* Leukotrienes)
LTD_4 antagonists (*see* Leukotrienes)
NOS inhibitors, 368, 369
PAF antagonists, 183–202, 368, 379
phosphodiestase inhibitors, 237–284, 378
"soft" inhaled steroids, 373
thromboxane antagonists, 368
TNF-α blockers, 368, 371
transcription factor blockers (*see also* Transcription factors), 373
tryptase inhibitors, 368
Anti-leukotrienes (*see* Leukotrienes)
Antioxidants, 7, 19, 368, 369
N-acetyl cysteine in asthma, 369
ascorbic acid, 369
release of oxidants from inflammatory cells, 369
spin-trap antioxidants, 374
inhibition of NF-κB, 374
Apafant, 368
APC-366, 61, 368
Arachidonic acid, 287
synthesis of leukotrienes (*see also* Leukotrienes), 287
Asthma
adverse effect of oral steroids, 165
airways remodeling in, 34, 35, 43, 68, 71, 286
definition, 285, 286
steroids, effects of, 169–170
allergic asthma, trials of anti-IgE antibodies in, 334–336
animal models
adenosine A1 antisense oligonucleotide, effect in rabbits, 249

[Asthma]
antigen-induced bronchoconstriction, effects of rolipram, 258
antigen-induced eosinophilia in rats, 261
antileukotriene agents in, 297–298
guinea pig, PAF-induced hyperresponsiveness, 260
ozone-induced hyperresponsiveness in guinea pigs, 260
predictive value of, 362
primate, ascaris-sensitive squirrel monkey, effect of CDP840 on, 259
primates, effect of anti-IL-5 antibodies on, 370
rabbit, antigen-induced bronchoconstriction after neonatal sensitization, 259
rabbit, antigen-induced hyperresponsiveness, 380
rat, effect of IL-12 on allergic inflammation, 372
aspirin-sensitive, 297
characteristic features, 28, 344
childhood, 1, 2, 13
allergens, 17, 18
infections, 15
PAF challenge, 194
pollution, 15, 16, 17
treatment with inhaled steroids, 160, 163–166, 170
variants, 13
clinical trials, 391
definition, 4, 27, 285, 391
as eosinophilic bronchitis, 58
epidemiology, 1–26
rapidly growing market for treatments, 362
exacerbation, 160–161
inflammation, effect of ozone on, 191
PAF levels in, 188, 191
steroids in, 160–161, 169
exercise-induced, effect of PAF antagonists on, 194

[Asthma]
fatal, findings in, 67, 68, 71
genetics, 5, 6, 10, 343, 348–350
twin studies, 8
growth rate, effect on, 163–165
health economic parameters, 398
IgE, role in allergic disease, 339
inflammation in (*see also* Airway inflammation), 28, 57
immunoregulation of, 62, 238
lung parenchyma, involvement of, 66
nocturnal, 66
BAL findings in, 66
outcome measures, 391, 392
pathology, 57–84
prenatal influences, 11, 12, 13
prevalence, 1, 2, 11
increase in, 1, 2
impact of Western lifestyle, 2, 19
relationship to IgE 11
tobacco smoke and 12
puberty, effect on onset, 164
questionnaires, 393, 396, 397
medical outcome survey short form with 36 units (SF36), 397
quality of life questionnaire (AQLQ), 397
severity, pathological determinants of, 64, 65
steroid-dependent, 169–170
symptom scores, 392
treatments
accolate (*see* Leukotrienes)
adverse effects
concerns about, 361
of steroids, 165, 361
anticholinergics (*see* Anticholinergics)
anti-IgE (*see* IgE)
azelastine, 186
beta$_2$-agonists (*see* Bronchodilators)
cetirizine, 188
cromolyn sodium, 161
cyclosporin A, 370, 373
cysLT$_1$ receptor antagonists (*see* Leukotrienes)

[Asthma]
effect of delay in initiation, 161
5-LO inhibitors (*see* Leukotrienes)
FLAP antagonists (*see* Leukotrienes)
guidelines, 161
inhaled glucocorticosteroids, 155–181
compliance issues, 361
isoprenaline, 242
lack of effect on natural history, 361
limitations of current agents, 361
LTB_4 antagonists (*see* Leukotrienes)
market for asthma therapies, growth, 362
montelukast (*see* Leukotrienes)
nedocromil sodium, 161, 165
neurokinin receptor antagonists (*see* Tachykinins)
oral prednisolone, 157, 160, 166, 169
PAF antagonists 183–202
phosphodiesterase 4 inhibitors (*see* PDE4 inhibitor pharmacology)
potential for new targets and treatments, 361–389
strategic approach to new targets 362
pranulukast (*see* Leukotrienes)
salbutamol (*see also* Bronchodilators), 120–122, 135–137, 160, 186, 190, 193, 242
salmeterol (*see also* Bronchodilators), 119, 120, 137, 146, 164, 186, 362–364
singulair (montelukast), 191
terbutaline, 160
terfenadine, 188
theophylline, 164, 186, 190, 238, 242, 244
zileuton (*see* Leukotrienes)
Atopy
definition, 343
genetics, 348–350
Atropa belladonna, 101
Atropine 86, 89, 96–101, 104
unwanted effects, 102
ATS-DLD (American Thoracic Society–Division of Lung Diseases), 393
Axon reflex, 203

B

B7-1 (CD80), 351, 353
B7-2 (CD86), 351, 353
Basophils, leukotriene synthesis, 289–290
BAY X1005, 28, 368
BAY X1015, 288
Bepafant, 368
$Beta_2$-agonists (*see also* Bronchodilators)
functional selectivity after inhalation, 363
long-acting, inhaled, 119
as needed, 146
combined with corticosteroids, 129–131
compared with corticosteroids, 128, 129, 131, 132
compared with cromoglycate, 133
compared with ketotifen, 133
compared with nedocromil, 133
compared with salmeterol, 128
compared with theophylline, 133
compliance, 142, 143
duration of action, 122, 125
effects on airway hyperresponsiveness, 141
effects on airway inflammation, 133–135
exacerbations, 141, 142
hypokalemia, 135
long-term use, 126, 127
mechanism of action, 122–124
mortality, 143–145
nonresponders, 128
pharmacokinetics, 125
pharmacology, 119, 120

[Beta$_2$-agonists]
potency, 120, 121
protection against bronchoconstrictor stimuli, 125, 126
recommended use, 145, 146
safety, 135
side effects, 135–137
tolerance, 137–141
long-term use of, 71
receptor, 120, 123
partial agonists, 120, 121
short-acting, inhaled, 119, 126
comparison to long-acting beta$_2$-agonists, 126, 127
unwanted effects, 363
B-lymphocytes, 285, 289, 345, 346, 354
role of CD23 in IgE production, 332
Bombesin, 260
Bone metabolism and osteoporosis, effects of steroids on, 161, 165, 171
Bosentan, 368
Bradykinin, 61
receptor antagonists, 368
FR167344, 368
icatibant, 368
WIN64338, 368
BRL3491 (cromakalim), 366
mechanism of action, 366–367
BRL38227 (levcromakalim), 367
Bronchial biopsy, 27, 190, 396
artefacts of, 69
assessment of epithelial damage by, 69
eosinophils, 239
IL-8 in, 66
neutrophils in, 66
steroids, study of action, 159
Bronchial rings in vitro
anaphylaxis after passive sensitization, 338
effect of nonanaphylactogenic anti-IgE antibodies on, 338
Bronchoalveolar lavage
alveolar macrophages in, 187
ECP in, 65
[Bronchoalveolar lavage]
eosinophils in, 59, 65, 239
LTB$_4$ in, 66
mast cells in, 59, 61, 159
mediators in, 59, 60
mice, findings in allergic airways, 186, 332
PAF antagonist effects, 186
neutrophils in, 66, 185
in nocturnal asthma, 66
PAF acetylhydrolase in, 187
PAF levels, 185
steroids, study of effects, 159
Th2 cytokine mRNA in, 67
Bronchoconstrictor agents
acetylcholine, 90
adenosine 5′-monophosphate (AMP), 31, 125, 140, 210, 395
allergen, 125, 133, 140, 215, 216, 297, 298, 352
aspirin, 297
bradykinin, 31, 36, 215, 216, 221
carbachol, 218
citric acid, 99, 216, 220
cold dry air, 31, 99, 140, 297
cyclooxygenase products, 184
dust, 99
endothelin, 368-369
exercise, 31, 32, 99, 101, 140, 221, 297, 395
histamine, 30, 60, 125, 133, 134, 140, 158, 184–185, 209, 215, 218, 296, 352, 377, 394, 395
hypertonic saline, 216, 221
hyperventilation, 125
leukotrienes, 31, 36, 60, 184, 289
methacholine, 30, 125, 140, 193, 218, 377, 394, 395
neuropeptides, 32
nonisotonic aerosols, 31
PAF, 183–202
parasympathetic nerves, 87
vagally mediated bronchospasm, 99
PDGF, 60
sodium metabisulfite, 31
sulfur dioxide, 99

[Bronchoconstrictor agents]
 tachykinins, 31, 36
 toluene diisocyanate, 218
Bronchodilators
 ANP
  bronchocontrictor challenges, effects on, 365
  stimulation of particulate guanylyl cyclase, 365
 anticholinergics, 86–98
  tiotropium, differentiating features, 366
 beta$_2$-agonists
  bronchodilator potency relative to PDE4 inhibitors, 253
  functional selectivity after inhalation, 243, 363
  unwanted effects, 363
 fundamental mechanisms of action and targets (schematic), 362
  cAMP elevation, 92, 362, 364–365
  cGMP elevation, 365
  cytosolic calcium, reduction, 362
  G protein stimulation, 365
  maxi-K+ channel openers, 362
  potassium channel openers (KCOs), 366–367
 nitrovasodilators, 365
  disadvantages in asthma, 366
  mechanism of action, 365
 PGE$_2$
  effect on early and late asthmatic responses, 364
  protussive effects, 364
  subtypes of EP receptors, 364
 potassium channel openers, 366–367
  BRL3491 (cromakalim), 366
  BRL38227 (levcromakalim), 367
  BRL55834, 367
  EMD52692 (bimakalim), 367
  HOE234, 367
  maxi-K channel openers, 367
  RP49356 (aprikalim), 367
  SCA40, 368
  spectrum of activity and limitations, 367
[Bronchodilators]
 relaxation of airway smooth muscle, 362
  potential for additional effects, 362
 salbutamol, 120–122, 135–137, 160, 242
 salmeterol, 119, 120, 137, 146, 362–364
 terbutaline, 120, 121, 160
 VIP profile in vitro and in vivo, 364
Bronchoprovocation tests, 30, 31

C

C fibers, 220
Capsaicin, 205, 215, 217, 218
 depletion of neuropeptides, 220
CC chemokines (*see also* Cytokines/chemokines/interleukins), 352
CCAAT (5-LO gene promoter), 291
CDP840, 373
 antigen-induced bronchoconstriction in rabbits and guinea pigs, inhibition, 259
 antigen-induced eosinophilia in guinea pigs, inhibition, 261
 eosinophil degranulation in vivo, inhibition, 263
 ozone-induced hyperresponsiveness in guinea pigs, inhibition, 260
 squirrel monkey, inhibition of early and late allergic responses, 259
 toleration in clinical trials, 265
 vagal bronchoconstriction in guinea pigs, inhibition, 261
CD28, 351, 353
CD40/CD40L, role in costimulation of lymphocytes, 62
CD80, 351
CD86, 351
CGP56901
 pharmacodynamics of IgE after treatment, 334–336
 serum IgE, effects on, 333–334
 trials in allergic rhinitis, 336
CGRP, 203

Cholinergic hypothesis, 85, 97
  nerves, 38, 97
  receptors, 86
Clenbuterol, 123
CI-930, inhibition of PDE3, 252
Corticosteroids (*see also* Inhaled glucocorticosteroids)
  anti-inflammatory effect, 65
  denditic cells, effects upon, 63
  long-term use of, 71
  mechanisms of, 67
  neutrophils, effects upon, 66
  resistance to, 67
  Th2 cytokines, impacts on, 67
Cortisol
  serum, 162, 170
  stimulation of, 162
  urine, 162, 170
CP80633, 251
Cromones, 376, 377
CTLA-4, 353
CXC chemokines, 352
Cyclesonide, 373
Cyclic AMP
  action on multiple cell functions, 237
  airway smooth muscle tone change, 92
    PKA-dependent, 240
  alveolar macrophages, cytokine release, inhibition by theophylline, 242
  catabolism, isoforms of phosphodiesterase (*see also* PDE enzymes), 237
  eosinophils, inhibition of cellular functions, 257
  formation
    adenylate cyclase and G protein coupled receptors (scheme 241), 240
    downstream signaling targets, 240
    isoforms of adenylate cyclase, 237
    second messenger role, 237
  lymphocytes
    cytokine synthesis, inhibition of, 243
[Cyclic AMP]
    IL-2 induced proliferation, inhibition by theophylline, 243
  neutrophils, inhibition of cellular functions by adenylate cyclase stimulants, 243
Cyclosporin A, 370, 373
CysLT1 and CysLT2 receptors, 289
Cytokines/chemokines/interleukins
  antagonism of chemokines, 372
  antagonism of cytokines as anti-inflammatory strategy, 370–373
  anti-IL-5 antibodies, effects in primates, 370
    autocrine actions on eosinophils, 59
    humanized anti-IL5 antibodies, 371, 373, 377, 378
    IL-4 as target for novel therapy, 371, 373
    IL-5 as target for novel therapy, 370
    novel approaches, 371
    transcription, effects of steroids, 371
    transcription factors, 371, 373
  BFGF, 70
  CCR3 receptor, 353, 372, 378
  Eotaxin, 239, 353, 372, 378
  GM-CSF, 59, 61, 70, 158–159, 238, 344, 346, 350, 372, 374, 377
  IFN-γ, 63, 100, 344–348, 351, 352, 372
    asthma, effects on, 372
  IL-1α, 64, 158, 217, 351, 372
    asthma, effects, 372
    hyperresponsiveness, effects in animals, 372
  IL-1β, 64, 70, 368, 372,
  IL-2, 59, 64, 67, 158, 217, 344, 350–355, 374
    receptor, 355, 396
  IL-3, 59, 61, 64, 158, 238, 290, 295, 344, 346, 348

[Cytokines/chemokines/interleukins]
IL-4, 59, 61, 64, 70, 158, 238, 285, 295, 344–350, 352, 354, 355, 368, 371, 373, 374, 378
eosinophils, 295
leukotriene synthesis, 290
promoter region, 349
receptors, 350, 355
role in IgE isotype switching (*see also* IgE), 349
Th2 response, 347, 348
IL-5, 43, 59, 61, 67, 95, 158, 218, 238, 285, 295, 344, 345, 352, 368, 370, 371, 374, 378
antibody against, 295
leukotriene synthesis, 290
role in eosinophil functions (*see also* Eosinophils), 295
IL-6, 61, 64, 70, 158, 217, 345
Th2 response, 351
IL-8, 61, 64, 70, 217, 290
IL-9, 345, 349
IL-10, 59, 344, 354, 372–384, 380
action via NFκB, 372, 374
effects in human inflammatory bowel disease, 372
inhibition of production of multiple cytokines, 372
IL-11, 70
IL-12, 63, 346–348, 350, 351, 372, 380
allergic rats, effects on inflammation, 372
defect in asthmatics, 372
regulation of Th subset balance (*see also* Lymphocytes), 346, 351, 372
IL-13, 63, 158, 285, 344, 346, 348, 349
IL-16, 59, 64, 70, 352, 353
IL-18, 70, 347
Th1 response, 351
MCP variants, 64, 70, 346, 352, 372, 378,
MIP-1α, 64, 70, 352
MIP-1β, 64

[Cytokines/chemokines/interleukins]
PDGF, 70
RANTES, 59, 64, 70, 346, 352, 372, 378
recruitment of eosinophils, 59
TGF-β, 43, 63, 70, 354
Th1/Th2 cell subsets and, 63
TNF-α, 62, 70, 158, 290, 344, 368, 371, 372
antagonists, 368, 371
blocking antibodies, 371
release ex vivo, 189
soluble receptors, 371

D

Dale's postulates, in asthma, 286
Darifenacin, 87, 102, 103
Datura plant, anticholinergic effects of, 96
Deep breath
bronchodilation, 34, 39
effect on bronchoconstriction responses, 39
Denbufylline
clinical trials for dementia, 250
preclinical models of asthma, 258
selective inhibition of PDE4, 250
Dendritic cells (*see also* Antigen-presenting cells), 346
as antigen-presenting cells, 63
macrophages, association with, 63
T cells, effects on, 63
Dipyridamole, inhibition of adenosine uptake, 250
Dose-response curve to bronchoconstrictors, 30, 43
maximum response plateau, 31–33, 43
position, 30
slope, 30

E

EMD52692 (bimakalim), 367
E-selectin, 58

Early asthmatic response
  definition, 298
  effect of long-acting beta$_2$-agonists, 133, 134
  effect of PAF antagonist, 194
  mediators contributing to, 60, 195
  PGE$_2$, inhibitory effect after inhalation, 364
  rhuMAb-E25, effect in humans, 336–338
  squirrel monkey, effect of CDP840, 259
Endothelin, 70
  constrictor of airway smooth muscle, 369
  proliferation of airway smooth muscle, 369
  receptor antagonists, 368, 369
    bosentan, 368, 369
    SB209670, 368, 369
Eicosanoids (*see* Lipid mediators)
Eicosapentaenoic acid, 298
  effect on asthma, 298
Elastic load, reduction in, 35
Eosinophils
  activation by PAF, 184
  activation state, 59
  allergen challenge, effect of in humans, 337–338
    rhuMAb-E25, effect upon, 337–338
  antiapoptotic effects of cytokines, 378
  catabolism of mediators by, 58
  CCR3 receptor, 372, 378
  chemoattraction by PAF, 184
  chemotaxis by leukotrienes, 295, 296
  cytokines, autocrine actions of, 59
  degranulation in vivo, 263
  determinants of asthma severity (scheme), 239, 295
  effector cells, 58
  GMCSF, 295, 344, 346, 350
  induction by allergen challenge, 58, 238
  interleukin-4 protein in, 62
[Eosinophils]
  interleukin-5, role in multiple aspects of function, 370, 371, 377, 378
  leukotriene release, 289, 290, 291
    effect of PDE4 inhibitors, 243, 257
  long-acting beta$_2$-agonists, effects on, 134, 135
  mediators of inflammation in asthma, 243, 377
  mice, recruitment in allergic airways, 332
    PAF antagonist effects, 186
  nocturnal asthma, 101
  PAF receptors, density, 187
    change after PAF inhalation, 189, 194
  proaptotic effects of steroids, 378
  products of, 59
    ECP, 59, 64, 190, 239, 396
    EPO, 59
    inhibition of release by PDE4 inhibitors, 257
    lipid mediators, 191
    MBP, 59, 158, 239
    TGF-β, 71
  proposed role in muscarinic receptor dysfunction, 95, 96
  proposed role in parasitic infections, 243
  sputum, 337–338
  steroids, reduction in number in airways, 159, 169
  tachykinins, effects on, 216, 218
  target for novel therapy, 377
  Th2 response element, 345, 352
Epithelium
  antigen-presenting cells, role as, 63
  antioxidant enzymes in, 70
  assessment by biopsy, 69
  collagen deposition, 70
  composition of, 69
  Creola bodies, 69
  damage to, 37, 67
    in fatal asthma, 68
    implications of, 68, 70

[Epithelium]
ICAM-1 expression on, 61, 70
injury by inflammatory mediators, 59
interleukin-8 in, 61
mechanisms of injury, 69
mediators released from, 70
mucosal edema, effect of, 59
myofibroblasts beneath, 70
neutral endopeptidase in, 70
regeneration of, 69
adhesion molecules in, 70
shedding in asthma, 69
source of secretory IgA, 70
steroids, effects on, 159
tight junctions in, 69
Excessive airway narrowing, 30, 32
airway narrowing, 36
airway smooth muscle growth, 34, 35
airway wall swelling, 35
mechanisms, 33–36, 41
prevention, 32, 33
reduction in elastic load, 35
steroids, effects of, 40
Excitatory postsynaptic potential
fast, 92
slow, 92

F

FACET study, 138
Fenoterol, 120–122, 135
FLAP (*see* Leukotrienes)
Forced expiratory volume in 1 second (FEV_1), 29, 30, 160, 394
fall after PAF challenge in humans, 189, 190
measurements, 29, 30
outcome measure in asthma, 394
Formoterol (*see also* Bronchodilators), 119, 120, 135, 146, 362–364
FR167344 368
Furosemide (frusemide) 362, 376, 377

G

Gallamine, 86, 93
blockade of M_2 receptors, 93
induced tachycardia, 86

H

Health-related quality of life, 396, 398
Heparin
antigen challenge, 95
inhibition of vagally induced hyperresponsiveness, 104
Histamine (*see* Bronchoconstrictors)
Histamine H_1 antagonists, 61
HOE234, 367
5HPETE, 288
Hyperresponsiveness, 4, 5, 30, 42, 43, 184, 190, 194, 238, 259, 285
acetylcholine challenge, 94
definition, 30
distribution in population, 16
IL-1 receptor antagonist, effect in animals, 372
inhaled steroids, effect of, 43
inflammation after allergen challenge, 36–38, 43, 184
outcome measure, 394
ozone, 191, 260
PAF antagonist, effect of, 190, 194
PAF receptor transgenic mice, 187
parasympathetic nerves, 99
plasma PAF, relationship, 185
pollution, 15, 16, 17
relationship to severity, 160–161
respiratory viral infections, 31, 43
rhuMAb-E25, effect in humans, 336–338
steroids, effects on, 159–160
Hypersensitivity
definition, 30, 36
mechanisms, 36–38
Hypothalamic-pituitary-adrenal axis
significance of, 163–164, 170
suppression by inhaled steroids, 156, 162, 167–168, 170–171

Hysteresis (*see also* Airway smooth muscle), 34

I

ICAM-1
on epithelial cells, 61
on inflammatory cells, 61
in mucosa, 58
soluble form, 61
Icatibant, 368
IFN-γ, 100, 344–348, 351, 352
leukotriene synthesis, 290
reduction in release by rolipram from lymphocytes, 255
Th1 response, 347, 351
IgE, 285, 343, 344
allergen-specific, 9
and atopy, 5, 11
CGP51901, 330, 334, 336
CGP56901, 330, 331, 333
concentrations in serum in relation to total IgE, 331
discovery, 329
evidence for role in allergic reactions, 329
FcεR1
cells possessing, 331
density change in response to serum IgE, 339
density on human basophils, 339
kinetics of removal of IgE, 331
number required for activation of basophils, 339
regulation of, by serum IgE, 339
FcεR2 (CD23)
cells possessing, 332
effect of anti-CD23 in allergic mice, 332
knockout mice, 332
role in antigen presentation, 332
humanization of anti-IgE monoclonal antibodies, 332
immunotherapy of allergy, 354, 355, 373, 379
IL-4, role in IgE production, 371
[IgE]
mast cells, degranulation, 184, 238, 254
mice, effects of anti-IgE, 332
PAF, IgE triggered release from rabbit basophils, 183
response to allergen, 329
through FcεR1, 329
through FcεR2, 330
rhuMAb-E25, 330
role in allergic asthma, 43, 329–342
rationale for, 332
safety concerns, 332
strategy for development of nonanaphylactogenic antibodies, 330
schematic, 332
therapeutic anti-IgE monoclonal antibodies, 329–342, 373, 379
target for novel therapy, 329–342
Th2 response, 345, 349, 351
and viruses, 14
IL-4 inhibitors, 368, 371, 373
IL-5 inhibitors, 43, 95, 362, 368, 370, 371, 378
reduction in release by rolipram from lymphocytes, 255
Induced sputum, 58
epithelial cells in, 69
MPO in, 66
neutrophils in, 66
soluble ICAM-1 in, 61
tryptase in, 60
Inhaled glucocorticosteroids, 155–181, 364
advantages over systemic administration, 155, 159, 160, 168
adverse effects
bone metabolism and osteoporosis, 161, 165–167, 171
biochemical markers for evaluation, 165
confounding influences in study of, 166
densitometry, 166
dermal thinning, 162, 167
determinants, 162, 168, 171

[Inhaled glucocorticosteroids]
dose size and frequency, influence, 161–162, 166–167
eye, effects, 162, 167
HPA axis suppression, 156
hypoglycemia, 162, 167
immunosuppression, 161, 167
growth suppression, 161, 163–165, 167
confounding effects of asthma on detection of, 164
methods for evaluation, 163
pediatric studies, 163–165, 167, 171
oral candidiasis, 156, 162
aerosolized cortisone, 156
aerosolized hydrocortisone, 156
aerosolized prednisolone, 156
beclomethasone diproprionate, 129–131, 157, 159, 164–166, 168, 170–171
beta$_2$-receptors, effects on, 138
budesonide, 132, 157, 159–161, 164–166, 168, 171
cyclesonide, 373
''dissociated'' steroids, 374
RU24858, 374
RU40066, 374
flunisolide, 157, 168
fluticasone proprionate, 129, 157, 163, 168–172
history, 155–157
hyperresponsiveness, 43
long-term use, 160–161, 163–168, 170
mechanisms of action, 158
methods for evaluation of systemic effects, 162
mometasone, 373
mouth rinsing, 162
oral steroids sparing activity, 157, 164, 169
RP106541, 373
spaced devices, 157, 162
topical-to-systemic potency, 157, 161, 168
determinants, 161–162, 168
[Inhaled glucocorticosteroids]
transcription factors, mediation of action of corticosteroids (*see also* Transcription factors), 373–374
triamcinolone acetonide, 157, 168
Interleukin-1 (*see also* Cytokines/chemokines/interleukins)
antagonism by recombinant soluble receptor, 368, 372
release by peripheral blood mononuclear cells, 189
Ipratropium (*see also* Anticholinergics), 96–98, 102, 104, 211
Isoprenaline (*see also* Beta$_2$-agonists), 120–122
IUATLD (International Union against Tuberculosis and Lung Disease), 392

J

JAK, 350

L

Langerhans cells, 346
LAR (*see* Late asthmatic response)
LAS31025
adenosine receptor antagonism, 250
preclinical models of asthma, 250
selective inhibition of PDE4, 250
Late asthmatic response, 61, 298
APC366, effect in humans, 61
PAF antagonist, effect in humans, 184, 194, 195
PGE$_2$, inhibitory effect after inhalation, 364
predictive value of effects on, 338
rhuMAb-E25, effect in humans, 336–338
squirrel monkey, effect of CDP840, 259
Leukotrienes
airway remodeling 294, 295

[Leukotrienes]
alveolar macrophages, release from, 238
antileukotriene agents, 307
comparative studies in asthma, 307
positioning in asthma management, 306–309
aspirin-sensitive asthma, 297
basal airway tone, 294
cellular sources, 289, 290
chemotaxis, 295, 296
contraction of airway smooth muscle, 292, 294
contribution to acute airway responses, 60
cysLT$_1$ receptors, 289
anti-inflammatory effects, 305, 306
early compounds, 301, 302
effects in human asthma models, 302, 303
MK571, 294, 295, 301, 302, 304
MK679, 301, 303
montelukast (*see also* MK-0476; Singulair), 301
pranlukast (*see also* ONO-1078; SB-205312; Ultair), 301
zafirlukast (*see also* ICI-204219; Accolate), 301
cysLT$_2$ receptors, 289
cytokine synthesis, 291, 292
eosinophils, 295, 296
FLAP (*see also* 5-LO activating protein), 287, 288
gene promoter, 291
FLAP inhibitors, 288
BAY X1005, 288, 300, 301, 368
BAY X1015, 288, 301
MK0591, 288, 300, 304
MK886, 288–300
hyperresponsiveness, 292, 294, 295
inactivation by eosinophils, 58
inhalation of LTD$_4$, 189, 297
inhibitors of formation, 288, 297, 298–300, 307–309, 362, 368
ABT761, 299
anti-inflammatory effects, 305, 306

[Leukotrienes]
piriprost, 298
ZD2138, 299, 368
zileuton, 288, 298, 299, 303–304, 368
involvement in inflammation, 66
leukocyte proliferation, 291, 292
LTB$_4$, 287–289
chemotaxis, 288, 295
cytokine synthesis, 291
effects on airways, 288
LTB$_4$ receptor, 288
LY293111, 288, 368
LTE$_4$, 287, 289, 292
effect on airway hyperresponsiveness, 294
synthesis, 287–289
mediation of effects of PAF, 191–193
mucus secretion, 293
peptidoleukotriene receptor antagonists, 287, 288, 301, 307, 308, 309, 368
bronchodilator properties, 307
montelukast, 368
responder and nonresponder subjects, 301, 309
steroid-sparing effects, 308
unwanted effects, 308
zafirkulast (accolate), 289, 301, 368
skin, effects on, 293
synthesis pathway, 287–289
urinary LTE$_4$, 296, 297
inhibition of increase by UK74505, 191
PAF challenge, effects on, 191, 193
vascular smooth muscle, 293
Lipid mediators (*see also* Leukotrienes)
cyclooxygenase 1 and 2 products, 287
15-HETE, 58
PAF (*see also* PAF antagonists), 58, 158, 183–202
PGD$_2$, 60, 133, 287, 296

[Lipid mediators]
PGE$_2$, 70, 287, 351
airway smooth muscle, relaxation, 240
cytokine release from T lymphocytes, inhibition, 243
mast cell degranulation, inhibition, 241
PGF$_{2\alpha}$, 287
Thromboxane, 242
5-Lipoxygenase (*see also* Leukotrienes), 287–288
expression in airways, 60
gene disruption, 295
gene promoter, 290, 291
polymorphism, 309
inhibitors of (*see* Leukotrienes)
LY293111, 368
Lymphocytes
accessory cell surface molecules, 62
anergy, 353, 354
asthma versus nonasthma, 352
chemoattractants for, 64
differentiation of Th0 cells
costimulation, effects of, 63
role of IL-4 in, 62
inflammation and allergy in asthma (*see also* Cytokines/chemokines/interleukins), 378
long-acting beta$_2$-agonists, 134, 135
memory T cells, 63
recruitment by cytokines/chemokines, 59, 64
regulatory, 354
regulatory cytokines of, 59
IL-2, 59
IL-4, 59, 62
IL-10, 59
subsets, 344–346
cytokine profiles (*see also* Cytokines), 344–346
differential sensitivity to PDE4 inhibitors, 257
polarization, 346, 350, 351
Th1 cells, 63, 343–355
Th2 cells, 62, 63, 345, 350, 351
Th1-to-Th2 switch, 354
[Lymphocytes]
CD4+ **T** cells, 63, 345, 346, 350, 352, 354
CD8+ **T** cells, 64, 345, 346, 352
regulation of balance by IL-12, 372
regulatory, 354
vaccination, altering subset balance, 380

M

Macrophages, 346
leukotriene synthesis, 289, 290
Major basic protein, muscarinic receptor dysfunction, 95, 96
Mast cells
activation via IgE cross-linking, 59, 184
in bronchoalveolar lavage, 59, 61, 159
contribution to early asthmatic response, 60
cytokines released by, 61
IL-4 protein in, 62
fatal asthma, changes in, 68
FcεRI upon, 59
granules in, 60
leukotriene release from, 289, 290
long-acting beta$_2$-agonists, 134, 135
mediators released in allergy, 60, 184, 191, 242, 254
patterns of degranulation, 60
tachykinin effects, 212
tryptase in bronchial biopsy, 189
Medical Research Council (MRC), 392, 393
Methoctramine, 87
MK-0476 (*see also* Montelukast), 301
MK-0591, 288
effects on clinical asthma, 304
effects in human asthma models, 300
MK-0679, 301
effects in human asthma models, 303
MK-571, 294, 295, 301
effects on clinical asthma, 304
effects in human asthma models, 302

MK-886, 288, 289
Modipafant, 368
Mofetil, 373
Mometasone, 373
Monitoring peak flow, 395
Montelukast (*see also* Singulair), 287, 289, 301, 368
  anti-inflammatory effect, 306
  effect on clinical asthma, 305
  effect on eosinophils, 306
  effects in human asthma models, 303
  steroid-sparing effect, 305
Mucus
  airway plugging by, in fatal asthma, 67
  effect of eosinophils, 68
  gland hyperplasia, 71
  inhibitory action by potassium channel openers, 367
  leukotrienes, release by, 191, 293
  neuropeptides, role in, 240
  PAF, release by, 191
  release by histamine, 61
Muscarine, 86
Muscarinic receptors, 38, 85
  antagonists, 86, 87, 99
    selective, 99
  distribution within the lungs, 88–92
  dysfunction of M_2 receptors, 94
  subtypes, 86
Mycophenolate, 373

N

NANC (*see also* Nonadrenergic noncholinergic neural activity), 203
  e-NANC, 203, 218
  i-NANC, 203
Nasal lavage
  LTB_4 in, 191
  PAF in, 191
Natural killer cells, 346
NEP (neutral endopeptidase), 205
Neurokinin A, 203, 205, 207
  effects in the airways, 203, 204, 209–211
  tachykinin effects, 217
Neurokinin B, 203, 207
Neuropeptide γ, 203, 207
Neuropeptides, 203
  catabolism by epithelium, 70
  depletion by capsaicin, 220
  sensory, 203
    bronchoconstrictor effect, 209, 210
    inhibition of, 205
  VIP, 60
Neutral endopeptidase, 205
  impairment, 37
  inhibition, 218
    by phosphoramidon, 216, 218
    by thiorphan, 215, 218
  upregulation, 37
Neutrophils
  allergen challenge, effects on circulating cells, 194
  blockade of a range of functions by PDE4 inhibitors, 256
  CD marker upregulation by fMLP, 256
  LTB4 released by, 191, 289-291
  nocturnal asthma, 101
  PAF, effects on circulating cells, 191
  PAF released by, 191
  zileuton, effect on, 192
NFκB (*see* Transcription factors)
Nicotine, 86
Nitric oxide, 32
  constitutive isoform of NO synthase, 369
  effects of inhaled steroids, 159
  exhaled NO in asthma, 369
  inducible isoform of NO synthase, 369
  inhibitors of nitric oxide synthase 368, 369
    aminoguanidine, 368, 369
    1400W, 368
  parameter of airway inflammation, 396
Nitrovasodilators, 363
NK-1, -2, -3 receptors, 204, 205, 208, 209
NKA, 203

NKB, 203
NO (*see* Nitric oxide)
Nocturnal asthma, role of parasympathetic nerves, 101
Nonadrenergic noncholinergic neural activity, 37, 203
  in airway hyperresponsiveness, 38
NPγ (*see also* Neuropeptide γ), 203
Nuclear transcription factors (*see* Transcription factors)

O

Onon (*see also* Pranlukast and Ultair), 289
Opioid receptors, 205
Oxitropium, 90, 100, 211
Ozone
  inflammation of airways, 191
  muscarinic receptor dysfunction, 95, 96
  tachykinins involvement, 218
Oxeclosporin, 373
Ozagrel, 368

P

PAF, 218, 219, 287, 295
  antagonists of receptor, 183–202, 368, 372
  binding protein, 186
  cellular sources, 185
    factors influencing release, 185
    intracellular retention, 185
    lysoPAF acetylhydrolase, 188
    transport protein, 186
  challenge studies in humans, 188-189
  discovery, 183
  levels in bronchoalveolar lavage fluid, 185, 185
  levels in plasma or serum, 184, 185, 187, 190
  metabolism, 184, 185
    acetylhydrolase from alveolar macrophages, 187
    in plasma, 187
  as PAF-acether, 183
[PAF]
  pharmacological effects, 184
    blood gas abnormalities, effects of 5-LO inhibitor, 192–193
    bronchial hyperresponsiveness, 189, 190
    bronchoconstriction, 187–190
    chemotaxis of eosinophils, 186
    degranulation of human blood eosinophils, 187
    flare after intradermal injection, 188
    hyperresponsiveness to bombesin in guinea pigs, 260
    neutropenia, 188
    neutrophil CD upregulation, 256
    potential mediation by leukotrienes, 191–193
    relative activity compared with methacholine, 193
    superoxide release from human blood eosinophils, 186
    tachyphylaxis to, 190, 193
  potential as intracellular messenger, 185
  rationale for development of receptor antagonists, 184
  receptors
    characterization, 186–187
    density on human blood eosinophils' relationship to leukotrienes, 191
  structure, 183
PAF antagonists
  animal models, activity in, 184
  apafant, 368
  bepafant, 368
  BN52063, effects on exercise-induced asthma, 193–194
  characterization of receptors with, 186
  hyperresponsiveness in humans, effects, 190
  modipafant, 368
  RP59227, effect in humans of allergen challenge, 194

[PAF]
SCH37370, effects on histamine and PAF challenge, 195
SR27417A, inhibition of late-phase response to allergen, 195
summary of effects in asthma, 195
UK74505
hyperresponsiveness in humans, effects, 194
urinary LTE_4, effects in humans, 191
UK80067, moderate asthma trials, 194
WEB2086 (apafant)
allergic mice effects, 186
eosinophil chemotaxis, effect on, 186
PAF challenge, effect on, 194
Y24180
allergic mice effects, 186, 195
hyperresponsiveness, effects in humans, 195
Papaverine, inhibition of adenosine uptake, 250
Parafluorohexahydrosiladifenidol, 87
Parainfluenza virus, muscarinic receptor dysfunction, 95, 96, 100
Parasympathetic nerves, 38, 85, 87
distribution within the airways, 87
mechanisms of action, 87
muscarinic receceptors, 92, 93
role in airway hyperresponsiveness, 99
role in antigen challenge, 99, 100
role in asthma, 97
Pathophysiology of airway narrowing, 29
Patient compliance, 397
PC_{20} (provocative concentration causing a 20% fall in FEV_1), 36
corticosteroids, effects of, 40
marker of airway inflammation, 394, 395
outcome measure of asthma, 394
PDE4 inhibitor pharmacology
adverse effects
[PDE4 inhibitor pharmacology]
CNS mediated effects in animals, 264
emesis in dogs, correlation with high affinity binding to PDE4, 265
emesis in ferrets, correlation with PDE4 inhibition, 264
gastric acid secretion in rabbit isolated tissues, augmentation, 265
nausea in clinical trials with rolipram, 264
bronchoconstriction
antigen-induced hyperresponsiveness, inhibition by CDP840, 260
inhibition of antigen induced airway responses in guinea pigs, 258
rolipram inhibition of antigen responses at nonbronchodilator doses, 258
edema, inhibition, 263
eosinophils
correlation of inhibition with binding of inhibitors to high affinity site, 256
coupling of PDE4 to $beta_2$ receptors, 256
inhibition of a range of cellular functions, 256, 257
PDE4D as predominant isoform, 256
recruitment after antigen inhibition, 261, 263
lymphocytes
cAMP PDE activity resistant to RO201724, 257
inhibition of a range of cellular functions, 257
PDE3, role in control of functions, 257
PDE7 in, 257
macrophages
augmentation of IL10 synthesis, 255

[PDE4 inhibitor pharmacology]
IL1 regulation, 255
TNF release inhibition, 255
mast cells
differential sensitivity of stored and newly synthesised mediators, 254
inhibition of degranulation, 254
neutrophils, antigen-induced recruitment, species dependent inhibitory effects, 263
neonatally sensitized rabbit, effect on antigen bronchoconstriction, 259
relaxation of airway smooth muscle, 252
correlation with high affinity binding, 253
dependency on mode of action of inhibitor, 254
potency relative to beta$_2$-agonists, 253
role of PDE3 and PDE4, 252
sensory neuropeptides
inhibition by CDP840 of vagal bronchoconstriction in guinea pigs, 261
inhibition by rolipram of neural bronchoconstriction in isolated airways, 261
squirrel monkey, early and late responses, effects of CDP840, 259
synergy between circulating catecholamines and PDE inhibitors 258
therapeutic potential and challenges (summary), 268–270
Peak expiratory flow (PEF)
ambulatory monitoring, 395
measurements, 29, 30
Peptidases, 205
angiotensin-converting enzyme, 205
neutral endopeptidase, 205
Phosphodiesterase inhibitors, 237–284, 363, 373, 378
dependency on level of cAMP tone, 253
[Phosphodiesterase inhibitors]
identification of isoforms (historical perspectives), 245
methylxanthines, 248
additional properties beyond PDE inhibition, 248
antagonism of adenosine receptors, 248, 249
denbufylline, 249, 250, 258
IBMX, 241, 250
LAS31025, 249, 250
RS25344, 249, 250
theophylline (*see also* Theophylline), 249
unspecific inhibition of PDE isoforms, 249
molecular diversity, 245
cloning of isoforms, 246
PDE subgroups, 245
non-xanthines, 250
CDP840, 251
CP80633, 251
RO201724, 250, 255, 256
rolipram (ZK62711), 250, 25, 256
RP73401, 251, 255
PDE3
inhibition by CI930, 252
role in regulation of cardiovascular system, 252
PDE4 (*see also* PDE4 inhibitor pharmacology)
distribution of subtypes, 248
inhibition by rolipram, 248
subtypes, 247, 248
RP73401, 373
SB207499, 373
sensory nerves, inhibition of neural bronnchoconstriction in isolated airways, 244
substrate preference for cAMP or cGMP, 245
targets for multiple indications, 238
theophylline, 368
tissue distribution, 247
tissue homogenate activity, disguising existence of isoforms, 245

[Phosphodiesterase inhibitors]
vascular endothelial cells, 244
vacular smooth muscle, elevation of cAMP as mechanism of some vasodilators, 244
Phosphoinositol 3 kinase, 350
Phospholipase A_2, 287, 290
Phospholipase C, bronchoconstiction, 91
Phospholipids, 287
Phosphoramidon (*see also* NEP), 216, 217, 218
PI-3 kinase (*see also* Phosphoinositol 3 kinase), 350
Pilocarpine, 93, 94
Pirenzepine, 86, 90
Platelets (*see* PAF antagonists)
Potassium channel openers (*see* Bronchodilators)
Potential for new targets and treatments in asthma, 361–389
anti-inflammatories, novel approaches, 373
bronchodilators, novel approaches, 362
gene therapy, 380
strategic approach to new targets, 362
Pranlukast (*see also* Ultair), 287, 289, 293–295, 301
anti-inflammatory effect, 306
effects on clinical asthma, 305
effect on eosinophils, 306
effects in human asthma models, 303
steroid-sparing effect, 305
Preprotachykinin A, 219
Prostacyclin, 287
PGI_2, 287
Prostaglandins (*see also* Lipid mediators)
PGD_2, 133, 287, 296
PGE_2, 287, 351
Th2 response, 351
$PGF_{2\alpha}$, 287
Prostanoids (*see also* Prostaglandins), 287
receptors, 287
synthesis, 287
Psychogenic asthma, 101
Pulmonary function tests, 29, 30, 393, 394

Q

Quality-Adjusted Life Years (QALYs), 398

R

RANTES, 59, 64, 70, 346, 352, 372, 378
Rapamycin, 373, 378
Respiratory virus infections, and increase in airway hyperresponsiveness, 31
Revatropate (*see also* Anticholinergic agents), 102, 103
Reversibility, measurements of airway obstruction in asthma, 29, 30
rhuMAb-E25
dose selection, rationale, 336, 339
FcεR1 density, influence, 339
lack of antibodies to in humans, 333
pharmacodynamics against allergen challenge, 337
pharmacodynamics against serum IgE, 334
pharmacokinetics in humans, 333-335
routes of administration, 336
serum IgE, effects on, 334
RO201724
adenosine uptake and monoamine oxidase inhibition, 250
augmentation of emesis in dogs, 265
cytokine induced eosinophilia in guinea pigs, inhibition, 263
RO251553, 363
Rolipram, 250, 255, 256
antigen-induced bronchoconstriction in rabbits, inhibition, 259
antigen-induced eosinophilia in rats, rabbits and monkeys, inhibition, 261
clinical trials for depression, 251

[Rolipram]
gastric acid secretion in rabbit isolated tissues, augmentation, 265
ozone induced hyperresponsiveness in guinea pigs, inhibition, 260
preclinical airway models, 258
RP1056541, 373
RP49356 (aprikalim), 367
RP73401, 251, 255, 260, 373
RS25344
high-affinity binding site and catalytic site activity on PDE4, 250
selective inhibition of PDE4, 250
RU24858, 374
RU40066, 374

S

Salbutamol (*see also* Bronchodilators), 120–122, 135–137, 160, 242
Salmeterol (*see also* Bronchodilators), 119, 120, 137, 146, 362–364
Salmeterol Nationwide Surveillance Project, 143
Salmeterol Surveillance Study, 127, 128, 142
Sampling of airways
bronchial biopsy, 58
bronchoalveolar lavage (BAL), 58
bronchoscopy, 58
induced sputum, 58
eosinophilia in, 337–338
histamine in, 61
SB207499, 373
results of early clinical trials, 265
SB209670, 368
SCA40, 368
Scopolamine (*see also* Anticholinergic drugs), 102
Sensitizing agents
allergen, 31
occupational sensitizers, 31
Sensory nerves, 240
neuropeptide release from, 240
Sensory neuropeptides (*see* Neuropeptides)
SGRQ (St. George Respiratory Questionnaire), 397
Singulair (*see also* Montelukast), 289
Slow-reacting substance of anaphylaxis (*see also* SRS-A), 289, 292
Smooth muscle, 32
contraction, 91
Sotalol, 123
Sputum, induced, 396
SRS-A (*see also* Slow-reacting substance of anaphylaxis), 289, 292
Steroids (*see also* Inhaled glucocorticosteroids)
iNOS, 8
molecular mechanisms, 158
cellular level, 158-159, 169
GC receptors, 158, 168
GRE, 158
transcription factors, 8
AP-1, 158
IκBα, 158
NFκB, 158
St. George Respiratory Questionnaire, 397
Stramonium, anticholinergic effects of, 96
Substance-P, 203, 205–207
in airways, 207, 208
effects of, 203, 204, 209–211

T

TA2005, 363
Tachykinins, 203
bronchoconstrictor effects, 209–211
chemotaxis of, 216, 217
growth factors, 217
mechanisms, 211–212
receptor agonists, 207
receptor antagonists, 203, 205, 206, 207
classification, 212–214
effects on airway inflammation, 215–218
effects on bronchoconstriction, 214, 215

[Tachykinins]
effects on cough, 219, 220
effects on hyperresponsiveness, 218, 219
effects in models of asthma, 221
receptors, 204, 205, 207
Tacrolimus, 370, 373, 378
TATA, 291
T cells (*see* Lymphocytes)
TCR, 350, 351, 353
Terbutaline, 120, 121, 160
TGF-β (*see* Cytokine/chemokines/interleukins)
T-helper cells (*see also* T-lymphocytes), 343–355
antigen presentation, 350, 351
Th-1 response, 345, 350, 351
Th-2 response, 345, 350, 351
Th-subsets, 344–346
cytokine profiles, 344–346
polarization, 346, 350, 351
regulatory subsets, 354
Theophylline
adverse effects, 244
antigen induced bronchoconstriction in rabbits, inhibition, 259
asthma therapy (historical perspectives), 238
augmentation of emesis in dogs, 265
bronchodilator mechanism, 238
lymphocytes, effects on proliferation and cytokine synthesis, 243
mediator release from alveolar macrophages, inhibition of, 242
Thiorphan (*see also* NEP), 215, 218
Thromboxane
ozagrel, 368
TXA_2, 287
TXB_2, 296
Tiotropium (*see also* Anticholinergic agents), 102, 362, 363, 366
TNF-α (*see* Cytokines/chemokines/interleukins)
TNF-β (*see* Cytokines/chemokines/interleukins)
Transcription factors
AP-1, 8, 373–375
in actions of glucocorticosteroids, 373
CREB, 8
inhibition by antioxidants, 374
mediation of action of anti-inflammatories, 373
NFAT, 373, 374
in actions of cyclosporin, 373
NFκB, 7, 8, 291
in actions of corticosteroids, 373, 375
antioxidants, inhibition by, 374
IκB-α, inhibition of gene expression by elevation of by IL10, 374
IκB, target for gene therapy, 380
IκB kinases as targets for novel anti-inflammatory therapy, 374
role in immune and host defense responses, 374
specific effects on gene expression, 373
PPARα, 291
retinoic acid, mediation of actions of, 375
Transforming growth factor-β (*see also* Cytokines/chemokines/interleukins)
Transpulmonary pressure, 33
Tryptase, 296
airway effects, 60, 61
eosinophil effect, 61
induced sputum levels, 60
inhibitor APC366, 61, 368
in remodeling airways, 70
therapeutic target potential, 60

U

Ultair (*see also* Pranlukast), 289, 301

V

Vagally mediated bronchospasm, 99
Vagotomy, 97, 99, 100

Vagus nerves, 94, 96
  role in asthma, 97
Variability in airway obstruction, 29, 43
VIP, 203, 207, 363
  Ro-25-1553, 363
VCAM-1, 295, 352
Viral infections
  muscarinic receptor dysfunction, 96
  role of parasympathetic nerves in, 100, 101
Viral neuraminidase, 96
VLA-4, 295, 352

W

Wheeze
  in childhood, 13
  genetics, 5, 6, 10
  prevalence, 1, 2, 3 (figure)
WIN64338, 368

Z

Zafirlukast, 191, 287, 289, 301, 368
  anti-inflammatory effects, 306
  effects on clinical asthma, 305
  effect on eosinophils, 296
  effects in human asthma models, 302
  steroid-sparing effect, 305
Zileuton, 288, 294, 295, 298, 299, 368
  effect on clinical asthma, 303, 304
  effect on eosinophils, 296, 306
  effect in human asthma models, 298, 299
ZD2138, 368